Contents

The Royal Marsden NHS Trust Manual of Clinical Nursing Procedures

Fourth Edition

Edited by

Jane Mallett

PhD, MSc, BSc, RGN

Research and Practice Development Manager
The Royal Marsden NHS Trust, London

and

Christopher Bailey

MSc, BA, RGN, Onc Cert

Study Co-ordinator
Centre for Cancer and Palliative Care Studies
Institute of Cancer Research, London

b

Blackwell
Science

© 1996 The Royal Marsden NHS Trust

Blackwell Science Ltd
Editorial Offices:
Osney Mead, Oxford OX2 0EL
25 John Street, London WC1N 2BL
23 Ainslie Place, Edinburgh EH3 6AJ
350 Main Street, Malden
  MA 02148 5018, USA
54 University Street, Carlton
  Victoria 3053, Australia
10, rue Casimir Delavigne
  75006 Paris, France

Other Editorial Offices:

Blackwell Wissenschafts-Verlag GmbH
Kurfürstendamm 57
10707 Berlin, Germany

Blackwell Science KK
MG Kodenmacho Building
7-10 Kodenmacho Nihombashi
Chuo-ku, Tokyo 104, Japan

First Edition published by Harper and Row Ltd 1984
Second Edition published 1988
Reprinted by HarperCollins 1990
Third Edition published by Blackwell Scientific Publications
1992
Reprinted 1993, 1994 (twice)
Fourth Edition published by Blackwell Science 1996
Reprinted 1997, 1998

Set in 9½/11 pt Ehrhardt
by Best-set Typesetter Ltd., Hong Kong
Printed and bound in Great Britain
by The Bath Press, Bath

DISTRIBUTORS
Marston Book Services Ltd
PO Box 269
Abingdon
Oxon OX14 4YN
(Orders: Tel: 01235 465500
        Fax: 01235 465555)

USA
Blackwell Science, Inc.
Commerce Place
350 Main Street
Malden, MA 02148 5018
(Orders: Tel: 800 759 6102
        781 388 8250
        Fax: 781 388 8255)

Canada
Login Brothers Book Company
324 Saulteaux Crescent
Winnipeg, Manitoba R3J 3T2
(Orders: Tel: 204 224-4068)

Australia
Blackwell Science Pty Ltd
54 University Street
Carlton, Victoria 3053
(Orders: Tel: 03 9347-0300
        Fax: 03 9347-3016)

A catalogue record for this title
is available from the British Library

ISBN 0-632-04068-8

Library of Congress
Cataloging-in-Publication Data

The Royal Marsden NHS Trust manual of clinical nursing
    procedures.— 4th ed. / edited by Jane Mallett and
    Christopher Bailey.
        p.   cm.
    Rev. ed. of: The Royal Marsden Hospital manual of
clinical nursing procedures / edited by A. Phylip Pritchard
and Jane Mallett. 3rd ed. 1992.
    Includes bibliographical references and index.
    ISBN 0-632-04068-8 (alk. paper)
    1. Nursing—Technique.   I. Mallett, Jane, RGN.
II. Bailey, Christopher.   III. Royal Marsden Hospital
manual of clinical nursing procedures.
    [DNLM: 1. Nursing Care—methods.   2. Nursing
Process.   3. Nursing Theory.   4. Patient Care Planning.
WY 100 R8885 1996]
RT42.R68   1996
610.73—dc20
DNLM/DLC
for Library of Congress
                                        96-19076
                                        CIP

Quick Reference to the Guidelines

Contributors to Fourth Edition

Edited by

Jane Mallett, *MSc, BSc, RGN*
Research and Practice Development Co-ordinator, The
Royal Marsden NHS Trust

Christopher Bailey, *BA, RGN, Onc Cert*
Macmillan Research Practitioner, Macmillan Practice
Development Unit, Centre for Cancer and Palliative
Care Studies, Institute of Cancer Research

Contributors

Caroline Badger, *BA, RGN, Onc Cert*, Macmillan
Nurse Consultant (Lymphoedema)
(CHAPTER 19, pp. 268–274)

Christopher Bailey, *BA, RGN, Onc Cert*, Macmillan
Research Practitioner, Institute of Cancer Research
(CHAPTER 16)

Amanda Baxter, *RGN, RMN, Onc Cert*, Clincal Nurse
Specialist (Pelvic Cancer)
(CHAPTERS 6, 8, 21, 39 with Mave Salter, 45)

Chris Berry, *RGN, ONC, Cert Ed, ENB100, MRSH*,
Back Care Advisor (CHAPTER 27)

Peter Blake, *MD, FRCR*, Consultant Clinical
Oncologist (CHAPTER 37)

Yannette Booth, *BSc, RGN, PGCEA, RNT*, Lecturer
in Cancer Nursing (CHAPTER 42)

Nancy Burnett, *RGN, Onc Cert*, Senior Nurse
Manager
(CHAPTER 34)

Jill Carter, *RGN, Onc Cert, Dip Pall Care, FEATC*,
Clinical Nurse Specialist (Palliative Care)
(CHAPTERS 17, 24, 31, 40)

Gay Curling, *RGN, Onc Cert*, Clinical Nurse
Specialist (Breast Diagnostic Unit)   (CHAPTER 9)

Tonia Dawson, *MSc, RGN, Onc Cert, Gynae Cert*,
Clinical Nurse Specialist (Pelvic Cancer)
(CHAPTER 37)

Shelley Dolan, *MSc, BA, RGN, ENB100, ENB ITU,
Onc Cert*, Clinical Nurse Specialist (High Dependency
and Critical Care Services)
(CHAPTERS 3, 10, 18, 22, 33, 35)

Lisa Dougherty, *MSc, RGN, RM, Onc Cert*, Clinical
Nurse Specialist/Manager (Intravenous Services)
(CHAPTERS 11, 13, 23, 36, 46)

Jean Edwards, *MSc, RGN, Onc Cert, PG(Dip), FETC*,
Senior Nurse Manager/Private Patient Co-ordinator
(CHAPTER 25)

Sara Faithfull, *MSc, BSc, RGN, Onc Cert*, CRC
Nursing Fellow, Institute of Cancer Research
(CHAPTER 30)

Deborah Fenlon, *MSc, BSc, RGN, Onc Cert*, Group
Clinical Nurse Specialist (Breast Care Services)
(CHAPTERS 2, 9)

Jacqueline Green, *BSc, SRD*, Senior Dietitian
(CHAPTER 29)

Douglas Guerrero, *MSc, BSc, RGN, NDN, Onc Cert*,
Clinical Nurse Specialist/Ward Manager
(Rehabilitation and Neuro-oncology)
(CHAPTERS 28, 44)

Sarah Hart, *MSc, BSc, RGN, FETC, Onc Cert*,
Clinical Nurse Specialist (Infection Control and
Radiation Protection)   (CHAPTERS 2, 4, 5, 37, 38)

Pauline Hill, *BA, RGN, RM, HV Cert, Onc Cert*,
Clinical Nurse Specialist (Community Liaison)
(CHAPTER 14)

Siân Horn, *BA, RGN, Onc Cert, ENB249, ENB980,
ENB998*, Lecturer in Biological Sciences Applied to
Professional Studies   (CHAPTER 12)

Penelope A. Jones, *MSc, BA, RGN, Onc Cert,*
ENB931, ENB998, formerly Clincal Nurse Specialist
(Community Liaison/Palliative Care)
(CHAPTER 14)

Margareta Johnstone, *RGN, Onc Cert,* formerly
Clinical Nurse Specialist (High Dependency Unit)
(CHAPTER 3)

Danny Kelly, *MSc, BSc, RGN, NDN Cert, Onc Cert,*
PGCE, RNT, Lecturer in Cancer Nursing, Institute of
Cancer Research
(CHAPTER 1 – Assessment)

Diane Laverty, *BSc, RGN, Onc Cert,* Clinical Nurse
Specialist (Palliative Care)
(CHAPTER 34, 48)

Nicholas Lodge, *RGN, EN(G), Onc Cert,* Clinical
Group Research Nurse (Gynaecology)
(CHAPTER 37)

E. Lopez-Verdugo, *B Tech,* Senior Technician/
Theatre Manager   (CHAPTER 7)

Jane Machin, *BA, Dip CCS, Reg MCSLT, DALF,*
Senior Oncology Speech and Language Therapist
(CHAPTERS 29, 41)

Elizabeth MacKenzie, *RGN, Onc Cert,* Manager (High
Dependency Unit)
(CHAPTER 35)

Lorraine Paxton, *RGN, Onc Cert, DPSN,* Sister
(Intravenous Services)   (CHAPTER 15)

Helen Jayne Porter, *MSc, RGN, Onc Cert,* Clinical
Nurse Specialist (High Dose Chemotherapy)
(CHAPTERS 7, 26, 43)

Frances Rhys-Evans, *MSc, RGN, Onc Cert, ENB100*
(Critical Care), Clinical Nurse Specialist/Ward
Manager (Head & Neck and Thyroid Cancer)
(CHAPTERS 20, 30, 41)

Tim Root, *BSc, MR PHARMS Soc,* Chief Pharmacist
(CHAPTER 15)

Lena Salter, *BSc, SRN, DipN, CNI, Neurology Cert,*
Patient Services Manager   (CHAPTERS 28, 44)

Mave Salter, *MSc, BSc, RGN, DN Cert, Cert ED, Onc*
Cert, ENB216, Counselling Cert, Clinical Nurse
Specialist (Community Liaison)
(CHAPTER 39)

Kate Scott, *BSc, RGN, RMN, Onc Cert, Counselling*
Cert, ENB870, ENB998, Clinical Nurse Specialist/
Lecturer/Practitioner (Psychological Care)
(CHAPTERS 1-Communication, 47)

Clare Shaw, *BSc, SRD,* Chief Dietitian
(CHAPTER 29)

James Smith, *MA, STL, SRN, RMN, Onc Cert,*
formerly Chaplain   (CHAPTER 24)

Val Speechley, *MA, RGN, RCNT, Onc Cert,* Patient
Information Officer
(CHAPTER 1 – Consent)

Mavis Stork, *BSc, RGN, RM,* Theatre Services
Manager   (CHAPTER 32)

Jennie Treleaven, *MD, FRCP, FRCPath,* Consultant
Haematologist   (CHAPTER 7)

Jane Wilson, *RGN, ENB176, ENB998,* formerly
Group Theatre Manager   (CHAPTER 7)

Mary Woods, *BSc, RGN, Onc Cert,* Clinical Nurse
Specialist (Lymphoedema Services)
(CHAPTER 19, pp. 274–283)

Miriam Wood, *BSc, RGN, Onc Cert,* Ward Manager
(Breast Care Services)
(CHAPTER 48)

Karen Young, *ONC,* Physiological Measurement
Technician   (CHAPTER 30)

Contributors to Previous Editions

First Edition edited by
A. Phylip Pritchard, *BA, RGN, RMN*
Research Assistant, Department of Nursing Research

Valerie-Anne Walker, *BSc, RGN*
Research Assistant, Department of Nursing Research

Second Edition edited by
A. Phylip Pritchard, *BA, RGN, RMN*
Assistant to the Director of In-Patient Services/Chief
Nursing Officer

Jill A. David, *MSc, RGN, HV Cert, Cert Ed, MI BIOL*
Director of Nursing Research

Third Edition edited by
A. Phylip Pritchard, *BA, RGN, RMN*
Formerly Co-ordinator of European Educational
Initiatives, The Royal Marsden Hospital, and
Executive Secretary, European Oncology Nursing
Society

Jane Mallett, *MSc, BSc, RGN*
Research and Practice Development Co-ordinator

Contributors
Caroline Badger, *BA, RGN*, formerly Senior Nurse
(Lymphoedema)

Sophia Baty, *RGN*, Sister (Recovery Theatre)

Judith Bibbings, *RGN, DipN, FETC*, formerly Sister
(Gastro-intestinal/Genito-urinary)

Derryn Borley, *RGN, RCNT*, formerly Assistant
Director of Nursing Services

Monica Burchall, *RGN*, formerly Sister (High
Dependency)

Antoinette Byrne, *DipDiets, CMS, COPQ*, formerly
Dietitian

Patrick Casey, *RGN*, formerly Clinical Nurse
Specialist/Unit Manager (Gastro-intestinal/
Genito-urinary)

Lisa Curtis, *BSc, RGN*, formerly Macmillan Lecturer,
Institute of Cancer Research

Tonia Dawson, *MSc, RGN*, Clinical Nurse Specialist
(Pelvic Cancer)

Barbara Dicks, *MBA, BA, RGN, RM, FETC*,
Director of Patient Services/Chief Nursing Officer

Emma Dilnutt, *RGN, RSCN, RCNT*, formerly
Clinical Nurse Specialist (Palliative Care)

Anne Doherty, *RGN*, formerly Staff Nurse (Operating
Theatres)

Shelley Dolan, *MSc, BA, RGN*, Clinical Nurse
Specialist (High Dependency and Critical Care)

Lisa Dougherty, *MSc, RGN, RM*, Clinical Nurse
Specialist/Manager (Intravenous Services)

Nuala Durkin, *RGN*, formerly Clinical Nurse
Specialist/Unit Manager (High Dependency)

Sara Faithfull, *MSc, BSc, RGN*, CRC Nursing
Fellow, Institute of Cancer Research

Douglas Guerrero, *MSc, BSc, RGN, NDN*, Clinical
Nurse Specialist/Ward Manager
(Rehabilitation and Neuro-oncology)

Rachel Hair, *RGN, DipN, FETC*, formerly Senior
Nurse (Neuro-oncology)

Sarah Hart, *MSc, BSc, RGN, FETC*, Clinical
Nurse Specialist (Infection Control/Radiation
Protection)

Cathryn Havard, *BA, RGN, DipN*, formerly Senior
Nurse (Gastro-intestinal/Genito-urinary)

Pauline Hill, *BA, RGN, RM, HV Cert*, Clinical Nurse
Specialist (Community Liaison)

Sian Horn, *BA, RGN,* formerly Sister (High Dependency)

Elizabeth Houlton, *BNurs, RGN, NDH, HV,* formerly Senior Nurse (Community Liaison/Self-Care Unit)

Nest Howells, *BSc, RGN, DipN,* formerly Information Officer, CancerLink

Jennifer Hunt, *MBA, MPhil, RGN, FRCN,* Director, Nursing Research Initiative for Scotland

Maureen Hunter, *BSc, SRD,* Rehabilitation Services Manager

Elizabeth Janes, *BSc, RGN, SRD,* formerly Dietitian

Annie Leggett, *RGN,* formerly Clinical Nurse Specialist (Intravenous Therapy)

Anne Lister, *RGN,* formerly Clinical Nurse Specialist/Unit Manager (Palliative Care)

Jane Mallett, *MSc, BSc, RGN,* Research and Practice Development Co-ordinator

Glynis Markham, *RGN, RMN, FETC,* formerly Director of Nursing Services

Catherine Miller, *RGN, FETC,* formerly Senior Nurse (Continuing Care)

Marion Morgan, *RGN,* formerly Research Sister (Gynaecology)

Katrina Neal, *RGN, FETC,* formerly Clinical Nurse Specialist/Unit Manager (Palliative Care)

Helen Jayne Porter, *MSc, RGN,* Clinical Nurse Specialist (High Dose Chemotherapy)

Judith Pretty, *RGN, RCNT,* formerly Clinical Nurse Specialist (Head and Neck)

Frances Rhys-Evans, *MSc, RGN,* Clinical Nurse Specialist/Ward Manager (Head & Neck and Thyroid Cancer)

Helen Roberts, *RGN,* formerly Senior Nurse (Head and Neck)

Tim Root, *BSc, MR PHARMS Soc,* Chief Pharmacist

Ray Rowden, *RGN, RMN, ONC MBIM,* formerly Director of Nursing Services

Miriam Rushton, *MSc, RGN, DipN, FETC,* formerly Senior Nurse (Gynaecology)

Lena Salter, *BSc, SRN, DipN,* Patient Services Manager

Mave Salter, *MSc, BSc, RGN, DN Cert,* Clinical Nurse Specialist (Community Liaison)

Kate Scott, *BSc, RGN, RMN,* Clinical Nurse Specialist/Lecturer/Practitioner (Psychological Care)

Clare Shaw, *BSc, SRD,* Chief Dietitian

Val Speechley, *MA, RGN, RCNT,* Patient Information Officer

June Toovey, *RGN,* formerly Sister (Intravenous Therapy Team)

Anne Topping, *BSc, RGN,* formerly Senior Nurse (Gastro-intestinal/Genito-urinary)

Robert Tunmore, *BSc, RGN, RMN,* formerly Clinical Nurse Specialist (Psychological Support)

Beverley van der Molen, *BSc, RGN, FETC,* formerly Clinical Nurse Specialist/Unit Manager (General Oncology)

Richard Wells, *BA, RGN, RMN, FETC,* formerly Rehabilitation Services Manager

Isabel White, *MSc, BEd, RGN, RSCN, DipLScN, RNT,* Head of Undergraduate Cancer Care Studies

Karen Wright, *RGN, RCNT, DipN, FETC,* formerly Research Assistant, Nursing Research Unit

Foreword

It is with great pleasure that I write the foreword to this, the fourth edition of *The Royal Marsden NHS Trust Manual of Clinical Nursing Procedures*.

Since the first publication in 1984 not only have we seen the advent of the 'health market', but also significant changes have occurred in the form of nursing's contribution to the organization of health care. Possibly one of the most notable changes is the growth of nurse-led care where nurses in community, and hospital in-patient and outpatient settings have shown beyond a doubt that skilled nursing practice does not merely make economic sense, but can make a unique contribution to the way patients experience disease.

Proof of the Manual's success has to lie in its widespread use, and every effort has been made to ensure that this fourth edition is an improvement on its forerunners. New and revised chapters will, we trust, guarantee its continued popularity as nursing rises to the challenges which the new millennium will inevitably bring.

Barbara Dicks
Director of Patient Services/Chief Nursing Officer

THE ROYAL MARSDEN NHS TRUST PHILOSOPHY OF NURSING

We believe that people with cancer should be nursed by staff with specialist knowledge and skills who are able to recognize the impact of cancer on patients' lives.

Specialist care is planned and given in response to physical, emotional, psychosocial, cultural and spiritual needs as expressed by the individual.

Nurses at The Royal Marsden NHS Trust pursue clinical excellence in cancer care by evidence based practice and accepting responsibility for their professional development.

Acknowledgements

The Royal Marsden NHS Trust Manual of Clinical Nursing Procedures is made possible by the commitment and expertise of a multidisciplinary team of professionals, some of whom are contributing for the first time, while others have been involved since the first edition in 1984. Something of the belief of each of those individuals in the continuing development of excellence in patient care is reflected throughout. Each chapter represents not only nursing in theory, but also nursing in practice, and the perceptions and ideals of nurses who are specialists in their fields.

We extend our many thanks to our contributors for producing procedures that complement and develop the material contained in the previous three editions of the Manual. Many colleagues, both medical and paramedical, have generously given their advice and support. Particular thanks must go to Phylip Pritchard, to whose very special talents this work is a continuing tribute. Others have also led the development of the Manual from its initial conception to the work it is today. Therefore thanks must go to Jennifer Hunt (now Director, Nursing Research Initiative for Scotland), who was involved in the beginning and collected and collated the hospital's procedures, and to Valerie-Anne Walker (formerly Research Assistant, The Royal Marsden NHS Trust) and Jill David (Director Officer (Education), Marie Curie Cancer Care) who were joint editors of, and contributors to, the second and third editions, and to the many health care professionals who have contributed over the years. However, without the vision to support this project from its conception to realization *The Royal Marsden NHS Trust Manual of Clinical Nursing Procedures* would not be at the leading edge of practice today and for this our gratitude must go to Mr Robert Tiffany who was the Director of Patient Services and Chief Nursing Officer during its development.

In an effort to strive for excellence this book is reviewed by external referees who are expert in the relevant areas and we are greatly indebted to Bridie Asquith (Occupational Health and Safety Manager, Worthing Southlands Hospitals), Walter Brennan (Course Facilitator for Care and Responsibility, Ashworth Hospital), Elizabeth Grimsey (Clinical Nurse Specialist, Breast Care, St George's NHS Trust, Tooting), Peter Davis (Principal Lecturer, Royal National Orthopaedic Hospital, Stanmore), Jill Hampson (Practice Nurse/Practice Nurse Trainer, Putney), Andreas Macris (Senior Registrar, Radiotherapy, The Royal Marsden NHS Trust), Tom Swan (Lecturer Practitioner, Ashworth Hospital) and other reviewers who remained anonymous, for their constructive, critical and helpful comments.

To Anne McLean, Ruby Rambaran and Anna Orlowska we owe a substantial debt for the care and skill with which the complex process of assembling and preparing manuscripts has been handled.

Finally, our thanks go to Lisa Field, Griselda Campbell and Julie Musk at Blackwell Science for their sure hand and judgement in all aspects of the publishing process.

Jane Mallett
Christopher Bailey

Introduction

The Royal Marsden NHS Trust Manual of Clinical Nursing Procedures embodies the principle that the highest standards in nursing practice depend upon recognizing and critically appraising the expanding body of nursing research and nursing knowledge. Indeed, detailed and appropriate evidence based procedures are an important part of that body of knowledge, providing benchmarks for clinical nursing practice, and becoming themselves the subject of research.

In an important sense, this book has become part of a dialogue within the nursing community, reflecting and responding to change and development within the profession. It is both a resource for nurses starting out on their training, and a comprehensive reference work for nurses with extensive experience. Nursing procedures are sometimes quite rightly challenged and may be exposed as ritual rather than reason (Adams, 1984; Gould, 1985; Wright, 1985), and it is vital that they are continually tested and proved both intellectually and practically. In the years since its third edition, The Royal Marsden Hospital Manual of Clinical Nursing Procedures has figured in discussion and debate over aspects of nursing practice (Campbell, 1993; Briggs, 1994; Castledine, 1994; Gittins, 1994; Hancock, 1994; Thurgood, 1994), and its place in this process of refinement is to be welcomed. The new edition includes additional chapters which place the procedures within a holistic framework and drive the 'leading edge' of nursing. 'Care in Context: Assessment, Communication and Consent' (Chapter 1) provides the professional, social and ethical context in which procedures rightly operate. 'Breast Aspiration' (Chapter 9) is also a practice in which nurses are taking on new challenges in the care of women. All other procedures have been reviewed, chapters updated and many have been extensively revised.

The fourth edition sets out to take forward the work of the previous three editions, and to contribute to the continuing development of a conceptual framework for nursing care.

The format remains substantially unchanged. Every procedure has two sections: (1) reference material, and (2) guidelines. Some procedures also have a third section devoted to nursing care plans.

REFERENCE MATERIAL

The reference material section consists of a review of the literature and other relevant material. Whenever possible, research findings have been utilized. A list of references and further reading is included at the end to indicate the source of the information and to assist the reader to follow up the topic if more detail is required.

GUIDELINES

The guidelines section provides a list of the equipment needed, followed by a detailed step-by-step account of the procedure and the rationale for the proposed action.

NURSING CARE PLAN

The nursing care plan section gives a list of the problems that may occur, their possible causes, and suggestions for their resolution and prevention. Items from this sheet can be used on the patient's own nursing care plan.

Procedures have been arranged in alphabetical order although some have been grouped together. The procedures on 'Blood Pressure', 'Respirations', 'Temperature', 'Urinalysis' and 'ECGs' will be found under the general heading of 'Observations' (Chapter 30). Many of the procedures associated with wound care (such as the care of pressure ulcers and fungating wounds) will be found under the general heading of 'Wound Management' (Chapter 48). Chapter 37, 'Sealed and Unsealed Radioactive Sources Therapy', offers detailed information on a range of radio-therapeutic options, including iodine-131 and brachy-therapy for gynaecological cancer.

All relevant procedures begin with the action 'Explain and discuss the procedure with the patient', the rationale for this being 'To ensure that the patient understands the procedure and gives his/her valid consent'. This is intended to reflect a patient-focused approach to obtaining appropriate consent and is addressed in depth in Chapter 1.

Extensive literature searches by the contributors have highlighted the lack of research and guidelines in important areas of practice. Little research has been conducted on the efficacy of various methods of gastric decontamination or the use of Entonox for different types of pain. Much work has yet to be conducted into how to manage fungating wounds, a cause of so much distress to patients and relatives. There are no detailed national guidelines for physically managing violent patients and effective methods of restraint. There is even a debate on the use of lubrication in urinary catheterization. These are all aspects of basic practice and yet we still do not have many of the answers which enable us to provide the best possible care. This will probably remain a major challenge for nurses as different and more complex treatments become available. Where no research evidence has been available the procedures have been based on extensive experience and systematic review. However, it is hoped that in the future more aspects of best practice will be defined by researchers and practitioners to allow *The Royal Marsden NHS Trust Manual of Clinical Nursing Procedures* to become fully research based.

The book is intended as a reference and guide to quality care and not as a replacement for education. None of the procedures in this book, from the most basic to the most technical, should be undertaken without appropriate instruction and supervision.

We hope that The Royal Marsden NHS Trust

Manual of Clinical Nursing Procedures will continue to stimulate further debate. To this end the editors welcome the opportunity to respond to specific points from readers.

Jane Mallett
Christopher Bailey

References

Adams, J. (1984) Soap opera . . . outdated nursing procedures . . . frequency of bathing. *Nursing Mirror*, 159(22), 31–2.

Briggs, M. (1994) Examining equipment for wound care: the use of forceps and cotton wool in dressing packs. *Accident and Emergency Nursing*, 2(4), 237–9.

Campbell, J. (1993) Making sense of blood groups. *Nursing Times*, 89(22), 36–8.

Castledine, G. (1994) Security and nurses' uniforms. *British Journal of Nursing*, 3(15), 784–5.

Gittins, B. (1994) Too important to miss out? Documentation of care in critical care nursing. *Professional Nurse*, 9(12), 820–22, 824–5.

Gould, D. (1985) Areas of dispute . . . outdated nursing procedures . . . prevention and treatment of pressure sores. *Nursing Mirror*, 160(1), 19.

Hancock, B. (1994) Self-administration of medicines. *British Journal of Nursing*, 3(19), 996–9.

Thurgood, G. (1994) Nurse maintenance of oral hygiene. *British Journal of Nursing*, 3(7), 332–4.

Wright, S. (1985) The red peril . . . mercurochrome on pressure areas . . . outdated nursing procedures. *Nursing Mirror*, 160(4), 30.

CHAPTER 1
Care in Context:
Assessment, Communication and Consent

INTRODUCTION

Meeting the needs of patients requires nurses to solve problems with accuracy. These problems will vary depending on the patient's condition and current status. Nursing practice encompasses a process of judgement which begins with assessment of health related needs and problems and requires continuous evaluation of the decisions made to resolve them.

This first section explores the role of assessment, the basis upon which nursing intervention rests. The assessment of the needs of individual patients is a key skill central to the delivery of high quality nursing care.

The second and third sections of this chapter highlight interpersonal skills necessary to allow patients to express their needs during the experience of illness and the importance of treating patients as individuals with unique rights. The main aims of this chapter are to focus on the individual behind the disease and encourage an awareness of some of the research and theory guiding nursing towards an individualized approach to care.

ASSESSMENT

The nature of assessment

The essence of individualistic approaches to nursing care is accurate assessment of patients' health status and changing needs. McFarlane (1988) identifies caring for the person as an important component of the nurse's role. Taking time to explore patients' needs is one way of demonstrating caring in everyday practice. The wide range of technical procedures that patients undergo should act as a reminder not to lose sight of the person undergoing such procedures. Caring for a person involves respect for their rights, using communication that is open, honest and facilitative.

Accurate assessment is vital in achieving an individualized approach. Campbell *et al.* (1985) summarize the nature of assessment as follows:

'Nursing is the diagnosis and treatment of human responses to actual or potential health problems. Nurses assess clients to ascertain these human responses, to which they will direct their actions.' (page 111)

Assessment, therefore, lies at the heart of clinical judgements and dictates whether or not patients' needs are met with skill and accuracy. Nurses also focus on making the patient 'feel better' despite a prognosis which may mean they will not 'get better' in terms of achieving cure (Kitson, 1988).

The decisions that nurses make in everyday practice have been the subject of recent research (Benner, 1984; Hurst. *et al.*, 1991; Dowie & Elstein, 1991). It is suggested that recognizing problems, and using the skills of assessment, is an art, which improves and becomes more accurate with experience and education. Benner's (1984) work is particularly relevant: she identifies assessment as an expert activity that has not always been sufficiently highly valued in clinical settings. The skills which nurses use to recognize problems include cognitive, situational and predictive elements and have some similarities with the process used by doctors in reaching a medical diagnosis. The major difference, however, seems to be that whilst medicine may look for the cause of the condition, nurses focus more on the effects of the condition on the patient (Crow *et al.*, 1995).

Assessment in cancer nursing practice

Assessing the needs of cancer patients is a dynamic activity which is not performed on admission only. It is ongoing and a central component of everyday care which nurses provide by using skills of observation and communication, and by applying relevant theoretical knowledge (Tanner *et al.*, 1987). The procedures outlined in this book, therefore, should be seen as part of a larger picture, which encompasses sensitive assessment of patients' and families' needs, and an appreciation of the experience of illness.

Illness brings many demands and patients with cancer

have complex needs which often change rapidly. Their illness may be life-threatening; the diagnosis of cancer is stressful in itself, and nurses may find relating to patients as people in severe distress especially challenging (Harris *et al.*, 1990).

In modern health care there is increasing pressure on professionals to deliver high quality care efficiently, which may mean a more rapid turnover of patients. This in turn increases the demand for the assessment skills and strategies that are crucial to patients' well-being. Teamwork is considered to be an essential component of holistic care and the person with cancer will require support from a range of skilled professionals during the course of their illness (Beddar & Aitken, 1994).

Assessment is often described as having physical, psychological, emotional, social and cultural dimensions. In reality, however, it may be impossible to make clear distinctions between dimensions when caring for an individual patient (Yura & Walsh, 1988). Problems or needs identified in one domain have direct effects on other domains. It may, therefore, be more useful to view assessment as a holistic process with particular aspects demanding more focus on specific occasions.

Assessment of this kind can be illustrated by an example. A non-English-speaking patient has received high dose chemotherapy. The nurse may note signs of infection in the patient's mouth, a situation complicated by the patient's poor understanding of mouth care regimens and poor nutritional intake. Pain and depression due to social and cultural isolation may be compounding the problems. Assessment of the patient's needs requires a holistic approach to identify appropriate interventions, improve the patient's quality of life, and minimize the risk of life-threatening infection. When viewed in this light, assessment, with the implementation of appropriate interventions, is a highly skilled activity which can have a dramatic effect on outcome for the individual patient as well as on job satisfaction for the nurse (Derdiarian, 1990).

Methods of assessment

Formal checklists and documents are available to guide nursing assessment. They can be useful for gathering baseline data, and as ongoing measures of patients' needs. Ongoing assessment of need is particularly important when disease processes are unpredictable and characterized by repeated admissions to hospital. During these times the patient will experience disruption in every aspect of their life including work and relationships. Whilst assessment schedules may allow these issues to be addressed, they must be used in a way which allows ongoing changes to be noted and regular evaluations to be taken into account (Hurst *et al.*, 1991).

The Multidisciplinary Care Plan and Patient Assessment Form in use at the Royal Marsden NHS Trust is shown in Fig. 1.1. This includes sections to assess physical health, such as nutritional needs or sleep patterns, social assessment, covering issues of employment and religious observances, and psychological status including sources of support and current concerns.

Other approaches to assessment have recently been described. One of these utilizes patient held records, which facilitate the transfer of information when a patient is discharged from hospital either to their own home or to another health care setting (Williams *et al.*, 1994). These authors identify five dimensions of assessment, addressing the emotional, spiritual, physical, social and intellectual needs of the patient.

A key requirement is an approach that staff find useful and appropriate in their particular area of practice. It must be sensitive enough to discriminate between different clinical needs, and flexible enough to be updated on a regular basis. Information technology is likely to revolutionize the record-keeping aspect of assessment, but nurses' clinical skills will remain vital to the effective application of assessment strategies.

Sources of assessment data

The information that is used in the assessment of patients is derived from a wide range of diverse sources. It is frequently classified as either objective or subjective in nature. Objective data are measurements or observations such as body temperature, weight or oral status, which can be purposefully gathered by the nurse.

Nurse researchers and clinicians have developed a wide range of specific tools to assess the problems frequently encountered by patients. A summary of recent examples of assessment tools developed to be used with patients with cancer is given in Table 1.1. Whilst it is unrealistic to assume that the use of tools like these is always feasible in everyday practice, motivated nurses

Table 1.1   Examples of assessment tools in cancer care.

Author	Date	Topic
Daut, R.L. *et al.*	1983	Measurement of acute, brief pain in cancer and non-cancer patients.
Eland, J.	1985	Assessment of pain in children.
Waterhouse, J. and Metcalf, M.C.	1986	Risk of sexual dysfunction after surgery.
Eilers, J. *et al.*	1988	Oral status.
Ganz, P.A. *et al.*	1992	Measuring health-related quality of life in cancer patients.

should be aware that an appropriate tool may be necessary to assess a particular patient's needs.

For example, a nurse caring for a leukaemic patient after chemotherapy and radiotherapy may use the assessment tool described by Eilers *et al.* (1988), which provides a baseline assessment of the patient's normal oral status and allows regular and ongoing evaluation. Daily changes can be observed, medication prescribed and referrals made quickly and efficiently. Benner (1984) suggests that inexperienced nurses find assessment tools particularly helpful, but this does not mean that they are without merit for expert clinicians.

Subjective data are derived primarily from patients' perceptions of their problems. Eliciting this kind of information requires a high standard of interpersonal skills on the part of the nurse, and may be gathered over time as the nurse–patient relationship develops (Vaughan, 1992). Asking patients to describe their needs and difficulties may be particularly helpful when dealing with complex problems such as anxiety and stress.

Information of this kind can also be collected in a health diary, which patients can use to record their needs and experiences since their last appointment (Faithfull, 1991). Feeling that someone is listening to your point of view makes it easier to develop a sense of control. This is important as chronic illnesses such as cancer are often said to take over a person's life (Quigley, 1989).

The collection of both 'objective' and 'subjective' assessment data requires motivation on the part of the nurse and the health care team: time and sensitivity are needed to listen to the patient and act upon the needs identified by the assessment process.

The essence of skilled nursing lies in recognizing patients' problems, sometimes in advance, and directing appropriate interventions towards their resolution (Aggleton & Chalmers, 1990). Patients' needs are diverse and can change quickly, making it important for nurses to utilize assessment skills regularly and appropriately. Without a constant awareness of the importance of assessment, standards of care will suffer.

Approaching patient assessment

Assessment of the patient may take place in the context of a model of nursing adopted in a particular clinical area. Walsh (1991) describes models as mapping out the boundaries and framing the values of nursing in a given area. Nurses may find themselves working with a particular model of nursing within which they frame or define their assessment strategies. Different models emphasize different perspectives on illness and nursing. Self-care, for example, is the basis of the model developed by Dorothea Orem (Orem, 1985). The concept of self-care may be particularly attractive when negotiating interventions with the patient, but may be less appropri-

ate for other areas where patients are most dependant, such as intensive care.

It is vital that nurses are aware of the rationale for choosing to implement a particular nursing model for their area of practice, because this choice will largely determine the nature of patient assessment in their day-to-day work. If the model is inappropriate, it may well follow that the assessment data collected are less effective than they could be. Whatever philosophy or model is in use, the best source of assessment data will always be the patient.

Nurses and patients meeting for the first time are essentially strangers who build up a relationship over time and may use this relationship to help them deal with the many challenges which illness may bring. Peplau (1952) sees this relationship as important in its own right, and McMahon & Pearson (1991) see it as demonstrating the therapeutic value of nursing.

Effective assessment means gathering both objective and subjective data from patients. Chipman (1991) describes the importance of 'engaging' with patients, communicating with them and respecting their rights as individuals, in achieving this objective. Assessment also involves families, partners, friends and other members of the health care team. Some patients, if they are confused for example, may be unable to provide accurate verbal information, and nurses may have to rely on secondary sources (such as the patient's partner) to a greater degree (Yura & Walsh, 1988).

Information from other members of the health care team is frequently valuable, and may help to avoid repeating assessments unnecessarily. Multidisciplinary care plans and regular multidisciplinary team meetings are an important part of planning and evaluating holistic care (Kerstetter, 1990). A multidisciplinary care plan may be used to enhance a team approach and the example of this format used at The Royal Marsden NHS Trust demonstrates this philosophy in a practical format.

The planned assessment interview, which often takes place when a patient is admitted, is an opportunity to collect detailed, specific information. Patients often see this planned interaction as a time to obtain clear answers to questions about their illness and treatment, especially if they are experiencing chronic illness. The assessment interview allows the nurse–patient relationship to be established on the basis of a mutual concern for the patient's well-being. Wilkinson (1991) demonstrates the importance of facilitating communication at this time, rather than blocking patients' concerns or using inappropriate information giving. She also confirms that nurses can find talking to patients about cancer an uncomfortable experience. Data collected during the assessment interview may reflect physical, emotional, spiritual, edu-

1

MDCP/IS

THE ROYAL MARSDEN NHS TRUST
MULTI-DISCIPLINARY CARE PLAN
INFORMATION SHEET

NAME:

HOSPITAL NO.

ADDRESS:

TEL:

DOB: AGE:

RELIGION:

PREFERRED NAME:

DIAGNOSIS:

ALLERGIES:

GP NAME:

ADDRESS:

TEL:

LANGUAGE SPOKEN:

INTERPRETER INFO.:

PERSON(S) TO CONTACT (plus next of kins if different)

NAME:

ADDRESS:

TEL:

NAME:

ADDRESS:

TEL:

DATE OF ADMISSION/ATTENDANCE:

REASON FOR ADMISSION/ATTENDANCE:

DATE OF DISCHARGE:

CLINICAL UNIT: NAMED NURSE:

SIGNATURE: DATE:

F16

2

SUBSEQUENT ADMISSIONS / ATTENDANCE

DATE OF RE-ADMISSION/RE-ATTENDANCE:

REASON FOR RE-ADMISSION/RE-ATTENDANCE:

PATIENT INFORMATION CHECKED [ ]   PATIENT ASSESSMENT CHECKED [ ]

HEIGHT: ....   WEIGHT: ....

INDICATE NEW AND ON-GOING AREAS OF CARE:

SIGNATURE: DATE:

DATE OF RE-ADMISSION/RE-ATTENDANCE:

REASON FOR RE-ADMISSION/RE-ATTENDANCE:

PATIENT INFORMATION CHECKED [ ]   PATIENT ASSESSMENT CHECKED [ ]

HEIGHT: ....   WEIGHT: ....

INDICATE NEW AND ON-GOING AREAS OF CARE:

SIGNATURE: DATE:

DATE OF RE-ADMISSION/RE-ATTENDANCE:

REASON FOR RE-ADMISSION/RE-ATTENDANCE:

PATIENT INFORMATION CHECKED [ ]   PATIENT ASSESSMENT CHECKED [ ]

HEIGHT: ....   WEIGHT: ....

INDICATE NEW AND ON-GOING AREAS OF CARE:

SIGNATURE: DATE:

3
MDCP/A

NAME: HOSP. NO:

ASSESSMENT
TO BE UNDERTAKEN BY NURSING STAFF WITHIN 24 HOURS OF ADMISSION

RELEVANT HEALTH HISTORY:
Previous (incl. cancer therapy)

CURRENT:

INFECTIOUS DISEASE HISTORY: (eg. hepatitis, tuberculosis, measles)

MEDICATIONS TAKEN ON ADMISSION/ATTENDANCE (if unable to self-administer, reason must be stated).

RELIGIOUS NEEDS (eg. importance, local minister, communion)

HEALTH STRATEGIES UNDERTAKEN (ie. for maintenance and health and supportive therapies).

PATIENT INFORMATION LITERATURE OBTAINED:

3a   HOSP. NO.

NAME:

COMMUNICATION SHEET

4
MDCP/PA

NAME: HOSP. NO:

PHYSICAL ASSESSMENT

HEIGHT: WEIGHT:

VITAL SIGNS:
Temperature   BP:
Respiration: Pulse:
                     Urine:

REFERRAL INFORMATION

RESPIRATION: (eg. pattern, variation on exertion or at rest, cough or wheeze):

SENSATION: (eg. recent changes, aids/prosthesis)

VISION:

HEARING:

SMELL:

TASTE:

TOUCH:

SPEECH:

HYDRATION & NUTRITION: (eg. weight: changes, appetite changes, swallowing, special diet and fluid imbalance, thirst, skin turgor, dry tongue):

ELIMINATION: (eg. changes in frequency, nature):

Figure 1.1 The Royal Marsden NHS Trust Multidisciplinary Care Plan and Patient Assessment Form.

NAME:

HOSP. NO:

5
MDCP/PA

PHYSICAL ASSESSMENT CONT.

REFERRAL INFORMATION

SLEEP/REST: (eg. position, time, relation to fatigue/relaxation, recent changes in pattern, usual pattern, aids to sleep):

MOVEMENT: (eg. balance, co-ordination, posture, energy level, musculo-skeletal disorders, pain oedema):

MOBILISATION: (eg. level of independence - mobility aids/orthoses used):

MOVEMENT IN BED: (eg. turning, sitting up):

Bed to Chair:
Walking Indoors:
On & Off Toilet:
Stairs:
Walking Outdoors:

MOVING AND HANDLING

Patient Ability Rating
Clinical Restrictions
Handling Task Rating

(please score according to category headings. If total score is greater than four please complete the PATIENT HANDLING RISK MANAGEMENT FORM)

PATIENT ABILITY RATING
0 - Patient able to move independently
1 - patient needs minimal assistance supervision
2 - Patient able to co-operate
3 - Patient aware of surroundings, may have moderate ability to assist
4 - Patient able to assist in a limited way, but may be unco-operative or likely to behave unpredictably
5 - Patient unable to assist in any way

CLINICAL ASSESSMENT
0 - No attachments
1 - 1 attachments eg. catheter (v) Oxygen (please state)
2 - Multiple attachments &/or special bed/chair (please comment)

HANDLING TASK RATING
0 - No assistance
1 - Moves under supervision
2 - Minimal human assistance
3 - Moving aids required

PERSONAL HYGIENE: (eg. teeth/dentures present, toothache, bleeding, soreness, dry mouth, inflammation):

SKIN (eg. integrity, dryness, colour, broken areas, sensitivity, bruising - especially if recent, treatment, marks, hair loss):

SKIN APPLIANCES/TOPICAL AGENTS (eg. stoma and/or special dressings):

6
MDCP/PA/SA

PHYSICAL ASSESSMENT CONT.

REFERRAL INFORMATION

ANATOMICAL CHANGES: (eg. through surgery, treatment side effects):

REPRODUCTION & FERTILITY: (eg. menstrual cycle, contraception, sperm banking):

SIGNATURE: DATE:

SOCIAL ASSESSMENT

CULTURAL NEEDS (eg. diet, dress, custom):

FAMILY DETAILS (eg. who lives in the family, responsibility for children under 18 and/or adult dependents who are vulnerable due to disability or frailty):

ACCOMMODATION (eg. house, flat, sheltered housing, nursing or residential home):

WORK: (occupation, previous occupation, likely or actual problem):

FINANCE: (would patient and/or carer like advice on income or disability-related DSS benefits?

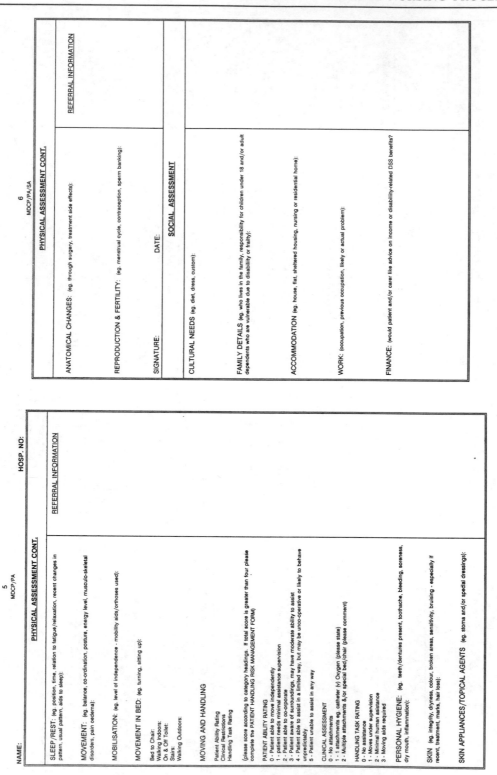

TRIGGERS FOR INITIAL ASSESSMENT BY SOCIAL SERVICES

8

Triggers for community care assessment by social services

These trigger questions are designed for use by nursing staff to screen out patients with potentially high social care needs whose eligibility for community care services has to be assessed in more detail by a hospital-based social worker. If you tick any of the boxes under "Care Needs", please refer immediately. If you tick any of the boxes under "Social Network" and "Environment", the patient should be discussed at the multi-disciplinary team meeting.

Care Needs

1. Significant change in ability to look after self due to the effects of treatment or the debilitating symptoms of progressive disease

2. Patient has, and is aware of limited prognosis, requiring a complex package of palliative and community care.

3. Patient appears to have very high social and nursing care needs which suggest a residential or nursing home as a placement option

4. Patient appears to be in need of NHS-funded Continuing Care (ie. has a score of 3 and less on Barthel ADL index)

Social Network

5. High dependency on a carer for all or most aspects of physical care

6. Carer is worried about his/her ability to continue caring

7. Patient is carer for partner, vulnerable adult dependent and/or child(ren) under 18

Environment

8. Housing unsuitable, access problems of inadequate heating, electricity, water supplies

9. Patient is homeless or threatened with homelessness

Please tick the appropriate box(es) and **telephone** the social services department with information **established** in the Social Assessment if a referral is indicated

Date of completion:

Referral made to social services department: Yes/No

Date of referral:

Signature:

NAME: HOSP. NO:

8a
MDCP/K1

KNOWLEDGE OF ILLNESS

This section asks you about your knowledge of your illness and treatment so that we can help you stay as informed as you'd like to be.

NAME: HOSP, NO:

7
MDCP/SA

SOCIAL ASSESSMENT CONT.

	REFERRAL INFORMATION
SPIRITUAL NEEDS (eg. attitudes towards illness, family, world, God)	

COMMUNITY SERVICES PRIOR TO ADMISSION/ATTENDANCE: (eg. home help, meals on wheels, district nursing)

TYPE OF SERVICE	CONTACT PERSON INCLUDING ADDRESS AND TELEPHONE NUMBER	NOTIFIED OF ADMISSION

ASSESSMENT COMPLETED BY: DATE:

Figure 1.1 *Continued*

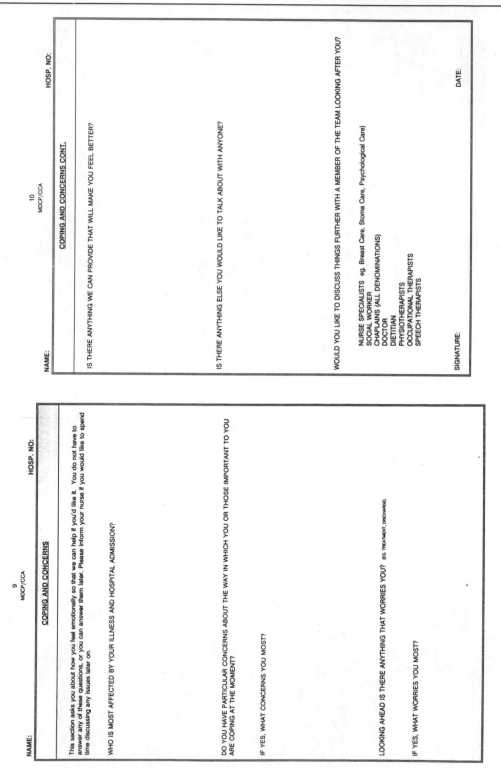

NAME: HOSP. NO:

10
MDCP/CCA

COPING AND CONCERNS CONT.

IS THERE ANYTHING WE CAN PROVIDE THAT WILL MAKE YOU FEEL BETTER?

IS THERE ANYTHING ELSE YOU WOULD LIKE TO TALK ABOUT WITH ANYONE?

WOULD YOU LIKE TO DISCUSS THINGS FURTHER WITH A MEMBER OF THE TEAM LOOKING AFTER YOU?

NURSE SPECIALISTS   eg. Breast Care, Stoma Care, Psychological Care)
SOCIAL WORKER
CHAPLAINS (ALL DENOMINATIONS)
DOCTOR
DIETITIAN
PHYSIOTHERAPISTS
OCCUPATIONAL THERAPISTS
SPEECH THERAPISTS

SIGNATURE: DATE:

NAME: HOSP. NO:

9
MDCP/CCA

COPING AND CONCERNS

This section asks you about how you feel emotionally so that we can help if you'd like it. You do not have to answer any of these questions, or you can answer them later. Please inform your nurse if you would like to spend time discussing any issues later on.

WHO IS MOST AFFECTED BY YOUR ILLNESS AND HOSPITAL ADMISSION?

DO YOU HAVE PARTICULAR CONCERNS ABOUT THE WAY IN WHICH YOU OR THOSE IMPORTANT TO YOU ARE COPING AT THE MOMENT?

IF YES, WHAT CONCERNS YOU MOST?

LOOKING AHEAD IS THERE ANYTHING THAT WORRIES YOU?   (EG. TREATMENT, DISCHARGE)

IF YES, WHAT WORRIES YOU MOST?

DISCHARGE NOTES

NAME: HOSP. NO.

Agreed D/C Co-ordinator

Agreed D/C Date

Agencis Contacted	Arrangements Made	Signature	Date
District Nurse Name: Telephone No.			
Hospice Home Care/ MacMillan Team Name: Telephone No.			
Social Services (Community Care) Name: Telephone No.			
Home Care Name: Telephone No.			
TTOs Prescribed With Patient	YES/NO YES/NO		
Transport booked for D/C	YES/NOT REQUIRED		
Date OPA/ reacmission	YES/NOT REQUIRED		
OPA given to patient	YES/NO Date: Time		
Respite Booked	YES/NO Date:		
District Nurse Referral Letter Completed/phones	YES/NOT REQUIRED		
Hospice Home Care/ MacMillan Letter/phoned	YES/NOT REQUIRED		
M.D. Interim D/C Summary	YES/NOT REQUIRED		

MDCP/DS

NAME: HOSP. NO:

DATE	SUMMARY OF CARE ON DISCHARGE	SIGNATURE

NAME: HOSP. NO:

11
MDCP/AC

AREAS OF CARE

FROM ASSESSMENT AND ASSESSMENT CHECKS, PLEASE LIST OR MODIFY PROBLEMS OR AREAS OF CARE WHICH NEED ATTENTION.

PROBLEM/AREA OF CARE	DATE IDENTIFIED	DATE OF FINAL REVIEW OR RESOLVED

NAME: HOSP. NO:

MDCP/RC

RECORD OF CARE

DATE	AREA OF CARE	SIGNATURE
	ANTICIPATED OUTCOME:	
	ACTION:	
	CONTINUOUS EVALUATION AND REVIEW:	

Figure 1.1 *Continued*

cational and social needs, but this is also a time when nurses have the opportunity to observe the patient from a holistic perspective. An awareness of the patient's relationship with their partner, and of their mood and body language, can provide nurses with information on how patients are coping with their illness and their treatments. Miaskowski & Nielson (1985) emphasize the importance of a structured approach to nursing assessment in reducing the risk of omitting key questions when time is short.

Whatever method is adopted to guide formal assessment, it remains a crucial part of effective nursing practice, alongside the less structured approach to ongoing daily assessment. In 1991 the Royal College of Nursing of the United Kingdom Cancer Nursing Society published standards of care as a guide to cancer nurses, acknowledging the crucial role of assessment in modern cancer nursing.

Summary
Nurses have a central role to play in helping patients to manage the demands of the procedures described in this book. The key to success in this role is accurate assessment of patients' needs and a commitment to meeting them with sensitivity. By assisting patients to communicate these needs, nurses can move towards care that is truly patient centred. These issues will now be explored in more depth.

COMMUNICATION
Good communication is regarded as being an integral and essential part of nursing (Macleod Clark & Sims, 1988; Wilkinson, 1991). Both verbal and non-verbal communication are required to assess, convey information and help meet emotional needs of patients and their families. The purpose of communication is to ensure appropriate social contact and professional interaction to meet patients' needs (Macleod Clark et al., 1991). In linking the importance of communication with patient assessment, this section will explore the need for, and effect of, communication in a cancer setting. It then describes adjustment styles of patients and the importance of good communication skills in differing circumstances.

The need for clear communication
The topic of communication in health care has been widely researched and evaluated and the beneficial effects of good communication have been clearly demonstrated. The provision of clear information and explanation on admission to hospital and prior to medical procedures has been shown to reduce pain, anxiety and side-effects of treatment (Wilson-Barnett, 1977; Watson, 1983; Byrne et al., 1993). It was found that knowledgeable patients expressed a desire for further

information to support their beliefs (Cassileth et al., 1980). This is substantiated by Eardley's three studies looking at questions that radiotherapy staff were asked and patients' reactions to this treatment. The studies state that meeting patients' needs for information, both prior to and during radiotherapy, would make the experience less traumatic (Eardley, 1983, 1986a,b).

Partners or family members may have even greater communication needs than the person with cancer (Bluglass, 1991). They are often responsible for the majority of care given to the cancer patient in the community and may wish to talk to the doctor or nurse but may not receive the information they require through inhibition or uncertainty (Macleod Clark & Sims, 1988).

The value to patients of good communication may be related to the degree of importance that this holds for them in the clinical environment (Mallett, 1997). King (1971) says that verbal communication is effective when it satisfies basic desires for recognition, participation and self-realization by direct personal contact between persons. It would appear from this that good communication is not only tangibly beneficial but is perceived by patients to be a necessary intervention.

Verbal and non-verbal communication
Communication is complex and involves more than the spoken word. Both verbal and non-verbal activity are integral to the process of communication and should be given consideration whenever nurse–patient interactions are studied (Mallett, 1997). Factors such as voice tone, volume and inflection form vocal content. However, the research into communication in nursing is often deductive, pre-categorized and pays little attention to the organization of naturally occurring non-verbal communication. This may result in a lack of consideration of the importance of factors such as gaze and gestures in nurse–patient interactions (Mallett, 1997).

Distancing, body movements and touch are other examples of non-verbal communication which may be crucial in assessing patients' needs (Porchet-Munro, 1991). This author states that 'body language gives away our uncertainties' and 'unmasks words'. Thus, in a clinical situation it may be possible to give one verbal message whilst transmitting an incongruous non-verbal one. For example, a nurse may adopt an inappropriate, cheerful expression whilst conveying bad news to a relative. Touch is another important aspect of non-verbal communication which can be directed and used in a meaningful manner. However, McCann & McKenna (1993) indicate that most of nursing touch may be task orientated rather than expressive in nature, but some patients may not perceive any touch positively.

It is important to recognize the differences in nonverbal communication across different cultures. Pease

(1981) shows that we do not necessarily have to look to other continents or countries to find differences; people from rural communities have variances in their behaviour from city dwellers. Other differences may also arise due to social background, family upbringing, sexuality, gender and past experience (Davitz *et al.*, 1976).

Skills of communication

There is a clear distinction to be made between communication which could be considered therapeutic and skilled communication, as the two are not necessarily synonymous (Mallett, 1989). This next section focuses on those skills which may be considered central to effective communication in nursing care.

Macleod Clark *et al.* (1991) describe a model of a hierarchy of communication skills in the form of a pyramid with information giving and allowing expression of feelings amongst the basic skills in the broad base. With self-awareness and training, specialist skills such as building a trusting relationship over time improve towards the peak.

Considering first the more basic skills, some examples of these are clarification, reflection, silence, probing and summarizing (Macleod Clark & Sims, 1988; Burton, 1991). For example, clarification can be illustrated as:

(Patient)   'I don't think I can cope with chemotherapy.'
(Nurse)   'What would be most difficult about the chemotherapy for you to cope with?'

Here the nurse is seeking to understand more specifically what the patient means.

Reflection may be used to invite the patient to elaborate, such as:

(Patient)   'I'm finding things really hard at the moment.'
(Nurse)   'Really hard?'

Silence, although uncomfortable at times, can also be a powerful communication skill used to encourage the patient to reflect on what has been said (Faulkner & Maguire, 1984; Burnard, 1990). At times probing may be employed to invite the patient to expand on a particular issue and clarify any vagueness, for instance:

(Nurse)   'You mentioned you were having trouble sleeping. Can you tell me more about that?'

Summarizing helps the nurse and the patient draw the main issues of the interaction together. It is especially useful to help the patient and nurse focus and move on and also allows for clarification of mutual understanding (Hargie *et al.*, 1987).

The use of open questions can be considered one of the simplest and yet most effective means of encouraging patients to communicate, as many research studies confirm (Hargie *et al.*, 1987; Macleod Clark & Sims, 1988; Burnard, 1990). An open question is prefixed by words such as 'When', 'What' or 'How', and will help to discourage a 'Yes' or 'No' response. In this way, open communication may be facilitated. Questions should not begin with the word 'Why', which may be perceived as threatening or provocative (Brennan & Swan, 1995).

Some advanced skills that require more practice and self-awareness are challenging, empathy and unconditional positive regard (Rogers, 1967, 1980; Egan, 1994). Challenging is defined by Egan (1994) as 'an invitation to examine internal or external behaviour that seems to be self-defeating, harmful to others or both and to change the behaviour if it is found to be so'. Rogers (1980) said of empathy that it 'means entering the private perceptual world of the other and becoming thoroughly at home in it'. Kalisch (1971) defines empathy as 'the ability to perceive accurately the feelings of another person and to communicate this understanding to him' (cited in Burnard, 1990). However, confusion arises from the distinction between empathy as a way of being and empathy as a communication process or skill (Egan, 1994). Rogers' phrase 'unconditional positive regard' (Rogers, 1967) means that the patient is viewed with dignity and value as a worthwhile human being. The regard is offered without preconditions or demand for reciprocity and so involves a deep and positive feeling for the person. It was once assumed that good communicators were born not made, but nurses may develop these advanced skills with appropriate preparation and training (Macleod Clark & Sims, 1988).

Counselling could also be viewed as an advanced skill. However, Macleod Clark *et al.* (1991) indicate that nurses using advanced communication skills may not be counselling in the formal sense. Some required conditions for counselling are undergoing a recognized training programme and having appropriate supervision. The definition of counselling is given by the British Association for Counselling (1989a) as:

'An interaction in which one person offers another person time, attention and respect, with the intention of helping that person to explore, discover and clarify ways of living more resourcefully and toward greater well-being'.

Skills of counselling differ from listening skills or formal counselling and can be summarized in the following quote from the British Association for Counselling (1989b):

'What distinguishes the use of counselling skills from these other two activities are the intentions of the user, which are to enhance the performance of their functional role and the recipient will, in turn, perceive them in that role'.

Thus it can be deduced that for nurses to be formally counselling they have to be perceived by patients to be in that role and must be adequately prepared. Counselling must not be seen as a panacea but may be a preferred option for consenting patients or family members who will need to be referred to suitably qualified staff. If the person referred has refused to consent then they are unlikely to be able to engage in the counselling process. Egan (1994), who provides one model of counselling, states that outcomes depend on the competence and motivation of the helper and client and that the client has to be willing to take part.

There are some patient groups who may not be appropriate for counselling, for example severely brain-damaged patients or those with psychotic symptoms. This stresses the importance of assessment of the patient's individual needs and the implications for nurses to consider referral to appropriate agencies if necessary. Nurses need to communicate with every patient, but only a few patients will require formal counselling. Therefore there is a clear distinction to be made between good communication and formal counselling.

Barriers to communication

There is some evidence in the literature on the subject to support the theory that nurses often lack basic communication skills, resulting in frustration and anxiety for patients and their families. Hewison (1995) suggests that much of nurses' communication with patients is still superficial, routinized and related to tasks. In another study conducted involving 54 nurses in cancer care it was shown that nurses frequently use blocking tactics to prevent patients divulging their problems (Wilkinson, 1991). This obviously has implications when assessing patients, especially in terms of psychosocial needs. It is important to bear in mind that communication is a two-way process and a criticism of both these studies is that the influence of the patient on the communication process is missing. In an earlier report Webster (1981) describes how nurses avoid communicating with dying patients in seven different ways such as an abrupt change of the subject of conversation and withdrawing from a stressful situation. Although some studies highlight a requirement for nurses to be more aware of the importance of communication skills, greater self-awareness may in itself lead to increased emotional needs (Vachon, 1995). This may then necessitate further support from their peers and/or colleagues.

Nurses are expected to be able to cope with their own emotional reactions as well as those of patients and families. In communicating with patients there is always the risk that difficult issues may arise, and nurses may not feel equipped to deal with them effectively or fear that they themselves may become affected. Avoidance behav-

iours such as those highlighted by Wilkinson (1991) and Webster (1981) may consequently be employed. Although avoidance and distancing are natural defence mechanisms in stressful situations, nurses who develop increased self-awareness may recognize those obstructive defence mechanisms employed in their everyday work (Burnard, 1990). Maguire (1985) highlights barriers such as distancing, giving false reassurance and selective attention used by staff to prevent them getting close to patients' psychological suffering. He suggests that regular psychological support, opportunities for taking time out and short training courses may enable staff to relinquish these distancing tactics. Burnard (1990) defines self-awareness as:

'the gradual and continuous process of noticing and exploring aspects of the self, whether behavioural, psychological or physical, with the intention of developing personal and interpersonal understanding'.

He goes on to argue that the benefits of increased self-awareness extend outwards to facilitate meaningful relationships with others.

Avoidance behaviours may also be employed by patients and family members either by choice or as a consequence of denial. They may wish not to have information regarding, for instance, the extent of the disease or may unconsciously avoid meaningful communication. This highlights the need for an individual approach. Glaser & Strauss (1965) studied terminally ill patients and identified four awareness contexts which may apply to patients and those close to them:

- Closed
- Suspected
- Mutual pretence and
- Open awareness.

With closed and suspected awareness there is an imbalance of information as the family, nursing or medical staff act as custodians of information that the patient does not have. There is more potential for misunderstandings and distress to all parties than when communication is open and mutual. It is important to recognize that these categories are not absolute; the patient and family may move between levels of awareness at different stages of the illness experience and may be influenced by their perceived ability to cope at the time. The nurse's role is to recognize the difficulties that may arise from misunderstandings between the people involved and offer clarification and support where required (Macleod Clark & Sims, 1988).

Awareness and recognition of the patient's mental adjustment to cancer may enable nurses to communicate more effectively with them. Factors such as the stage of illness, available support, physical symptoms and so on will affect the fluctuation between adjustment styles (Moorey & Greer, 1989). The primary role of the nurse in communication is to assess, identify and help prioritize the needs of patients and families as well as facilitating their expression of feelings (catharsis). Moorey & Greer (1989) state that the thought process of the person with cancer incorporates three key factors:

• The view of the diagnosis
• Perceived control and
• The view of the prognosis.

In addition, there are five adjustment styles identified by Greer & Watson (1987) which indicate how patients may react to the experience of cancer. These are:

(1) Fighting spirit
(2) Avoidance or denial
(3) Fatalism
(4) Helplessness and hopelessness
(5) Anxious preoccupation.

In the first of these, the diagnosis is seen as a challenge, the person can exert some control over the stress and the prognosis is seen as optimistic. With avoidance or denial the threat from the diagnosis is minimal, the issue of control is irrelevant and the prognosis is seen as good. For the fatalist, the diagnosis represents a relatively minor threat, there is no control that can be exerted over the situation and the consequences of lack of control can and should be accepted with equanimity. In the fourth adjustment style, the diagnosis is seen as a major threat, no control can be exerted over the situation and the inevitable negative outcome is experienced as if this has already come about. With anxious preoccupation, where the person compulsively searches for reassurance, the diagnosis represents a major threat and there is uncertainty over the possibility of exerting control over the situation or the future. Similar to the awareness contexts, patients may change adjustment styles according to their circumstances and there is a danger in assuming patients may fall into specific categories. The adjustment styles are perhaps most helpful in enabling the nurse to assess patients' emotional reactions over time.

There may be many barriers to good communication present for the nurse and patient besides denial. The psychological impact of cancer may cause great mental anguish and patients and families may suffer symptoms of anxiety, depression and hopelessness. Findings on the levels of distress in cancer patients vary widely but as many as 44% have been found to have clinically significant psychiatric disorders (Derogatis et al., 1983). Depression may result in somatic symptoms such as insomnia and loss of appetite or behavioural effects such as social withdrawal. Cognitive symptoms include negative thoughts and loss of self–esteem (Moorey & Greer,

1989). Anxiety may impair the ability of the patient to retain information, as may pain or drowsiness (Nichols, 1984). Where possible the nurse should endeavour to minimize or eliminate physical discomfort prior to giving information or conducting a meaningful conversation.

There are many factors in the hospital setting which inhibit therapeutic communication such as noise, excessive heat, harsh lighting, interruptions and lack of privacy. It is helpful if the patient and/or family can be seen in a private room where interruptions can be minimized by an engaged sign on the door and the telephone silenced. Screens round the patient's bed are not sufficient as they only provide visual privacy. It is also useful to both patient and nurse if the nurse sets a time limit on the conversation, thereby giving a clear indication of boundaries (Phillips, 1992).

Psychosexual needs of adults

The importance of nurses addressing psychosexual needs has been reflected in the increasing amount of literature describing sexuality as an integral part of nursing care (Waterhouse & Metcalfe, 1991). Patients may experience a wide variety of problems from reduced ability to express themselves sexually due to alopecia, for example, to sexual dysfunction (Webb & O'Neill, 1988). Cancer treatments frequently create altered body image which may in turn lead to loss of libido and depression (Webb & O'Neill, 1988; Roberts et al., 1992). These needs can be assessed by putting them on the agenda through open communication.

There is anecdotal evidence to suggest that there are often misinterpretations of communication signals, such as a woman who is distanced by her partner post-mastectomy. The partner thinks that he or she is causing pain and the woman feels rejected. There is a clear need for openness in such situations to help avoid misunderstandings. Waterhouse & Metcalfe (1991) explored attitudes toward nurses discussing sexual concerns with patients and found that 92% of subjects thought that nurses should discuss sexual concerns with patients. However, Webb (1988) found that gynaecology nurses were less knowledgeable about sexuality than non-gynaecology nurses. As far back as 1988, Wilson & William's (1988) highlighted a positive relationship between nurses' attitudes towards sexuality in cancer patients and the number of nursing care practices related to alterations in sexuality. They suggest that as it is also demonstrated that lack of knowledge was given as a reason for not addressing sexual concerns, more initiatives to incorporate sexuality in the nursing curriculum could ease the discomfort. In some specialist areas these educational needs are being addressed. Nurses with more years of education and experience reported more nursing practices in this area. It would appear then from the literature that nurses' knowledge, attitudes and educational experience are inextricably linked when addressing psychosexual needs of patients.

Communication needs of children with cancer

Children with cancer have special communication needs highlighted by several factors given in the literature. There are different fears at different ages for the child. Sepion (1988) states that for young children, fears of abandonment and isolation are most prevalent while for the teenager, peer group rejection may be the greatest fear (Thompson, 1988). There is an intensified need to truth-tell to avoid confusion arising out of myths and secrecy (Sepion, 1988). Bluebond-Langner (1978) substantiates this by demonstrating that if parents and children resist communicating the mutual pretence used as a defence mechanism may deny children the opportunity to express their fears. Also, there may be iatrogenic educational problems for the child and physical and emotional disruption for siblings (Lansdown & Goldman, 1991). It can be seen from this that there is a need to involve the whole family in the treatment of the child which gives a greater sense of control for each family member (Lansdown & Goldman, 1991). Readers are referred to more specialized texts which explore this issue in greater depth (Douglas, 1993; Eiser, 1993; Koocher & O'Malley, 1991; Last & VanVeldhuizen, 1992; Muller *et al.*, 1992).

Summary

Communication can be seen to be a vital part of nursing and is one of the means of enabling ongoing assessment of patient individual needs as part of skilled cancer care. It is hoped that this brief review will put into perspective the most salient concerns, aims and difficulties present for the nurse wishing to explore the use of good communication skills. It can be seen that there are certain difficulties when researching communication but this remains essential in order to promote this key aspect of patient care.

Using an individualized care approach, patients have unique needs which may be met through careful assessment and good communication skills. However, promoting a patient-focused approach will inevitably raise moral and ethical dilemmas which require discussion and debate. In the following part of this chapter, some of these dilemmas will be explored in the context of consent to examination and treatment.

CONSENT TO EXAMINATION AND TREATMENT

Consent is an individual's freely given agreement to examination, treatment or an act of care based on informa-tion about, and an understanding of, what is proposed. In order to give consent, a person must be deemed to be competent (Kennedy & Grubb, 1994). Obtaining valid consent prior to a clinical procedure is both a legal and an ethical imperative. The process requires sophisticated assessment and communication skills, together with a profound respect for the rights of the individual. The health care professional, in order to demonstrate their respect for another person, the patient, and to avoid committing a civil wrong in law, must obtain that individual's consent prior to any procedure.

The nurse's responsibilities towards patients are clearly laid down in the *Code of Professional Conduct* (United Kingdom Central Council for Nursing, Midwifery and Health Visiting, 1992) and *Exercising Accountability* (UKCC, 1989). These are essential reading for all practitioners and form a useful introduction to the detailed information presented here. First, consideration is given to a possible ethical framework to be applied to the consent process. Second, the law is examined to determine what is required of the practitioner. Finally, a brief mention is made of consent in a research setting, with provision of further references.

An ethical basis for consent

The law and the Department of Health (DoH) in its documents *Patient Consent to Examination or Treatment* (1990) and *The Patient's Charter* (1995) use the language of rights to describe a patient's claims on, or expectations of, health care. 'Rights' is also a term which is used widely by society in general in the 1990s. It is necessary to consider the nature of these rights particularly in relationship to the health care professional's duties.

Health care professionals have a special relationship with their patients. On entering this relationship the practitioner assumes certain special duties towards the patient, over and above those which ordinary human beings have to each other such as a duty not to kill them, a duty to keep a promise or a duty not to tell a lie. The features of this relationship are described generally as a duty of care which contains the following:

- a duty to respect the patient's autonomy;
- a duty to act in the patient's best interests;
- a duty to promote health and prevent harm (United Kingdom Central Council for Nursing, Midwifery and Health Visiting, 1992).

The patient can then be said to have certain rights, as mirror images of those duties, that is the right to expect the practitioner to respect their autonomy, the right to expect the practitioner to act in their best interests and the right to expect the practitioner to promote their health and not cause them harm.

There also exists on behalf of the practitioner a duty to

advise the patient and to inform them of what is proposed. This duty may be seen as part of the duty to respect autonomy as the information imparted will enable the patient to determine what action should be taken, or it could be viewed by the practitioner as part of their duty to act in the best interests of the patient, in which case only selected information may be forthcoming (Speechley, 1992).

Duties, and therefore rights, may be ordered in more than one way and this order is dependent on the opinion of the individual practitioner – one duty may be given greater or lesser weight in a particular circumstance. Respect for autonomy may be overridden in order to act in the best interests, or vice versa. The professional is in control and, therefore, the patient's rights are restructured in order of importance by them. Consideration of rights from this perspective loses much of the force normally given to the term, as the patient's rights are decided and prioritized by another. Because rights mirror duties, they are negative rights which the patient does not own or have control of, for example they may not be waived or alienated. The right may only be exercised in one way, the way determined by the professional. For example, information to the patient may be controlled so that the action (choice of treatment) is what the practitioner regards as in the patient's best interests (the most medically efficacious) (Speechley, 1992).

The humanist principles of biomedical ethics formulated and developed by Beauchamp & Childress (1994) contain similar elements to those embodied within a duty of care – respect for autonomy, nonmaleficence, beneficence – plus the concept of justice. Justice may be applied on an individual basis as fair, equitable and appropriate treatment or at a societal level as fair, equitable and appropriate distribution of health care in society. These principles may also be ranked in different orders, so that once again the respect for autonomy may not be uppermost.

Of the three components of valid consent, information is the one which can be best used to illustrate the different ways in which the duty of care and the principle of respect for autonomy can be used. Selective information giving is justified using a number of possible arguments.

- In seeking help, the patient has demonstrated a willingness to undergo the recommended treatment and explicit consent, demanded as a respect for autonomy, is not required.

- The patient, given their vulnerability and anxiety, is not autonomous and, therefore, cannot rationally decide between treatment options. There is no autonomy to be respected.

- Withholding information is in the patient's best interests as full knowledge of the situation and/or treatment may cause distress and may even lead to the patient refusing the recommended treatment.

- The patient will not be able to understand the rationale and complexities of the treatment given that she/he has not had the training and experience of the professional and there is not sufficient time to explain the intricacies of therapy, if the desired outcome is to be achieved.

- Full disclosure, particularly of any uncertainty, will cause confusion and distress resulting in loss of trust and confidence and, once again cannot be considered as compatible with a duty of care.

The theory of positive patient's rights to make a valid consent to examination, treatment or act of care originates from the North American doctrine of the informed consent theorists (Beauchamp & Childress, 1994), which is supported in part by law. The assertion that patients have a prima facie right to make an informed choice about treatment is grounded in the principle of autonomy or self-determination and levels a positive duty to inform upon the professional.

There are several practical difficulties within informed consent theory due to the burden which it places on the professional or that which rests with the patient. However, it is a useful concept within which to consider what rights are exercised during the consent process and what kind of rights they are. In order for a competent person to make a voluntary decision two rights need to be exercised:

- the right to self determination;
- the right to information to enable autonomous action.

Rights-based moral theorists adopt slightly differing views depending on whether those rights are grounded in autonomy (Hart, 1984) or equal respect (Dworkin, 1984). The autonomy-based theorist proposes that a natural right is discretionary, that is it may be exercised as we please within the limits of the rights of others. Discretionary rights are alienable in that they can be waived temporarily or relinquished permanently provided only that the decision to do this is fully informed, well considered and fully voluntary.

When equal respect is used as the central premise, rights are again regarded as discretionary but inalienable, that is always retained. However, that to which the right pertains is alienable. For example, the right to life is discretionary and inalienable, to live or die as we choose within the boundaries of autonomy. However, that to which we have the right is alienable, that is life. Therefore the right to life may be exercised as the right to die, unimpeded by others.

Both these views of rights place control firmly with

the individual and, in addition, allow them to decide to what extent they wish to control a situation such as information giving or decision making. The individual is further respected if one incorporates the view of Mackie (1984) that rights provide a 'persistent defence of . . . certain vital interests of people', which are largely determined by that person to protect the 'choice of how to live [one's life]'.

All rights-based theories stress autonomy and therefore can only be valid in circumstances where the individual is, or has been, autonomous (legally competent). However, if autonomous, the individual's wishes are paramount and should be respected even if they appear to conflict or lack congruence with the health care professional's opinions, or current thought. This requires careful assessment of the person's needs and use of verbal and non-verbal communication skills to elicit the degree of control they wish to exercise and how much information is desired.

This model provides a flexible framework in which the patient always leads but which is not onerous to themselves or the practitioner, and also enables joint or negotiated decision making to occur. A schematic representation is found in Fig. 1.2 (Speechley, 1992).

Lack of autonomy, refusal of treatment and advance directives

Problems arise, however, when an individual is not, or has never been, autonomous as they are accorded no rights. In this situation an autonomous proxy may enter consent on behalf of a minor using a 'best interests' approach as required by law, or the incompetent adult may be treated within the health care professional's duty of care using the same criteria (Law Commission, 1995).

If a patient has been autonomous but is no longer, the right to self-determination may be exercised using an advance directive. The ethical issues surrounding the right to anticipatory decision making, particularly related to refusal of treatment and rejection of life-prolonging procedures, have been widely discussed but mainly in the context of actively withdrawing treatment (Scowen, 1993, 1994; Craig, 1994; Ashby & Stoffell, 1995; Dunlop *et al.*, 1995) or with people who have AIDS (Schlyter, 1992), including 'do not resuscitate' orders.

An instruction by the patient fits comfortably within a rights-based theoretical framework and this view has recently been accepted in English law (*Re T* 1992; *Re C* 1993). Although these cases dealt primarily with refusal of treatment in both instances, advance directives are acknowledged and commented upon.

In *Re T* Lord Donaldson, Master of the Rolls, states that the patient must express his wishes 'in clear terms', preferably in writing. It is Grubb's opinion (1992) that *Re T* had 'undoubtedly given the "green light" for advance directives in the form of "living wills"'.

In *Re C* this stance was reinforced as C did not just wish to prevent amputation of his leg at the time he was competent but also in the future when he might become incompetent. Once again Grubb's view (1993) is that 'The injunction granted by Thorpe, J. only gave court backing to what was already legally binding upon the doctors'. Competency (autonomy) was an issue in this case and Grubb welcomes the three stage approach adopted by Mr Justice Thorpe as 'it is important . . . that the law does not make the hurdle of competence too onerous otherwise the law will effectively deprive all but the most "comprehending" of their right of self determination'.

Nevertheless this view is disputed by some (Stauch, 1995) and endorsed by others, namely the Law Commission in its report on mental incapacity (1995). This includes a section on advance statements in health care which 'embraces anticipatory decision-making by the person while competent to make arrangements for future incapacity'.

Summary

Exploration of moral theory and principles enables the discovery of an approach which places the patient at the centre of decision making, but in a flexible and pragmatic way. Rights emerge as positive claims which

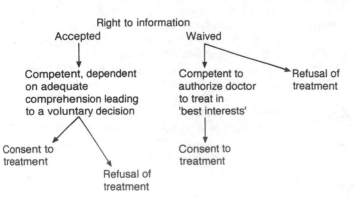

Figure 1.2 The right to information and self-determination: treatment. (Speechley, 1992)

are enduring. The non-autonomous (legally incompetent) individual is protected within the professional's duty of care.

Conflict between the wishes of the patient, the professional and occasionally the relatives may be resolved more easily within this framework and the process of allocating pre-eminence to one duty or principle unnecessary.

The legal basis for consent

'A patient has the right under common law to give or withhold consent prior to examination or treatment. . . . This is one of the basic principles of health care.' (DoH, 1990).

English common law identifies three components of a valid consent:

(1) Competency
(2) Information
(3) Voluntrariness

If an examination, procedure or treatment is carried out without these requirements being fulfilled then a civil action may be brought in the tort of battery, which protects a person from unwanted touching, or in the tort of negligence, where harm results directly from the procedure. It is the health care professional's duty to ensure that a person is competent to consent, has sufficient information on which to base their decision and that the decision is voluntary and uncoerced (DoH, 1990).

Competency

Competency or capacity to consent to a procedure must be considered in all situations. It should not be assumed that an adult or a child is competent, or incompetent, without a full assessment of that individual. The law provides some guidance here.

Minors, that is children under the age of 16 years: following *Gillick* v. *West Norfolk and Wisbech AHA* (1986), in which the lawfulness of prescribing contraceptives to a minor was considered, a competent child is defined as one who '. . . is capable of understanding what is proposed, and of expressing his or her wishes' . . .' (Lord Justice Fraser). In practice, most children are accompanied by their parents or legal guardians who will formally consent after discussion with the child and health care professional. In the case of a child who is not competent, a parent will usually offer a proxy consent on behalf of their child. Others who may be empowered to act as proxy for a child are laid down in the Children Act 1989 (in Scotland, the Age of Legal Capacity (Scotland) Act 1991). All proxies must adopt a 'best interests' approach, that is they act in the child's best interests, inherent in which is that the examination, procedure or

treatment is therapeutic and intended to benefit the particular individual.

Persons between the ages of 16 and 18 years: The Family Law Reform Act 1969 states in section 8 (1)

'The consent of a minor who has attained the age of sixteen years to any surgical, medical or dental treatment which, in the absence of consent, would constitute a trespass to his person, shall be as effective as it would be if he were of full age; and where a minor has by virtue of this section given an effective consent to any treatment it shall not be necessary to obtain any consent for it from his parent or guardian.'

If a person between 16 and 18 years is not competent, using the 'Gillick' definition, a proxy consent will be appropriate, as for minors.

Although statute law and common law indicate who is competent to consent, there is a contradiction regarding competency to refuse treatment. Recent cases, *Re R* (a minor) (wardship: medical treatment) 1991 and *Re W* (minor: refusal of treatment) 1992, one concerning a child under 16 and one over, have given both a parent and a court the power to override a refusal of treatment by a competent child.

Adults: when considering if an adult is competent to consent to a clinical procedure, an individual approach is, once again, necessary as Lord Donaldson, Master of the Rolls, pointed out (*Re T* 1992)

'. . . every adult is presumed to have . . . capacity [to consent], but it is a presumption which can be rebutted.'

This was stated in a contrasting way by Skegg (1984)

'The fact that a person is suffering from a mental disorder, as defined in the Mental Health Act 1983, does not in itself preclude that person from giving a legally effective consent.'

There are several circumstances within health care, and more specifically cancer care, where capacity to consent may be wrongly perceived to be present or absent. Examples include:

(1) Persons with mental disabilities or learning disorders, where capacity may be dependent solely on the communication skills of the health care professional.
(2) Patients with cerebral tumours where a physical disability or speech impediment does not necessarily indicate an impairment of comprehension.
(3) Patients who are in pain, emotionally distressed or shocked and temporarily lacking competency which may by restored by pain relief, time, patience and psychological support.

Competency, as defined by the courts and for the purposes of this section, is based on the capability of a person to understand and express a view. Therefore, all measures to assist this process must be employed, such as provision of interpreters, including those proficient in British sign language, and the involvement of speech and language therapists for people with communication difficulties. Examples of legal, health and social services cases where choices have been influenced by communication can be found in *Access to Justice* (Nuffield Foundation, 1993).

With regard to proxy consent on behalf of an incompetent adult, the view put forward by Professor Skegg is

'. . . there is no general doctrine whereby a spouse or near relative is empowered to give legally effective consent to medical procedures to be carried out on an adult.'

The common law appears to support this view and Lord Goff (*Re F* 1990), concerning sterilization, uses the principle of necessity to solve the practical problems related to this. He says '. . . the doctor must then act in the best interests of his patient, just as if he had received his patient's consent to do so'. However, the decision will most frequently be taken after discussion with relatives, carers and other health care professionals. In cases of conflicting views or doubt, the courts should be consulted.

Information

'Patients are entitled to receive sufficient information in a way that they understand about proposed treatments, the possible alternatives and any substantial risks, so that they can make a balanced judgement.' (DoH, 1990)

As Kennedy and Grubb point out (1994)

'The aphorism "informed consent" has entered the language as being synonymous with valid consent. . . . The requirement that consent be informed is only one, albeit a very important ingredient of valid consent. Furthermore, the expression informed consent begs all the necessary questions . . . for example, how informed is informed?'

So how much information is required by English law to be given to the patient? Various medical negligence cases provide a background to the current requirements and some clarification of the Department of Health's statement which opens this section. These legal cases also provide the definition of the standard of care which patients may expect from all health care professionals carrying out procedures such as those contained in this manual.

In *Hills* v. *Potter* (1984) Mr Justice Hirst states

'. . . on any view English law does require the surgeon to supply to the patient information to enable the plaintiff to decide whether or not to undergo the operation'.

He continues

'. . . In my judgement, McNair, J. in *Bolam* v. *Friern Barnet Hospital Management Committee* (1957) applied the medical standard to advice prior to an operation, as well as to diagnosis and to treatment. . . . In every case the court must be satisfied that the standard contended for on their behalf accords with that upheld by a substantial body of medical opinion, and that this body of medical opinion is both respectable and responsible, and experienced in this particular field of medicine.'

The amount and quality of information became the point at issue once again in *Sidaway* v. *Board of Governors of the Bethlem Royal Hospital* (1985). The majority judgement in the House of Lords confirmed the view expressed in *Hills* v. *Potter*. However, two new elements were identified in Sidaway. First was the need to warn of risk which Lord Bridge described as a 'substantial risk of grave adverse consequences'. Lord Templeman offered a similar but slightly more specific definition:

'There is no doubt that a doctor ought to draw the attention of a patient to a danger which may be special in kind or magnitude or special to the patient.'

Despite these statements it was acknowledged that this remains an area where clinical judgement is the prime determinant.

Second was the duty to answer questions which, again, was addressed by Lord Bridge who said

'when questioned specifically by a patient of apparently sound mind about the risks involved in a particular treatment proposed, the doctor's duty must, in my opinion, be to answer both truthfully and as fully as the questioner requires'.

The importance of assessment – what is important, or likely to be important, to the patient – and communication of information is reinforced here. Sometimes the content of an answer may not be in doubt but the means of communicating it may be vital to understanding, and the subsequent decision.

There have been several 'failure to warn' cases since Sidaway in the mid-1980s, all of which have supported the views expressed by one or other of their Lordships. However, courts in other common law jurisdictions have challenged the judgement in Sidaway, notably Australia in 1992 (Kirby, 1995).

In 1994 three cases of actions for negligence addressed the issue of information in the English courts. In *Smith* v. *Barking, Havering and Brentwood Health Authority*, the surgeon was found to be negligent in having failed to warn of the risks inherent in the operation and failing to inform the plaintiff of the possible consequences of not having the operation (Stern, 1995). Also in *Smith* v. *Salford Health Authority* the surgeon was found to be negligent in his pre-operative assessment of the patient and his explanation of the risks of both treatment and non-treatment (Stern, 1995). However, in neither instance did the actions succeed on the basis of this alone, as in both it was found that even if given the appropriate information, the patients would have consented to the operations and, therefore, the outcome would have been unchanged. In the third case, *Smith* v. *Tunbridge Wells Health Authority* (1994) negligence was proven based on non-disclosure of information. Mr Justice Morland considered that the patient would have been acting reasonably in refusing to follow the surgeon's advice and have the operation if he had known of the risk of impotence associated with it. Therefore, the harm was caused by lack of information.

Provision of information to patients to achieve a valid consent to examination, treatment and care requires the health care professional to use their clinical judgement:

- To assess the amount of information needed by the patient and carers.
- To explain the procedure clearly and accurately.
- To provide honest answers to the patient's questions in a sympathetic manner.

These require considerable communication skills and, perhaps most important of all, time.

Kirby (1995) concludes with a criticism of the differing standards of information between England and other countries, saying

'. . . at the heart of the difference is an attitude to the fundamental rights of the particular patients. Those rights should take primacy both in legal formulae and in medical practice.'

Voluntariness

'Consent to treatment must be given freely and without coercion . . .' (DoH, 1990).

In the USA the President's Commission report on making health care decisions (1983) (in Kennedy & Grubb, 1994) considered voluntariness in decision making thus:

'The patient's participation in the decision making process and ultimate decision regarding care must be voluntary. A choice that has been coerced, or that resulted from serious manipulation of a person's ability to make an intelligent and informed decision, is not the person's own free choice. This has long been recognised in law: a consent forced by threats or induced by fraud or misrepresentation is legally viewed as no consent at all.'

Within this statement three issues are identified – force, coercion and manipulation.

The nature of cancer, the vulnerability of an individual faced with an unfamiliar and frightening environment and the disproportionate amount of power and perceived inequality between health care professional and patient may all, to varying degrees, intrude into the decision making process.

Force is not a concept normally associated with health care. However, the subtle features of this are explained by the President's Commission (1983) (in Kennedy & Grubb, 1994):

'Although it is typically not viewed as forced treatment, a good deal of routine care . . . is provided without explicit and voluntary consent by patients. The expectation on the part of professionals is that patients, once in such a setting, will simply go along with such routine care.'

This far reaching report included a survey of treatment refusals and observational studies in care settings where the communications which accompanied the care offered no choice, compliance was expected and enforced. In addition the routine tests or acts of care were those most likely to be refused.

Coercion is

'. . . when the person is credibly threatened by another individual, either explicitly or by implication, with unwanted and avoidable consequences unless the patient accedes to the specified course of action.' (President's Commission (1983) in Kennedy & Grubb, 1994).

Coercion is typically perceived to be associated with an imbalance of power between professional and patient, and this may indeed be so. However, the motivation may be benevolent when conflicts arise as to the best course of action to be taken but, even so, this cannot be condoned.

Pressure may also be exerted by family or carers, acting with the patient's best interests in mind or from an ulterior motive to further their own ends. All members of the caring team need to be aware of this possibility and, if the situation arises, support the patient and assist them to overcome such pressure.

Manipulation is often a more subtle way of influencing the voluntary nature of choice. For example, while on one hand information may be withheld or distorted, alternatives may not be presented and risks may be minimized, on the other hand '. . . a professional's careful choice of words or nuances of tone and emphasis might present the situation in a manner calculated to heighten the appeal of a particular course of action' (President's Commission 1983).

Many legal cases relate to institutional settings where it could be said that there is no freedom to exercise choice. However in *Re T* (adult: refusal of treatment) 1992 Lord Donaldson offered guidance as to what could be considered undue influence by English law:

'. . . (t)he doctors have to consider whether the decision is really that of the patient . . . (d)oes the patient really mean what he says or is he merely saying it for a quiet life, to satisfy someone else, or because the advice and persuasion to which he has been subjected is such that he can no longer think and decide for himself?'

Lord Donaldson went on to say that consideration should also be given to the strength of will of the patient and the relationship between the patient and the persuader, whether personal or professional. In *Re T* it was found that using these criteria T's decision (to refuse a blood transfusion) was not her own but that of her mother.

In cancer care health professionals have several responsibilities related to the voluntary nature of decision making:

• To recognize the vulnerability of patients and to be alert to circumstances when undue influence may be exerted by colleagues or relatives.
• To gain consent for all investigations, treatment or acts of care and not to assume that 'routine' procedures will be carried out automatically.
• To communicate effectively and impartially with patients to enable them to reach a voluntary decision, and to offer support for that decision.

'Since voluntariness is one of the foundation stones of . . . consent, professionals have a high ethical obligation to avoid coercion and manipulation of their patients. The law penalises those who ignore the requirements of consent or who directly coerce it.' (President's Commission (1983) in Kennedy & Grubb, 1994).

Summary
'The ethical principle that each person has a right to self determination finds its expression in law through the concept of consent' (Kennedy & Grubb, 1994). The authors go on to quote the definitive statement of Mr Justice Cardoza in *Schloendorff* v. *Society of New York Hospitals* (1914):

'Every human being of adult years and sound mind has a right to determine what shall be done with his own body; and a surgeon who performs an operation without his patient's consent commits an assault . . .'

The scope of this statement has now been expanded as health care has become increasingly sophisticated and personnel performing invasive procedures have become multidisciplinary. The consent procedure is formalized and explicit and continuing consent should be obtained throughout all stages of management.

Issues relating to consent

Waiver
Within the rights-based ethical framework outlined, rights are perceived as discretionary and therefore, can be waived or relinquished. There is little opinion expressed in English law regarding the legal validity of waiver. Kennedy & Grubb (1994) are of the view that 'while the patient may waive the right to information as to risks or whatever, it would be against public policy to allow him to waive the right to be informed of the "nature and purpose" of the proposed procedure'.

The North American view was expressed by the President's Commission (1983) (in Kennedy & Grubb, 1994) as follows:

'it is questionable whether patients should be permitted to waive the professional's obligation to disclose fundamental information about the nature and implications of certain procedures (such as, "when you wake up, you will learn that your limb has been amputated" or "that you are irreversibly sterile"). In the absence of explicitly legal guidance, health care professionals should be quite circumspect about allowing or disallowing, encouraging or discouraging, a patient's use of waiver.'

However, within its report it also comments

'The impact of the waiver exception is that if a waiver is properly obtained the patient remains the ultimate decision maker, but the content of his decision is shifted . . . from the equivalent of "I want this treatment (or that treatment or no treatment)" to "I don't want any information about the treatment" . . .'

which allows the patient to exercise his rights. As previously described, the health care professional may proceed with treatment using the 'best interests' approach.

Treatment without consent
As is clear from both the legal and ethical basis for consent, treatment without consent is only permissible

in an emergency situation where there is no explicit refusal, oral or written, which has been entered by the patient.

Emergency treatment has been defined as that which is both necessary and cannot be reasonably delayed. Lord Goff in *Re F* states

'Where, for example, a surgeon performs an operation without his consent on a patient temporarily rendered unconscious in an accident, he should do no more than is reasonably required, in the best interests of the patient, before he recovers consciousness. I can see no practical difficulty arising from this requirement, which derives from the fact that the patient is expected before long to regain consciousness and can then be consulted about longer term measures.'

In many situations the relatives may be consulted but the onus is on the health care professional to assess the need for examination or treatment and proceed accordingly.

The more troublesome issue of what is permissible when a secondary condition is discovered during the course of an operative procedure – whether a surgeon should proceed with treatment or await the patient's recovery and gain consent – requires the practitioner to differentiate between necessity and convenience.

The form and scope of consent

Consent may be implied or explicit. Implied consent may be illustrated by a patient who rolls up their sleeve to allow their blood pressure to be measured or a blood sample to be taken. This is regarded by many commentators as unsatisfactory (Kennedy & Grubb, 1994) and at best should be regarded only as the absence of any objection. This form of consent may only be acceptable if a procedure is negligible in terms of risk and non-invasiveness.

Explicit or express consent may be verbal or, more commonly, written. Which form is employed will depend on the relationship between professional and patient, the nature of the procedure – invasiveness, degree of physical or psychological risk or harm – and local policy. The Department of Health has extended the necessity to obtain written consent from operative procedures alone to examinations, investigations and non-surgical treatments. Written consent is increasingly becoming the norm in most areas of clinical practice.

However, a written consent form is merely evidence of what was agreed between practitioner and patient. The process by which that consent was obtained is by far the more important dimension, as discussed previously. Moreover, consent can be said to be valid only at the time at which it is given. It is the professional's responsibility to reaffirm that the patient has not changed his mind between the signature being placed on

the form and the procedure occurring. This is particularly important when a series of treatments (or course of treatment), investigations or procedures is embarked upon, often with intervals of days or weeks in between each one.

Research

The clinical procedures within this book may be carried out in either a treatment or research setting. The research will usually be therapeutic but it is not the sole intention to benefit the patient, the demands of science are also served. There is currently no statute law which governs the conduct of research generally, but considerable guidance has been produced in recent years (Gilbert Foster, 1994) and regulatory bodies exist to consider research proposals and advise NHS bodies (DoH, 1991). Consent to research is of equal importance with consent to treatment, and many would argue more so, but it is not within the brief of this chapter to discuss these issues in detail. Consent to research, however, must be explicit and well informed. From the legal perspective a health care professional cannot justify any action without this by using a 'best interests' defence when these are unknown. From an ethical point of view the patient is asked to consent not only to therapy but to agree to be used as a means to the ends of research. Briefly these are just two of the differences between consent to treatment and consent to research which require greater debate and are fully discussed in other references (Baum, 1990; Botros, 1990; Williams, 1992). A schematic representation is shown in Fig. 1.3 (Speechley, 1992).

Conclusion

The procedures in this book affect the whole person. They range from those which are observational and physically non-invasive to those involving intrusion into both the physical body and the psychological persona. The intent also varies; some are diagnostic, others therapeutic and some are supportive with the aim of increasing well-being. Finally, there are those where the purpose is to resuscitate the individual or to prolong their life.

This introductory chapter has emphasized, and reiterated, the need for the patient to be the central focus, whatever the situation and whatever the procedure or activity. It is essential to recognize that the differing lengths of the sections in this chapter do not mean that one topic is more important than another. Assessment is the starting point, to ascertain the patient's attitudes, beliefs and values, and to discover their needs – the amount of involvement they wish to have in their care, how much information they require and what is acceptable to them, particularly as their disease experience progresses.

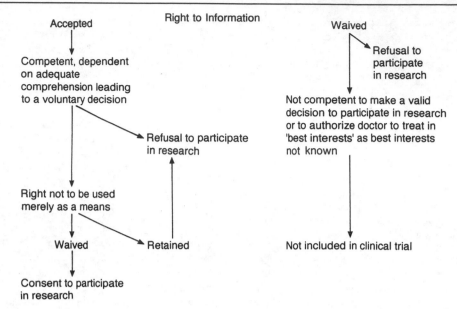

Figure 1.3   The right to information and self-determination: research. (Speechley, 1992)

Assessment is impossible without the ability to communicate, using both verbal and non-verbal skills to explore, and allow expression of, the patient's feelings. Fear of many of the procedures described here may exist – because they are unknown, because of previous experiences or because of what may be revealed. Good, clear communication may be able to allay fears, minimize discomfort and enable individual adjustment.

The nature and complexity of the consent process, required for all procedures, relies greatly on both assessment and communication skills in order to be conducted in a responsible manner. Both the ethical and legal background emphasize the need for dynamic assessment and the importance of not making assumptions or dismissing what the patient says or expresses.

Conflicts due to lack of congruence between professionals' and patients' beliefs or priorities are not uncommon and can be painful for both parties, for example leading to refusal of treatment. It is hoped that this chapter will help to avoid, minimize or resolve such dilemmas.

REFERENCES

Aggleton, P. & Chalmers, H. (1990) Model future. *Nursing Times*, 86, 41–3.

Alderson, P. (1993) *Children's consent to surgery*. Open University Press, Buckingham.

Ashby, M. & Stoffell, B. (1995) Artificial hydration and alimentation at the end of life: a reply to Craig. *Journal of Medical Ethics*, 21(3), 135–40.

Baum, M. (1990) The ethics of clinical research. In: *Ethics and Law in Health Care and Research*, (ed. P. Byrne). Wiley, Chichester.

Beauchamp, T. L. & Childress, J. F. (1994) *Principles of Biomedical Ethics*, 4th edn. Oxford University Press, Oxford.

Beddar, S. M. & Aitken, J. L. (1994) Continuity of care: A challenge for ambulatory oncology nursing. *Seminars in Oncology Nursing*, 10, 254–63.

Benner, P. (1984) *From Novice to Expert*. Addison-Wesley, California.

Bluebond-Langner, M. (1978) *The Private Worlds of Dying Children*. Princeton University Press, Princeton, New Jersey.

Bluglass, K. (1991) Care of the cancer patient's family. In: *Cancer Patient Care: Psychosocial Treatment Methods*, (ed. M. Watson). BPS Books and Cambridge University Press, Cambridge.

Botros, S. (1990) Equipoise, consent and the ethics of randomised clinical trials. In: *Ethics and Law in Health Care and Research*, (ed. P. Byrne). Wiley, Chichester.

Brennan, W. & Swan, T. (1995) *Managing Violence and Aggression. Royal College of General Practitioners, Members' Reference Book*, pp. 443–5. Sabrecrown Publishing, London.

British Association for Counselling (1989a) *BAC Training Directory*. BAC, 1 Regent Place, Rugby, CV21 2PJ.

British Association for Counselling (1989b) *Code of Ethics and Practice for Counselling Skills*. BAC, 1 Regent Place, Rugby, CV21 2PJ.

Burnard, P. (1990) *Learning Human Skills: An Experiencial Guide for Nurses*, 2nd edn. Heinemann Nursing, Oxford.

Burton, M. (1991) Counselling in routine care: A client-centred approach. In: *Cancer Patient Care: Psychosocial Treatment Methods*, (ed. M. Watson). BPS Books and Cambridge University Press, Cambridge.

Byrne, D. *et al.* (1993) Evaluation of the efficacy of an instructional programme in the self-management of patients with asthma. *Journal of Advanced Nursing*, 18, 637–46.

Campbell, J. *et al.* (1985) A theoretical approach to nursing assessment. *Journal of Advanced Nursing*, 10, 111–15.

Cassileth, B. *et al.* (1980) The effect of experience on radiation therapy patients' desire for information. *International Journal of Radiation Oncology, Biology, Physics*, 6, 493–6.

Chipman, Y. (1991) Caring: its meaning and place in the practice of nursing. *Journal of Nursing Education*, 3, 171–5.

Craig, G. M. (1994) On withholding nutrition and hydration in the terminally ill: has palliative medicine gone too far? *Journal of Medical Ethics*, 20(3), 139–43.

Crow, R. *et al.* (1995) The cognitive component of nursing assessment: an analysis. *Journal of Advanced Nursing*, 22, 206–12.

Daut, R. L. *et al.* (1983) Development of the Wisconsin brief pain questionnaire to assess pain in cancer and other diseases. *Pain*, 17, 197–210.

Davitz, L. *et al.* (1976) Suffering as viewed in six different cultures. *American Journal of Nursing*, 76(8), 1296–7.

Department of Health (1990) *Patient Consent to Examination or Treatment*. HC (90)22. HMSO, London.

Department of Health (1991) *Local Research Ethics Committees*. HSG 91(5). HMSO, London.

Department of Health (1995) *The Patient's Charter*. HMSO, London.

Derdiarian, A. K. (1990) Effects of using systematic assessment instruments on patient and nurse satisfaction with nursing care. *Oncology Nursing Forum*, 17(1), 95–101.

Derogatis, L. *et al.* (1983) The prevalence of psychiatric disorder among cancer patients. *Journal of the American Medical Association*, 249, 751–7.

Douglas, J. (1993) *Psychology and Nursing Children*, (ed. D. Muller). BPS Books, Leicester.

Dowie, J. & Elstein, A. (1991) *Professional Judgement: A Reader in Clinical Decision Making*. Cambridge University Press, Cambridge.

Dunlop, R. J. *et al.* (1995) On withholding nutrition and hydration in the terminally ill: has palliative medicine gone too far? A reply. *Journal of Medical Ethics*, 21(3), 141–3.

Dworkin, R. (1984) Rights as trumps. In: *Theories of Rights*, (ed. J. Waldron). Oxford University Press, Oxford.

Eardley, A. (1983) What do radiotherapy patients want to know? The results of a staff survey. *Radiography*, 49(581), 122–4.

Eardley, A. (1986a) Expectations of recovery. *Nursing Times*, 23 April, 53–4.

Eardley, A. (1986b) After the treatment's over. *Nursing Times*, 30 April, 40–41.

Egan, G. (1994) *The Skilled Helper: A Systematic Approach to Effective Helping*, 5th edn. Brooks/Cole, Belmont, CA.

Eilers, J. *et al.* (1988) Development, testing, and application of the Oral Assessment Guide. *Oncology Nursing Forum*, 15, 325–30.

Eiser, C. (1993) *Growing up with a Chronic Disease: The Impact on Children and Their Family*. J. Kingsley Publications, London.

Eland, J. N. (1985) The child who is hurting. *Seminars in Oncology Nursing*, 1(2), 116–22.

Faithfull, S. (1991) Patients' experiences following cranial radiotherapy: A study of the somnolence syndrome. *Journal of Advanced Nursing*, 16, 939–46.

Faulkner, A. & Maguire, P. (1984) Teaching assessment skills. In: *Recent Advances in Nursing 7, Communication*, (ed. A. Faulkner). Churchill Livingstone, Edinburgh.

Ganz, P. A. *et al.* (1992) The CARES: A generic measure of health-related quality of life for patients with cancer. *Quality of Life Research*, 1, 19–29.

Gilbert, Foster, C. (1994) *Manual for Research Ethics Committees*, 3rd edn. Centre for Medical Law and Ethics, King's College, London.

Gillick v. West Norfolk and Wisbech AHA 1986 AC 112, 1985 3 All ER 402, 1985 2 BMLR 11 (HL). In: *Medical Law: Text with Materials*, 2nd edn, (I. Kennedy & A. Grubb), p. 111. Butterworths, London, Dublin and Edinburgh.

Gillon, R. (1986) *Philosophical Medical Ethics*, 2nd edn. Wiley, Chichester. (For an introduction to ethical theory and principles.)

Glaser, B. & Strauss, A. (1965) *Awareness of Dying*. Weidenfeld and Nicolson, London.

Greer, S. & Watson, M. (1987) Mental adjustment to cancer: Its measurement and prognostic importance. *Cancer Surveys*, 6, 439–53.

Grubb, A. (1992) Refusal of medical treatment I – the competent adult. *Dispatches*, 3(1), 1–4.

Grubb, A. (1993) Refusal of medical treatment II – the competent child. *Dispatches*, 3(2), 6–8.

Hargie, O. *et al.* (1987) *Social Skills in Interpersonal Communication*, 2nd edn. Routledge, London.

Harris, R. D. *et al.* (1990) Nursing stress and stress reduction in palliative care. *Palliative Medicine*, 4, 191–6.

Hart, H. L. A. (1984) Are there any natural rights? In: *Theories of Rights* (ed. J. Waldron). Oxford University Press, Oxford.

Hewison, A. (1995) Nurses' power in interactions with patients. *Journal of Advanced Nursing*, 21(1), 75–82.

Hills v. Potter (1984) 1 WLR 641n. In: *Medical Law: Text with Materials*, 2nd edn, (I. Kennedy & A. Grubb), pp. 172–3. Butterworths, London, Dublin and Edinburgh.

Hurst, K. *et al.* (1991) The recognition and non-recognition of problem-solving strategies in nursing practice. *Journal of Advanced Nursing*, 16, 1444–55.

Kennedy, I. & Grubb, A. (1994) *Medical Law: Text With Materials*, 2nd edn. Butterworths, London, Dublin and Edinburgh. (See subject of 'Waiver', pp. 232–3; 'Implied Consent', p. 101; 'Making Health Care Decisions', pp. 233–5.)

Kerstetter, N. C. (1990) A stepwise approach to developing and maintaining an oncology multidisciplinary conference. *Cancer Nursing*, 13, 216–20.

King, I. (1971) *Towards a Theory of Nursing*. John Wiley and Sons, New York.

Kirby, M. (1995) Patients' rights – Why the Australian courts have rejected *Bolam*. *Journal of Medical Ethics*, 21, 5–8.

Kitson, A. (1988) On the concept of nursing care. In: *Ethical Issues in Caring*, (eds G. Fairbairn & S. Fairbairn). Avebury, Aldershot.

Koocher, G. & O'Malley, J. (1991) *The Damocles Syndrome*.

McGraw Hill, New York.

Lambe, N. (1995) The law on mental incapacity: a major overhaul. *Dispatches*, 5(3), 3–5.

Lansdown, R. & Goldman, A. (1991) Children with cancer. In: *Cancer Patient Care: Psychosocial Treatment Methods*, (ed. M. Watson). BPS Books and Cambridge University Press, Cambridge.

Last, B. & VanVeldhuizen, A. (1992) *Developments in Paediatric Oncology*. Taylor and Francis, Washington DC.

Law Commission (1995) Report on mental incapacity. In: *Bulletin of Medical Ethics*, 106, pp. 13–18.

Mackie, J. L. (1984) Can there be a right-based moral theory? In: *Theories of Rights*, (ed. J. Waldron). Oxford University Press, Oxford.

McCann, K. & McKenna, H. (1993) An examination of touch between nurses and elderly patients in a continuing care setting in Northern Ireland. *Journal of Advanced Nursing*, 18, 838–46.

McFarlane, J. (1988) Nursing: a paradigm of caring. In: *Ethical Issues in Caring*, (eds G. Fairbairn & S. Fairburn). Avebury, Aldershot.

Macleod Clark, J. & Sims, S. (1988) Communication with patients and relatives. In: *Oncology for Nurses and Health Care Professionals*, Vol. 2, (eds R. Tiffany & P. Webb), 2nd edn. Harper and Row, Beaconsfield.

Macleod Clark, J. *et al.* (1991) Progression to counselling. *Nursing Times*, 87(8), 41–3.

McMahon, R. & Pearson, A. (eds) (1991) *Nursing as Therapy*. Chapman and Hall, London.

Maguire, P. (1985) Barriers to psychological care of the dying. *British Medical Journal*, 291, 1711–13.

Mallett, J. (1989) Taking patients round. *Nursing Times*, 85(38), 37–9.

Mallett, J. (1997) *Nurse – Patient Haemodialysis Sessions: Orchestrated Institutional Communication and Mundane Conversations*. Unpublished PhD thesis.

Miaskowksi, C. A. & Neilson, B. (1985) A cancer nursing assessment tool. *Oncology Nursing Forum*, 12(6), 37–42.

Moorey, S. & Greer, S. (1989) *Psychological Therapy for Patients with Cancer: A New Approach*. Heinemann Medical Books, Oxford.

Muller, D., Harris, P. & Wattley, L. (1992) *Nursing Children: The Psychology, Research and Practice*, 2nd edn. Chapman & Hall, London.

Nichols, K. (1984) *Psychological Care in Physical Illness*. Croom Helm, Beckenham.

Nuffield Foundation (1993) Access to Justice: Non-English Speakers in the Legal System. Nuffield Interpreter Project, The Nuffield Foundation, London.

Orem, D. (1985) *Nursing: Concepts of Practice*. McGraw-Hill, New York.

Pease, A. (1981) *Body Language: How to Read Others' Thoughts by their Gestures*. Sheldon Press, London.

Peplau, H. (1952) *Interpersonal Relationships in Nursing*. Putnam, New York.

Phillips, J. (1992) Breaking down the barriers. *Nursing Times*, 88(35), 30–31.

Porchet–Munro, S. (1991) Aspects of non-verbal communication. *Recent Results in Cancer Research*, 121, 313–20.

Quigley, K. M. (1989) The adult cancer survivor; psychosocial consequence of cure. *Seminars in Oncology Nursing*, 5, 63–9.

Re C (Adult: refusal of treatment) 1993 in Law Update (1993). *Dispatches*, 4(1), 10–12.

Re F (Mental patient: sterilisation) 1990 2 AC1, 1989 4 BMLR 1 (HL). In: *Medical Law: Text with Materials*, 2nd edn, (I. Kennedy & A. Grubb), pp. 317–20. Butterworths, London, Dublin and Edinburgh.

Re R (1991) and Re W (1992) in Grubb, A. (1993) Refusal of medical treatment II – the competent child. *Dispatches*, 3(2), 6–8.

Re T (Adult: refusal of treatment) 1992 4 All ER 649 (CA).

Roberts, C. *et al.* (1992) Psychosocial impact of gynecologic cancer: A descriptive study. *Journal of Psychosocial Oncology*, 10(1), 99–109.

Rogers, C. (1967) *On Becoming a Person*. Constable, London.

Rogers, C. (1980) *A Way of Being*. Houghton Mifflin, Boston.

Schlyter, C. (1992) *Advance Directives and AIDS*. Centre for Medical Law and Ethics, King's College, London.

Scowen, E. (1993) The case of Anthony Bland – Reflections. *Dispatches*, 4(1), 1–4.

Scowen, E. (1994) The case of Anthony Bland – Further reflections. *Dispatches*, 4(2), 10–11.

Sepion, B. (1988) Children with cancer. In: *Oncology for Nurses and Health Care Professionals*, Vol. 2, (eds R. Tiffany & P. Webb), 2nd edn. Harper and Row, Beaconsfield.

Sidaway v. Board of Governors of the Bethlem Royal Hospital 1985 AC 871; 1985 1 All ER 643. In: *Medical Law: Text with Materials*, 2nd edn, (I. Kennedy & A. Grubb), pp. 173–84. Butterworths, London, Dublin and Edinburgh.

Skegg, P. D. G. (1984) Law ethics and medicine. In: *Medical Law: Text with Materials*, 2nd edn, (I. Kennedy & A. Grubb), p. 116. Butterworths, London, Dublin and Edinburgh.

Smith v. Tunbridge Wells Health Authority 1994 5 Med LR 334 in Law Notes (1995). *Dispatches*, 5(3), 8–10.

Speechley, V. (1992) *Provision of an information service for people with cancer: legal and ethical issues*. MA thesis, King's College, London.

Stauch, M. (1995) Rationality and the refusal of medical treatment: a critique of the recent approach of the English Courts. *Journal of Medical Ethics*, 2(3), 162–5.

Stern, K. (1995) What might have happened? Causation in cases of negligent medical omission. *Dispatches*, 5(2), 1–3.

Tanner, C. A. *et al.* (1987) Diagnostic reasoning strategies of nurses and student nurses. *Nursing Research*, 36(6), 358–63.

The Age of Legal Capacity (Scotland) Act 1991. HMSO, London.

The Children Act 1989. HMSO, London.

The Family Law Reform Act 1969. HMSO, London.

The Mental Health Act 1983. HMSO, London.

The Royal College of Nursing of the United Kingdom Cancer Nursing Society (1991) *Standards of Care for Cancer Nursing*. Scutari, London.

Thompson, J. (1988) Adolescents with cancer. In: *Oncology for Nurses and Health Care Professionals*, Vol. 2, (eds. R. Tiffany & P. Webb), 2nd edn. Harper and Row, Beaconsfield.

United Kingdom Central Council for Nursing, Midwifery and Health Visiting (1992) *Code of Professional Conduct*. UKCC,

London.

United Kingdom Central Council for Nursing, Midwifery and Health Visiting (1989) *Exercising Accountability*. UKCC, London.

Vachon, M. (1995) Staff stress in hospice/palliative care: a review. *Palliative Medicine*, 9, 91–122.

Vaughan, B. (1992) The nature of nursing knowledge. In: *Knowledge for Nursing Practice*, (eds K. Robinson & B. Vaughan). Butterworth-Heinneman, Oxford.

Walsh, M. (1991) *Models in Clinical Nursing – The Way Forward*. Balliere Tindall, London.

Waterhouse, J. & Metcalfe, M. C. (1986) Development of the sexual adjustment questionnaire. *Oncology Nursing Forum*, 13, 53–9.

Waterhouse, J. & Metcalfe, M. (1991) Attitudes toward nurses discussing sexual concerns with patients. *Journal of Advanced Nursing*, 16, 1048–54.

Watson, M. (1983) Psychosocial interventions with cancer patients: a review. *Psychological Medicine*, 13, 839–46.

Webb, C. (1988) A study of nurses' knowledge and attitudes about sexuality in health care. *International Journal of Nursing Studies*, 25(3), 235–44.

Webb, C. & O'Neill, J. (1988) Sexuality and cancer. In: *Oncology for Health Care Professionals*, Vol. 2, (eds R. Tiffany & P. Webb), 2nd edn. Harper and Row, Beaconsfield.

Webster, M. (1981) Communicating with dying patients. *Nursing Times*, 4 June, 999–1002.

Wilkinson, S. (1991) Factors which influence how nurses communicate with cancer patients. *Journal of Advanced Nursing*, 16, 677–88.

Williams, C. (ed.) (1992) *Introducing New Treatments for Cancer: Practical, Ethical and Legal Problems*. Wiley, Chichester.

Williams, C. *et al.* (1994) A framework for patient assessment. *Nursing Standard*, 8(38), 29–33.

Wilson, M. & Williams, H. (1988) Oncology nurses' attitudes and behaviours related to sexuality of patients with cancer. *Oncology Nursing Forum*, 15(1), 49–53.

Wilson-Barnett, J. (1977) *Patients' emotional reactions to hospitalisation*. PhD thesis, University of London.

Yura, H. & Walsh, M. (1988) *The Nursing Process*. Appleton Century-Crofts, New York.

CHAPTER 2
Abdominal Paracentesis

Definition

Abdominal paracentesis is the puncture of the abdominal wall with an abdominal trochar and cannula, usually for the relief of ascites (Hoerr & Osol, 1956). The cannula may also be used for the insertion of solutions into the peritoneal cavity.

Indications

Abdominal paracentesis is indicated under the following circumstances:

(1) To obtain a specimen of fluid for analysis.
(2) To relieve pressure when abdominal fluid interferes with respiration or bladder function or is compressing the abdominal viscera and blood vessels.
(3) To insert substances such as radioactive gold colloid or cytotoxic drugs (e.g. bleomycin) into the peritoneal cavity; to achieve regression of serosae deposits responsible for fluid formation.

REFERENCE MATERIAL

Abdominal ascites is an 'abnormal accumulation of serous (oedematous) fluid within the peritoneal cavity' (Weller, 1989). It can be caused by non-malignant conditions such as advanced congestive heart failure, chronic pericarditis and cirrhosis of the liver, or by malignant conditions such as metastatic cancer of the ovary, stomach, colon or breast (Macleod, 1977; Weller, 1989).

Abdominal paracentesis is not undertaken lightly because of the risk of inducing hypovolaemia, hypokalaemia or hyponatraemia. It provides only short term relief, as ascites tends to re-accumulate. Because ascitic fluid contains proteins, repeated paracentesis may cause protein depletion (Zehner & Hoogstraten, 1985). Further possible complications include perforation of the bowel and introduction of infection during insertion of the ascitic drain.

However, the degree of distress experienced by some patients with ascites is such that drainage of fluid by abdominal paracentesis is a valuable treatment option. In one study, the amount of ascitic fluid drained ranged from 250 ml to 11.4 litres (Lifschitz, 1982). Large amounts of fluid in the peritoneal cavity cause an increase in intra-abdominal pressure. There may be pain as a result of pressure on internal structures. Gastric pressure may cause anorexia, indigestion or hiatus hernia. Intestinal pressure may result in constipation, bowel obstruction or decreased bladder capacity. Pressure on the diaphragm decreases the intra-thoracic space and causes shortness of breath.

The relief of symptoms following paracentesis can be dramatic. Many cancer patients with ascites have a prognosis of only a few months (Zehner & Hoogstraten, 1985), and the procedure is often justified by the relief offered. The insertion of cytotoxic agents such as bleomycin may delay or prevent recurrence of malignant effusions (Ostrowski, 1986).

Nursing care

Nursing care of patients with abdominal ascites is aimed at relief of the suffering caused by the symptoms. Care of the patient undergoing abdominal paracentesis is directed at prevention of discomfort and complications. The procedure is usually performed by a doctor assisted by a nurse. It is an invasive procedure performed at the patient's bedside.

There is much debate about whether it is safe to drain large volumes of fluid rapidly from the abdomen. Profound hypotension may follow because of the sudden release of intra-abdominal pressure and consequent possible vasodilation. Kearney (1990) recommends a rate of 1 litre every 2 hours up to a maximum of 4 litres, states that removing large amounts of ascitic fluid from frail patients can be debilitating and suggests that a 'partial' paracentesis may be enough to relieve symptoms. Regnard & Mannix (1989) state that it is usual to drain to dryness over 6 hours. Reports exist of rapid removal of up to 21 litres of fluid (Ratcliff *et al.*, 1991), and it is suggested that the mechanism of malignant ascites may be different to that of non-malignant ascites, as lymphatic drainage from the diaphragm may be obstructed by tumour.

Smith & Powles (1993) recommend that no more than 2 litres are drained initially, then 1 litres every 4 hours for 24 hours, and finally free drainage. They also recommend that if ascitic protein content exceeds 20 g/l, protein should be replaced by intravenous infusion of 4.5% human albumin.

Nursing interventions for patients undergoing abdominal paracentesis include education about the nature of the procedure, about what results can realistically be expected, and about the importance of diet and fluid intake to replace proteins and fluid lost in the ascitic fluid. Regular observations must be carried out to detect early signs of shock and infection, which can then be treated quickly. Drainage of the fluid must be monitored frequently, volumes recorded and blockages dispersed. Patients may require assistance to move and position themselves, and may experience pain requiring careful repositioning or appropriate analgesia (see the Nursing Care Plan).

Anatomy and physiology

The peritoneum is a semi-permeable serous membrane consisting of two separate layers:

(1) Parietal layer: this layer lines the wall of the abdominal cavity.
(2) Visceral layer: this layer covers the organs contained within the abdominal cavity (Figure 2.1).

Those organs completely surrounded by peritoneum will be suspended from the posterior abdominal wall by a double fold of the membrane. It is in this way that a mesentery or fold of the peritoneum by which the intestine is attached to the posterior abdominal wall is formed. It is between these two layers that the blood vessels reach the organs, for the abdominal aorta and its branches lie outside the peritoneal cavity (Hinchliff & Montagne, 1988).

The stomach, intestines (except for the duodenum and rectum), liver and spleen are almost completely surrounded by peritoneum. The duodenum, rectum and pancreas are covered only on their anterior surfaces.

The pelvic peritoneum is continuous with that of the rest of the abdominal cavity. It covers the front aspects of the rectum. In the male it passes forwards over the posterior and anterior surfaces of the bladder to become continuous with that on the anterior abdominal wall. In the female it passes from the rectum over the posterior and anterior surfaces of the uterus before reaching the bladder.

Functions of the peritoneum

(1) The peritoneum is a serous membrane which enables the abdominal contents to glide over each other without friction.

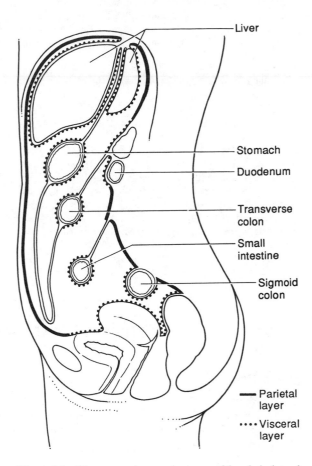

PERITONEAL CAVITY

Liver
Stomach
Duodenum
Transverse colon
Small intestine
Sigmoid colon
—— Parietal layer
···· Visceral layer

Figure 2.1 Diagram to show peritoneum of female in lateral view.

(2) It forms partial or complete cover for the abdominal organs.
(3) It forms ligaments and mesenteries which help keep the organs in position.
(4) The mesenteries contain fat and act as a store for the body.
(5) The mesenteries can move to engulf areas of inflammation and this prevents the spread of infection.
(6) It has the power to absorb fluids and exchange electrolytes.

References and further reading

Alban, C. J. et al. (1990) Postoperative chylous ascites: diagnosis and treatment. A series report and literature review. *Archives of Surgery*, 125(2), 270–73.

Hinchliff, S. & Montagne, S. (1988) *Physiology for Nursing Practice*. Ballière Tindall, London.

Hoerr, N. & Osol, A. (1956) (eds) *Blakiston's New Gould Medical Dictionary*. McGraw Hill, New York.

Kearney, M. (1990) Gynaecological malignancy: Care of the terminally ill. In: *Clinical Gynaecological Oncology*, (eds J. H. Shepherd & J. M. Monaghan), 2nd edn. Blackwell Scientific Publications, Oxford.

Lentz, S. S. *et al.* (1990) Chylous ascites after whole-abdomen irradiation for gynaecologic malignancy. *International Journal of Radiation, Oncology, Biology and Physics*, 19(2), 435–8.

Lifschitz, S. (1982) Ascites: pathophysiology and control measures. *International Journal of Radiation, Oncology, Biology and Physics*, 8, 1423–6.

Macleod, J. (ed.) (1977) *Davidson's Principles and Practice of Medicine*. Churchill Livingstone, Edinburgh.

Marieb, E. N. (1989) *Human Anatomy and Physiology*. The Benjamin/Cummings Publishing Co Inc, Redwood City.

Ostrowski, M. (1986) An assessment of the long-term results of controlling the re-accumulation of malignant effusions using intracavitary bleomycin. *Cancer*, 57, 721–7.

Phipps, W. J. *et al.* (1986) *Medical-Surgical Nursing: Concepts and Clinical Practice*, 3rd edn. C. V. Mosby, St Louis.

Ratcliff, C., Hutchinson, M. & Conner, C. (1991) Rapid paracentesis of large volumes of ascitic fluid. *Oncology Nursing Forum*, 18(8), 1416.

Regnard, C. & Mannix, K. (1989) Management of ascites in advanced cancer: a flow diagram. *Palliative Medicine*, 4, 45–7.

Sears, W. G. & Winwood, R. S. (1985) *Anatomy and Physiology for Nurses*, 6th edn. Edward Arnold, London.

Smith, I. E. & Powles, T. J. (1993) Specific medical problems: effusions, brain, spinal and meningeal disease. In: *Medical Management of Breast Cancer*, (eds T. J. Powles & I. E. Smith). Dunitz, London.

Twycross, R. G. & Lack, S. A. (1990) *Therapeutics in Terminal Cancer*, 2nd edn. Churchill Livingstone, Edinburgh.

Weller, B. F. (1989) (ed.) *Baillière's Encyclopaedic Dictionary of Nursing and Health Care*. Baillière Tindall, London.

Wolff, L. (1983) *Fundamental Nursing: the Humanities and the Sciences in Nursing*, 7th edn. J. B. Lippincott, Philadelphia.

Zehner, L. C. & Hoogstraten, B. (1985) Malignant effusions and their management. *Seminars in Oncology Nursing*, 1(4), 259–68.

GUIDELINES: ABDOMINAL PARACENTESIS

EQUIPMENT

1 Sterile abdominal paracentesis set containing forceps, scalpel blade and blade holder, swabs, towels, suturing equipment, trocar and cannula (or other approved catheter and introducer), rubber tubing to attach to the cannula and guide fluid into the container.
2 Sterile dressing pack.
3 Sterile receiver.
4 Sterile specimen pots.
5 Local anaesthetic.
6 Needles and syringes.
7 Chlorhexidine 0.5% in 70% isopropyl alcohol.
8 Plaster dressing or plastic spray dressing.
9 Large sterile drainage bag or container.
10 Gate clamps.
11 Sterile gloves.

PROCEDURE

Action	Rationale
1 Explain and discuss the procedure with the patient.	To ensure that the patient understands the procedure and gives his/her valid consent.
2 Ask the patient to void bladder.	If the bladder is full there is a chance of it being punctured when the trocar is introduced.
3 Ensure privacy.	

4 | The patient should lie supine in bed with the head raised 45–50 cm with a back rest.

Normally the pressure in the peritoneal cavity is no greater than atmospheric pressure but, when fluid is present, pressure becomes greater than atmospheric pressure. This position will then aid gravity in the removal of fluid and the fluid will drain of its own accord until the pressure is equalized.

5 | The procedure is performed by a doctor:
(a) The abdomen is prepared aseptically and draped with sterile towels.
(b) Local anaesthetic is administered

To reduce the risk of local and/or systemic infection. The peritoneal cavity is normally sterile.
To minimize pain during the procedure and thus maximize patient comfort and facilitate cooperation.
To avoid puncturing the colon.

(c) Once the anaesthetic has taken effect the doctor makes an incision approximately halfway between the umbilicus and the symphysis pubic on the midline of the abdomen.
(d) The trocar and cannula are inserted via the incision and the rubber tubing is attached to the cannula.
(e) The trocar is removed.

6 | If the cannula is to remain in position, sutures will be inserted and a supportive dry dressing applied and taped firmly in position.

To prevent trauma to the patient.
To prevent local and/or systemic infection.

7 | A closed drainage system is now attached to the cannula.

A sterile container with a non-return valve is necessary to maintain sterility.

8 | Monitor the patient's blood pressure, pulse and respirations and observe drainage. A clamp should be available on the tubing to reduce the flow of fluid if necessary.

To observe for signs of shock and/or infection, and to ensure unobstructed drainage.

9 | Monitor the patient's fluid balance. Encourage a high-protein and high-calorie diet.

After removal of large amounts of peritoneal fluid, fluid moves from the vascular space and reaccumulates in the peritoneal cavity. Ascitic fluid contains protein in addition to sodium and potassium. Problems of dehydration and electrolyte imbalance may be present.

10 | When the cannula is withdrawn, apply a sterile dry dressing to the wound.

To maintain asepsis and protect the wound.

NURSING CARE PLAN

Problem	Cause	Suggested action
Patient exhibits shock.	Major circulatory shift of fluid or sudden release of intra-abdominal pressure, vasodilatation and subsequent lowering of blood pressure.	Clamp the drainage tube with a gate clamp to prevent further fluid loss. Record the patient's vital signs. Refer to the medical staff for immediate intervention.

Nursing Care Plan (cont'd)

Problem	Cause	Suggested action
Cessation of drainage of ascitic fluid.	Abdomen is empty of ascitic fluid.	Check with the total output of ascitic fluid given on the patient's fluid balance chart. Measure the patient's girth; compare this measurement with the pre-abdominal paracentesis measurement. Suggest to medical staff that the cannula should be removed. Discontinue the drainage system.
	Patient's position is inhibiting drainage.	Change the patient's position, i.e. move the patient upright or onto his/her side to encourage flow by gravity.
	The ascitic fluid has clotted in the drainage system.	'Milk' the tubing. If this is unsuccessful, change the drainage system aseptically.
Signs of local or systemic infection.	Bacterial invasion at site of abdominal paracentesis cannula.	Obtain a swab from the site of the cannula for cultural review. Apply a dry dressing. Refer to the medical staff.
Cannula becomes dislodged.	Ineffective sutures or trauma at the puncture site.	Apply a dry dressing. Inform the medical staff.
Pain.	Pressure of ascites or position of drain.	Identify cause. Anchor drain securely to avoid pulling at insertion site or movement within abdomen. Assist patient with repositioning. Administer appropriate prescribed analgesic, monitor the patient's response and inform medical staff.

CHAPTER 3

Arterial Lines

Definition

Placement of a catheter into a peripheral artery (most frequently the radial or dorsalis pedis). If it is not possible to access a peripheral site the femoral artery may be used.

Reasons for arterial cannulation

Ease of access thereby avoiding the discomfort of frequent punctures of the artery, e.g. blood gases, serial blood lactate levels, full blood count, urea and electrolytes. To gain continuous and accurate direct measurement of intra-arterial blood pressure.

Indications

(1) During and following major surgery involving prolonged anaesthesia.
(2) Monitoring of acid–base balance and respiratory status in:
   (a) acute respiratory failure;
   (b) mechanical ventilation;
   (c) the period during and after cardio-respiratory arrest;
   (d) severe sepsis;
   (e) shock conditions;
   (f) major trauma;
   (g) acute poisoning, particularly with carbon dioxide, salicylates and paracetamol;
   (h) acute renal failure;
   (i) severe diabetic ketoacidosis.
(3) Patients who require continuous arterial monitoring, e.g. those who are critically ill, or after cardiac surgery. Such patients typically receive numerous inotropic drugs i.e. catecholamines such as dopamine or adrenalin, which have a direct effect on mean arterial pressure (MAP), making accurate measurement of MAP essential.

REFERENCE MATERIAL

Direct haemodyamic monitoring is performed more frequently than ever before and one particular method,

intra-arterial pressure monitoring, is used with increasing frequency in operating theatres, recovery rooms, intensive care units, acute general wards and during inter-hospital transfer of acutely ill patients (Allan, 1984).

The most convenient site for arterial cannulation is the right or left radial artery (the cannula should not be positioned close to an adjoining intravenous cannula) and vice versa. The radial artery passes down the radial or lateral side of the forearm to the wrist. Just above the wrist it lies superficially and can be felt in front of the radius, where the radial pulse is palpable. The artery then passes between the first and second metacarpal bones and enters the palm of the hand (Ross & Wilson, 1990).

Note: Before the insertion of a radial artery cannula, circulation to the hand should be evaluated by assessing the circulation of the palmar arch using the Allen test. The Allen test consists of simultaneously compressing both the ulnar and radial arteries for approximately one minute. During this time, the patient rapidly opens and closes the hand to promote exsanguination.

Approximately 5 seconds after release of the artery (usually the ulnar), the extended hand should blush due to capillary refilling. This reactive hyperaemia indicates adequate circulation in the hand. If blanching occurs, palmer arch circulation is inadequate, and a radial cannula could lead to ischaemia of the hand (Hinds, 1987).

Direct arterial cannulation to ensure continuous monitoring of the patient's haemodynamic performance is now an established and essential procedure. The monitoring systems necessary limit its use to intensive care units, coronary care units, theatre and recovery areas and, increasingly, high dependency areas. Direct cannulation of the artery has been carried out safely in these settings for at least 15 years (Oh, 1995).

An additional advantage of the indwelling arterial cannula is that sampling, for example for blood gas analysis, serum electrolytes or drug levels, can be performed without repeatedly puncturing the artery, which may be more traumatic than prolonged cannulation (Hinds, 1987).

Complications

There are three main areas of concern:

(1) Accidental intra-arterial injection of drugs intended for administration through a central or peripheral venous line. This has been shown to cause distal ischaemia and necrosis, with sometimes permanent damage (Teplitz, 1990; Tinker & Zapol, 1991; Marieb, 1992).

(2) Hypovolaemia. Accidental disconnection of tubing from the cannula or one of the connections can result in severe haemorrhage and hypovolaemia. Patients in shock and children are particularly vulnerable. The risk can be minimized by clearly labelling the arterial line (Zideman & Morgan, 1981).

(3) Local damage to artery. Local damage is the most common complication of arterial cannulae (Hinds, 1987). Signs include change in temperature in the distal limb and mottling and blanching of the limb when the cannula is flushed. Frequent observation of the site and local digits (fingers/toes), and early removal of the cannula is necessary to minimize permanent damage.

Debate continues about whether the fluid used to flush the tubing and cannula should contain heparin. Some authors (e.g. Oh, 1995; Clifton et al., 1991) claim that heparin prolongs the patency of the line.

If the dorsalis pedis site is chosen to locate the artery find the mid-point between the two malleoli on the dorsal surface of the foot. Then follow the mid-line down to the space between the first and second metatarsal.

References and further reading

Allan, D. (1984) Care of the patient with an arterial catheter. *Nursing Times*, 14 November, 80(46), 40–41.

Clifton, G. D. et al. (1991) Comparison of 0.9% sodium chloride and heparin solutions for maintenance of arterial catheter patency. *Heart and Lung*, 20(2), 115–18.

Hinds, C. J. (1987) *Intensive Care*. Baillière Tindall, Gillingham, Kent.

Marieb, E. N. (1992) *Human Anatomy and Physiology*. Benjamin/Cummings Publishing Co, Wokingham.

Oh, T. E. (1995) *Intensive Care Manual*. Butterworths, Sydney, Australia.

Ross, J. S. & Wilson, K. J. (1990) *Anatomy and Physiology and Illness*, 7th edn. Churchill Livingstone, Edinburgh.

Santolla, A. & Weckel, C. (1983) A new closed system for arterial lines. *RN*, June, 46(6), 49–52.

Teplitz, L. (1990) Arterial line disconnection: first aid procedure. *Nursing*, 20(5), 33.

Tinker, J. & Zapol, W. (1991) *Care of the Critically Ill Patient*. Springer Verlag, London.

Zideman, D. A. & Morgan, M. (1981) Inadvertent intra-arterial injection of Flucloxacillin. *Anaesthesia*, 36(6), 296–8.

GUIDELINES: SETTING UP AN ARTERIAL LINE

EQUIPMENT

1 500 ml pressure infuser cuff.
2 500 ml bag of 0.9% sodium chloride or prescribed solution.
3 Heparin as prescribed, plus additive label.
4 22 SWG cannula or other available arterial catheters.
5 Sterile intravenous pack.
6 Gloves.
7 70% isopropyl alcohol.
8 Semi-occlusive dressing.
9 Syringes – various.
10 Arterial identification label.
11 1% lignocaine injection.
12 Pressure monitoring system equipment.

PROCEDURE

Action	Rationale
1 Explain and discuss the procedure with the patient.	To ensure that the patient understands the procedure and gives his/her valid consent.

(*Note*: Most arterial cannulas are inserted when patients are anaesthetized.)

2	Prepare infusion and additive (e.g. heparin 1 unit per ml) as prescribed. Apply additive sticker to front of bag.	To prevent duplication of treatment. To maintain accurate records. To provide a point of reference in the event of any queries.
3	Check that all luer lock connections are secure. Do not force because they may crack.	To prevent disconnection.
4	Connect giving set to bag.	
5	Open intravenous controller fully.	
6	Squeeze the flush device-actuator (see instructions with set).	To prime the giving set and three-way tap ports.
7	Check thoroughly for air bubbles in the circuit.	To prevent an air embolus.
8	Insert bag of heparinized saline into pressure infuser cuff. Inflate to 300 mm Hg.	This pressure is higher than arterial blood pressure, therefore an automatic flush mode is activated in the system which delivers 3 ml/hour, which maintains patency of circuit, cannula and artery (Allan, 1984).
9	Wash your hands with bactericidal soap and water or bactericidal alcohol hand rub before leaving clinical room.	To reduce the risk of cross-infection.
10	Prepare trolley near the patient as described in Chapter 4, Aseptic Technique.	
11	Radial site (or other site chosen by doctor) is prepared aseptically by doctor, hair removed where necessary, cleaned with 70% isopropyl alcohol and a sterile towel is placed under the arm.	To maintain asepsis.
12	Complete Allen test.	To assess if palmar arch circulation is adequate.
13	Local anaesthetic is administered if cannulation is performed while the patient is conscious.	To minimize pain during the procedure.
14	Nurse and doctor apply gloves. See Chapter 4, Aseptic Technique, for safe technique and practice guidelines.	To prevent contamination of hands if blood spillage occurs.
15	The nurse holds the patient's arm in suitable position.	To prevent movement and facilitate insertion.
16	Cannula is inserted by the doctor.	
17	Pressure is applied to artery in which cannula is inserted.	To prevent blood spillage.
18	Open infusion controller fully.	To prevent back-flow of blood.

Guidelines: Setting up an arterial line (cont'd)

Action	Rationale
19 Tape the line and cannula securely, and apply semi-occlusive dressing. Clearly label 'arterial' (Fig. 3.1).	Leaving the site visible allows the observer to recognize immediately any dislodgement or disconnection. Clear labelling prevents accidental injection of drugs.
20 When the patient is awake, loop the tube around the thumb.	To minimize movement of cannula and damage to vessel.
21 Inform patient of amount of movement permitted, e.g. arm may be moved gently and fingers may be exercised. Discourage any stress on arm and connections.	To prevent dislodgement.

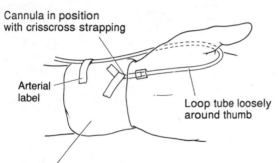

Figure 3.1   Positioning, securing and labelling of the cannula.

GUIDELINES: TAKING A BLOOD SAMPLE FROM AN ARTERIAL LINE

This should be carried out by a nurse who is skilled in the procedure. Care must be taken not to introduce air or infection.

EQUIPMENT

1 Intravenous sterile dressing pack.
2 Gloves.
3 Appropriate syringes and blood sample bottles.
4 Sterile Luer lock connection.
5 70% isopropyl alcohol.
6 Bactericidal alcohol hand rub.

PROCEDURE

Action	Rationale
1 Explain and discuss the procedure with the patient.	To ensure that the patient understands the procedure and gives his/her valid consent.
2 Prepare the trolley.	To ensure all equipment is ready.

3	Wash hands with bactericidal soap and water or bactericidal alcohol hand rub before leaving clinical room.	To prevent cross-infection.
4	Check that the three-way tap (Fig. 3.2a) is closed to air.	To prevent back-flow of blood and blood spillage.
5	Clean hands with bactericidal alcohol hand rub.	Hands have been contaminated by touching three-way tap.
6	Prepare trolley as described in Chapter 4, Guidelines: Aseptic Technique.	
7	Apply gloves. See Chapter 4 for safe technique and practice guidelines.	To prevent contamination of hand with blood.
8	Remove cap from three-way tap (Fig. 3.2a) and clean open port with 70% isopropyl alcohol.	To reduce risk of infection.
9	Connect 5 ml syringe to open port.	
10	Turn three-way tap to artery and port (Fig. 3.2b).	To prevent contamination of blood sample with heparinized infusion fluid.

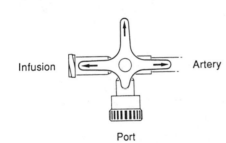

Figure 3.2a   Three-way tap closed to port.

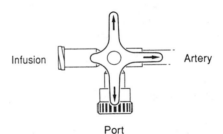

Figure 3.2b   Three-way tap turned to artery and port.

11	Gently withdraw 5 ml of blood or until line is clear of infusion fluid.	To prevent contamination of blood with infusion fluid.
12	Turn three-way tap diagonally to close off infusion, artery and port (Fig. 3.2c).	To prevent back-flow of blood from artery, contamination with infusion fluid and blood spillage.
13	Remove syringe.	
14	Connect appropriately sized syringe for sample.	
15	Turn three-way tap to artery and port (Fig. 3.2b).	To prevent contamination with infusion fluid.
16	Gently remove amount of blood required.	
17	Turn three-way tap to infusion and artery (Fig. 3.2a).	To prevent back flow of blood and blood spillage.
18	Remove syringe.	

Guidelines: Taking a blood sample from an arterial line (cont'd)

Action   **Rationale**

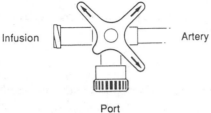

Figure 3.2c Three-way tap turned diagonally to close off infusion, artery and port.

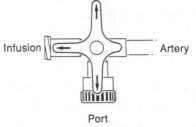

Figure 3.2d Three-way tap turned to infusion and port.

19	Turn three-way tap to infusion and port (Fig. 3.2d). Flush line hourly by squeezing actuator.	To prevent blood clotting in port.
20	Turn three-way tap to infusion and artery (Fig. 3.2a). Flush line gently by squeezing actuator (see instructions with set).	To clear blood from line.
21	Clean port with antiseptic.	To reduce the risk of infection.
22	Apply sterile Luer lock cap and check it is secure.	To prevent haemorrhage or blood spillage.
23	Check pressure infuser cuff is inflated to 300 mm Hg.	To prevent back-flow of blood into circuit.
24	Empty blood from syringe into appropriate sample bottle, and immediately label or record blood gas.	To ensure identity of sample is correct.

GUIDELINES: REMOVAL OF AN ARTERIAL LINE

EQUIPMENT

1 Intravenous sterile dressing pack.
2 Gloves.
3 Hypo-allergenic tape.
4 Antiseptic alcoholic cleanser.
5 Bactericidal skin cleanser.

PROCEDURE

Action   **Rationale**

1	Explain and discuss the procedure with the patient.	To ensure that the patient understands the procedure and gives his/her valid consent.

2	Prepare trolley as described in Chapter 4, Guidelines: Aseptic Technique.	
3	Wash hands with bactericidal soap and water or bactericidal alcohol hand rub before leaving clinical room.	To reduce the risk of cross-infection.
4	Prepare trolley by patient as described in Chapter 4, Guidelines: Aseptic Technique.	
5	Turn three-way tap diagonally (Fig. 3.2c).	To prevent back-flow of blood into line.
6	Turn off intravenous set.	To prevent spillage when removing cannula.
7	Deflate pressure cuff.	Pressure no longer required.
8	Remove semi-occlusive dressing and tape from cannula site.	To enable easy removal of cannula.
9	Clean hands with a bactericidal skin cleanser solution.	
10	Apply gloves. See Chapter 4 for safe technique and practice guidelines.	To prevent contamination of hands with blood.
11	Clean cannula site area with 70% isopropyl alcohol.	To reduce the risk of infection.
12	Place sterile piece of gauze over area and gently remove cannula.	To minimize bleeding.
13	Apply pressure to site for a minimum of 5 minutes or until bleeding stops.	To prevent a haematoma and blood loss.
14	Apply a clean, sterile, dry dressing using a non-touch technique.	To maintain asepsis.
15	Apply strapping.	To ensure pressure and prevent haematoma or blood loss.

Following this procedure, check the patient's hand hourly or as frequently as required for warmth, colour, swelling and signs of bleeding. Ask the patient to inform staff if feeling faint or if there is oozing from dressing. The medical staff must be informed immediately if the hand or forearm becomes discoloured or swollen, or if the patient complains of pain in the limb.

NURSING CARE PLAN

Problem	Cause	Suggested preventative care
Haemorrhage.	Luer lock connections are loose or cracked. Blood will be lost from open connection.	Check that Luer locks are fitted securely. Do not force because the locks may crack.
	Blood may ooze around the cannula site.	Place a semi-occlusive dressing over the cannula site and observe hourly.

Nursing care plan (cont'd)

Problem	Cause	Suggested preventative care
	Cannula may have become dislodged.	Inform the patient about the amount of movement that is preferred. Take care when moving the patient. Avoid putting stress on the arm and connections. Secure the line well (Fig. 3.1).
Back-flow of blood into the line.	The pressure infusor cuff may not be inflated to the optimal pressure.	Ensure that the pressure infusor cuff is inflated to 300 mm Hg. This pressure is higher than arterial blood pressure and an automatic flush mode is activated in the system which delivers 3 ml/hour. This maintains patency of circuit, cannula and artery (Allan, 1984).
Ischaemia.	A thrombosis may form in the circuit cannula or artery.	Ensure that heparin is added to the saline infusion (Clifton, 1991). Assess limb pulse, colour and temperature hourly, or more frequently as required. Absent pulses, pallor, cyanosis and coldness denote occlusion. If this occurs medical advice must be sought and the cannula removed promptly (Hinds, 1987).
Erythema or inflammation around the insertion site.	Phlebitis due to sepsis, chemical irritation or mechanical irritation.	Refer to the Nursing Care Plan in Chapter 23, Intravenous Management.
Hypotension, tachycardia, cyanosis, unconsciousness.	Embolism: air particle	Refer to the procedure in Chapter 23, Intravenous Management.
Arterial spasm.	Forceful flushing or aspiration when withdrawing blood.	Avoid forceful flushing and maintain a slow even pressure when withdrawing blood.
Cerebral vascular accident (CVA).	Large flush volumes can cause back-flow of arterial blood leading to central artery emboli and subsequent CVA (Santolla & Wechel, 1983).	Manual flushing should be kept to a minimum if cerebral vascular accidents are to be prevented.
Gangrene.	Accidental injection of a drug into the artery.	Label the arterial cannula and circuit clearly (Fig. 3.1). In the event of accidental injection of any drug, report the error immediately to medical staff and senior nurse and perform the following:

(a) Gently withdraw blood from the three-way tap to try and withdraw the drug.
(b) Stop the infusion and wait for instructions from the medical staff.
(c) Assess limb pulse, colour and temperature hourly, or more frequently if required.
(d) Complete an accident form and/or other relevant documentation.

CHAPTER 4

Aseptic Technique

Definition

Aseptic technique is the effort taken to keep the patient as free from hospital micro-organisms as possible (Crow, 1989). It is a method used to prevent contamination of wounds and other susceptible sites by organisms that could cause infection. This can be achieved by ensuring that only sterile equipment and fluids are used during invasive medical and nursing procedures. Potter & Perry (1992) suggest that there are two types of asepsis: medical and surgical asepsis. Medical or clean asepsis reduces the number of organisms and prevents their spread; surgical or sterile asepsis includes procedures to eliminate microorganisms from an area and is practised by nurses in operating theatres and treatment areas.

Indications

An aseptic technique should be implemented during any invasive procedure that bypasses the body's natural defences, e.g. the skin and mucous membranes, or when handling equipment such as intravenous cannulae and urinary catheters that have been used during these procedures.

REFERENCE MATERIAL

Hospital acquired infection (also called nosocomial infection) is defined as infection occurring in patients after admission to hospital that was neither present nor incubating at the time of admission. Infections acquired in hospital but not manifest until after the patient is discharged are included in the definition (Ayliffe et al., 1992).

The cost of nosocomial infections to the NHS in 1992 was an estimated £110 million (Chapman et al., 1993). Health authorities recognize the significance of nosocomial infections and employ infection control teams to:

(1) Reduce the likelihood of patients being exposed to infectious micro-organisms whilst in hospital.
(2) Provide adequate care for patients with communicable infections.

(3) Minimize the likelihood of employees, visitors and communicable contacts being exposed to infectious micro-organisms.
(4) Develop policies for appropriate management of patients with communicable infections.
(5) Provide surveillance systems which give adequate feedback to appropriate staff.
(6) Provide education in techniques to prevent the emergence and spread of infection.

A 10 year study in the USA found that an infection control team reduced the incidence of nosocomial infection by up to 32%. Hospitals in the study with no infection control programme experienced an increase in infection rates of up to 18% (Haley et al., 1985). A 3 year study reported a reduction in the infection rate from 10.5% to 5.6% following the introduction of an infection control team (French et al., 1989). It has been estimated that a reduction by one fifth of the UK nosocomial infection rate of 5% would save the NHS £15.6 million, even if the costs of infection control teams and programmes are taken into account (Chaudhuri, 1993).

When cross-infection does occur the cost of investigating and controlling even a small outbreak is high. Mehtar et al. (1989) estimated the cost of a small outbreak of methicillin resistant staphylococcus aureus (MRSA) to be £13 000, emphasizing how important it is to prevent infection. The Infection Control Standards Working Party has prepared standards for practice to make prevention, detection and control of infection in hospitals as effective as possible (Infection Control Standards Working Party, 1993). Surgical wound infections are the second most common nosocomial infection in England and Wales, which is directly related to wound contamination at the time of operation (Table 4.1) (Cruse & Foord, 1980).

Similarly, urinary tract infections continue to be the most common hospital acquired infections. The prevalence study in 1980 by the Public Health Laboratory showed that urinary tract infection caused 30.3% of all

Table 4.1 Category of wound and infection rate.

Category of wound	Infection rate (%)
Clean	1.5
Clean contaminated	7.7
Contaminated	15.2
Dirty	40.0

infections; of the 8.6% of patients catheterized, 21.2% had infections, compared with 2.9% in non-catheterized patients (Meers *et al.*, 1981), illustrating the association between invasive procedure and infection.

The diagnosis of infection relies on classic signs of inflammation such as local redness, swelling and pain. Although decreased numbers of neutrophils produce minimal or atypical clinical signs of infection (Candell & Whedon, 1991). These local signs and symptoms can precede a further sequence of events, which can be lymphangitis, lymphadenitis, bacteraemia and septicaemia which, if not promptly recognized and treated, can result in death (Laurence, 1991).

The cost of infection is high, both to the patient and the hospital. Nosocomial infections increase mortality and morbidity and cause an increase in pain and suffering experienced by the patients (Sproat & Inglis, 1992). The patient may be inconvenienced by a prolonged period of hospitalization, which can cause economic and social hardships to the whole family. The hospital will have increased waiting lists and increased hospital costs. It is essential that when aseptic techniques are used as a method of preventing infection that these procedures are sound in theory and are carried out correctly.

Gwyther (1988) discusses how most teaching occurs on the hospital ward and questions whether this teaching is based on knowledge of the principles of, for example, wound care, or simply on experience. Jenks & Ferguson (1994) reviewed the discrepancy between what is taught in the classroom and what nurses experience in the clinical setting. This suggested that collaboration is needed between education and service staff to integrate learning within the nursing curricula. Thomlison (1990) emphasises the importance of replacing infection control procedures which involve unnecessary ritual with sound, cost efficient and environmentally responsible practices to encourage a greater understanding of the principles of asepsis.

Principles of asepsis

Infection is caused by organisms which invade the host's immunological defence mechanisms, although susceptibility to infection may vary from person to person (Gould, 1994). The risk of infection is increased if the patient is immunocompromised (Hart, 1990) by:

(1) Age. Neonates and the elderly are more at risk due to their less efficient immune systems.
(2) Underlying disease. For example, those patients with severe debilitating or malignant disease.
(3) Prior drug therapy, such as the use of immunosuppressive drugs or the use of broad-spectrum antimicrobials.
(4) Patients undergoing surgery or instrumentation.

The following factors must be considered when nursing immunocompromised patients (Trester, 1982):

(1) Classic signs and symptoms of infection are often absent.
(2) Untreated infection may disseminate rapidly.
(3) Infections may be caused by unusual organisms or organisms which, in most circumstances, are non-pathogenic.
(4) Some antibiotics are less effective in immunocompromised patients.
(5) Repeated infections may be caused by the same organism.
(6) Superimposed infection is a frequent occurrence requiring nursing care of the highest standard to prevent infection (Gurevich *et al.*, 1986), which includes strict adherence to aseptic techniques.

Sproat & Inglis (1992) suggest that a basic principle of infection control for all patients is to assess the risk of infection from one patient to another and to plan nursing care accordingly before action is taken. Haley *et al.*, (1985) add that if each patient is evaluated individually it is possible to focus more closely on those patients who are most susceptible to infection. The most usual means for spread of infection include:

(1) Hands of the staff involved.
(2) Inanimate objects, e.g. instruments and clothes.
(3) Dust particles or droplet nuclei suspended in the atmosphere.

Hand washing

Hand washing is the single most important procedure for preventing nosocomial infection as hands have been shown to be an important route of transmission of infection (Casewell *et al.*, 1977). Jacobson *et al.* (1985) demonstrated that wearing rings increases the number of micro-organisms on the hands. However, studies have shown that hand washing is rarely carried out in a satisfactory manner (Taylor, 1978a), with the most important factor inhibiting hand washing being busyness (Larson *et al.*, 1982) or inaccessible sinks (Albert *et al.*, 1981). Studies have shown that up to 89% of staff miss some part of the hand surface during hand washing (Taylor, 1978a) (Fig. 4.1).

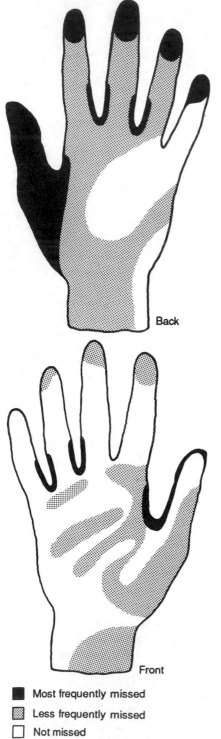

Back

Front

■ Most frequently missed

▨ Less frequently missed

□ Not missed

Figure 4.1 Areas most commonly missed following hand washing. (Reproduced by kind permission of *Nursing Times*, where this article first appeared in 1978.)

Taylor (1978b) and Phillips (1989) use Feldman's criteria for hand washing, which include the following:

(1) Roll up sleeves, remove rings and wrist watches.
(2) Use soap.
(3) Use continuously running water.
(4) Position hands to avoid contaminating arms.
(5) Avoid splashing clothing or floor.
(6) Rub hands together vigorously.
(7) Use friction on all surfaces.
(8) Rinse hands thoroughly with hand held down to rinse.
(9) Dry hands thoroughly.

Paper towels have been shown to be a quick, convenient and reliable method of drying hands (Blackmore, 1987) and are preferable to a roller towel which could be a source of cross-infection (Rowland & Alder, 1972). Hot air dryers which dry hands slowly and, in some cases inadequately (Matthews & Newman, 1987), may discourage some people from washing their hands (Blackmore, 1987). Hand washing should be undertaken after patient contact and before an aseptic technique is performed (Centre for Disease Control, 1986).

Transient bacteria can be almost completely removed from the hands by soap and water washing (Lowbury *et al.*, 1974a). Conversely, soap and water do not reduce the number of resident bacteria by any significant amount. Resident skin flora, such as *Staphylococcus aureus*, are removed most effectively by rubbing the hands with a bactericidal alcoholic solution of chlorhexidine. Lowbury *et al.* (1974b) showed that rinsing the hands with alcoholic chlorhexidine 0.5% removed more resident skin flora than did washing the hands with a chlorhexidine 4% detergent wash.

It is suggested that a preparation such as chlorhexidine 4% detergent wash is used for cleaning physically dirty or contaminated hands, while a bactericidal alcoholic hand rub should be used for disinfecting clean hands immediately before carrying out an aseptic technique. A nurse with 'socially clean' hands will not need to wash them during the aseptic procedure, but should use a bactericidal alcoholic hand rub whenever disinfection is required, e.g. after opening the outer wrappers of dressings. This will also remove the need for the nurse to leave the patient during the procedure to wash the hands at a basin, as it is unlikely that nurses' hands will become soiled with blood or body fluids as long as blood and body fluid precautions are adopted at all times (Hart, 1991).

No-touch technique

A no-touch technique is essential to ensure that hands, even though they have been washed, do not contaminate the sterile equipment or the patient. This can be achieved either by the use of forceps or sterile gloves

(Lascelles, 1982). However, it must be remembered that gloves can become damaged and allow the passage of bacteria (Rowland *et al.*, 1985), while forceps may damage tissue (David, 1991).

Inanimate objects

All instruments, fluids and materials that come into contact with the wound must be sterile if the risk of contamination is to be reduced. The sterile supplies department should normally provide all sterile instruments. In the event of supplies being short in an emergency, it is acceptable to disinfect a clean instrument, such as a pair of scissors, by immersing it completely in 70% ethanol alcohol for 10 minutes. This will destroy vegetative bacteria, mycobacteria and viruses but not bacteria spores (Ayliffe *et al.*, 1984).

Most disinfectants have a limited antimicrobial spectrum and must be used only on clean surfaces or equipment, e.g. instruments, as they may fail to penetrate blood or pus (Ayliffe *et al.*, 1984). Any equipment that becomes contaminated during a procedure must be discarded. On *no* account should it be returned to the sterile field. Care must also be taken to ensure that equipment and lotions are sterile and that packaging is undamaged before use.

While following aseptic techniques, it is also important to evaluate the whole procedure to ensure the principles are being followed during the whole process; errors such as taking adhesive tape from a contaminated roll (Oldman, 1987) or using dressings left over from a previous dressing (Roberts, 1987) must be avoided.

The dressing trolley

Most disinfectants are not sporicidal and also fail to penetrate organic matter. Therefore it is essential that equipment such as trolleys are cleaned daily and when contaminated with a detergent solution and dried carefully with paper towels. This will remove a high proportion of micro–organisms, including bacterial spores (Ayliffe *et al.*, 1992). Prior to use for aseptic technique, trolleys should be wiped over with chlorhexidine in 70% ethanol alcohol using a clean paper towel (Ayliffe *et al.*, 1984). Trolleys used for aseptic procedures must not be used for any other purpose.

Protective clothing

Protective clothing may be worn for a variety of reasons, including the need to proclaim the identity of the wearer (Sparrow, 1991). Generally, however, protective clothing is worn for the following reasons:

(1) To prevent the user's clothing becoming contaminated with pathogenic micro–organisms which may subsequently be transferred to other patients in their care.

(2) To prevent the user's clothing becoming soiled, wet or stained during the course of their duties.
(3) To prevent transfer of potentially pathogenic micro-organisms from user to patient.
(4) To prevent the user acquiring infection from the patient (Ayton *et al.*, 1984).

There is evidence that transfer of organisms can occur from one room to another on clothing (Hambraeus, 1973). An impermeable apron offers better protection than a cotton gown, which allows bacteria and moisture to pass through because of the weave (Mackintosh *et al.*, 1980). It is therefore recommended that a disposable plastic apron, which is impermeable to bacteria, is worn during aseptic procedures. Aprons should be changed or removed after each dressing.

Masks are worn to prevent the dissemination of organisms from the nose and mouth during breathing, talking, sneezing or coughing, and to protect the wearer from inhaling airborne micro-organisms disseminated from infected patients. Studies have shown that not wearing a mask does not alter infection rates (Orr, 1981) and that masks contribute little or nothing to the protection of people in wards. Therefore the routine use of masks for aseptic ward procedures is unnecessary (Taylor, 1980). However, there is some justification for wearing masks when giving prolonged close care to major burn patients (Ayton *et al.*, 1984).

The patient's skin flora is an important source of infection following invasive procedures (Goodinson, 1990). Patient hygiene will reduce this hazard (Mackenzie, 1988). Studies comparing washing with soap or chlorhexidine solution demonstrated a marked decrease in bacteriuria in patients washing with chlorhexidine (Sanderson, 1990). Other research has shown that the use of chlorhexidine solution for bathing or showering pre- and post-operatively reduces the incidence of wound infections (Randall *et al.*, 1984).

Studies to establish whether the incidence of infection or prolonged or delayed healing occurred when stitches became wet during washing, showed that getting stitches wet was not detrimental to wound healing (Noe *et al.*, 1988). Therefore, a patient with, for example, an indwelling intravenous Hickman catheter, while showering with stitches still *in situ* should wear a protective dressing, and after showering any non-waterproof dressing should be changed immediately (Mitchell, 1984).

Airborne contamination

The spread of airborne infection is most likely to occur following procedures such as bed making and cleaning, which can disperse organisms into the air. Ideally such activities should cease 30 minutes before a dressing is to be undertaken. To reduce further the risk of airborne contamination of open wounds curtains should be drawn round the bed 10 minutes before the dressing is to be changed and the wound should be exposed for as short a time as possible (Ayliffe *et al.*, 1992). Dirty dressings should be placed carefully in a yellow clinical waste bag, which is sealed before disposal (Lowbury *et al.*, 1981). Clean wounds should be dressed before contaminated wounds. Colostomies and infected wounds should be dressed last of all to minimize environmental contamination and cross-infection.

Air movement should be kept to a minimum during the dressing. This means that adjacent windows should be closed and the movement of personnel within the area discouraged.

References and further reading

Albert, R. K. *et al.* (1981) Handwashing patterns in medical intensive care units. *New England Journal of Medicine*, 304, 1465–6.

Ayliffe, G. A. J. *et al.* (1984) *Chemical Disinfection in Hospitals.* Public Health Laboratory Service, London, pp. 7–8.

Ayliffe, G. A. J. *et al.* (1992) *Control of Hospital Infection. A Practical Handbook*, 3rd edn. Chapman & Hall Medical, London.

Ayton, M. *et al.* (1984) *Report of a Working Party on Ward Protective Clothing.* Infection Control Nurses Association, London.

Blackmore, M. (1987) Hand drying methods. *Nursing Times*, 83(37), 71–4.

Candell, K. A. & Whedon, M. B. (1991) Haematopoietic complications found in bone marrow transplantation. In: *Principles, Practices and Nursing Insight*, (ed. M. B. Whedon), pp. 135–157. Jones & Bartlett, Boston.

Casewell, M. *et al.* (1977) Hands as route of transmission for *klebsiella* species. *British Medical Journal*, 2, 1315–17.

Centre for Disease Control (1986) Guidelines for handwashing and hospital environmental control. *Infection Control*, 7(4), 233–5.

Chapman, R. *et al.* (1993) Surveillance and feedback of hospital acquired infection rates in the USA. *Public Health Laboratory Service Microbiology Digest*, 11(1), 35–7.

Chaudari, A. K. (1993) Infection control in hospitals: Has its quality enhancing and cost effective role been appreciated? *Journal of Hospital Infection*, 25, 1–6.

Crow, S. (1989) Asepsis: an indispensable part of the patient's care plan. *Critical Care Nurse Questions*, 11(4), 11–15.

Cruse, P. J. E. & Ford, R. (1980) The epidemiology of wound infection – a 10-year prospective study of 62,939 wounds. *Surgical Clinics of North America*, 60(1), 27–40.

David, J. (1991) Letters. *Wound Management*, 1(2), 15.

French, G. L. *et al.* (1989) Repeated prevalence surveys for monitoring effectiveness of hospital infection control. *Lancet*, 11, 1021–3.

Goodinson, S. M. (1990) Keeping the flora out. *Professional Nurse*, 5(11), 572–5.

Gould, D. (1994) Understanding the nature of bacteria. *Nursing Standard*, 8(28), 29–31.

Gurevich, I. *et al.* (1986) The compromised host deficit specific infection and the spectrum of prevention. *Cancer Nursing*, 9, 263–75.

Gwyther, J. (1988) Skilled dressing. *Nursing Times*, 84(19), 60–61.

Haley, R. W. *et al.* (1985) Identifying multivariate index of patients' susceptibility and wound contamination. *American Journal of Epidemiology*, 121(2), 206–15.

Haley, R.W. *et al.* (1985) The efficiency of infection surveillance and control programmes in preventing nosocomial infections in US hospitals. *American Journal of Epidemiology*, 121, 182–205.

Hambracus, A. (1973) Transfer of *Staphylococcus aureus* via nurses' uniform. *Journal of Hygiene*, 71, 799–814.

Hart, S. (1990) The immunosuppressed patient in infection control. In: *Guidelines for Nursing Care* (eds M. A. Worsley *et al.*), pp. 15–20. Surgikos Ltd.

Hart, S. (1991) Blood and body precautions. *Nursing Standard*, 5(25), 25–8.

Infection Control Standards Working Party (1993) *Standards in Infection Control in Hospitals.* HMSO, London.

Jacobson, G. *et al.* (1985) Handwashing: ring-wearing and number of microorganisms. *Nursing Research*, 34(3), 186–8.

Jenks, A. M. & Ferguson, K. E. (1994) Intergrating what is taught with what is practised in the nursing curriculum, a multi dimensional model. *Journal of Advanced Nursing*, 20, 687–95.

Larson, E. *et al.* (1982) Factors influencing handwashing behaviour of patients' care personnel. *American Journal of Infection Control*, 10(3), 93–9.

Lascelles, I. (1982) Wound dressing technique. *Nursing*, 2(8), 217–19.

Laurence, C. (1991) Bacterial infection of wounds. *Wound Management*, 1(1), 13–15.

Lowbury, E. J. *et al.* (1974a) Disinfection of hands: removal of transient organisms. *British Medical Journal*, 2, 230–33.

Lowbury, E. J. *et al.* (1974b) Preoperative disinfection of surgeons' hands: Use of alcoholic solutions and effects of gloves on skin flora. *British Medical Journal*, 4, 369–72.

Lowbury, E. J. *et al.* (1981). *Control of Hospital Infection – A Practical Handbook*, 2nd edn. Chapman & Hall, London.

Mackenzie, I. (1988) Pre-operative skin preparation and surgical outcome. *Journal of Hospital Infection*, Suppl. B., pp. 27–32.

Mackintosh, C. A. *et al.* (1980) The evaluation of fabric in relation to their use as protective garments in nursing and surgery. *Journal of Hygiene*, 85, 393–403.

Matthews, J. A. & Newman, S. W. B. (1987) Hot-air electric driers compared with paper towels. *Journal of Hospital Infection*, 9, 85–8.

Meers, P. D. *et al.* (1981) Report on the National Survey of Infection in Hospital 1980. *Journal of Hospital Infection*, 2(Supplement), 1–53.

Mehtar, S. *et al.* (1989) Expenses incurred during a five week epidemic methicillin resistant *Staphylococcus aureus* outbreak. *Journal of Hospital Infection*, 13, 199–203.

Mitchell, N. J. (1984) Whole-body disinfection with chlorhexidine in shower bathing more effective than bathing. *Journal of Hospital Infection*, 5, 96–9.

Noe, J. M. *et al.* (1988) Can stitches get wet? *Plastic and Reconstructive Surgery*, 81(1), 82–4.

Oldman, P. M. (1987) An unkind cut. *Nursing Times*, 83(48), 71–4.

Oldman, P. (1991) A sticky situation – microbiological study of adhesive tape used to secure IV cannulae. *Professional Nurse*, February, 265–9.

Orr, N. W. M. (1981) Is a mask necessary in the operating theatre? *Annals of the Royal College of Surgeons*, 63, 390–92.

Phillips, C. (1989) Hand hygiene. *Nursing Times*, 85(37), 76–9.

Potter, P. A. & Perry, A. G. (1992) *Fundamentals of Nursing*, 3rd edn. Mosby, London.

Randall, P. E. *et al.* (1984) Prevention of wound infection following vasectomy. *British Journal of Urology*, 57, 227–9.

Roberts, J. (1987) Pennywise, pound foolish. *Nursing Times*, 83(37), 68–9.

Rowland, A. J. & Alder, V. G. (1972) Transmission of infection through towels. *Community Medicine*, 5, 71–3.

Rowland, C. *et al.* (1985) In the surgeons' hands. *Nursing Times*, Supplement, 5–7.

Sanderson, P. J. (1990) A comparison of the effect of chlorhexidine antisepsis, soap and antibiotics on bacteriuria, perineal colonization and environmental contamination in spinally injured patients. *Journal of Hospital Infection*, 15, 235–43.

Sparrow, S. (1991) An exploration of the role of the nurses' uniform through a period of non-uniform wear on an acute medical ward. *Journal of Advanced Nursing*, 16, 116–22.

Sproat, L. J. & Inglis, T. J. J. (1992) Preventing infection in the intensive care unit. *British Journal of Intensive Care*, September, 277–85.

Stronge, V. L. (1984) Principles of Wound Care. *Nursing*, 2(26), Supplement, 7–10.

Taylor, L. (1978a) An evaluation of handwashing techniques 1. *Nursing Times*, 74(2), 54–5.

Taylor, L. (1978b) An evaluation of handwashing techniques 2. *Nursing Times*, 74(3), 108–10.

Taylor, L. J. (1980) Are masks necessary in operating theatres and wards? *Journal of Hospital Infection*, 1, 173–4.

Thomlinson, D. (1990) Time to dispense with the rituals. *Professional Nurse*, May, 421–4.

Trester, A. (1982) Nursing management of patients receiving cancer chemotherapy. *Cancer Nursing*, 6, 206–10.

Webster, M. (1986) Control measures. *Nursing Times*, 82(5), 26–8.

GUIDELINES: ASEPTIC TECHNIQUE

EQUIPMENT

1 Sterile dressing pack* containing gallipots or an indented plastic tray, low-linting swabs and/or medical foam, disposable forceps, gloves, sterile field, disposable bag.
2 Fluids for cleaning and/or irrigation.
3 Hypo-allergenic tape.
4 Appropriate dressing (see Chapter 48, Wound Management).
5 Appropriate hand hygiene preparation.

Any other material will be determined by the nature of the dressing: special features of a dressing should be referred to in the patient's nursing care plan.

PROCEDURE

Action	Rationale
1 Explain and discuss the procedure with the patient.	To ensure that the patient understands the procedure and gives his/her valid consent.
2 Clean trolley with chlorhexidine in 70% spirit with a paper towel.	To provide a clean working surface.
3 Place all the equipment required for the procedure on the bottom shelf of a clean dressing trolley.	To maintain the top shelf as a clean working surface.
4 Take the patient to the treatment room or screen the bed. Position the patient	To allow dust and airborne organisms to settle before the sterile field (and in the case of a

Guidelines: Aseptic technique (cont'd)

Action	Rationale

comfortably so that the area to be dealt with is easily accessible without exposing the patient unduly.

dressing, the wound) is exposed. Maintain the patient's dignity and comfort.

5 If the procedure is a dressing and the wound is infected or producing copious amounts of exudate, put on a disposable plastic apron.

To reduce the risk of spreading infection.

6 Take the trolley to the treatment room or patient's bedside, disturbing the screens as little as possible.

To minimize airborne contamination.

7 Wash your hands with bactericidal soap and water or a bactericidal alcohol hand rub.

To reduce the risk of wound infection.

8 Check the pack is sterile (i.e., the pack is undamaged, intact and dry. If autoclave tape is present, check that it has changed colour from beige to beige and brown lines), open the outer cover of the sterile pack and slide the contents onto the top shelf of the trolley.

To ensure that only sterile products are used.

9 Open the sterile field using only the corners of the paper.

So that areas of potential contamination are kept to a minimum.

10 Check any other packs for sterility and open, tipping their contents gently onto the centre of the sterile field.

To prepare the equipment and in the case of a wound dressing reduce the amount of time that the wound is uncovered. This reduces the risk of infection and a drop in temperature of the wound which will delay wound healing (Stronge, 1984).

11 Wash hands with a bactericidal alcohol rub.

Hands may become contaminated by handling outer packets, etc.

12 Using the forceps in the pack, arrange the sterile field with the handles of the instruments in one corner or around the edge of the sterile field. Where appropriate, swab along the 'tear area' of lotion sachet with chlorhexidine in 70% spirit/swab saturated with 70% isopropyl alcohol. Tear open sachet and pour lotion into gallipots or on indented plastic tray (see Table 48.3).

To minimize risk of contamination of lotion.

13 If appropriate, put on sterile gloves, touching only the inside wrist end.

To reduce the risk of infection. Gloves provide greater sensitivity than forceps and are less likely to cause trauma to the patient.

Carry out procedure

14 Make sure the patient is comfortable.

15 Dispose of waste in yellow plastic clinical waste bags.

To prevent environmental contamination. Yellow is the recognized colour for clinical waste.

16 If necessary, draw back curtains or, if
    appropriate, help the patient back to the bed
area and ensure the patient is comfortable.

17 Check that the trolley remains dry and   To reduce the risk of spreading infection.
    physically clean. If necessary, wash with
liquid detergent and water and dry throughly with
a paper towel.

18 Wash hands with soap and water.   To reduce the risk of spreading infection.

* Please note that for some procedures it may be more appropriate to use different types of sterile packs
(e.g. intravenous packs). Since usage of these will vary locally reference is generally made to 'sterile
dressing pack'.

CHAPTER 5

Barrier Nursing: Nursing the Infectious or Immunosuppressed Patient

BARRIER NURSING

Definition

Barrier nursing involves the use of practices aimed at controlling the spread of, and destroying, pathogenic organisms. These practices may require the setting up of mechanical barriers to contain pathogenic organisms within a specified area.

Indications

Barrier nursing is required under the following circumstances:

(1) To prevent the spread of infection from patients with communicable diseases (i.e. contagious diseases such as glandular fever, or infectious diseases such as chicken pox).
(2) To prevent the spread of infection from patients infected with organisms which are resistant to the usual range of antibiotics; such as methicillin-resistant *Staphylococcus aureus* (MRSA).
(3) To protect those patients whose susceptibility to infection is increased (protective isolation or reverse barrier nursing). Susceptibility to infection varies from individual to individual, and depends on many factors. It is often associated with invasive procedures (Bowell, 1992).

REFERENCE MATERIAL

Surveys of the prevalence of hospital infection show that about one in ten patients will acquire a nosocomial infection whilst in hospital (Meers *et al.*, 1981; Mayon-White *et al.*, 1988). Most precautions against transferring infection demand more effort, take more time and cost more than the comparable procedures in normal circumstances. However, the cost of an outbreak of infection can be far more. In 1991, 175 patients developed nosocomial *Clostridium difficile* diarrhoea. As a direct result 17 patients died and the organism was a contributing factor in a further 43 deaths. The cost of managing the outbreak was at least £75 000 (Worsley, 1993).

For the infected patient the consequences can be considerable and may include the following:

(1) Delayed or prevented recovery.
(2) Increased pain, discomfort and anxiety.
(3) Extended hospitalization, which has implications for the patient, the family and the hospital.
(4) Psychological stress as a result of long periods spent in isolation (Knowles, 1993).

Sources of infection

Self-infection (endogenous infection)

Self-infection results when tissue becomes infected from another site in the patient's body. The normal microbial flora of the human body consists largely of the organisms in the alimentary tract, upper respiratory tract and female genital tract and on the skin. This flora may include versatile pathogens (e.g. *Staphylococcus aureus*) that may cause disease in almost any tissue as well as others (e.g. micrococcus species and diphtheroids) which are usually of very low pathogenicity; many organisms exist with capabilities between these extremes (Mims *et al.*, 1993).

Cross-infection (exogenous infection)

Cross-infection may be caused by infection from patients, hospital staff or visitors who are suffering from the relevant disease (cases) or who are symptomless carriers. Food and the environment may also be factors in cross-infection.

Routes and reservoirs of infection

A reservoir of infection is anywhere where organisms can survive and multiply. For infection to occur there has to be a route of transmission between the reservoir and the susceptible host. Routes of spread include:

Direct contact

Organisms can be transmitted directly to susceptible people by contaminated equipment or by the hands of health care attendants (Casewell *et al.*, 1977). Washing the skin removes harmful organisms quickly. However, studies of hand washing by nurses and others have shown that this procedure is generally not carried out efficiently (Gidley, 1987). The use of disinfectants improves the cleaning process, although no method of chemical disinfection will produce a sterile hand. Soaps and detergent emulsions containing hexachlorophane build a protective barrier in the skin against gram-positive organisms (Mackenzie, 1988). A widely used solution is one containing 4% chlorhexidine. Washing in running water is essential. Basins should be deep enough to contain any splashing water and should be plugless. Taps should not be operated by hand but by elbow, knee or foot as appropriate.

A quick, convenient and effective disinfectant for clean hands, without the use of soap and water, is an alcoholic hand rub containing 70% isopropyl and a bactericidal agent such as 2.5% chlorhexidine, with the addition of enough glycerine to prevent excessive drying of the skin (Lee *et al.*, 1988). Such solutions may not be effective against viruses, therefore if contamination is likely, for example when leaving a source isolation room, washing the hands with soap and water before using the alcoholic hand rub is advised (Ayliffe *et al.*, 1992).

Hands must be washed after direct patient contact or contact with contaminated material, e.g. toys, bed linen etc., and before contact with susceptible patients (Gidley, 1987), and dried thoroughly using a good quality disposable paper towel (Rowland, 1972). (See Chapter 4, Aseptic Technique.)

Airborne

Organisms can be transmitted in dust or skin scales carried by air. This is likely to occur during procedures such as bed making when particles may land directly on open wounds or puncture sites (Glenister, 1983). Airborne infection may also occur through droplets. Water from nebulizers or humidifiers may be contaminated by *Pseudomonas* species (Redding, *et al.*, 1980). Fine droplet spray from ventilation cooling towers or showers contaminated with *Legionella pneumophila* has also been shown to be a hazard (Alderman, 1988).

Food borne

Food poisoning occurs when contaminated foods are ingested, with *Salmonella* species being one of the most common causes (White, 1986).

Blood borne

Blood, or blood-stained material, is potentially hazardous, transmitting infection through inoculation accidents, existing breaks in the skin, gross contamination of mucous membranes, sexual activity or, prenatally, from mother to baby (Hart, 1991).

Insect borne

Although disease transmitted by biting insects is not a major problem in the UK, insects such as cockroaches can carry pathogenic organisms on their bodies and in their digestive tracts. This may infect the hospital environment, which includes food and sterile supplies (Burgess, 1979). Storage of supplies in dry, clean, well ventilated areas is therefore essential.

Types of barrier nursing

(1) Protective isolation.
(2) Source isolation.

Protective isolation protects the patient from the hospital enviroment. Protective isolation techniques have also been referred to as reverse barrier nursing and reverse isolation, and include laminar air flow rooms (Caudell & Bakitas Whedon, 1991) (see Protective isolation, below).

Source isolation is designed to prevent the spread of pathogenic microrganisms from an infected patient to other patients, hospital personnel and visitors. The need for isolation is determined by the ease with which the disease can be transmitted in hospital and, if it is transmittable, by its severity. As infectious diseases are transmitted by different routes, isolation procedures must, in order to be effective, provide appropriate barriers to the route of transmission. In addition, the procedures imposing these barriers must be adhered to universally by all hospital staff entering the isolation unit.

SOURCE ISOLATION

The decision to isolate a patient will be influenced by the availability of facilities as well as by the physical condition of the area where the isolation is to take place. In determining the most suitable area, a number of criteria need to be met. Among these are the relative cleanliness of the ward, the standard of domestic services support, the microbiological status of the other patients and the anticipated length of the isolation.

Source isolation may be achieved by:

(1) Purpose-built infectious disease wards.
(2) Plastic isolators found in high security units and used only for infections such as viral haemorrhage fever (Bowell, 1986).
(3) Single rooms on general wards.

Effective barrier nursing practice is achieved most easily

by isolating the patient in a single room with the following:

(1) An anteroom area for protective clothing.
(2) Hand washing facilities.
(3) Toilet facilities.

However, with good technique, an area in the ward away from especially vulnerable patients can be used. In some instances where cross-infection has occurred it may be more appropriate to care for these patients together in a small ward with designated staff, so containing the infection to one area, rather than using side rooms on different wards (Duckworth, 1990). Uninfected patients must not be admitted into this area until all the infected patients have been discharged and the area thoroughly cleaned.

General principles of barrier nursing

The main emphasis for successful barrier nursing procedures is on hand washing and protection of clothes. Several general principles need to be adhered to if effective barrier nursing is to occur. Every effort must be made to ensure that instructions are kept simple and realistic. Regular assessment and evaluation of the situation must take place to ascertain whether barrier nursing continues to remain the most appropriate form of care.

Protective clothing

Gowns or aprons

The wearing of a protective gown or apron is an accepted part of barrier nursing technique to prevent the spread of micro-organisms from one patient to the next on clothing (Hambraeus, 1973).

Disposable plastic aprons are cheap, impermeable to bacteria and water (Babb *et al.*, 1983), are easy to put on, protect the probable area of maximum contamination and are preferable to cotton gowns, which provide increased cover but are *readily penetrated* by moisture and bacteria (Mackintosh, 1982).

Caps

Although the wearing of disposable caps while nursing infected patients is still practised, hair that is clean and tidy has not been implicated in cross-infection. Therefore, unless heavy contamination or splashing is present, the wearing of caps is not justified (Gaya, 1980).

Masks

Masks are sometimes worn to protect the patient, for example when a large burn is being dressed. Studies indicate that masks are generally of little value outside the operating theatre (see Chapter 32, Peri-operative Care) whilst the improper use of a mask can increase hand contamination (Ayton, 1984). Masks can also be worn to protect the wearer, for example when caring for patients with untreated meningococcal meningitis, or for patients with smear positive pulmonary tuberculosis who have a productive cough and are unable to cover their mouth and nose when sneezing and coughing (Joint Tuberculosis Committee of the British Thoracic Society, 1983). The organism which causes meningococcal meningitis is found at the back of the throat, and can be passed from person to person by droplet spread from the mouth and nose (Department of Health and Social Secuity, 1987a). More recent guidelines suggest that if the infected patient is cared for in a room ventilated by a mechanical extraction system, staff need not wear a mask (Joint Tuberculosis Committee of the British Thoracic Society, 1994). If masks are worn, they must be a filter type and fit the face closely.

Overshoes

The floors of hospital wards become easily contaminated by large numbers of bacteria (Ayliffe *et al.*, 1967). However, the wearing of overshoes has little value and there could even be an increased risk of cross-infection by contaminating the hands while putting on overshoes, making it necessary for the hands to be washed after putting on or taking them off (Jone *et al.*, 1988).

If airborne transmission of micro-organisms is a potential risk, a dry dust control mat placed at the patient's door, which is vacuumed daily and washed weekly, will be an effective means of limiting spread of infection by feet and trolley wheels (Meddick, 1977).

Gloves

Boxed, clean non-sterile gloves are adequate for routine non-invasive nursing care (Rossoff *et al.*, 1993). Clean gloves must be worn when handling blood or body fluids, or cleaning (Hart, 1991), but are not a substitute for hand washing. Therefore, hands must be washed with bactericidal soap and water or bactericidal alcohol hand rub after removing gloves.

Cleaning

Scrupulous daily cleaning of the barrier nursing room is essential. All furniture must be damp dusted to remove organisms dispersed into the air from bed making. The floor must be either vacuum cleaned with a machine fitted with a filter or damp mopped with hot, soapy water (the mop head must be laundered daily). Dry dusting or the use of a broom should be forbidden as studies have shown this method of cleaning simply redisperses the organisms into the air (Ayliffe, 1982). The cleaning equipment must be kept for sole use in this room.

Patient hygiene

The numbers of some micro-organisms on the skin will be reduced by using an antiseptic detergent for skin and hair washing (Mitchell, 1984) and this has been shown to be effective in eradicating the carriage of MRSA (Duckworth, 1990). The antiseptic should be applied directly to the flannel and rinsed off thoroughly.

Studies comparing standard baths with shower baths showed no overall significant difference between the two bathing techniques. However, one study indicated that shower baths were more effective in disinfecting axillae, and standard baths more efficient in reducing microbes in the perineum (Mitchell, 1984). Assessment and evaluation of the patients must be made to establish which patients will benefit most from a standard bath and which patients will benefit from a shower bath.

It is essential that baths are cleaned and dried between patients with a non-abrasive cleaning agent, ideally incorporating a hypochlorite (Austin, 1988), as viable organisms can survive in bath scum (Ayliffe et al., 1975). It is recommended that all hospital showers are fitted with automatic drain valves to reduce the the risk of nosocomial Legionnaire's disease (Humphrey, 1988). Bathing and showering are preferrable to bed baths, as organisms can be redistributed over the body during bed bathing (Greaves, 1985). If bed bathing is unavoidable the patient should be supplied with their own bowl which is washed and dried after use and stored at the bedside to prevent cross-infection.

Waste

Infected rubbish must be disposed of in yellow clinical waste bags. Full bags must be sealed securely within the room before being sent for incineration (Health and Safety Commission, 1982). Sharps must be placed immediately into a sharps disposal box (Department of Health and Social Security, 1983) which, when full, must be sealed before being sent for incineration (Health and Safety Commission, 1982).

Linen

Infected linen must be placed in a red alginate polythene bag. The bag is tied shut and then placed in a red linen bag to be sent in a safe manner to the laundry for barrier washing. This entails placing the full alginate bag in the washing machine where it dissolves, allowing the hot water to wash and disinfect the linen. In this way staff and the environment are protected from contamination (Department of Health and Social Security, 1987b).

Cutlery, crockery

All crockery must be machine washed in a dishwasher with a final rinse of 82°C to disinfect it (Collins, 1981).

Disposable crockery and cutlery are needed only when gross contamination has occurred or if a dishwasher is not available.

Urine, faeces and vomit

These are to be disposed of immediately down a heat-disinfecting bedpan washer.

Notification of infection

If a patient develops signs and symptoms of infection or if bacteriological analysis identifies an organism which necessitates barrier nursing, swift communication and action are needed to instigate this. Any problems may be discussed with the microbiologist or infection control nurse.

Informing the patient and visitors

Giving careful explanation to the patient is essential so that he/she can cooperate fully with the restrictions. (Wilson-Barnett et al., 1983). The nurse should be sensitive to the psychological implications of being labelled 'infectious' and of being confined in isolation. Wilkins et al. (1988) examined the psychological effects of being admitted to a barrier nursing room, and found that patients were unlikely to have significant psychological problems unless there was a previous history of mental illness. Many patients in fact preferred a single room, and adapted well to any subsequent loneliness and boredom. Other research has indicated that patients' needs are sometimes neglected when they are barrier nursed (Knowles, 1993). The patient's visitors must also be informed why the barrier nursing restrictions are necessary. Visitors will generally be allowed into the room at the discretion of the infection control team. They must be taught to observe the correct procedures for entering and leaving the room. As children are more susceptible to infection than adults, any visit by a child should be discussed with the appropriate personnel.

Domestic staff

The domestic manager must be informed as soon as barrier nursing is commenced. He or she will then provide the ward domestic with written instructions.

The ward domestic staff must understand clearly why barrier nursing is required and should be instructed on the correct procedure. The nursing staff must check that the ward domestics understand and are following their instructions correctly. If the patient is in a single room, a mop, bucket, cleaning fluid and disposable cloths should be kept solely for this patient's use. If the patient is in a general ward, special care must be taken with the cleaning so that potentially infectious material is not transferred from the area around the infected patient to other patient areas. The infected patient's area must be cleaned last and separately.

Staff allocation

A minimum number of staff should be involved with an infected patient. The nurse concerned with the infected patient should not also attend to other susceptible patients. If barrier nursing is for an infectious disease, it is preferable that only personnel who have already had the disease should attend this patient.

The protection of staff against the risk of infection is one of the main functions of the occupational health department. This department offers an immunization and counselling service.

References and further reading

Alderman, C. (1988) The cooler culprits. *Nursing Standard*, 2(33), 22.

Austin, L. (1988) The salt bath myth. *Nursing Times*, 84(9), 79–83.

Ayliffe, G. A. J. (1982) Airborne infection in hospital. *Journal of Hospital Infection*, 3, 217–40.

Ayliffe, G. A. J. *et al.* (1967) Ward floors and other surfaces as reservoirs of hospital infection. *Journal of Hygiene*, 65, 515–36.

Ayliffe, G. A. J. *et al.* (1975) Disinfection of baths and bath water. *Nursing Times*, 71(37), 22–3.

Ayliffe, G. A. J. *et al.* (1992) *Control of Hospital Infection: A Practical Handbook*. Chapman & Hall, London.

Ayton, M. (1984) Protective clothing: what do we use and when? *Nursing Times*, 80(19), 68–70.

Babb, J. R. *et al.* (1983) Contamination of protective clothing and nurses' uniforms in an isolation ward. *Journal of Hospital Infection*, 4, 149–57.

Bowell, B. (1992) Protecting the patient. *Nursing Times*, 88(13), 32–5.

Bowell, E. (1986) Nursing the isolated patient, Lassa fever. *Nursing Times*, 82(33), 72–81.

Burgess, N. R. H. (1979) Cockroaches and the hospital environment. *Nursing Times*, 75(11) (Contact), 5–7.

Casewell M. *et al.* (1977) Hands as route of transmission of *Klebsiella* species. *British Medical Journal*, 2, 1315–17.

Caudell, K. A. & Bakitas Whedon, B. (1991) Hematopoietic complications. In: *Bone Marrow Transplantation*, (ed. M. Bakitas Whedon). Jones and Bartlett, Boston.

Collins, B. (1981) Infection and the hospital environment. *Nursing*, 1, Supplement, 1–3.

Department of Health and Social Security (1983) *Containers for the Disposal of Used Needles and Sharp Instruments*. DHSS Specifications TSS/8/330, DHSS, London.

Department of Health and Social Security (1987a) *Meningococcal Meningitis*, DA(87)26. DHSS, London.

Department of Health and Social Security (1987b) *Hospital Laundry Arrangements For Used and Infected Linen*, HC(87)30. DHSS, London.

Duckworth, G. (1990) Revised guidelines for the control of epidemic methicillin-resistant *Staphylococcus aureus*. *Journal of Hospital Infection*, 16, 351–77.

Gaya, H. (1980) Questions and answer section. Is it necessary for staff and visitors in an intensive care unit to wear masks, hats, gowns and overshoes? *Journal of Hospital Infection*, 1, 369–71.

Gidley, C. (1987) Now wash your hands. *Nursing Times*, 83(29), 40–42.

Glenister, H. (1983) The passage of infection. *Nursing Mirror*, 12 January, 79, 28–30.

Greaves A. (1985) We'll just freshen you up, dear. . . . *Nursing Times*, 81(9), Supplement, 3–8.

Hambraeus, A. (1973) Transfer of *Staphylococcus aureus* via nurses' uniform. *Journal of Hygiene*, 71, 799–814.

Hart, S. (1991) Blood and body fluid precautions. *Nursing Standard*, 5(25), 25–8.

Health and Safety Commission (1982) *The Safe Disposal of Clinical Waste*. HMSO, London.

Humphrey, T. J. (1989) Microbial contamination of hospital showers and shower water: the effect of an automatic drain valve. *Journal of Hospital Infection*, 13, 55–61.

Joint Tuberculosis Committee of the British Thoracic Society (1983) Control and prevention of tuberculosis: a code of practice. *British Medical Journal*, 287, 1118–21.

Joint Tuberculosis Committee of the British Thoracic Society (1994) *Control and Prevention of Tuberculosis in the United Kingdom: Code of Practice*.

Jones, M. *et al.* (1988) Over-estimating overshoes. *Nursing Times*, 84(41), 66–71.

Knowles, H. E. (1993) The experience of infectious patients in isolation. *Nursing Times*, 89(30), 53–6.

Lee, M. G. *et al.* (1988) A comparison of two bactericidal handwashing agents containing chlorhexidine. *Journal of Hospital Infection*, 12, 59–63.

Mackenzie, I. (1988) Pre-operative skin preparation and surgical outcome. *Journal of Hospital Infection II*, Supplement B, 27–32.

Mackintosh, C. A. (1982) A testing time for gowns. *Journal of Hospital Infection*, 3, 5–8.

Mayon-White, R. T. *et al.* (1988) An international survey of the prevalence of hospital acquired infection. *Journal of Hospital Infection*, 11, Supplement A, 43.

Meddick, H. M. (1977) Bacterial contamination: control mats: – a comparative study. *Journal of Hygiene*, 79, 133–40.

Meers, P. D. *et al.* (1981) Report on the national survey of infection in hospital 1980. *Journal of Hospital Infection*, Supplement 2, 1–51.

Mims, C. A. *et al.* (1993) *Medical Microbiology*. Mosby, London.

Mitchell, N. J. (1984) Whole-body disinfection with chlorhexidine in shower bathing more effective than bathing. *Journal of Hospital Infection*, 5, 96–9.

Redding, R. J. *et al.* (1980) *Pseudomonas fluorescens* cross-infection due to contaminated humidifier water. *British Medical Journal*, 26 July, 281, 275.

Rossoff, L. J. *et al.* (1993) Is the use of boxed gloves in a intensive care unit safe? *American Journal of Medicine*, 94, 602–7.

Rowland A. J. (1972) Transmission of infection through towels. *Community Medicine*, 5 May, 71–2.

White, P. M. B. (1986) Food poisoning in a hospital staff canteen. *Journal of Infection*, 13, 195–8.

Wilkins, E. G. L. *et al.* (1988) Does isolation of patients with infection induce mental illness? *Journal of Infection*, 17, 43–7.

Wilson-Barnett, J. *et al.* (1983) Studies evaluating patient teaching implication for practice. *International Journal of Nursing Studies*, 20(1), 33–40.

Worsley, M. A. (1993) A major outbreak of antibiotic associated diarrhoea. *Public Health Laboratory Service Microbiology Digest*, 10(2), 97–9.

GUIDELINES: SOURCE ISOLATION

EQUIPMENT

1 Isolation suite if possible.
2 All items required to meet the patient's nursing needs during the period of isolation, e.g. instruments to assess vital signs.

PROCEDURE

Preparation of the isolation room

Action	Rationale
1 Place a barrier nursing sign outside the door.	To inform anyone intending to enter the room of the situation.
2 List requirements for personnel before entering and after leaving the isolation area.	To decrease entries and exits to the room.
3 Remove all non-essential furniture. The remaining furniture should be easy to clean and should not conceal or retain dirt or moisture either within or around it.	To minimize the risk of furniture harbouring microbial spores or growth colonies.
4 Stock the hand basin with a suitable antibacterial detergent preparation and paper towels for staff use.	Facilities for hand washing within the infected area are essential for effective barrier nursing.
5 Place yellow clinical waste bag in the room on a foot-operated stand. The bag must be sealed with tape before it is removed from the room.	For containing contaminated rubbish within the room. Yellow is the recognized colour for clinical waste.
6 Place a container for 'sharps' in the room.	To contain contaminated 'sharps' within the infected area.
7 When the 'sharps' container is two-thirds full it must be firmly shut and sent for incineration.	To minimize the risk of leakage from the 'sharps' safe.
8 Keep the patient's personal property to a minimum. Advise him/her to wear hospital clothing. All belongings taken into the room should be washable, cleanable or disposable.	The patient's belongings may become contaminated and cannot be taken home unless they are washable or cleanable. Anything else may have to be destroyed.
9 Provide the patient with his/her own thermometer and sphygmomanometer, water jug, glass and tray, and all items necessary for attending to personal hygiene.	Equipment used regularly by the patient should be kept within the infected area to prevent the spread of infection.

Guidelines: Source isolation (cont'd)

Action

10 Keep dressing solutions, creams and lotions, etc. to a minimum and store them within the room.

11 Set up a trolley outside the door to hold plastic aprons and bactericidal alcoholic hand rub (this is contraindicated if the trolley causes an obstruction or is a hazard to staff and others).

Rationale

All partially used materials must be discarded when barrier nursing ends (sterilization is not possible), therefore unnecessary waste should be avoided.

Staff are more likely to use the equipment if it is readily available.

Entering the room

Action

1 Collect all equipment needed.

2 Roll up long sleeves to the elbow.

3 Put on a disposable plastic apron when there is no risk of airborne transmission of organisms or when close contact with the patient is not anticipated.

4 Put on a disposable, impermeable gown for close work (e.g. lifting, nursing neonates).

5 Put on a disposable well-fitting mask if there is a risk of airborne contamination, i.e.
(a) Meningococcus meningitis.
(b) Blood and body fluids.

6 Safety glasses, visors and goggles should be put on when it is likely that aerosoled droplets of blood or body fluids are present in the air.

7 Put on disposable gloves only if you are intending to deal with blood, excreta or contaminated material.

8 Enter the room, shutting the door behind you.

Rationale

To avoid entering and leaving the infected area unnecessarily.

To protect clothing from contamination.

A plastic apron is inexpensive, quick to put on and protects the front of the uniform which is the most likely area to come in contact with the patient.

To protect clothing from contamination to shoulders, arms and back. Cotton gowns are an ineffective barrier against bacteria, particularly when wet.

To reduce the risk of inhaling organisms and to comply with safe techniques and practices.

To give protection to the conjunctiva from blood and body fluid splashes.

To reduce the risk of contaminating your hands.

To reduce the risk of airborne organisms leaving the room.

Attending to the patient

Action

1 *Meals.* Meals should be served only on disposable crockery and eaten with disposable cutlery if deemed necessary by the infection control team. Disposables and uneaten food should be discarded in the appropriate bag.

Rationale

Contaminated crockery is a potential disease vector.

2 *Non-disposable crockery.* A personal water jug, glasses and tray should be kept at the bedside. These, and any other non-disposable crockery, should be washed in a dishwasher with a hot disinfecting cycle.

Water at 80°C for 1 minute in a dishwasher will disinfect crockery and cutlery.

3 *Excreta.* Ideally, a toilet should be kept solely for the patient's use. If neither this nor disposable items are available, a separate bedpan or urinal and commode should be left in the patient's room. Gloves must be worn by staff when dealing with excreta. Bedpans and urinals should be bagged in the isolation room, emptied and then washed in a bedpan washer, then dried and returned immediately to the patient's room.

To minimize the risk of infection being spread from excreta, e.g. via a toilet seat or a bedpan.

4 *Accidental spills.* Any suspected contaminated fluids must be mopped up immediately and the area cleaned with disinfectant.

Damp areas encourage microbial growth and increase the risk of spread of infection.

5 *Bathing.* An infected patient must be bathed last on the ward. Clean and dry the bath after the previous patient and after the infected patient. If the patient has infected lesions, disinfectant (e.g. Savlon) may be added to the bath water. Salt is not a disinfectant and has little antibacterial effect (Austin, 1988).

Leaving the bath dry after disinfection reduces the risk of microbes surviving and infecting others. Bacteria will not grow on clean, dry surfaces.

6 *Dressings.* Aseptic technique must be used for changing all dressings. Waste materials and dirty dressings should be discarded in the appropriate bag. Used lotions, creams, etc. must be kept in the room and not used for other patients.

Aseptic procedure minimizes the risk of cross-infection. Lotions and creams can become easily contaminated.

7 *Linen.* Place infected linen in a red alginate polythene bag, which must be secured tightly before it leaves the room. Just outside the room, place this bag into a red linen bag which must be secured tightly and not used for other patients. These bags should await the laundry collection in a safe area.

Placing infected linen in a red alginate polythene bag confines the organisms and allows staff handling the linen to recognize the potential hazard.

8 *Waste.* Yellow clinical waste bags should be kept in the room for disposal of all the patient's rubbish. The bag's top should be sealed and labelled with the name of the ward or department before it is removed from the room.

Yellow is the international colour for clinical waste.

Leaving the room

Action

Rationale

1 If wearing gloves, remove and discard them in the yellow clinical waste bag. Wash hands with an appropriate antiseptic solution.

To remove pathogenic organisms acquired during contact with patient before removing gown, so preventing contamination of uniform.

Guidelines: Source isolation (cont'd)

Action	Rationale
2 Remove apron and discard it in the appropriate bag. Wash hands again with an appropriate antiseptic solution.	Hands may be contaminated by a dirty gown.
3 Used gowns should not be re-used.	Mistakes are made if gowns have to be re-used, particularly as staff find it hard to distinguish the inside/outside of a gown. If the gown is worn inside out, uniforms can be contaminated.
4 Leave the room, shutting the door behind you.	
5 Rinse hands with a bactericidal alcohol-based hand wash solution.	To remove pathogenic organisms acquired from such items as the door handle.

Cleaning the room

Action	Rationale
1 Domestic staff must understand why barrier nursing is required and should be instructed on the correct procedure.	To reduce the risk of mistakes and to ensure that barrier nursing is maintained.
2 The area where barrier nursing is being carried out must be cleaned last.	To reduce the risk of the transmission of organisms.
3 Separate cleaning equipment must be kept for this area.	Cleaning equipment can easily become infected. Cross-infection may result from shared cleaning equipment.
4 Members of the domestic services staff must wear gloves and plastic aprons.	To reduce the risk of cross-infection.
5 *Floor* (hard surface). This must be washed daily with a disinfectant as appropriate. All excess water must be removed.	Daily cleaning will keep bacterial count reduced. Organisms, especially Gram-negative bacteria, multiply quickly in the presence of moisture.
6 After use, the bucket must be cleaned, dried and stored within the barrier nursing area.	Bacteria will not survive on clean dry surfaces.
7 Ideally, mop heads should be laundered in a hot wash daily, when this is not possible, the mop must be washed, rinsed, all excess water removed and stored with the mop head uppermost to allow for quick drying within the barrier nursing area.	Mop heads become contaminated easily.
8 *Floor* (carpet). An infected patient may have been admitted into a room with a carpet. A vacuum cleaner should be used which is fitted with an efficient filter. After use the dust bag must be changed and the brush head washed and dried.	Vacuum cleaning reduces the dust thus reducing organisms.
9 On discharge, the carpet must be steam cleaned.	Bacteria can survive in dust trapped in the carpet fibres. The heat of the steam will kill these bacteria.

	Action	Rationale
10	Furniture and fittings should be damp dusted using a disposable cloth and a detergent solution or a disinfectant if appropriate.	To remove any organisms.
11	The toilet, shower and bathroom area must be cleaned at least once a day using a non-abrasive hypochlorite powder or cream. A disinfectant will only be required if soiling of the area has occurred.	Non-abrasive powders or creams preserve the integrity of the surfaces. These areas recontaminate rapidly after cleaning and routine chemical disinfection is of little value and should be saved for terminal cleaning.

Transporting infected patients outside the barrier nursing area

	Action	Rationale
1	Inform the department concerned about the diagnosis.	To allow other departments time to make their own arrangements.
2	Arrange for the patient to have the last appointment of the day.	The department concerned will then be empty of other patients; time can be allowed for special cleaning or disinfecting; hospital corridors, lifts, etc. are usually less busy at this time of day.
3	Any porters involved must be instructed carefully. The trolley or chair should be cleaned after use.	Protection and reassurance of porters are necessary to allay fear and to minimize the risk of the infection being spread to them.
4	It may be necessary for the nurse to escort the patient.	To ensure the necessary precautions are maintained.

Discharging the patient

	Action	Rationale
1	Inform the microbiologist when the patient is due for discharge.	The microbiologist will advise on any special precautions.
2	The room should be stripped and aired. All textiles must be changed and curtains sent to the laundry.	Curtains readily become colonized with bacteria.
3	Impervious surfaces, e.g. lockers, stools, blinds and thermometer holders, should be washed with soap and water.	Wiping of surfaces is the most effective way of removing contaminants. Relatively inaccessible places, e.g. ceilings, may be omitted; these are not generally relevant to any infection risk.
4	The floor must be washed and dried thoroughly.	To remove any organisms present.
5	If the room is known to be contaminated with blood or blood-stained excreta from hepatitis B positive or human immunodeficiency virus (HIV) antibody positive individuals, a hypochlorite solution should be used.	To remove the source of potential contamination.
6	If the room has been used used by a patient with an enteric infection a clean, soluble phenolic should be used.	To remove the source of potential contamination.

ANTIBIOTIC-RESISTANT ORGANISMS

Definition
The term *antibiotic resistance* denotes a strain of bacteria that is not killed or inhibited by antimicrobial agents to which the species is generally sensitive.

REFERENCE MATERIAL
The importance of antibiotic-resistant organisms cannot be overemphasized. Patients who are immuno-compromised, debilitated or with open wounds are at particular risk and deaths have occurred (Cox *et al.*, 1995). Bacterial resistance to antibiotics may take many years to develop, as in the case of the gonococcus. Strains resistant to penicillin G only appeared after 25 years of use (Sparling *et al.*, 1976). Methicillin-resistant *Staphylococcus aureus* (MRSA), however, was first reported in 1961 (Jevons), only two years after the drug's clinical introduction. MRSA is now increasing with some hospitals reporting its frequenty as high as 20–40% of all *Staphylococcus aureus* identified (Ayliffe, 1986).

The widespread and often indiscriminate use of anti-biotics for prophylactic and veterinary purposes, as well as the inappropriate selection of antibiotics, are believed to be important factors in the development of resistant forms of bacteria (Swan Joint Committee, 1969; Garrod, 1972). The transmission of genetic material between bacteria by conjugation has been well documented (Jaffe *et al.*, 1980; Mendoza, 1985) and this conjugation accounts in part for the rapid spread of resistance, with mutation, transformation and transduction also being involved (Sande & Mandell, 1980).

The consequences of a patient being infected with a resistant form of bacteria are demanding in terms of increased length of stay, costs of care and treatment (Grazebrook, 1986).

The North East Thames Microbiology Sub-Committee MRSA Working Party (1987) estimated the annual cost to a hospital with a large MRSA infection problem to be £250000 (Duckworth, 1990).

A recent study from Hong Kong showed that the average cost of antimicrobial therapy per patient with MRSA bacteraemia was £440, compared with £60 for patients with methicillin-sensitive *Staphylococcus aureus* bacteraemia. The extra cost reflected the increased cost of antimicrobials and the longer treatment required (Cheng *et al.*, 1988).

Theoretically, any organism can develop antibiotic resistance. In practice, however, two groups present the major problem: Gram-negative bacteria and *Staphylococcus aureus* (Mimms *et al.*, 1993).

Gram-negative bacteria
Gram-negative bacteria normally inhabit the gut but cause infections in the urinary tract, respiratory tract and wounds. Outbreaks of resistant forms have been reported (Casewell, 1982; Dance, 1987) which may be the consequence of excessive use of broad-spectrum antibiotics. *Pseudomonas* species may cause particular problems (Jarvis & Martone, 1992) being ubiquitous in the hospital environment (Laa Poh & Yeo, 1993). This organism can multiply in warm, moist conditions and has been identified in eye drops, soap solutions, lotions and in the tubing used for ventilators and incubators. This is particularly difficult because of the shortage of drugs which are effective against resistant forms of *Pseudomonas* species (Mimms *et al.*, 1993).

Gram-negative bacteraemia
Gram-negative bacteraemia is associated with septic shock (Ferguson, 1991), which occurs primarily in debilitated, hospitalized patients who are the group that also develops the resistant form of Gram-negative bacteraemia (Bryant *et al.*, 1971).

The major problem regarding Gram-negative-resistant organisms is that shock progresses before antibiotic sensitivities are known, with increased clinical manifestations which can result in death (Glauser *et al.*, 1991; Truett, 1991).

Staphylococcus aureus
Staphylococcus aureus is part of the normal human flora, with large numbers of the organism being found on the skin and mucosa. Colonization or infection by MRSA is therefore more likely to occur in the nose, lesions and sites of abnormal skin, and in indwelling devices such as catheters and tracheostomies (Ayliffe, 1986).

There are many distinguishable strains of MRSA which may or may not be epidemic in character, i.e. epidemic MRSA (EMRSA) (Cox *et al.*, 1995). Phage typing of the strain to establish strain and epidemiology is important (Richardson *et al.*, 1988) as increased barrier nursing precautions will be required for epidemic strains (Cox *et al.*, 1995). Outbreaks of clinically significant MRSA have been a particular problem in special units with highly dependent patients (Simpson, 1992). These patients tend to have frequent contact with staff which increases the risk of cross-infection. A high level of compliance with infection control strategies is necessary to minimize the risk to patients.

Carriers and infected patients need to be identified and the extent of colonization must be established. Prompt barrier nursing may limit the spread of MRSA (Selkon *et al.*, 1980). Patients transferred from hospitals and countries known to have an MRSA problem should be screened on admission and treated as suspect until the results of screening specimens are known (Duckworth, 1990). These restrictions may be minimal, with nursing care involving just good hand washing following patient contact. However, if the patient is obviously ill with, for example, a discharging wound then this would necessitate barrier nursing (see beginning of this chapter).

Any patients in contact with infected patients must be screened to detect cross-infection. This would include nose swabs, and swabs from skin lesions, catheters and intravenous lines (Cox et al., 1995).

If cross-infection occurs it may be necessary to close a ward to new admissions, particularly to surgical or intensive care patients. Once patients have been discharged, the ward must be cleaned thoroughly before patients are readmitted. The use of a phenolic disinfectant for surface disinfection in cross-infection incidences has been advised (Duckworth, 1990).

Screening of staff contacts must include medical, nursing, paramedical and domestic staff. There is no evidence that MRSA poses a risk to healthy staff, but staff may become colonized and could transmit MRSA to other patients (Locksley, 1982). *All* staff in contact with the infected patient should be screened and, if working in a high-dependency unit, may need to be removed from duty if widespread carriage develops. Generally, only nasal carriage occurs, which can be treated with mupirocin ointment, while staff continue at work (Hill et al., 1988). The psychological effects of MRSA on patients and on staff who provide care are significant (Tuffnall, 1988). Knowles (1993) suggests that patients with infections can feel stigmatized and lonely. The MRSA load on skin can be reduced by twice-weekly hairwashing and daily showering for one week, using an antiseptic detergent such as chlorhexidine povidone iodine or triclosan (Bartzokas et al., 1984). Serious clinical infection should be treated with vancomycin. New agents such as teicoplanin and ciprofloxacin are still being evaluated (Duckworth, 1990). Unfortunately resistance to teicoplanin has already been seen (Cunnery et al., 1993).

Agency staff are a particular problem with respect to cross-infection, and may transmit MRSA between hospitals. It is preferable to use a central agency and make it known that staff who have recently worked in an infected hospital will not be employed until negative screening swabs are available (Cookson et al., 1989). Infected patients must be identified quickly and barrier nursing commenced (Duckworth, 1990; Cox et al., 1995). Unfortunately in many cases nursing patients with MRSA in side-rooms in general wards has not prevented cross-infection (Beedle, 1993).

Eradication of carriage sites other than the nose is difficult and may often fail. Mupirocin nasal ointment in paraffin base for mucous membranes and mupirocin cream in a miscible macrogol base for non-mucous membrane intact skin has been seen to be most effective (Duckworth, 1990).

Relapses may occur, especially in debilitated patients and particularly in sites such as tracheostomies (Cox et al., 1995). This means that barrier nursing must be maintained even after three negative cultures have been obtained. The presence of MRSA should be documented in the patient's records in order to alert staff should readmission be necessary (Cookson et al., 1986).

Inter-hospital movement should be restricted to the absolute minimum. If the patient must be transferred to another hospital, the receiving hospital must be informed in plenty of time for the necessary arrangements to be made. The ambulance service should be notified if it is being used to transfer an MRSA patient, mainly to prevent another patient being placed in the same vehicle before it is cleaned. Hand washing by the ambulance service staff and cleaning of local areas of patient contact, i.e. chair or stretcher, is all that is required after transport of an affected patient.

References and further reading

Ayliffe, G. A. J. (1986) Guidelines for the control of epidemic methicillin-resistant *Staphylococcus aureus*. *Journal of Infection*, 7, 193–201.

Bartzokas, C. A. et al. (1984) Control and eradication of methicillin-resistant *Staphylococcus aureus* on a surgical unit. *New England Journal of Medicine*, 311, 1422–5.

Beedle, D. (1993) Beating the bug. *Nursing Times*, 89(45), *Journal of Infection Control Nursing*, Supplement, i–vi.

Bryant, R. E. et al. (1971) Factors affecting mortality of Gram-negative rod bacteraemia. *Archives of International Medicine*, 127, 120.

Casewell, M. W. (1982) The role of multiply resistant coliforms in hospital acquired infection. *Recent Advances in Infection*, 2, 31–50.

Cheng, A. F. et al. (1988) Methicillin-resistant *Staphylococcus aureus* bacteraemia in Hong Kong. *Journal of Hospital Infection*, 12, 91–101.

Cookson, B. D. et al. (1986) A hospital computer system as a tool for infection control. In: *Current Perspectives in Health Care Computing*, (eds J. Bryant, J. Roberts & P. Windson), pp. 126–31. British Computer Society Health Information, Specialist Group, and *British Journal of Health Care Computing*, London.

Cookson, B. D. et al. (1989) Staff carriage of epidemic methicillin-resistant *Staphylococcus aureus*. *Journal of Clinical Microbiology*, 27, 1471–6.

Cox, R. A. et al. (1995) A major outbreak of methicillin-resistant *Staphylococcus aureus* caused by a new phage-type (EMRSA-16). *Journal of Hospital Infection*, 29, 87–106.

Cunnery, R. J. et al. (1993) Failure of teicoplanin therapy in *Staphylococcus* septicaemia. *Journal of Hospital Infection*, 3, 325–7.

Dance, D. A. B. (1987) A hospital outbreak caused by a chlorhexidine and antibiotic resistant *Proteus mirabilis*. *Journal of Hospital Infection*, 10, 10–16.

Duckworth, G. (1990) Revised guidelines for the control of epidemic methicillin-resistant *Staphylococcus aureus*. *Journal of Hospital Infection*, 16, 351–77.

Ferguson, J. (1991) Septic shock in the critically ill patient. *Surgical Nurse*, 4(2), 21–4.

Garrod, L. P. (1972) Causes of failure in antibiotic treatment. *British Medical Journal*, 4, 473–6.

Glauser, M. P. *et al.* (1991) Septic shock: pathogenesis. *Lancet*, 338, 732–5.

Granzebrook, J. (1986) Counting the cost of infection. *Nursing Times*, 83(6), 24–6.

Hill, R. L. R. *et al.* (1988) Elimination of nasal carriage of methicillin-resistant *Staphylococcus aureus* with mupirocin during a hospital outbreak. *Journal of Antimicrobial Chemotherapy*, 22, 377–84.

Hughes, W. T. (1971) Fatal infections in childhood leukaemia. *American Journal of Diseases in Childhood*, 122, 283–7.

Jaffe, H. W. *et al.* (1980) Identity and interspecific transfer of gentamicin resistant plasmids in *Staphylococcus aureus* and *Staphylococcus epidermidis*. *Journal of Infectious Diseases*, 141, 738.

Jarvis, W. R. & Martone, W. J. (1992) Predominant pathogen in hospital infection. *Journal of Antimicrobiology and Chemotherapy*, 29, Supplement A, 19–24.

Jevons, M. P. (1961) Celberin resistant staphylococci, *British Medical Journal*, 1, 124–5.

Knowles, H. E. (1993) The experience of infectious patients in isolation. *Nursing Times*, 89(30), 53–6.

Laa Poh, C. & Yeo, C. C. (1993) Recent advances in typing *Pseudomonas aeruginosa*. *Journal of Hospital Infection*, 24, 175–81.

Locksley, R. M. (1982) Multiple antibiotic resistant *Staphylococcus aureus*: introduction, transmission and evaluation of nosocomial infection. *Annals of Internal Medicine*, 97, 317–24.

Mayet, F. (1989) The microbe file, *Nursing Standard*, 3, 57–8.

Mendoza, M. C. (1985) Evidence for the dispersion and evolution of R. plasmids from *Serratia marcescens* in hospital. *Journal of Hospital Infection*, 6, 147–53.

Mims, C. A. *et al.* (1993) *Medical Microbiology*. Mosby, London.

Peters, G. *et al.* (1983) Antibacterial activity of teichomycin – a new glycopeptide antibiotic in comparison to vancomycin. *Journal of Antimicrobial Chemotherapy*, 11, 94–5.

Richardson, J. F. *et al.* (1988) Another strain of methicillin-resistant *Staphylococcus aureus* epidemic in London. *Lancet*, 2, 748–9.

Sande, M. A. & Mandell, G. L. (1980) Chemotherapy of microbial diseases. In: *The Pharmacological Basis of Therapeutics*, (eds L. S. Goodman *et al.*). Macmillan, London.

Selkon, J. B. *et al.* (1980) The role of an isolation unit in the control of hospital infection with multi-resistant *Staphylococcus aureus*. *Journal of Hospital Infection*, 1, 41–6.

Simpson, S. (1992) Methicillin resistant *Staphylococcus aureus* and its implications for nursing practice. A literature review. *Nursing Practice*, 5(2), 2–7.

Smith, S. M. *et al.* (1989) Ciprofloxacin therapy for methicillin-resistant *Staphylococcus aureus* infection or colonizations. *Antimicrobial Agents and Chemotherapy*, 33, 181–4.

Sparling, F. P. *et al.* (1976) Antibiotic resistance in the gonococcus. In: *Microbiology*, (ed. D. Schlessinger). American Society of Microbiology.

Swan Joint Committee (1969) *Use of Antibiotics in Animal Husbandry and Veterinary Medicine*. HMSO, London.

Truett, L. (1991) The septic syndrome. *Cancer Nursing*, 14(4), 175–80.

Tuffnall, C. (1988) MRSA: isolating the patients and nurses. *New Zealand Nursing Journal*, 1, 21–3.

PROTECTIVE ISOLATION

Definition

Immunosuppression is a generalized depression of the immune system, which increases the risk of acquiring an infection. This necessitates protecting immunosuppressed patients from micro-organisms carried in the environment, from health care workers providing care, from visitors and from other patients.

Protective isolation provides a safe environment for patients who are susceptible to infection and can be an appropriate form of care for many patients, e.g. burns patients, children with immunodeficiency disease and patients receiving bone marrow transplantation. The aim of protective isolation is to prevent and treat infection until the period of immunosuppression is past.

Indications

Immunosuppression can be caused by many factors including:

(1) Primary disease such as leukaemia, lymphoma (Field *et al.*, 1977), acquired immune deficiency syndrome (AIDS) (Centre of Disease Control, 1988), severe combined immunodeficiency disease (SCID) (Hill, 1989).

(2) Secondary disease, such as diabetes, which may complicate primary disease (Reeves, 1980).

(3) Drugs, in particular, cytotoxic drugs and corticosteroids (Reheis, 1985).

(4) Antimicrobial therapy causing changes in the patient's microbial flora (Hahn *et al.*, 1978).

(5) Irradiation therapy: the degree of immunosuppression is related directly to the area being treated (Strober *et al.*, 1981).

(6) Trauma (Maclean, *et al.*, 1975) and burns (Miller *et al.*, 1979).

(7) Age (Leonard, 1986).

The risk of infection will be increased by breaches in the body's natural defence mechanisms, for example:

(1) Skin by, for example, indwelling catheters; repeated venepuncture; pressure ulcers (Wade *et al.*, 1982).

(2) Mucous membranes, from oral ulceration (Richardson, 1987).

(3) Body cavities by urinary catheters (Meers *et al.*, 1981) or endotracheal tubes.

Nursing care of the highest standard is required when involved in such procedures to reduce the risk of infection as much as practically possible.

Infection risk is also related to the absolute level of circulating granulocytes (Bodey *et al.*, 1966) with the frequency of infection rising as the granulocytes count drops below 500/µl, with a dramatic increase as the granulocyte count reaches zero (Schimpff *et al.*, 1978).

Granulocytopenia, occurring rapidly, is more likely to be associated with an increased risk of infection than is a slow decline or a stable granulocytopenia (Dale *et al.*, 1979).

Some patients have an increased risk of infection due to a combination of immunosuppressive factors. For example, in the case of a patient with leukaemia who is undergoing bone marrow transplantation and who develops graft-versus-host disease (GVHD), which requires treatment with increased doses of immuno-suppressive drug (Van Der Meer, 1994).

Therefore, the severity and expected length of immunosuppression should be assessed to decide the level of protective isolation which is required (Meyer, 1986). Generally, the greater the state of immuno-suppression, the greater the need for protection (Rubin *et al.*, 1990). Russell *et al.* (1992) discuss the probable number of naturally occurring infections and describe how institutional care affects the risk of acquiring an infection. They suggest that intensive treatment programmes can be safely completed without protective isolation is some cases. On the other hand, Poe *et al.* (1994) describe a survey of infection prevention practices on bone marrow transplant units which indicates that there is little standardization of practice. They conclude that efforts should be made to test the benefits of various infection control measures to allow national standards to be developed.

REFERENCE MATERIAL
Protective isolation may be achieved by:

(1) Purpose-built units (Borley, 1982).
(2) Plastic isolators (Bowell, 1986).
(3) Single rooms on a general ward (Nauseef *et al.*, 1981).
(4) Shared rooms within a controlled environment on a general ward.

Purpose-built units
A purpose-built unit will include:

(1) Filtered air supply.
(2) Single rooms with integral toilet, shower, a hatch system for the aseptic transfer of equipment into the room, an entry area for visitors and staff where protective clothing can be donned and hands washed.
(3) Facilities to provide pathogen-free food.
(4) Gastrointestinal decontamination (Jameson *et al.*, 1971).

These units are expensive to build, maintain and staff. Although evidence shows that this form of protective isolation does reduce infection, Buckner *et al.* (1978) it does not affect long-term survival (Levine *et al.*, 1973; Schimpff *et al.*, 1975; Yates *et al.*, 1973) although it may reduce graft-versus-host disease (GVHD) (Storb *et al.*, 1983).

Opinion is also divided as to whether protective isolation causes psychological damage (Kohle, 1979), particularly among paediatric patients (Powazek *et al.*, 1978), necessitating such units to provide psychological support in the form of social workers, play therapists, teachers and psychologists.

Plastic isolators
An isolator consists of a framework erected around a bed from which a PVC tent is suspended. The tent has an air supply attached which keeps the whole apparatus inflated. A positive air pressure is usually maintained within the isolator. In some cases, for example, when nursing patients with Lassa fever, the pressure within the isolator is slightly below atmospheric pressure, which prevents the escape of any infected particles. Although patients may feel a strong sense of containment within the isolator, this system does have the advantage of achieving high standards of bacteriological control, and it can be assembled and dismantled rapidly.

Single rooms and shared rooms in general wards
The decision to isolate a patient will be influenced by the availability of facilities coupled to the general condition of the ward area where the isolation is to take place. In determining the most suitable area, a number of criteria need to be met. Among these are the relative cleanliness of the ward, the standard of domestic services support, the microbiological status of the other patients and the anticipated length of the isolation.

This less vigorous method of protective isolation is unlikely to greatly reduce the acquisition of potential pathogens, as only person-to-person transfer of infection is prevented, since facilities such as clean air and pathogen-free food are not usually available on general wards (Hann *et al.*, 1984).

The prevention of exogenous transmission of infection is important and can be achieved by careful monitoring of the environment to remove items which could predispose to infection, for example, flowers (Taplin *et al.*, 1973). Scrupulous cleaning with special attention to furniture and equipment within the room will also prevent transmission (Crane, 1980).

The limiting of endogenous transmission of infection, which is the major cause of infection in immunosuppressed patients (Schimpff *et al.*, 1970; Selden *et al.*, 1971), is difficult but good patient hygiene, restriction of invasive devices and procedures are useful.

A thorough and continuing assessment of the patient is essential in order to recognize the first signs of infection (see Chapter 30, Observations). The most common areas of early infection include the lung, pharynx, anorectal area, skin and subcutaneous tissue (Reheis, 1985). Unfortunately, signs and symptoms of infection are often absent in immunosuppressed patients (Sickles *et al.*, 1975).

Investigations to establish the cause of infection include chest X-ray, bacteriological and viral culture of blood, urine and sputum, and swabs obtained from any suspicious lesion (see Chapter 38, Specimen Collection).

As progression of infection in the immunosuppressed patient may be rapid and widespread, the earliest sign of infection must be looked for, and appropriate antimcirobial therapy commenced immediately. If an infection is left untreated, fatality rate ranging from 18% to 40% can occur within the first 48 hours (Schimpff, 1977).

Bacterial infections are generally caused by Gram-negative organisms, such as *Pseudomonas* species, *Escherichia coli* and *Klebsiella* species, normally found in the gastrointestinal tract. Gram-positive organisms causing infections are commonly *Staphylococcus epidermidis*, which is generally a skin contaminant (Bodey, 1975).

The most common fungal infection is by *Candida albicans*, which is most usually found in the oral cavity, but which may affect the oesophagus, bowel or vagina, and cause systemic infection, pneumonia and septicaemia.

Aspergillus infection, particularly associated with nearby building work has also been seen (see the Aspergillosis section later in this chapter). Viral infections, particularly by cytomegalovirus and herpes zoster may occur (see the section an herpes viruses, later in this chapter). Immunosuppressed patients are at increased risk of nosocomial infection, and bacteria that cause infection are particularly easily disseminated from health care workers' hands (Larson, 1988). Strict hand washing can reduce rates of infection (Gould, 1993). Hand washing can be said to be the most important means of infection control (Bowell, 1992).

Airborne infectious micro-organisms, notably staphylococci, may be inhaled or transferred to the patient via wounds, intravenous cannulae, etc. Patients may also infect themselves directly from their own micro-organisms (Elliot, 1993).

Food is a potential source of infection (Correa *et al.*, 1991). Generally, if non-absorbable gut antibiotics are prescribed, pathogen-free food must be provided (Patterson, 1993). Thoroughly cooked foods, canned foods and foods known to be pathogen-free such as cereal, should be served with sterile utensils on sterile trays. If these facilities are unavailable, then the diet should consist only of food that has been well-cooked; foods known to have high bacterial counts should be avoided (Roberts, 1982). This involves eliminating raw fruit and vegetables from the diet (Wright *et al.*, 1976). A recent review of practice related to clean diets found evidence of a move away from stringent sterile diets towards more relaxed regimes with rational, justifiable food hygiene guidelines (Patterson, 1993).

Protective isolation can cause increased stress for patients (Gaston-Johnson *et al.*, 1992). Nurses can reduce anxiety by assisting patients to learn about their situation and about health promoting activities (Belec, 1992). It is also suggested that nursing on a protective isolation unit, particularly with patients undergoing bone marrow transplantation, increases the stress suffered by nurses themselves (Borley, 1985). This can result in burn-out, producing symptoms such as fatigue, anxiety, depression and poor concentration (Scully, 1980), which can be detrimental to nurses, their colleagues and the patients in their care.

Nursing managers of intensive care units such as protective isolation units need to be aware of this risk and provide support and a treatment plan if burn-out does occur (McElroy, 1982).

Poe *et al.* (1994), in their survey of bone marrow transplant units across the USA, found that little standardization of infection prevention practices exists nationwide. Whilst most units used some type of protective environment, practices varied considerably.

The procedure described below (Guidelines: Nursing the neutropenic patient) is intended to protect the patient whose period of neutropenia can reasonably be expected to be measured in days. It does not involve the special precautions of full protective isolation with protection from commensal infection in patients whose neutropenia is likely to be prolonged.

References and further reading

Belec, R. H. (1992) Quality of life: perception of long-term survivors of bone marrow transplantation. *Oncology Nursing Forum*, 19(1), 31–7.

Bodey, C. P. *et al.* (1966) Quantitative relationships between circulating leukocytes and infection in patients with acute leukaemia. *Annals of International Medicine*, 64, 328–40.

Bodey, C. P. (1975) Infections in cancer patients. *Cancer Treatment and Review*, 2, 89–128.

Borley, D. (1982) A protected environment for bone marrow transplantation. *Pictures in Nursing Medical Education*, 156–8.

Borley, D. (1985) Bone marrow patients can plant extra stress on nurses. *Nursing Mirror*, 160(8), 6.

Bowell, B. (1992) Protecting the patient at risk. *Nursing Times*, 88(3), 32–5.

Bowell, E. (1986) Nursing the isolated patient. *Nursing Times*, 82(33), 72–81.

Buckner, C. D. *et al.* (1978) Protective environment for marrow transplant recipients. *Annals of Internal Medicine*, 89, 893–901.

Centre of Disease Control (CDC) (1988) Revision of CDC surveillance case definition of AIDS. *Morbidity and Mortality Weekly Report*, No 36, 1–15.

Correa, C. M. C. *et al.* (1991) Vegatables as a source of infection with *Pseudomonas aeruginosa* in a university and oncology hospital of Rio de Janeiro. *Journal of Hospital Infection*, 18, 301–306.

Crane, L. R. (1980) Prevention of infection on the oncology unit. *Nursing Clinics of North America*, 15(4), 843–55.

Dale, D. C. *et al.* (1979) Chronic neutropenia. *Medicine*, 58, 128–44.

Elliot, T. S. J. (1993) Line-associated bacteraemias. *Communicable Disease Report Review*, 3(7), R91–R95.

Field, R. *et al.* (1977) Infections in patients with malignant lymphoma treated with combination chemotherapy. *Cancer*, 39, 1018–77.

Gaston-Johnson, F. *et al.* (1992) Pain and psychological distress in patients undergoing autologous bone marrow transplantation. *Oncology Nursing Forum*, 19(1), 41–7

Gould, D. (1993) Assessing nurses' hand decontamination performance. *Nursing Times*, 90(25), 47–50.

Hahn, D. M. *et al.* (1978) Infection in acute leukaemia patients receiving oral, non-absorbable antibiotics. *Antimicrobial Agents and Chemotherapy*, 13, 958–64.

Hann, I. M. *et al.* (1984) Infection prophylaxis in the patient with bone marrow failure. *Clinics in Haematology*, 13(3), 523–46.

Hill, H. R. (1989) Infections complicating congenital immunodeficiency syndromes. In: *Clinical Approaches to Infection in the Compromised Host*, (eds R. H. Rubin & L. S. Young), 2nd edn, pp. 407–32. Plenum Medical Book Co, London.

Jameson, B. *et al.* (1971) Five-year analysis of protective isolation. *Lancet*, 1, 1034–40.

Kohle, K. (1979) Psychological aspects in isolated patients' experience during eight years. *Clinical and Experimental Gnotobiotics*, 7, 45–72.

Larson, E. (1988) A causal link between hand washing and risk of infection. *Infection Control and Hospital Epidemiology*, 9, 28–35.

Leonard, M. (1986) Handling infection. *Nursing Times*, 82(33), 81–4.

Levine, A. S. *et al.* (1973) Protective environment and prophylactic antibiotics – a prospective controlled study of their utility in the therapy of acute leukaemia. *New England Journal of Medicine*, 288, 477–83.

Maclean, L. D. *et al.* (1975) Host resistance in sepsis and trauma. *Annals of Surgery*, 182, 207–15.

McElroy, A. (1982) Burn-out: a review of the literature with application to cancer nursing. *Cancer Nursing*, June, 3(6), 211–17.

Meers, P. D. *et al.* (1981) Report on the Natural Survey of Infections in Hospitals, 1980. *Journal of Hospital Infection*, Supplement, 2, 1–53.

Meyer, I. D. (1986) Infection in bone marrow transplant recipients. *American Journal of Medicine*, 81, 27–8.

Miller, C. L. *et al.* (1979) Changes in lymphocyte activity after thermal injury. *Journal of Clinical Investigation*, 63, 202–10.

Mims, C. A. *et al.* (1993) *Medical Microbiology*. Mosby, London.

Nauseef, W. M. *et al.* (1981) A study of the value of simple protective isolation in patients with granulocytopenia. *New England Journal of Medicine*, 304(8), 448–53.

Patterson, A. J. (1993) Review of current practices in clean diets in the UK. *Journal of Human Nutrition and Dietetics*, 6, 3–11.

Poe, S. S. *et al.* (1994) A national survey of infection prevention practices on bone marrow transplant units. *Oncology Nursing Forum*, 21(10), 1687–93.

Powazek, M. *et al.* (1978) Emotional reaction of children to isolation in a cancer hospital. *Journal of Paediatrics*, 92(5), 834–7.

Reeves, W. G. (1980) Immunology of diabetes and insulin therapy. *Recent Advances in Clinical Immunology*, 2, 183–7.

Reheis, C. E. (1985) Neutropenia causes complications: treatment and resulting nursing care. *Nursing Clinics of North America*, 20(1), 219–25.

Richardson, A. (1987) A process standard for oral care. *Nursing Times*, 83(32), 38–40.

Roberts, D. (1982) Factors contributing to outbreaks of food poisoning in England and Wales, 1970–1979. *Journal of Hygiene*, 89, 491.

Rubin, R. H. *et al.* (1990) Therapy, both immunosuppressive and antimicrobial for the transplant patient in the 1990s. In: *Organ Transplantation – Current Clinical and Immunological Concepts*, (eds L. Brent & R. Sells), pp. 71–89. Baillière Tindall, Eastbourne.

Russell, J. A. *et al.* (1992) Allogeneic bone marrow transplantation without protective isolation in adults with malignant disease. *Lancet*, 339(8784), 38–40.

Schimpff, S. C. (1977) Therapy for infection in patients with granulocytopenia. *Medical Clinics of North America*, 61, 1101–18.

Schimpff, S. C. *et al.* (1970) Relationship of colonization with *Pseudomonas aeruginosa* to development of *Pseudomonas bacteraemia* in cancer patients. *Antimicrobials and Chemotherapy*, 10, 240–44.

Schimpff, S. C. *et al.* (1975) Infection prevention in acute non-lymphocytic leukaemia laminar air flow room reverse isolation with oral non-absorbable antibiotic prophylaxis. *Annals of International Medicine*, 82, 351–8.

Schimpff, S. C. *et al.* (1978) Infection prevention in acute leukaemia. *Leukaemia Research*, 2, 231–40.

Scully, R. (1980) Stress in the nurse. *American Journal of Nursing*, May, 80(5), 912–15.

Selden, R. *et al.* (1971) Nosocomial Klebsiella infections. Intestinal colonization as a reservoir. *Annals of International Medicine*, 74, 675–84.

Sickles, E. A. *et al.* (1975) Clinical presentation of infection in granulocytopenia patients. *Archives of International Medicine*, 135, 715–19.

Storb, R. *et al.* (1983) GVHD and survival in patients with asplastic anaemia treated by bone marrow grafts with HLA identifiable siblings. *New England Journal of Medicine*, 308, 302–7.

Strober, S. *et al.* (1981) Immunosuppressive and tolerogenic effect of whole-body total lymphoid regional irradiation. In: *Immunosuppressive Therapy*, (ed. J. R. Salaman). MTP Press, Lancaster.

Strom, T. B. (1990) Immunosuppression in graft rejection. In: *Organ Transplantation – Current Clinical and Immunological Concepts* (eds L. Brent & R. Sells) pp. 44–56. Baillière Tindall, Eastbourne.

Taplin, D. *et al.* (1973) Flower vases in hospital as reservoirs of pathogens. *Lancet*, 11, 1279–81.

Van Der Meer, J. W. N. (1994) Defects in the host immune mechanisms. In: *Clinical Approaches to Infection in the Compromised Host*, (eds R. H. Rubins & L. S. Young), 3rd edn. Plenum Medical Book Co, London.

Wade, J. C. *et al.* (1982) *Staphylococcus epidemidis*, an increasingly but frequently recognised cause of infection in granulocytopenia. *Annals of International Medicine*, 97, 503–8.

Wright, C. *et al.* (1976) *Enterobacteriaceae* and *Pseudomonas aeruginosa* recovered from vegetable salads. *Applied and Environmental Microbiology*, 31(3), 453–4.

Yates, J. W. *et al.* (1973) A controlled study of isolation and endogenous microbial suppression in acute myelocytic leukaemia patients. *Cancer*, 32, 1490–8.

GUIDELINES: NURSING THE NEUTROPENIC PATIENT

PROCEDURE

Preparation of the room and maintenance of general cleanliness

Action	Rationale
1 A single room should be used if possible.	To reduce airborne transfer of micro-organisms.
2 A toilet to be kept for the sole use of the patient.	To reduce the risk of cross-infection.
3 Area to be cleaned meticulously before the patient is admitted.	To reduce the risk of infection.
4 Equipment and supplies to be kept for the sole use of the patient. (This must also include any cleaning equipment used by domestic staff.)	To reduce the risk of cross-infection. Cleaning equipment can easily become colonized with micro-organisms which may cause cross-infection.
5 Surfaces and furniture to be damp dusted daily using disposable cleaning cloths and detergent solution.	Damp dusting and mopping removes micro-organisms without distributing them into the air.
6 Floor to be mopped daily using soap and water.	To reduce the risk of cross-infection.
7 Mop head to be laundered daily.	As above.
8 Bucket and mop handle to be cleaned and dried and stored in the isolation area.	As above.

Nursing procedure

Entering room

Action	Rationale
1 Hands must be washed thoroughly with bactericidal soap and water or bactericidal alcohol hand rub.	Hands are regarded as the principle source of transfer of micro-organisms. (For further information see Chapter 4, Aseptic Technique.)
2 A disposable plastic apron should be worn for all nursing procedures.	Staff clothing can easily become contaminated. A disposable plastic apron reduces the risk of transfer of organisms.
3 Door of room to be kept closed. Ideally the air in the room should be under slightly positive pressure. The air flow should be from the room into the corridor.	To reduce the risk of airborne transmission of infection by inhaling organisms from the rest of the ward when entering the protective isolation room.

Visitors

Action	Rationale
1 The patient should be asked to nominate close relatives and friends who may then, after instruction, visit freely. The patient or his or her representative should inform casual acquaintances or non-essential visitors that they should avoid visiting during the period of neutropenia.	The incidence of infection increases in proportion to the number of people visiting. Large numbers of visitors are difficult to screen and educate. Unlimited visiting by close relatives and friends diminishes the sense of isolation that the patient may experience.
2 Any visitor with an infection or who has been in contact with infection should be excluded.	Neutropenic patients are susceptible to infection.
3 Children, unless very close relatives, should be discouraged.	Children are more likely to have been in contact with infectious diseases which can have serious consequences if transmitted to a neutropenic patient.

Diet

Action	Rationale
1 Educate the patient to choose only cooked food from the hospital menu and avoid raw fruit, salads and uncooked vegetables, whether on the menu or brought in by visitors.	Uncooked foods are often heavily colonized by micro-organisms, particularly Gram-negative bacteria.
2 Food brought into the hospital by visitors must be: (a) Obtained from well-known, reliable firms. (b) In undamaged, sealed tins and packets. (c) Within expiry date.	Correctly processed and packaged foods are acceptable as they should not be unacceptably infected.
3 Water may be boiled and allowed to cool in a covered jug.	Tap water is safe to drink but can become colonized by organisms, particularly Gram-negative organisms found in the plug hole of sinks or overflow outlet when the water is being filled.

Guidelines: Nursing the neutropenic patient (cont'd)

Action

| | Rationale |

4 Bottled concentrated fruit drinks made from whole fruit and containing sugar are invariably pathogen-free.

Pathogens do not easily survive or multiply in a high sugar concentrate.

5 Sealed packets of fruit juice (long shelf-life varieties, particularly those rich in vitamins) are suitable. It should be poured directly into a clean jug and drunk the same day.

These juices have been pasteurized and remain pathogen-free until they are opened.

Discharging the patient

Action

Rationale

1 Crowded areas, for example shops, cinemas, pubs and discos, should be avoided.

Although the patient's white cell count is usually high enough for discharge, the patient remains immunocompromised for some time.

2 Pets should not be allowed to lick the patient, and new pets should not be obtained.

Pets are known carriers of infection (Mims *et al.*, 1993).

3 Certain foods, for example take-away meals, soft cheese and pâté, should continue to be avoided.

Take-away meals are subject to handling by a large number of individuals and are stored for longer periods, both of which increase the likelihood of contamination.

4 Salads and fruit should be washed carefully, dried and, if possible, peeled.

To remove as many pathogens as possible.

5 Any sign or symptoms of infection should be reported immediately to the patient's general practitioner or to the discharging hospital.

Any infection may continue to have serious consequences if left unlocated.

ACQUIRED IMMUNE DEFICIENCY SYNDROME (AIDS)

Definition

Acquired immune deficiency syndrome (AIDS) is a state of immunosuppression caused by the human immuno-deficiency virus 1 (HIV 1) and 2 (HIV 2). As no overall description can be made for AIDS, an internationally agreed case definition has been made (Communicable Disease Centre, 1987) and includes the following:

(1) Certain opportunistic infections.
(2) Certain cancers.
(3) Wasting syndrome.
(4) Encephalopathy.

The definition was revised in 1992 to include three new clinical conditions: pulmonary tuberculosis, recurrent pneumonia and invasive cervical cancer. The new definition provides uniform, simple criteria for categorizing HIV conditions to facilitate evaluation of treatment and care of persons with HIV (Centers for Disease Control and Prevention, 1992).

Since 1989 several investigators have independently reported cases of unexplained severe immunodeficiency without evidence of infection with HIV 1 or 2 (Pankhurst & Peakman, 1989; Jowitt *et al.*, 1991; Laurence *et al.*, 1992). In an extensive search for such cases, initiated in the USA by the Centers for Disease Control and Prevention (CDC), 80 widely scattered cases were identified. A review of these cases, however, did not reveal any epidemiological links between them. Other investigators have concluded that cases of unexplained severe immunodeficiency without HIV infection are rare, and that the available data do not show that unexplained severe immunodeficiency without HIV is endemic (WHO, 1993). Subsequently, a variant of HIV, presently classified as subtype O (HIV-1-0), has been found, and it is likely that others will follow (Communicable Disease Report, 1994).

A relatively small number of people claim that HIV does not cause AIDS (Stine, 1993). Duesberg (1990), for example, states that the disease is caused by 'lifestyle'. This explanation has been discounted by others (Weiss & Jaffe, 1990).

REFERENCE MATERIAL

The human immunodeficiency virus has been isolated in the blood (Gallo et al., 1984), semen (Zagury et al., 1984), tears and saliva (Fujikawara et al., 1985), breast milk (Thiry et al., 1985), genital secretions of women (Wofsy et al., 1986) and cerebrospinal fluid and the brain (Levy, 1985). In adults, transmission of the virus between individuals most often occurs during sexual activity (male to male (Kingsley et al., 1987); male to female (Padian et al., 1987a), female to male (Padian, 1987b); whereas female to female is rare (Cabane et al., 1984)). Other causes of transmission of virus are by needle sharing in drug abusers (Marmor et al., 1987) and by the administration of contaminated blood and blood products (Peterman, 1987). HIV transmission has been reported rarely by organ transplantation (Communicable Disease Centre, 1987), and following artificial insemination (Steward et al., 1985).

Most infants and children become infected as a result of vertical transmission of HIV from their infected mothers, either during pregnancy, at delivery or during the immediate post-partum period (Sprecher et al., 1986). HIV transmission to newborn infants from infected breast milk has occurred (Lepage et al., 1987), and it has also been recorded as a result of sexual abuse (Rubinstein et al., 1986). Zidovudine prophylaxis for HIV-antibody-positive pregnant women who have only mildly symptomatic HIV disease and who have had no prior anti-retroviral therapy has been seen to reduce transmission of HIV from mother to infant by approximately two-thirds (Conner et al., 1994).

Studies of prolonged social contact with HIV infection have failed to show that transmission has occurred, unless the transmission routes already mentioned are present (Jason et al., 1986), except in one case from a child to a mother who was providing health care (Communicable Disease Centre, 1986). Transmission has also occurred between children living in the same house (Communicable Disease Report, 1993).

Transmission of HIV infection to health care workers has occurred following needlestick injuries, contamination of mucous membranes or through breaks in the skin (Department of Health and Social Security, 1990a). 214 cases of occupationally acquired HIV infection have been reported in health care workers (Royal College of Pathologists, 1995). The overall risk with a single sharps injury is estimated to be approximately 0.3%, and prob-ably needs to involve a hollow needle, with an inoculation of greater than 0.1 ml of blood (Shanson, 1991).

Trials of prophylactic zidovudine following inoculation accidents involving HIV-antibody-positive blood have been undertaken (Henderson et al., 1989; Department of Health and Social Security, 1990b). Failure to prevent seroconversion has been seen (Lange, 1990), which emphasizes the need to adopt and promote safe practices at all times (Hart, 1991). Side-effects of zidovudine after occupational exposure to HIV-infected blood have also been identified (Schmitz et al., 1994). Experts in the USA and UK have not stipulated that zidovudine is to be used for chemoprophylaxis after exposure to HIV-infected blood, but have recommended that each district develop a local policy for its use (Report of the Working Group of the Royal College of Pathologists, 1992).

The period immediately following infection with HIV is termed the window period, during which time antibodies to the virus will be produced. This generally occurs within 3 months of exposure, although longer window periods have been reported (Ranki et al., 1987).

Generally, a negative antibody test six months after a known or expected exposure to HIV 1 will provide a reasonable basis for reassurance, although in a few reported cases detectable antibodies could not be recovered although detected virus was present (Groopman, et al., 1985). After the window period, seroconversion occurs, followed by an incubation period. Seroconversion is the point at which an individual exposed to HIV becomes serologically positive (Stine, 1993). Incubation periods in excess of 12 years have been recorded (Burger et al., 1990).

Antibodies to HIV are measured using an enzyme-linked immunosorbent assay (ELISA) (Arpadi et al., 1991). Usually a positive test is retested by ELISA and a confirmatory test using Western Blot Analysis is undertaken (Schochetman, 1990).

HIV 1 antigen tests are available and play a major contribution to the serological assessment of HIV infection (Allain, 1986). However, this test has not yet become generally available, as the expense and time involved render it unsuitable as a screening system.

The Department of Health and Social Security (1985) recommends that no patient should be tested for HIV antibodies without their informed consent, and that counselling should be offered to the patient before and after the test. Miller (1987) discusses the information which should be included in the counselling sessions. Carr & Gee (1986) discuss the significance of positive and negative test results, while Grimshaw (1987) suggests that the time spent on counselling not only provides psychological and emotional support, but is also a good basis for future communication.

Hospitals involved in anonymous HIV antibody screening must ensure that patients are aware of the ongoing research project. No post-test counselling is possible in these circumstances.

The World Health Organization (1993) estimates that 14 million people are infected with HIV worldwide, 13 million of whom are adults. It is not known how many people are infected with HIV in the UK, but the number continues to increase. Between January 1982 and February 1996 12 040 people were diagnosed as having AIDS; 8306 people in this group have died (Communicable Disease Report, 1996).

AIDS raises many ethical issues (Reisman, 1988). Mindel (1987) discusses the importance of confidentiality when dealing with any antibody-positive patient. This was supported by the United Kingdom Central Council for Nursing, Midwifery and Health Visiting (1986) and the Department of Health and Social Security (1990a) which also states that health care workers dealing with known or suspected seropositive patients or specimens must be made fully aware of the risk.

The Public Health (Infectious Diseases) Regulations 1985 make certain provisions to safeguard public health where a person is suffering from AIDS. It is stressed that these provisions are to be used only in exceptional circumstances where transmission of HIV may occur. One study has indicated that HIV remains viable for a considerable time in a cadaver. It is important, therefore, that careful procedures to avoid contamination are maintained after the death of an infected person (Ball et al., 1991).

Adler (1987) suggests that not all infected people go on to develop AIDS, but may develop persistant generalized lymphadenopathy (PGL) or AIDS-related complex (ARC). It is not clear why and when an infected person will develop full-blown AIDS. Prophylactic therapy for the prevention of opportunistic infections has been shown to improve the health and quality of life of people infected with HIV (Hewett & Hecht, 1993). Stine (1993) outlines how HIV causes a chronic, progressive disruption of the immune system, leading to signs and symptoms that indicate the progression of the disease towards AIDS. Survival appears to be related to a person's age, their initial diagnosis and the year that they were diagnosed (Lemp, 1990).

Much research is in progress to identify and evaluate treatments and vaccines for the treatment and prevention of HIV infection (Mayer, 1993). Several drugs have inhibited the action of reverse transcriptase, a viral enzyme which allows HIV to make a deoxyribonucleic acid (DNA) copy of its ribonucleic acid (RNA) genetic material. Zidovudine has been seen to be the most effective drug as yet, by prolonging survival and reducing mortality, but it is expensive and potentially toxic (Graham et al., 1992). Bone marrow transplantation as a treatment for AIDS is being evaluated in the USA (Holland et al., 1989).

HIV infection alone does not affect a person's ability to continue with regular employment (Department of Employment – Health and Safety Executive, 1987) unless injury to the worker could result in blood contaminating the patients' open tissues (UK Health Department, 1991). Following reports that an HIV-antibody positive dentist in the USA transmitted HIV to six of his patients (Centers for Disease Control and Prevention, 1990), concern was expressed about the hazards of HIV-antibody positive health care workers undertaking invasive procedures. In the UK the Department of Health has issued guidance for health care workers (Department of Health, 1991), and procedures to be followed when health care workers involved in invasive procedures are found to be HIV-antibody positive (Department of Health, 1993).

AIDS disease is changing all the time. At present, records show a decline in the incidence of Kaposi's sarcoma (Rutherford, et al., 1989) and a reduced mortality from *Pneumocystis carinii* pneumonia (Harris, 1990), but the emergence of new opportunist pathogens (Peters, et al., 1991). Neurological manifestations are seen in about 40% of patients with AIDS. At post-mortem involvement of the nervous system is seen in 10–80% of cases (Guiloff, 1992).

People with AIDS need specialized, often intensive nursing care (Swan et al., 1992). The support of a well informed community nurse is essential (Few, 1993). One small study demonstrated that community nurse supervision of patients receiving long-term treatment for cytomegalovirus (CMV) reduces the incidence of line infections and may increase survival (Reilly et al., 1992).

The psychosocial impact of being diagnosed as HIV-antibody positive is considerable. A high standard of assessment and skilled counselling is often required (Carlisle, 1994). It is also important to provide close psychosocial support for health care workers (Harvey, 1991).

Nurses must keep up to date with improved, earlier diagnosis of AIDS, with better treatments and with the increased use of prophylaxis. They must be ready to adapt to these changes and be prepared and able to provide good care. This process will be achieved only by good education (Armstrong-Esther et al., 1990) and management support.

Prevention of hospital acquired infection relies on the availability of resources for cleaning and where necessary sterilizing both equipment and the environment (Mims *et al.*, 1993). Patients' accommodation can be vacuum cleaned and washed with hot soapy water (Ayliffe *et al.*, 1992) unless contamination with blood or body fluids has occurred. In these circumstances, the statutory regulations require cleaning with fresh hypochlorite solution or granules (Health and Safety Commission, 1988). When non-disposable equipment is used, autoclaving is the method of choice for sterilization (Ayliffe *et al.*, 1992). Equipment likely to be damaged by autoclaving can be disinfected with glutaraldehyde in the manner specified by the 1988 *Control of Substances Hazardous to Health (COSHH)* guidelines. Glutaraldehyde inactivates vegetative bacteria, mycobacteria, spores and viruses (Ayliffe *et al.*, 1984).

References and further reading

Adler, M. N. (1987) Range and natural history of infection. *British Medical Journal*, 294, 1145–7.

Allain, J. P. (1986) Serological markers in early stages of human immunodeficiency virus infection in haemophiliacs. *Lancet*, 2, 1233.

Armstrong-Esther, C. *et al.* (1990) The effect of education on nurses' perception of AIDS. *Journal of Advanced Nursing*, 15, 638–51.

Arpadi, S. *et al.* (1991) HIV testing. *Journal of Pediatrics*, 199(1), Part 2, S8–S13.

Ayliffe, G. A. J. *et al.* (1984) *Chemical Disinfection in Hospitals.* Public Health Laboratory Service, London.

Ayliffe, G. A. J. *et al.* (1992) *Control of Hospital Infection. A Practical Handbook.* Chapman & Hall, London.

Ball, J. *et al.* (1991) Long lasting viability of HIV after patient's death. *Lancet*, 338, 63.

Burger, H. *et al.* (1990) Long HIV-1 incubation period and dynamics of transmission within a family. *Lancet*, 336, 134–6.

Cabane, J. *et al.* (1984) AIDS in an apparently risk-free woman. *Lancet*, 2, 105.

Carlisle, C. (1994) Psychosocial care of HIV-positive patients. *Nursing Standard*, 8(18), 37–40.

Carr, G. & Gee, C. (1986) AIDS and AIDS-related conditions: screening for populations at risk. *Nurse Practitioner*, 11(10), 25–46.

Centers for Disease Control and Prevention (1990) Possible transmission of HIV to a patient during invasive dental procedure. *Morbidity and Mortality Weekly Report*, 39, 489–93.

Centers for Disease Control and Prevention (1992) Revised classification system for HIV infection and expanded surveillance case definition for AIDS among adolescents and adults. *Morbidity and Mortality Weekly Report*, 41, 1–19.

Communicable Disease Centre (CDC) (1986) Apparent transmission of human T-lymphotropic type III/lymphadenopathy associated virus from a child to a mother providing health care. *Morbidity and Mortality Weekly Report*, 35, 76–9.

Communicable Disease Centre (1987) Human immunodeficiency virus infection transmitted from an organ donor screened for HIV antibody. *Morbidity and Mortality Weekly Report*, 36(20), 306–8.

Communicable Disease Centre (1990) Possible transmission of human immunodeficiency virus to a patient during an invasive dental procedure. *Morbidity and Mortality Weekly Report*, 39(29), 489–93.

Communicable Disease Report (1993) HIV transmission between children at home. *Communicable Disease Report*, 3(52), 1. Public Health Laboratory Service Communicable Disease Surveillance Centre.

Communicable Disease Report (1994) HIV-1-0: a variant of HIV-1. *Communicable Disease Report*, 4(24), 1. Public Health Laboratory Service Communicable Disease Surveillance Centre.

Communicable Disease Report (1996) AIDS and HIV 1 infections in the United Kingdom. Monthly Report. *Communicable Disease Report*, 6(7), 63–4. Public Health Laboratory Service Communicable Disease Surveillance Centre.

Conner, E. M. *et al.* (1994) Reduction of maternal infant transmission of HIV-1 with zidovudine treatment. *New England Journal of Medicine*, 331(18), 1173–80.

Department of Employment – Health and Safety Executive (1987) *AIDS and Employment.* Central Office of Information, London.

Department of Health and Social Security (1985) *The Public Health (Infectious Diseases) Regulations 1985 (HC(85)17) (LAC(85)10).* HMSO, London.

Department of Health and Social Security (1990a) *Advisory Committee on Dangerous Pathogens. HIV The Causative Agent of AIDS and Related Conditions. Second Revision of Guidelines HN(90)4.* HMSO, London.

Department of Health and Social Security (1990b) *Guidance for Clinical Health Care Workers. Protection Against Infection with HIVB and Hepatitis Viruses.* HMSO, London.

Department of Health (1991) *AIDS and HIV-infected Health Care Workers: Occupational Guidance for Health Care Workers, their Physicians and Employers.* Health Publication Unit, HMSO, London.

Department of Health (1993) *AIDS-HIV Infected Health Care Workers: Practical Guidance on Notifying Patients.* Health Publication Unit, HMSO, London.

Duesberg, P. H. (1990) Duesberg replies. *Nature*, 346, 788.

Few, C. (1993) Home care for AIDS. *Journal of Community Nursing*, November, 4–8.

Fujikawara, L. S. *et al.* (1985) Isolation of human T lymphotropic virus type III from tears of patients with AIDS. *Lancet*, 2, 529–30.

Gallo, R. C. *et al.* (1984) Frequent detection and continuous production of cytopathic retroviruses (HTLV III) from patients with AIDS. *Science*, 224, 497–500.

Graham, N. M. H. *et al.* (1992) The effects on survival of early treatment of HIV infection. *New England Journal of Medicine*, 326(16), 1037–42.

Grimshaw, J. (1987) Being HIV antibody positive. *British Medical Journal*, 295, 256–7.

Groopman, J. E. *et al.* (1985) Antibody seronegative human T lymphotropic virus type III (HTLV III) infected patients with acquired immunodeficiency syndrome or related disorders. *Blood*, 66, 742–4.

Guiloff, R. J. (1992) Neurological manifestation of AIDS. *Medicine International*, February, No 98, 4114–19.

Harris, J. E. (1990) Improved short-term survival of AIDS patients initially diagnosed with *Pneumocystis carinii* pneumonia 1984 through 1989. *Journal of the American Medical Association*, 263, 397–401.

Hart, S. (1991) Blood and body fluid precautions. *Nursing Standard*, 5, 25–7.

Harvey, N. (1991) The psychosocial context of HIV/AIDS. *Nursing Standard*, 5(27), 50–51.

Health and Safety Commission (1988) *Control of Substances Hazardous to Health and Control of Carcinogenic Substances (COSHH): Approved Codes of Practice*. HMSO, London.

Henderson, D. K. *et al.* (1989) Prophylactic Zidovudine after occupational exposure to the human immunodeficiency virus; an interim analysis. *Journal of Infectious Diseases*, 160, 321–7.

Hewett, J. F. & Hecht, F. M. (1993) Preventive health care for adults with HIV infection. *Journal of the American Medical Association*, 269(9), 1144–53.

Holland, H. K. *et al.* (1989) Allogeneic bone marrow transplantation, zidovudine and HIV-1 infection. *Annals of Internal Medicine*, 111(12), 973–81.

Hoover, D. R. *et al.* (1992) The progression of untreated HIV-1 infection prior to AIDS. *American Journal of Public Health*, 82(11), 1538–41.

Jason, J. M. *et al.* (1986) HTLV III/LAV antibody and immune status of household contacts and sexual partners of persons with haemophilia. *Journal of the American Medical Association*, 155, 212.

Jowitt, S. N. *et al.* (1991) CD4 lymphocytopenia without HIV in patients with cryptococcal infection. *Lancet*, 337, 500–501.

Kingsley, L. A. *et al.* (1987) Risk factors for seroconversion to human immunodeficiency virus among homosexuals. *Lancet*, 1, 345–8.

Lange, J. M. A. (1990) Failure of Zidovudine prophylaxis after accidental exposure to HIV. *New England Journal of Medicine*, 322(19), 1375–7.

Laurence, J. *et al.* (1992) AIDS without evidence of infection with HIV-1 and 2. *Lancet*, 340, 273–4.

Lemp, G. F. (1990) Survival trends for patients with AIDS. *Journal of the American Medical Association*, 263, 402–406.

Lepage, P. *et al.* (1987) Postnatal transmission of HIV from mother to child. *Lancet*, 2, 400.

Levy, J. A. (1985) Isolation of AIDS-associated retroviruses from cerobrospinal fluid and brain of patients with neurological symptoms. *Lancet*, 2, 586–8.

Marmor, M. *et al.* (1987) Risk factors for infection with human immune-deficiency virus among intravenous drug abusers in New York City. *AIDS*, 1(1), 39–44.

Mayer, D. L. (1993) Zidovudine and other antiretroviral agents including drug interactions and toxicities. *Current Opinions in Infectious Diseases*, 6(2), 210–17.

Miller, D. (1987) Counselling. *British Medical Journal*, 294, 1670–74.

Mindel, A. (1987) Management of early HIV infection. *British Medical Journal*, 294, 1145–7.

Padian, N. S. *et al.* (1987a) Male to female transmission of human immunodeficiency virus. *Journal of the American Medical Association*, 258, 788–90.

Padian, N. S. (1987b) Heterosexual transmission of acquired immunodeficiency syndrome. International perspectives and national projections. *Review of Infectious Diseases*, 9, 947–60.

Pankhurst, C. & Peakman, M. (1989) Reduced CD4 T-cells and severe candidiasis in absence of HIV infection. *Lancet*, 1, 672.

Peterman, T. A. (1987) Transfusion associated acquired immunodeficiency syndrome. *World Journal of Surgery*, 11(1), 36–40.

Peters, B. S. *et al.* (1991) Changing disease pattern in patients with AIDS in a referral centre in the United Kingdom. The changing face of AIDS, *British Medical Journal*, 302, 203–6.

Ranki, A. *et al.* (1987) Long latency periods precedes overt seroconversion in sexually transmitted human immunodeficiency virus infection. *Lancet*, 2, 589–93.

Reilly, G. *et al.* (1992) The role of a dedicated community liaison tean in the inpatient care of patients with AIDS. *International Conference on AIDS*, 19–24 July, 8(2), PGB 151, abstract POB 3385.

Report of the Working Group of the Royal College of Pathologists (1992) *HIV Infection: Hazards of Transmission to Patients and Health Care Workers during Invasive Procedures*. Royal College of Pathologists.

Reisman, E. C. (1988) Ethical issues confronting nurses. *Nursing Clinics of North America*, 23(4), 789–801.

Royal College of Pathologists (1995) *HIV and the Practice of Pathology*. Marks and Spencer Publication Unit of the Royal College of Pathologists, London.

Rubinstein, A. *et al.* (1986) The epidemiology of paediatric acquired immunodeficiency syndrome. *Clinical Immunology and Immunopathology*, 40, 115–21.

Rutherford, G. W. *et al.* (1989) The epidemiology of AIDS-related Kaposi's sarcoma in San Francisco. *Journal of Infectious Diseases*, 159, 567–71.

Schmitz, S. H. *et al.* (1994) Side-effects of AZT prophylaxis after occupational exposure to HIV-infected blood. *Annals of Hematology*, 69(3), 135–8.

Schochetman, G. (1990) Laboratory diagnosis of infection with the AIDS virus. *Lab. Medica*, April/May, 15–24.

Shanson, D. C. (1991) Current surgical controversies over HIV infection. *Journal of Hospital Infection*, 17, 77–81.

Sprecher, S. *et al.* (1986) Vertical transmission of HIV in a 15-week fetus. *Lancet*, 2, 288.

Steward, G. J. *et al.* (1985) Transmission of HTLV III by artificial insemination by donor serum. *Lancet*, 2, 581–4.

Swan, J. H. *et al.* (1992) Skilled nursing facility care for patients with AIDS: comparison with other patients. *American Journal of Public Health*, 82(3), 453–5.

Stine, G. J. (1993) *AIDS Update 1993*. Prentice Hall, New Jersey.

Thiry, L. *et al.* (1985) Isolation of AIDS virus from cell-free breast milk of three healthy virus carriers. *Lancet*, 1, 891–2.

UK Health Department (1991) *AIDS-HIV Infected Health Care Workers – Occupational Guidance for Health Care Workers, their Physicians and Employers*. Recommendations of the expert advisory group on AIDS. Copies from Health Publication Unit, Heywood Stores, Lancashire OL 10 2PZ.

United Kingdom Central Council for Nursing, Midwifery and Health Visiting (1986) *Confidentiality – An Elaboration of Clause 9 of the Second Edition of the UKCC's Code of Professional Conduct*. UKCC, London.

Weiss, R. A. & Jaffe, H. W. (1990) Duesberg, HIV and AIDS. *Nature*, 345, 659–60.

WHO (1993) *Report of a Scientific Meeting on Unexplained Severe Immunodeficiency without Evidence of HIV Infection*. GPA/RES/93.3. World Health Organization, Geneva.

WHO (1993) *Global Programme on AIDS. The HIV/AIDS Pandemic: 1993 Overview*. GPA/CNP/EVA 93.1. World Health Organization, Geneva.

Wofsy, C. B. *et al.* (1986) Isolation of AIDS associated retrovirus from genital secretions of women with antibodies to the virus. *Lancet*, 1, 527–9.

World Health Organization (WHO) (1990) *WHO Weekly Epidemiology Record*, 20 July. WHO, Geneva.

Zagury, D. *et al.* (1984) HTLV III cells culture from semen in two patients with AIDS. *Science*, 226, 449–51.

HUMAN IMMUNODEFICIENCY VIRUS 2 (HIV2)

Definition

HIV 2 was first recognized in 1986 (Clavel *et al.*, 1986), although evidence that HIV 2 infections were present in many West Africans as far back as 1966 (Karamura *et al.*, 1989) has been disputed (Mohammed *et al.*, 1989). Serological evidence supporting the existence of a second HIV was published in 1985 (Barin *et al.*, 1985). Today, HIV 2 is present in many West African countries and, in some, it is a more common cause of AIDS than HIV 1 (Naucler *et al.*, 1989).

REFERENCE MATERIAL

In the UK, screening of blood donors and people attending genitourinary medicine clinics shows that the occurrence of HIV 2 infection is rare. A few HIV 2 infections have been reported in many European countries, and 18 HIV 2 infections have been reported in the USA . Of these, over two-thirds of patients had contact with, or were from, Africa (Evans *et al.*, 1991).

Transmission of HIV 2 follows the same pattern as HIV 1 (Kroegal *et al.*, 1987), although the rate of vertical transmission from mother to child is uncertain, with some studies suggesting that it might be low (Morgan *et al.*, 1990).

Despite the high prevalence of HIV 2 infections in West Africa, there have been many fewer reported AIDS cases compared with East and Central Africa, where HIV 1 predominates, implying HIV 2 is less pathogenic than HIV 1 (Romieu *et al.*, 1990).

The range of opportunistic infections and malignancies and the wasting and dementia associated with progressive HIV 1 infections are also present in HIV 2 disease, although *Pneumocystis carinii* pneumonia (Clavel *et al.*, 1987) and active tuberculosis may be less common in HIV-2-infected people than in those infected with HIV 1. However, this may represent a difference in prevalence of opportunistic pathogens rather than being a direct effect of HIV infection (Kanki, 1989).

In May 1989, the AIDS laboratory diagnostic working group advised combined screening in diagnostic laboratories in the UK (Evans *et al.*, 1991).

Since July 1990, combined anti-HIV 1/HIV 2 testing of all donations of blood was introduced in the UK Blood Transfusion Service. Of the first 250 000 donations, only one HIV-2-infected donor was detected.

Since there is no difference in the method of transmission between HIV 1 and HIV 2, prevention and nursing care are the same.

References and further reading

Ayliffe, G. A. J. *et al.* (1992) *Control of Hospital Infection. A Practical Handbook*, 3rd edn. Chapman & Hall Medical, London.

Barin, F. *et al.* (1985) Serological evidence for virus related to Simian T-lymphotropic retrovirus III in residents of West Africa. *Lancet*, 2, 1387–9.

Clavel, F. *et al.* (1986) Isolation of a new human retrovirus from West African patients with AIDS. *Science*, 233, 343–6.

Clavel, F. *et al.* (1987) Human immunodeficiency virus type 2 infection associated with AIDS in West Africa. *New England Journal of Medicine*, 316, 1180–85.

Evans, B. G. *et al.* (1991) HIV 2 in the United Kingdom. A review. *Communicable Disease Report*, 1(2), R19–R232.

Kanki, P. J. (1989) Clinical significance of HIV 2 infection in West Africa. *AIDS Clin. Rev.*, 95–108.

Karamura, M. *et al.* (1989) HIV 2 in West Africa in 1966. *Lancet*, 1, 385.

Kroegal, C. *et al.* (1987) Routes of HIV 2 transmissions in Western Europe. *Lancet*, 1, 1150.

Mohammed, I. *et al.* (1989) HIV 2 West Africa in 1966. *Lancet*, 1, 385.

Morgan, G. *et al.* (1990) AIDS following mother to child transmission of HIV 2. *AIDS*, 4, 879–82.

Naucler, A. *et al.* (1989) HIV 2-associated AIDS and HIV 2 sero-prevalence in Bissau, Guinea-Bissau. *Journal of AIDS*, 2, 88–93.

Romieu, I. *et al.* (1990) HIV 2 link to AIDS in West Africa. *Journal of AIDS*, 3, 220–30.

GUIDELINES: ACQUIRED IMMUNE DEFICIENCY SYNDROME IN A GENERAL WARD

PROCEDURE

Action

Rationale

1   Staff suffering from eczema should not nurse patients who are HIV antibody positive.

Any break in staff members' skin should be covered with a waterproof dressing to prevent entry of HIV. This would be difficult to accomplish with eczema lesions and would exacerbate the eczema.

2   Immunodeficient-compromised staff, either through illness or therapy, should not nurse patients who are HIV antibody positive.

HIV antibody positive patients who present with generalized infection could put this category of staff at risk.

3   All staff should read and be familiar with government guidelines on AIDS and their own hospital's codes of practice.

To ensure all staff are aware of, and take, the necessary precautions.

4   Hospital staff should cover any broken skin with a waterproof dressing.

To prevent the entry of infectious material.

5   Accidental inoculations must be avoided at all cost.

Serious inoculation accidents have been seen to be a means of transmission of HIV.

6   In the event of gross contamination of intact skin the affected area must be washed thoroughly with soap under hand hot water. A scrubbing brush must not be used.

Intact skin is a natural barrier against infection. By thorough washing the infectious material can be removed. Scrubbing brushes can cause skin damage which allows infection to enter.

7   Puncture wounds or cuts must be made to bleed freely and washed under hot running water.

To flush out infectious material.

8   A waterproof dressing must be applied and medical advice sought for large wounds.

To prevent further infection.

9   An accident form must be filled in immediately and taken to bacteriology, the occupational health physician or other medical advisor as appropriate.

It is important to have accurate records of all accidents and incidents in order to monitor events.

Low-risk, HIV positive individuals

Nursing assessment of the risk of contamination of the environment with pathogenic organisms, blood or body fluids from a patient known to be HIV antibody positive allows care to be more accurately planned.

Action

Rationale

1   If the patient is not bleeding, incontinent, confused or infected with a contagious disease, he/she may be nursed on an open ward using all the patients' facilities as normal.

HIV cannot be transmitted by general social contact.

2   If a low-risk, HIV positive individual develops an infection, is undergoing invasive procedures or becomes incontinent nursing care will commence as for high-risk, HIV positive persons.

Incontinent, bleeding HIV antibody positive patients have the potential risk of transmitting the HIV virus to others.

Increased risk, HIV positive individuals

Action

| | |
|1| Known or strongly suspected HIV antibody positive patients who are bleeding, incontient, infected with a contagious disease or receiving invasive procedures should be nursed in a single room with its own toilet and hand-washing facilities.

Rationale

To minimize the risk of transmitting infection. HIV can be transmitted via blood and body fluid.

Entering the room

Action

| | |
|1| When the patient is not bleeding, coughing, incontinent or receiving procedures, protective clothing is not required.

Rationale

Transmission of HIV is not possible from general social contact.

|2| When the patient is incontinent, bleeding or undergoing invasive procedures, disposable well-fitting gloves and a plastic apron are needed. A specification for non-sterile, natural rubber latex examination gloves has been published by the Department of Health (Doc No TSS/D/300.010, October 1988, Supplies Technology Division, Procurement Directorate). Users should check that their supplier's products conform with this specification.

Transmission of HIV is possible from body fluids.

|3| If there is a possibility of airborne contamination, a correctly fitting theatre mask and safety spectacles should be worn.

Transmission of HIV is possible if contaminated material is allowed to contaminate mucous membrane.

Liquid waste

Action

|1| All liquid waste from AIDS patients must be disposed of in a bedpan washer immediately, taking care to avoid splashing.

Rationale

To prevent contamination of the environment.

|2| Areas without bedpan washers will need to use the slop hopper. Great care must be taken to pour waste slowly and carefully down the hopper to avoid splashing.

To prevent contamination of the environment.

Non-disposable equipment

Action

|1| Cleaning of non-disposable equipment needs to be performed thoroughly and in a safe manner.

Rationale

Careless cleaning, immersion, drying, etc. can increase contamination of the environment.

|2| Gloves/aprons must be worn, together with masks/eye protection if appropriate.

To prevent self-contamination.

Guidelines: Acquired immune deficiency syndrome in a general ward (cont'd)

Action	Rationale

3 Before disinfection, equipment must be cleaned with soap and water, avoiding splashing.

Disinfectants cannot completely penetrate organic matter.

4 The equipment must then be dried carefully.

Wet objects would alter the disinfectant's strength and could inactivate the solution if soap and soiling were still present.

5 If equipment will not be damaged by immersion in freshly activated 2% glutaraldehyde for 30 minutes, this is the method of choice.

Glutaraldehyde's bacteriostatic action is completely effective against the AIDS retrovirus.

6 If the equipment will be damaged by immersion in the glutaraldehyde solution, or is too big to fit into the disinfection container, these items must be first washed thoroughly with soap and water and dried, followed by washing and drying with a hypochlorite 1% solution.

Hypochlorite 1% solution has a non-corrosive action for delicate equipment and is less toxic to staff than glutaraldehyde.

7 If the equipment will be damaged by glutaraldehyde or hypochlorite solution, these items must be first washed thoroughly with soap and water and dried, and immersed in 70% ethanol.

70% ethanol is virucidal against most categories of viruses, but does not penetrate organic matter and is inflammable.

8 If the equipment can be autoclaved it must be placed in a sterile supplies department (SSD) bag, taped shut with biohazard tape and marked with a biohazard label. The bag must then be taken to SSD.

Autoclaving is the most effective sterilization method. Correct bagging and transportation of the equipment will prevent contamination of the environment.

9 Expensive, delicate items which have had prolonged, close contact with the patient, i.e. a ventilator, will require ethylene oxide disinfection.

Ethylene oxide disinfection is the second process of choice after autoclaving (Ayliffe *et al.*, 1992).

10 Before the ethylene oxide disinfection process, these items must have all their disposable parts, filters, etc. removed and the whole item cleaned completely and thoroughly with hypochlorite 1% solution and dried carefully.

To prevent contamination of the environment.

11 The transportation and ethylene oxide process will take at least one week. Thought must be given beforehand to the use of this equipment for actively bleeding, incontinent patients.

Ethylene oxide disinfection involves lengthy airing of equipment after the process to ensure it is safe to re-use. During this time other patients may be deprived of the item.

Other hospital departments

Action	Rationale

1 It is essential that all request cards for such items as specimens have the biohazard label attached.

To ensure all departments are informed that the sample is potentially dangerous.

2 All specimens must have the biohazard label attached and be double bagged in a specimen polythene biohazard bag with a

To ensure the laboratory is aware of potential risk and that the specimen is correctly contained to prevent cross-infection. (For further information on

Action	Rationale
biohazard label attached to the bag.	specimen collection see Chapter 38, Specimen Collection.)
3 The specimen should be taken to the laboratory in a washable, covered container.	To prevent contamination of the environment. If leakage does occur, it can be simply contained and cleaned up.
4 A nurse should accompany an antibody-positive patient to other departments. If there is not a departmental nurse in the department, the ward nurse should remain with the patient.	To give help and advice.
5 The patient will normally be given the first or last appointment of the day if invasive procedures are planned.	The department will be less crowded and busy, thus allowing time for appropriate precautions to be taken.

Domestic staff

Action	Rationale
1 The room must be prepared and cleaned. (For further information see Guidelines: Source Isolation, above.)	To minimize the risk of cross-infection.
2 A nurse must check the patient's room to establish that it is suitable for the domestic staff to clean.	To ensure the room is not contaminated with blood or body fluids.
3 If contamination of the environment with blood or body fluids occurs it must be treated with a hypochlorite solution or granules containing 10 000 ppm available chlorine.	To prevent cross-infection.

Terminal cleaning of the room

Action	Rationale
1 The room must be cleared of all equipment before it is cleaned.	It is impossible to clean thoroughly if potentially contaminated items are in the room.
2 The carpet must be steamed if contamination by blood or excreta has occurred.	Organisms have been known to survive in carpets. Steam cleaning destroys these.
3 The walls should only be cleaned if contamination is known to have occurred.	HIV does not survive on intact walls.
4 The curtains must be changed if contamination has occurred.	Discretion and assessment need to be used. If the room has only been used for a short time for a patient who has not contaminated the environment, curtains would not need changing.

The patient

Action	Rationale
1 As soon as possible, the probable/known diagnosis must be discussed with the patient and the hospital policy explained.	It is essential that the patient understands fully the reason for these restrictions which, while protecting contacts, also protect the patient from further risks of infection.

Guidelines: Acquired immune deficiency syndrome in a general ward (cont'd)

Action

2 Psychological support is essential.

3 It is necessary that all nurses caring for antibody positive patients are familiar with treatment and care procedures.

4 Staff should adopt a non-judgemental approach in their dealings with antibody positive patients.

5 It may be appropriate to recommend voluntary agencies to antibody positive patients.

Rationale

Psychological dysfunction is likely and should be recognized and treated early to alleviate and contain the mental distress which an AIDS patient may experience.

To ensure appropriate nursing care is delivered.

It is the responsibility of all health professionals to care for patients and not to pass moral judgements.

Support groups have knowledge and experience which can help HIV antibody positive individuals.

Visiting

Action

1 Visitors should be encouraged.

2 The diagnosis of AIDS is confidential and should not be disclosed.

Rationale

To prevent isolation.

To maintain confidentiality.

Discharging the patient

Action

1 Almost all patients with AIDS will require community services at some time during their illness.

2 If an AIDS patient requires community services, the patient must have given consent for HIV antibody positive diagnosis to be given to the general practitioner and community care personnel.

Rationale

AIDS patients will need to be admitted to hospital for the treatment of clinical illness, but will be encouraged to resume their normal activities when in remission.

Confidentiality must not be breached without the patient's consent. However, health care workers such as ambulance men and women and district nurses will need to take precautions if bleeding, incontinence or infections are present.

Disposal of waste in the community

Action

1 Excreta, infected fluids and such items as sanitary towels can be discarded into the toilet in the normal manner.

2 Infected waste such as dressings, gloves and aprons, must be burned or placed in yellow clinical waste bags and the local authority asked to collect them.

Rationale

To prevent contamination of the environment.

Yellow is the international colour for infected waste bags, and they are available on request from the local authority.

3 Sharps must be placed in a sharps box and stored in a safe place when full, and collected by the local health authority.	To prevent inoculation accidents.

Laundry in the community

Action	Rationale
1 Clothes and linen which are heavily soiled or bloodstained should be washed separately by washing machine at 71°C for 25 minutes. Wash as for above in a public launderette.	Heat is effective in destroying the HIV. If the temperature is increased, the duration of the wash may be decreased.
2 If the person is not fit enough, infected linen should be placed in red alginate polythene bags and the local authority asked to arrange collection and laundering.	Red alginate polythene bags are recognized internationally for infected linen.

Cookery and cutlery

Action	Rationale
1 Ideally, crockery and cutlery should be washed in a dishwasher with a final rinse temperature of at least 80°C.	Heat is effective in destroying the HIV.
2 There is no need to keep a separate store of crockery and cutlery.	Crockery and cutlery present no risk of contamination if washed in a dish washer with a final rinse temperature of at least 80°C.

Protective clothing in the community

Action	Rationale
1 Disposable apron and gloves need be worn only when blood or excreta are being handled.	There is no risk of acquiring infection from general social contact.
2 Disinfectants are required only if blood or excreta spillage has occurred. A strong hypochlorite solution (1 part household bleach to 10 parts water) is recommended.	Unnecessary use of disinfectants is expensive and may be potentially hazardous to staff and the environment (Health and Safety Commission, 1988).

Visitors in the community

Action	Rationale
1 Visitors should be encouraged.	There is no risk of acquiring infection from casual contact.
2 The patient should be encouraged to resume social activities.	Social activities will help to contain any symptoms such as stress and depression.

Prevention of further infection

Action	Rationale
 1 The patient should be encouraged to stay away from individuals with infections.	AIDS patients are susceptible to infections.

Guidelines: Acquired immune deficiency syndrome in a general ward (cont'd)

Action	Rationale
2 If the patient develops any signs and symptoms of ill health, the general practitioner or hospital must be informed immediately.	Early treatment of symptoms will enhance the chances of containing the disease.

(For further details on discharge planning see Chapter 14.)

Death

Action	Rationale
1 The body should be laid out as described in the Procedure, Last Offices (Chapter 24). In addition, the nurse should wear gloves and a plastic apron.	To prevent contamination.
2 All orifices must be packed.	The body continues to secrete fluids after death has occurred. Any leakage may contaminate the environment.
3 Any wounds, intravenous sites or skin breakages must be sealed with waterproof dressing.	To prevent leakage of contaminated fluids.
4 All documentation relating to this procedure must have a biohazard label attached.	To alert administration, portering and mortuary staff of the infection risks.
5 Once the body has been laid out and the room made presentable, family and friends may view the body.	Once the body has left the ward or home, viewing will be difficult if the funeral director adheres strictly to infectious diseases regulations.
6 The body must be placed in a cadaver bag and sealed securely with biohazard tape.	The cadaver bag will prevent leakage and ensures infectious diseases regulations are complied with.
7 Porters must be given help and support.	There is no infection risk when the body is sealed in a cadaver bag unless the bag becomes torn or damaged in transportation. Gloves and aprons will prevent contamination of the staff handling the body.

Funeral arrangements

Action	Rationale
1 Ideally, the hospital administration should have a list of funeral directors who will attend to an HIV antibody positive patient.	It is important that the bereaved relatives are given every help and support to prevent unnecessary distress.

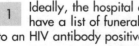

ASPERGILLOSIS

Definition

An infection caused by a fungus of the genus *Aspergillus*, causing inflammatory granulomatous lesions on or in any organ.

REFERENCE MATERIAL

Aspergillus are common saprophytic moulds, easily recognized by their conidiophores, which are swollen ends of hyphae, from which radiate large numbers of sterigmata which end in short chains of spores. Each *Aspergillus* conidiospore releases thousands of spores, which remain suspended in the air for long periods and are viable for many months in dry locations. They are among the most buoyant of fungal spores and are present in all unfiltered air (Rhame, 1991). Over 200 species of *Aspergillus* have been characterized, but less than 20 are reported as being pathogenic to man, the most common species causing allergic and invasive disease being *Aspergillus fumigatus* (Warren *et al.*, 1982). In recent years *Aspergillus flavus* has also emerged as an important pathogen (Bodey *et al.*, 1989).

Aspergillus spores are commonly found in soil, decaying vegetation, spices, potted plants and dried flowers. Cases of allergic and invasive disease have been reported among individuals working in close contact with such substances and who inhale large numbers of *Aspergillus* spores.

Generally, aspergillosis has been associated with building renovation, when large numbers of spores are often liberated into the environment (Arnow *et al.*, 1978). These spores are then inhaled and deposited in the lungs. Ear, cutaneous, sinus and dental infections have also been known to occur. Other reported modes of transmission include: airborne spread, which is associated with indwelling catheters, implants and contaminated bandages (Anaissie, 1992) and foodborne spread. *Aspergillus flavus* can generate a carcinogenic substance called aflotoxin in foodstuffs (Rhame, 1991).

Normal healthy people rarely develop invasive disease. Aspergillosis is primarily an infection of severely immune-compromised patients. The major predisposing factor of infection includes prolonged neutropenia, chronic administration of steroids, insertion of prosthetic devices and tissue damage due to prior infection or trauma (Khardoni, 1989).

The organism is capable of invasion across all natural barriers, including cartilage and bone, and has a propensity for invading blood vessels, causing thrombosis and infection. The major concern is the potential for severe haemorrhage, which may cause death and which occurs in about 10% of patients.

Generally, infection is chronic, causing symptoms directly related to the site of infection.

Diagnosis is difficult as *Aspergillus* spores are cultured infrequently from the respiratory tract secretions (Weiland, 1983), and there is considerable debate about the significance of isolation as this organism is a common contaminant. Diagnosis generally relies on serological (Trull *et al.*, 1985) or histocytochemical tests (Meyer *et al.*, 1973).

Therapy for invasive aspergillosis has been less than satisfactory, with amphotericin B being the only antifungal agent with established activity against the infection (Pizzo *et al.*, 1982). Newer antifungal agents such as Fluconazole and Itraconazole appear to exhibit good activity against a variety of fungi (Anaissie, 1992).

Control measures are essential. Air conditioning systems must be functioning and well maintained, and the environment kept scrupulously clean, with emphasis placed on vacuuming, damp dusting and mopping. Instruments, dressings equipment and linen must always be stored properly to prevent contamination by *Aspergillus*. This highlights the importance of removing wound dressings for the shortest period of time possible before dressing changes to prevent contamination of open wounds.

During structural work it is essential to provide and maintain impermeable barriers to ensure that spores from work areas do not enter ventilation systems or get carried to other wards. Ideally, relocation of immune-suppressed patients to unaffected areas is advisable, and thorough cleaning of work areas before the return of patients is essential (Arnow *et al.*, 1978).

Person-to-person spread has not been demonstrated, and therefore barrier nursing is not required. However, careful disposal of sputum, and encouraging patients to cover the mouth and nose when coughing, are necessary precautions.

References and further reading

Anaissie, E. (1992) Opportunistic mycoses in the immunocompromised host: experience at a cancer centre and review. *Clinical Infectious Diseases*, 14 (Suppl 1), S43–S53.

Arnow, P. M. *et al.* (1978) Pulmonary aspergillosis during hospital renovation. *American Review of Respiratory Disease*, 118, 49–53.

Bodey, G. P. *et al.* (1989) Aspergillosis. *European Journal of Clinical Microbiology and Infectious Disease*, 8(5), 413–37.

Khardoni, N. (1989) Host-parasite interactions in fungal infections. *European Journal of Clinical Microbiology and Infectious Diseases*, 8, 331–52.

Meyer, R. D. *et al.* (1973) Aspergillosis complicating neoplastic disease. *American Journal of Medicine*, 54, 6–54.

Pizzo, P. A. *et al.* (1982) Empiric antibiotic and antifungal therapy for cancer patients with prolonged fever and granulocytopenia. *American Journal of Medicine*, 72, 101–11.

Rhame, F. S. (1991) Prevention of nosocomial aspergillosis. *Journal of Hospital Infection*, 18 (Supplement A), 466–72.

Trull, A. *et al.* (1985) IgG enzyme linked immunosorbent essay for diagnosis of invasive aspergillosis: retrospective study over 15 years of transplant recipients. *Journal of Clinical Pathology*, 38, 1045–51.

Warren, R. E. *et al.* (1982) Clinical manifestations and management of aspergillosis in the compromised patient. In: *Fungal Infections in the Compromised Patient*, (eds D. W. Warnock & M. D. Richardson), pp. 119–53. John Wiley, New York.

Weiland, D. (1983) Aspergillosis in 25 renal transplant patients. *Annals of Surgery*, 198, 622–9.

CLOSTRIDIUM DIFFICILE

Definition

Clostridium difficile is a slender, Gram-positive anaerobic rod which is spore forming and motile. Bacteria of this type may be a normal component of gut flora and flourish when other gut organisms are eradicated by antibiotics. *Clostridium difficile* was first recognized in the late 1970s when it was identified as the causative organism for pseudomembranous colitis (PMC). In the 1980s it was identified as a major cause of antibiotic associated diarrhoea (AAD) (Duerden *et al.*, 1994). It is now one of the most commonly detected enteric pathogens and an important cause of nosocomial infection in nursing homes and hospitals (Kim *et al.*, 1981).

REFERENCE MATERIAL

Diarrhoea can be caused by disruption of the normal flora of the gut by antibiotics which allows *Clostridium difficile* to multiply. The colonic mucosa becomes covered with a characteristic fibrinous pseudomembrane. Signs and symptoms can be relatively mild, resolving when antibiotics are discontinued, or more severe, as in cases of pseudomembranous colitis, which may require surgical resection of parts of the colon and is associated with a significant mortality rate.

About 5% of healthy adults carry *Clostridium difficile* in their faeces, usually in small numbers. Infants are more likely to carry the organisms but are less likely to develop colitis (Fekety & Shah, 1993).

Diagnosis

Diagnosis is based on clinical findings, endoscopy and laboratory evalutaion. Clinical findings range from profuse, watery, green, foul smelling or bloody diarrhoea, with cramping abdominal pains, tenderness and high fever, to hypovolaemic shock and overwhelming sepsis. Endoscopy may reveal effects similar to those seen in non-specific colitis, or may show the yellow–white raised plaques which go on to form a membrane on the intestinal mucosa (Kofsky *et al.*, 1991).

Laboratory Diagnosis

Clostridium difficile is difficult to isolate in ordinary culture because of overgrowth by other organisms. To overcome this a selective culture medium is used. The presence of *Clostridium difficile* in culture is not by itself an indication of infection, it simply marks the organism's presence. Infection or disease is indicated by the presence of toxins produced by the organism which can be identified using screening tests. Approximately 75% of *Clostridium difficile* bacteria produce toxins which may cause disease, whilst the remainder are unlikely to lead to serious problems. The toxins produced by *Clostridium difficile* are exotoxins: enterotoxin (toxin A) and cytotoxin (toxin B) cause diarrhoea, disruption of cell membranes in the gut and the microfilaments and protein synthesis associated with PMC. A method of rapid 'fingerprint' analysis is under development to assist with the identification of cases of cross-infection. It will make it possible to establish whether cases of infection occurring in a ward over a short period of time are related, or whether patients are separate, individual carriers of the organism (Communicable Disease Report, 1993).

Treatment

Clostridium difficile is highly sensitive to oral vancomycin or metronidazole. Other antibiotics should be withheld if possible. Recurrence is seen in 10–20% of patients, often 1–4 weeks after initial treatment has been completed. It is due either to germination of spores not eradicated by treatment, or to re-infection through contact with organisms from other people or in the environment (Fekety & Shah, 1993).

Transmission

Pseudomembranous colitis develops from overgrowth of *Clostridium difficile* already present in the gut, or from exogenous organisms acquired via the person-to-person or faeco-oral route. *Clostridium difficile* can be transmitted on the hands of hospital personnel (McFarland *et al.*, 1989), and outbreaks in hospital have resulted in the deaths of a number of elderly people (Duerden *et al.*, 1994). One such outbreak affected 39 elderly patients, 5 of whom died. In this instance the ward was closed for thorough cleaning to eliminate the infection (Snell, 1992). Worsley (1993) describes a prolonged outbreak of *Clostridium difficile* involving 175 patients in three hospitals. The infection caused 17 deaths directly and contributed to a further 43. In addition to an estimated financial cost of £75 000, there was a loss of public confidence and an increase in staff sick leave.

Prevention

Prevention is only achieved by maintaining strict hygiene in the environment and by scrupulous attention to principles of hygiene by staff (Worsley, 1993). Johnson *et al.* (1990) demonstrated a decrease in the incidence of infection following the introduction of gloves for staff in contact with patients infected with *Clostridium difficile*. When an infected patient is discharged, the ward must be thoroughly cleaned before other patients are allowed into the area.

Nursing care

Careful barrier nursing is required for all patients with toxin producing *Clostridium difficile* or unexplained diarrhoea. Segregation from other patients must continue until stool cultures are clear of infectious organisms.

References

Communicable Disease Report (1993) Typing service for *Clostridium difficile*. *Public Health Laboratory Service*, 3(53), 1.

Duerden, B. I. *et al.* (1994) Report of the PHLS *Clostridium difficile* working party. *Public Health Laboratory Service Microbiology Digest*, 11(1), 22–4.

Fekety, R. & Shah, A. B. (1993) Diagnosis and treatment of *Clostridium difficile* colitis. *Journal of the American Medical Association*, 269(1), 71–5.

Johnson, S. *et al.* (1990) Prospective controlled study of vinyl glove use to interrupt *Clostridium difficile* transmission. *American Journal of Medicine*, 88, 137–40.

Kim, K. H. *et al.* (1981) Isolation of *Clostridium difficile* from the environment and contacts of patients with antibiotic associated colitis. *Journal of Infectious Disease*, 143, 42–4.

Kofsky, P. *et al.* (1991) *Clostridium difficile*: a common and costly colitis. *Diseases of the Colon and Rectum*, 34(3), 244–8.

McFarland, L. V. *et al.* (1989) Nosocomial acquisition of *Clostridium difficile* infection. *New England Journal of Medicine*, 320(4), 204–10.

Snell, J. (1992) Old die in clostridium outbreak. *Nursing Times*, 88(3), 6.

Worsley, M. (1993) A major outbreak of antibiotic associated diarrhoea. *Public Health Laboratory Service Microbiology Digest*, 10(2), 97–9.

CRYPTOSPORIDIOSIS

Definition

Cryptosporidium is a protozoan parasite, first isolated in 1907. The only species of the organism known to affect man is *Cryptosporidium parvum* (Department of Health, 1990).

Cryptosporidia species were initially considered a cause of severe protracted diarrhoea (Navin *et al.*, 1984) in immunocompromised patients (Wolfson *et al.*, 1985). Cryptosporidium is now being increasingly recognized as the cause of self-limiting enteritis in otherwise healthy people, with sporadic and epidemic cryptosporidiosis most commonly recorded in young children (Holley *et al.*, 1986).

REFERENCE MATERIAL

Cryptosporidium is rarely isolated in people with normal stools (Soave *et al.*, 1986). In Britain, the number of reported cases of crytosporidiosis has been increasing. This may reflect greater public awareness and improved detection methods, rather than a true increase (Department of Health, 1990).

The organism infects livestock, particularly calves and lambs, whose faecal matter infects water supplies, which then can infect man (Tzipori, 1983).

Two outbreaks of cryptosporidiosis traceable to swimming baths have been reported: in one case the cause was contamination of water in the pool by a swimmer, in the other a plumbing defect allowed sewage to enter the water circulating system (Hunt *et al.*, 1994).

Routine water disinfection by chlorination is ineffective in controlling the organism except in small numbers. Contamination of the water supply generally occurs when heavy rains follow drought (Peeters *et al.*, 1989), causing leakage of effluent or slurry into treated water.

Based on epidemiological evidence, consumption of certain foods (especially undercooked sausages, offal and unpasteurized milk) appears to be a risk factor (Casemore, 1987). Infection can also occur following direct contact with animals, and is easily transmitted from one person to another (Department of Health, 1990) which is probably the main mode of transmission in urban populations. Only a small innoculum of organism appears to be required to cause infection.

The incubation period is between 3 and 11 days, but may be as long as 25 days. Illness usually presents as acute offensive, non-bloody, diarrhoea, sometimes accompanied by fever. Acute illness may last for 2–3 weeks, with excretion of the organism in faeces for as long as a fortnight after symptoms have cleared. While infection is usually self-limiting in healthy people, it can cause intractable diarrhoea in immunocompromised people, who will need admission to hospital for care and rehydration. There is no effective antimicrobial agent available to treat this organism (Wolfson *et al.*, 1985).

Strict barrier nursing is required while diarrhoea persists, with segregation from other patients continuing until clear specimens of stool cultures are obtained.

Any sign of cross-infection must be pursued vigorously to prevent further spread. This will include close co-operation with health and local authorities, the appropriate water companies and the outbreak control team with the authority, as recommended by the Department of Health (1990).

The organism is unaffected by chlorine in the concentrations that can be used in the treatment of drinking water, and is inactivated only by being frozen or heated to temperatures of 65–85°C for 5–10 minutes or by exposure to boiling water. Prevention relies on compliance with safe practices by water companies and health authorities in water treatment processes.

References and further reading

Casemore, D. P. (1987) Cryptosporidiosis PHLS. *Microbiology Digest*, 4, 1–5.

Department of Health (1990) *Report of the Group of Experts on Cryptosporidium in Water Supplies* (Chairman, Sir John Badenock). HMSO, London.

Holley, H. P. *et al.* (1986) Cryptosporidiosis – a common cause of parasitic diarrhoea in otherwise healthy individuals. *Journal of Infectious Diseases*, 153, 365–7.

Hunt, D. A. *et al.* (1994) Cryptosporidiosis associated with a swimming pool complex. *Communicable Disease Report*, 4(2), R20–R22.

Navin, T. R. *et al.* (1984) Cryptosporidiosis – clinical, epidemiological and parasitologic review. *Review of Infectious Diseases*, 6, 313–27.

Peeters, J. E. *et al.* (1989) Effects of disinfection of drinking water with ozone or chlorine dioxide on survival of *Cryptosporidium parvum* oocysts. *Applied Microbiology*, 55(6),

1519–22.

Soave, R. *et al.* (1986) Cryptosporidium and cryptosporidiosis. *Review of Infectious Diseases*, 8, 1012–23.

Tzipori, S. (1983) Cryptosporidiosis in animals and humans. *Microbiological Review*, 47, 84–96.

Wolfson, J. S. *et al.* (1985) Cryptosporidiosis in immunocompetent patients. *New England Journal of Medicine*, 312, 1278–82.

HEPATITIS A

Definition

Hepatitis A is an acute infectious disease caused by the hepatitis A virus (HAV).

REFERENCE MATERIAL

HAV is a small, symmetrical RNA virus (enterovirus type 72) (Melnick, 1982). The virus is unusually stable, resisting heat at 60°C for 1 hour of 25°C for 3 months, indefinite cold storage (5°C), acidic conditions (pH 3) and non-ionic detergents (Siegl *et al.*, 1984; Sorbey *et al.*, 1988). It can survive for several months in sewage and the environment.

HAV is spread predominantly by the faecal–oral route, and viral replication probably occurs in the jejunum before transmission via the portal vein to the liver (Siegl, 1988) and has been associated with the following:

(1) Contaminated water, milk and food. Any uncooked foods and drinks could be responsible for infection. However, particular problems are due to contamination at the time of harvesting and packaging of uncooked frozen foods which are then thawed and used (Ramsey *et al.*, 1989).
(2) Poor general hygiene and low economic status (Ayoola, 1988).
(3) Contact with children in day centres (Hadler *et al.*, 1986) and neonatal intensive care units (Azimi *et al.*, 1986).
(4) Foreign travel to countries where HAV is endemic (Skinhof *et al.*, 1981).
(5) Blood transfusions (Noble *et al.*, 1984).
(6) Contact with a case of hepatitis A in the home (Maguire *et al.*, 1995).

The HAV antigen (HAAg) can be detected in stools early in the course of illness. HAAg levels decline rapidly with the onset of symptoms but can remain detectable for up to 2 weeks after the onset of clinical hepatitis (Coulepis *et al.*, 1980).

Diagnosis of acute HAV infection is usually confirmed serologically, by detecting IgM antibodies to HAAg which appear in serum 3–7 weeks after oral inoculation, and may persist for some time, occasionally for more than a year (Lemon *et al.*, 1980). Evidence of past infection and therefore immunity which can persist for life (Lemon, 1985) is obtained by detecting serologically the presence of IgG antibody to HAAg.

HAV usually causes a minor illness in children and young adults, with as few as 5% of cases being symptomatic (Eddleston, 1990). The illness often presents as an upper respiratory infection with the following signs and symptoms: anorexia; malaise; weight loss; pyrexia; diarrhoea and vomiting (Wright *et al.*, 1985); dark urine; and jaundice.

In total 7430 cases of hepatitis A were reported in England and Wales in 1991, with children and young adults most frequently affected (Maguire *et al.*, 1995). Symptomatic infection is more likely to occur with increasing age, with UK census data for 1979 to 1985 showing a positive correlation between age and death from HAV (Office of Population Censuses and Surveys, 1989). Control and prevention of HAV relies on provision of good sanitation facilities and clean drinking water, and supervision of food handlers. Passive immunization with intramuscular normal pooled immunoglobulin (HNIg) gives protection against clinical hepatitis for about 3 months in most people. However, it is probable that passive immunization allows HAV infection with greatly attenuating effects which could lead to life-long immunity (Gust *et al.*, 1988). Concern has been expressed that the decreasing prevalence of HAV infection in the general population of the UK might lead to inadequate levels of anti-HAV antibody in HNIg. However, no case of HNIg failing has been reported (Teo, 1992). It is advisable before travel, in endemic regions; post-exposure prophylaxis is advisable for household contacts during outbreaks of HAV infection (Department of Health, 1992).

The Department of Health (1992) has recommended that sewage workers, military personnel and foriegn diplomats should be considered for vaccination. In institutions for the care of the mentally ill, and in children's centres where the children are not toilet trained, vaccination policy should be formulated according to local circumstances (Department of Health, 1992). A study by Maguire *et al.* (1995) showed no clear evidence that health care workers are at increased occupational risk of aquiring hepatitis A.

References and further reading

Ayoola, E. A. (1988) Viral hepatitis in Africa. In: *Viral Hepatitis and Liver Disease*, (ed. A. J. Zuckerman), pp. 161–9. Alan R. Liss. New York.

Azimi, P. H. *et al.* (1986) Transfusion-acquired hepatitis A in a premature infant with second nosocomial spread in an intensive care nursery. *American Journal of Diseases of Childhood*, 140, 23–7.

Coulepis, A. C. *et al.* (1980) Detection of hepatitis A virus in the faeces of patients with naturally acquired infection. *Journal of Infectious Diseases*, 141, 151–6.

Department of Health (1992) *Immunisation against infectious diseases*. HMSO, London.

Eddleston, A. (1990) Modern vaccines. Hepatitis. *Lancet*, 335, 1142–5.

Gust, I. D. *et al.* (1988) Prevention and control of hepatitis A. In: *Viral Hepatitis and Liver Disease*, (ed. A. J. Zuckerman), pp. 77–80. Alan R. Liss, New York.

Hadler, S. C. *et al.* (1986) Hepatitis in day care centres. Epidemiology and prevention. *Review of Infectious Diseases*, 8, 548–57.

Lemon, S. M. (1985) Type A viral hepatitis. New developments in an old disease. *New England Journal of Medicine*, 313, 1059–67.

Lemon, S. M. *et al.* (1980) Specific immunoglobulin. A response to hepatitis A virus determined by solid phase radioimmunossay. *Infectious Immunology*, 28, 927–36.

Maguire, H. C. *et al.* (1995) A collaboration case control study of sporadic hepatitis A in England. *Communicable Disease Report*, 5(3), R33–R40.

Melnick, J.-L. (1982) Classification of hepatitis A virus as enterovirus type 72 and of hepatitis B virus as hepadnovirus type 1. *Intervirology*, 18, 105–6.

Noble, R. C. *et al.* (1984) Post-transfusion hepatitis A in a neonatal intensive care unit. *Journal of the American Medical Association*, 252, 2711–15.

Office of Population Censuses and Surveys (1989) *Mortality Statistics, Cause, 1979–1985. Series DH2 Nos. 6–12*. HMSO, London.

Ramsey, C. N. *et al.* (1989) Hepatitis A and frozen raspberries. *Lancet*, 1, 43–4.

Siegl, G. *et al.* (1984) Stability of hepatitis A virus. *Intervirology*, 22, 218–26.

Siegl, G. (1988) Virology of hepatitis. In: *Viral Hepatitis and Liver Disease*, (ed. A. J. Zuckerman), pp. 3–7. Alan R. Liss, New York.

Skinhof, P. *et al.* (1981) Travellers' hepatitis: origin and characteristics of cases in Copenhagen, 1976–1978. *Scandinavian Journal of Infectious Diseases*, 13, 1–4.

Sorbey, M. D. *et al.* (1988) Survival and persistence of hepatitis A virus in environmental samples. In: *Viral Hepatitis and Liver Disease*, (ed. A. J. Zuckerman), pp. 121–4. Alan R. Liss, New York.

Teo, C. G. (1992) The virology and serology of hepatitis: an overview. *Communicable Disease Report Review*, 2(10), R109–R114.

Wright, R. *et al.* (1985) Acute viral hepatitis. In: *Liver and Biliary Disease*, (eds R. Wright *et al.*), pp. 677–767. Baillière Tindall, London.

GUIDELINES: HEPATITIS A

Outpatient

Action	Rationale
1 It is not usually necessary to admit the individual to hospital.	Self-limiting disease.
2 Patient education is essential and must include advice on good personal hygiene and careful hand washing.	Limits the spread of the virus. Careful hand washing removes contamination from hands.
3 Separate soap, flannel and towel must be provided.	To minimize the risk of infection being spread via equipment used for hygiene purposes.
4 Meticulous cleaning of bath, wash basin and toilet with a cream cleaner and hot water.	To remove contamination.
5 Bath and wash basin must be allowed to dry after use.	Viruses will not survive on clean dry surfaces.
6 Soiled bed linen and underclothing should be washed.	To remove contamination.
7 Patient should refrain from intimate kissing and sexual intercourse while symptoms are present.	To prevent cross-infection.

Guidelines: Hepatitis A (cont'd)

Action	Rationale

 8 Avoid contact with susceptible people, i.e. very young, old or those with debilitating illness.

To reduce the likelihood of infection.

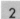 **9** Crockery and cutlery must be washed and rinsed in hot water.

Heat destroys the virus.

Inpatient

Action	Rationale

1 Whenever possible, the patient should have medical or surgical treatment postponed until he/she is symptom free.

Medical and surgical treatment will debilitate the patient further and recovery will be slower.

2 Ideally, the patient should be discharged.

Cross-infection is less likely to occur at home among fit, healthy people.

3 A single room with separate toilet should be made available for the patient, although barrier nursing is not necessary.

Although patients are no longer excreting the virus once they have become symptomatic, there are always exceptions.

4 Blood, secretions and excreta (particularly faeces) must be disposed of immediately in a heat-disinfecting bedpan washer.

To prevent cross-infection.

5 Careful hand washing after patient contact.

To prevent cross-infection.

HEPATITIS B

Definition

Hepatitis B is a serious infectious disease caused by the hepatitis B virus (HBV), which produces an inflammatory condition of the liver characterized by jaundice, hepatomegaly, anorexia, abdominal and gastric discomfort, abnormal liver function, clay-coloured stools and dark urine.

REFERENCE MATERIAL

HBV is a 42 nm double-shelled particle, termed initially Dane particle after its discoverer, which represents the intact infectious virion (Dane *et al.*, 1970). Contained within is a 27 nm inner core particle which contains the viral nucleic acid (Lau & Wright, 1993).

Epidemiology

HBV may be found in virtually all body secretions and excreta of patients with acute hepatitis B and carriers of the virus. Blood, semen and vaginal fluids are mainly implicated in the transmission of infection, which occurs by:

(1) Sexual transmission, both vaginal and anal.
(2) Accidental inoculation of blood following a sharps injury, for example, or by drug addicts sharing used needles and syringes (Shattock *et al.*, 1985).
(3) Contamination of mucous membranes, eye, nose or mouth.
(4) Contamination of non-intact skin.
(5) Perinatally at or about the time of birth.
(6) Blood transfusion. The frequency of post-transfusion HBV infection has decreased significantly since the exclusion of hepatitis B surface antigen (HBs Ag) seropositive blood donors in Britain (O'Grady *et al.*, 1988), but transfusions abroad are still implicated as sources of infection (Papaevangelou *et al.*, 1984).

This explains why high rates of infection occur in narcotic drug addicts, promiscuous homosexuals and prostitutes (Durante & Heptonstall, 1995). A high prevalence of HBV infection has been reported in areas of the world where socioeconomic conditions are poor, and in individuals requiring repeated transfusions of blood or blood products, in institutions for the mentally retarded and in some semi-closed institutions (Follett, 1987).

The number of male homosexuals and intravenous drug abusers developing HBV has decreased, suggesting the concerns about AIDS have influenced safe sex practices among promiscuous individuals and the use of clean needles and syringes among intravenous drug abusers (Polakoff, 1989).

The number of new cases of HBV infection in the UK is about 1000 reported cases a year. The prevalence of infection in the UK is not known, but has been suggested to be as low as one in 500 of the general adult population (Department of Health and Social Security, 1988).

Clinical response

HBV infection is clinically extremely variable, with the incubation period varying from 4 weeks to as long as 6 months. Approximately 60% of adult cases produce a subclinical infection with only mild symptoms such as fatigue and malaise, which often go unnoticed. Acute infection occurs in about 40% of adults, with spontaneous recovery usually within one month, although prolonged recovery can occur, accompanied by post-viral depression. Only about 5–10% of infected people become chronically infected and run the major risk of developing cirrhosis and liver cell cancer (Jacyna et al., 1990). This accounts for less than 1% of deaths due to HBV infection.

The incidence of chronic infection is higher in those in whom there is a relative deficit of T cell function, the young, the aged, those with Down's syndrome, those with malignancy and those receiving immunosuppressive or cytotoxic therapy (Alexander, 1990).

Infectivity

The progress of HBV can be monitored by serological testing. Hepatitis B surface antigen is detected in the blood approximately 3 to 4 weeks after exposure, with antibodies to hepatitis B core (HBc) antigen (HBc Ag) developing about 2 weeks after HBs Ag occurs.

Anti-HBc will eventually be replaced by anti-HBs, which is the antibody to HBs Ag, and marks the end of high infectivity and the development of immunity to subsequent HBV infection (Lau & Wright, 1993).

The antigen HBe Ag is an internal component of the core of HBs and is an indicator of high infectivity; it will be replaced eventually by anti-HBe, which correlates with loss of viral replication (Tedder, 1980). HBV is capable of surviving for at least 1 week in the environment (Trevelyan, 1991).

Diagnosis

Diagnosis is confirmed by a virological blood test with regular monitoring of antigen status to evaluate progress (Teo, 1992).

Screening policy for HBs Ag

Screening of the entire hospital patient population would be an effective way to identify hepatitis B infection, but this would be costly and time consuming in terms of the benefits derived. It is important, however, to screen patients before their admission to a transplant or renal unit (Tedder, 1980).

In general, the best compromise is to test those patients belonging to groups in which there is a high prevalence of hepatitis B. These include the following people:

(1) All new admissions who currently live or were born in countries where there is a high prevalence of hepatitis B, such as the developing countries.
(2) Drug addicts.
(3) Promiscuous heterosexuals and male homosexuals (i.e. individuals who frequently change sexual partners, particularly those who are prostitutes or male homosexuals).
(4) Mentally subnormal patients in institutions.
(5) Multiple transfusion patients.
(6) All patients acutely or recently jaundiced.

Transmission of HBV in the health care setting

Studies of health care workers who have sustained inoculation accidents involving HBs Ag positive blood indicates the risk of transmission to be approximately 20%, where the potential source of infection is an HBe Ag positive patient or carrier (Werner et al., 1982). Most carriers can be classified as low risk where blood contains anti-HBe. The chance of transmission from these patients is approximately 0.1%; overall, the chance of transmission of infection is probably of the order of 5%.

There is no evidence of transmission of HBV by inhalation of droplets, neither has faecal–oral transmission been demonstrated (UK Health Department, 1990). However, one study estimated that up to 94% of HBV infections among health care workers may have been acquired without any inoculation injury (Callender et al., 1982).

Immunization and vaccination

Passive immunization is achieved by hepatitis B immunoglobulin which is prepared from pooled plasma with a high titre of hepatitis B surface antibody, which confers temporary passive immunity under certain defined conditions (Department of Health, 1992), as follows:

(1) Administered preferably within 48 hours and no later than seven days following inoculated, ingested or splashed HBs Ag-infected blood. If the blood is HBe Ag positive, a second dose should be given 30 days later (Deinhardt et al., 1985). The Medical

Research Council report (1980) describes a low incidence (3%) of subsequent HBV infection when specific HBV immunoglobulin had been given prophylactically.

(2) Vertical and perinatal spread is the commonest method of spread of HBV world-wide, and accounts, for example, for the very high carrier rate in South East Asia and parts of Africa (Stevens *et al.*, 1975). Prophylactic immunoglobulin given as soon as possible after birth reduces by 70% the risk of the baby developing the persistent carrier state. Protection is increased to about 90% when given with active immunization (Zuckerman, 1990). Infants that acquire HVB infection despite vaccination are thought to do so as a result of an 'escape mutant' (Teo, 1992). The infection they develop appears to resolve promptly (Lau & Wright, 1993).

Active immunization is by hepatitis B vaccine. There are two HBV vaccines available:

(1) Human plasma derived from symptomless carriers which has been purified by a combination of ultracentrifugation and biochemical procedures.

(2) A genetically engineered vaccine from yeast. All health care staff who carry out procedures which involve exposure to blood and body fluids must receive hepatitis B vaccine (Department of Health, 1993). Their response to the vaccine must be checked: levels of 100 IU/ml and above indicate immunity; levels of 10–100 IU/ml indicate the need for a booster dose of vaccine; levels below 10 IU/ml indicate no response. Ten per cent of vaccinees will not respond at all to hepatitis B vaccine. Lack of response is more common in people aged 50 years and over, in people who are immunocompromised, and if the injection has been given into fatty tissue (Department of Health, 1992).

Indications for immunization include:

(1) Personnel including teaching, training and nursing staff directly involved over a period of time in patient care where there is a high prevalence of HBV or where blood and blood products are handled regularly.

(2) Laboratory workers.

(3) Dentists, dental personnel.

(4) Medical and surgical personnel.

(5) Health care personnel on secondment to work in areas of the world where there is a high prevalence of HBV.

(6) Patients on entry to residential institutions for the mentally handicapped where there is a high prevalence of HBV.

(7) Patients treated by maintenance haemodialysis.

(8) Sexual contacts of patients with acute HBV or carriers of HBV.

(9) Infants born to mothers who are HBs Ag positive.

(10) Health care workers who receive an inoculation accident from a needle used on a patient who is HBs Ag positive, either used alone or in combination with hepatitis B immunoglobulin.

Prevention of hepatitis B in health care workers

Dienstag & Ryan (1982) have shown that general ward nurses are at no greater risk of acquiring hepatitis B than the general population. However, it is important that health care workers adopt safe techniques when in contact with blood and body fluids of all patients, regardless of their hepatitis status.

Avoiding inoculation accidents is an essential component of safe techniques. Resheathing needles accounts for 15–41% of all needlestick injuries and must not be undertaken (McCormick *et al.*, 1981). Resheathing commonly occurs as a result of trying to ensure safe transit to a disposal sharps bin (Edmond *et al.*, 1990), suggesting that sharps bins should be either attached to trolleys or placed at the bedside (Hart, 1990).

Vickers *et al.* (1994) reviewed an outbreak of hepatitis B which involved three volunteers at a residential drug trial unit where blood samples were taken by staff who did not wash their hands after each patient contact, and whose hands, gloves, and equipment were visibly contaminated with blood. Such incidents demonstrate the importance of written policies that are regularly reviewed and updated.

Employment of HBs Ag people

Tedder (1980) discusses the problem of carriers of HBs Ag who want to return to full-time employment, particularly those whose carrier state lasts for many years or possibly for the rest of their lives. Prentice *et al.* (1992) report that between 1975 and 1990 there was on average one outbreak a year of hepatitis B which could be attributed to transmission from hospital staff to patients. Heptonstall's (1991) study indicates that infected surgical health care staff were associated with these outbreaks. New guidelines issued in 1993 by the Department of Health recommend that health care workers who are HBe Ag positive must not carry out procedures in which there is a risk that injury to the health care worker could result in their blood contaminating the open tissues of patients. Previously HBs Ag positive staff were excluded from renal dialysis units: now only HBe Ag positive staff are excluded (Department of Health, 1993).

Death of patients with hepatitis B

When infected patients die, their bodies are no more hazardous than when they were alive, providing that appropriate precautions against contamination with blood and body fluids are maintained (Young & Healing, 1995). Guidelines recommend that bodies of patients known to be infected with hepatitis B, C or non-A and non-B should be placed in a body bag. Relatives and significant others should be permitted to view, touch and spend time with the deceased person. However, embalming should not be undertaken (Healing *et al.*, 1995).

Patient education

The Department of Health and Social Security (1984) recommends that individuals found to be HBs Ag carriers should be educated about the ways in which hepatitis B may spread and the precautions which can be taken to reduce the risk to others. It is stressed that unnecessary restrictions and precautions may cause distress and should be avoided.

Anti-viral therapy

Alpha-interferon given subcutaneously or intramuscularly has been shown to be effective in terminating viral replication and in eradicating carrier status in patients with chronic HBV infection (Wong *et al.*, 1993). Long-term follow-up is required to establish whether interferon therapy influences the incidence of HBV related cirrhosis and carcinoma (Crowe, 1994).

References and further reading

Alexander, G. J. M. (1990) Immunology of hepatitis B virus infection. *British Medical Bulletin*, 46(2), 354–67.

Callender, M. E. *et al.* (1982) Hepatitis B virus infection in medical and health care personnel. *British Medical Journal*, 284, 423–6.

Crowe, H. M. (1994) Forum: a perspective on hepatitis. *Asepsis*, 16(2), 13–17.

Dane, D. S. *et al.* (1970) Virus-like particle in serum of patients with Australian antigen-associated hepatitis. *Lancet*, 1, 695–8.

Deinhardt, F. D. *et al.* (1985) Immunization against hepatitis B. Report on a WHO meeting on viral hepatitis in Europe. *Journal of Medical Virology*, 17, 209–17.

Department of Health (1992) *Immunisation against Infectious Diseases*. HMSO, London.

Department of Health (1993) Protecting health care workers and patients from hepatitis B. *Health Service Guidelines, HSG (93) 40*. Department of Health, London.

Department of Health and Social Security (1981) *Hepatitis B and NHS Staff (CMO (81)11)*. HMSO, London.

Department of Health and Social Security (1984) *Guidance for Health Service Personnel Dealing with Patients Infected With Hepatitis B Virus (CMO (84)11, CNO (84)7)*. HMSO, London.

Department of Health and Social Security (1993) *Immunization agaisnt infectious diseases*. DHSS, London.

Dienstag, J. L. & Ryan, D. M. (1982) Occupational exposure to hepatitis B virus in hospital personnel; infection or immunization. *American Journal of Epidemiology*, 115, 22–9.

Durante, A. J. & Heptonstall, J. (1995) How many people in England and Wales risk infection from injecting drug use? *Communicable Disease Report*, 5(3), R40–R44.

Edmond, M. *et al.* (1990) Effects of bedside needle disposal units on needle recapping frequency and needlestick injury. *Canadian Intravenous Nurses Association Journal*, 6(1), 10–11.

Follett, E. (1987) Psychiatric hospitals and the mentally handicapped – a special case. *Royal College of Nursing Wendsly Conference Report*, pp. 7–16.

Hart, S. (1990) Clinical hepatitis B; guidelines for infection control. *Nursing Standard*, 4(45), 24–7.

Healing, T. D. *et al.* (1995) The infection hazards of human cadavers. *Communicable Disease Report*, 5, R61–R69.

Heptonstall, J. (1991) Outbreak of hepatitis B virus infection associated with infected surgical staff. *Communicable Disease Report*, 1(8), R81–R85.

Jacyna, M. R. *et al.* (1990) Antiviral therapy – hepatitis B. *British Medical Bulletin*, 46(2), 368–82.

Lau, J. Y. N. & Wright, T. L. (1993) Molecular virology and pathogenesis of hepatitis B. *Lancet*, 342, 1335–9.

McCormick, R. D. *et al.* (1981) Epidemiology of needlestick injuries in hospital personnel. *American Journal of Medicine*, 70, 928–32.

Medical Research Council and Public Health Laboratory Service (1980) The incidence of hepatitis B infection after accidental exposure and anti-HBs immunoglobulin prophylaxis. *Lancet*, 1, 6–8.

O'Grady, J. G. *et al.* (1988) Early indicators of prognosis in acute liver failure and their applications of patients for orthotopic liver transplantation. *Gastroenterology*, 94, A578.

Papaevangelou, G. *et al.* (1984) Etiology of fulminant viral hepatitis in Greece. *Hepatology*, 4, 369–72.

Polakoff, S. (1989) *Acute Viral Hepatitis B in Laboratory Reports 1985–1988. Communicable Disease Report 89/92 3–6.* HMSO, London.

Prentice, M. S. *et al.* (1992) Infection with hepatitis B virus after open heart surgery. *British Medical Journal*, 304, 761–4.

Shattock, A. C. *et al.* (1985) Increased severity and morbidity of acute hepatitis in drug abusers with simultaneously acquired hepatitis B and hepatitis D infection. *British Medical Journal*, 290, 1377–80.

Stevens, C. F. *et al.* (1975) Vertical transmission of hepatitis B antigen in Taiwan. *New England Journal of Medicine*, 292, 771–4.

Tedder, R. S. (1980) Hepatitis B in hospitals. *British Journal of Hospital Medicine*, 23(3), 266–79.

Teo, C. G. (1992) The virology and serology of hepatitis: an overview. *Communicable Disease Report*, 2(10), R109–R113.

Trevelyan, J. (1991) Hepatitis B – who is at risk? *Nursing Times*, 87(5), 26–9.

UK Health Department (1990) *Guidance for Clinical Health Care Workers; Protection Against Infection With HIV and Hepatitis Viruses*. HMSO, London.

Vickers, V. *et al.* (1994) Hepatitis B outbreak in a drug trials unit: investigations and recommendations. *Communicable Diease Report*, 4(1), R1–R4.

Werner, B. G. *et al.* (1982) Accidental hepatitis B surface–

antigen–positive inoculations. *Annals of International Medicine*, 97, 367–9.

Wong, D. K. *et al.* (1993) Effects of alpha-interferon treatment in patients with hepatitis Be antigen positive chronic hepatitis B: a meta-analysis. *Annals of Internal Medicine*, 119, 312–23.

Young, S. E. J. & Healing, T. D. (1995) The management of the deceased with known or suspected infectious disease. *Communicable Disease Report*, 5, R69–R73.

Zuckerman, A. J. (1990) Immunization against hepatitis B. *British Medical Bulletin*, 46(2), 383–98.

GUIDELINES: HEPATITIS B

PROCEDURE

Action

Rationale

1 The patient may be nursed on an open ward using all the patients' facilities as normal unless there is a high risk of blood contamination of the ward environment.

If adequate precautions can be adhered to on an open ward, there is no need to isolate the patient.

2 The patient must be assessed daily to establish accurately any sites of bleeding. Changes in the patient's condition should be recorded in the care plan.

Sites of bleeding must be identified in order that the appropriate precautions can be taken.

3 An individual container for disposing sharps must be kept by the patient. When half full it must be securely sealed, marked 'high risk' and sent for incineration.

Contaminated sharps are a potential inoculation hazard to others, so particular caution must be taken in handling them. Overloaded sharps containers may cause needles to pierce the walls of the container or even protrude through the top.

4 A personal yellow clinical waste bag should be kept on a regular holder with a lid for the patient's disposable waste. When full this should be securely closed, marked 'high risk' and sent for incineration.

To confine potentially contaminated material, e.g. bloodstained tissues.

5 The patient's personal hygiene equipment must be kept at the bedside.

To prevent accidental use of equipment by others.

6 Used linen that is not bloodstained is placed in the ward linen bags in the usual way.

Linen free from blood stains is not contaminated and may be dealt with in the normal manner.

7 During venepuncture or other procedures likely to cause bleeding, furniture, bedding and clothing in the adjacent area should be protected with polythene sheeting.

To prevent contamination of the environment with spilled blood.

8 All staff involved with the patient should cover any cuts or grazes on their hands with waterproof dressings.

Broken skin provides a portal of entry for the hepatitis virus in the event of contact with the patient's blood.

9 Routine daily cleaning procedures may be carried out as normal. As part of universal safe technique and practices, domestic staff will be aware of the potential hazard associated with any blood contamination.

Education is necessary so the domestic staff can understand the hazards involved, otherwise they may over-react to the situation.

Accidental inoculation or spillage of blood

Action

Rationale

1   Any accident involving skin penetration or heavy contamination of abraded skin or mucosal surfaces of staff should be recorded on an accident form and this taken to bacteriology immediately. If the risk of infection from this incident is high, hepatitis B immunoglobulin must be given within 48 hours.

To protect personnel. To comply with legal and/or hospital requirements (Department of Health, 1993).

2   Blood spillage onto unbroken skin should be washed off with soap and running water. A scrubbing brush should not be used as this could break the skin. Complete an accident form, as above.

To remove the source of potential contamination.

3   Accidental inoculation sites should be cleaned under running water, encouraged to bleed freely and then sealed. Complete an accident form, as above.

Bleeding helps to expel the inoculated virus from the site.

4   Blood spilled on hard surfaces must be wiped up immediately with paper towels and the area washed well with a solution such as to hypochlorite.

To prevent viral spread. Dried blood remains infectious for several days.

5   Linen stained with blood should be treated as infected linen and placed in red alginate polythene bag before being placed in a red linen bag.

Bloodstained linen is highly infectious. All linen in red alginate polythene bags will be washed in a barrier wash at the laundry.

Precautions if bleeding is present

Action

Rationale

1   If serious bleeding is present in the mouth:
    (a) Use disposable crockery and cutlery and discard, with any uneaten food, into the disposal bag at the bedside.
    (b) Keep a personal food tray and water jug at the bedside.
    (c) Disposable mouth-care equipment, sputum pot and tissues should be kept at the bedside.

The sputum may be contaminated with blood from the mouth, therefore precautions must include avoiding contact with the patient's sputum.

2   If haematuria or melaena is present:
    (a) Wear plastic gowns and gloves when handling excreta.
    (b) Keep a toilet and handbasin for the patient's sole use, if practicable.
    (c) If a toilet is not available for the patient's sole use, bedpans or urinals must be used. These should be washed in the usual manner in the bedpan washer and dried carefully. They should then be placed in

Blood present in the urine or faeces makes the patient's excreta a potential source of hepatitis B contamination.

Guidelines: Hepatitis B (cont'd)

Action	Rationale
the appropriate bag, marked 'high risk', stapled securely and sent to the sterile supplies department for autoclaving. Disposable bedpans are dealt with in the routine manner.	
3 If the patient has a wound or a break in the skin:	To prevent the spread of the virus from dried or fresh blood. It should be remembered that dried blood can remain infectious for several days.
(a) Cover the area adequately so that there is no seepage.	
(b) Used dressings should be sealed securely in a plastic bag before being disposed of in the appropriate bag.	
(c) All tapes, lotions and creams are kept solely for the patient's use.	
(d) The dressing trolley must be cleaned carefully before re-use.	
(e) Non-disposable equipment should be emptied and wiped clean, placed in a central sterile supplies department bag, securely stapled shut, marked 'high risk', and sent to the sterile supplies department in a safe manner, to be resterilized.	

Other hospital departments

Action	Rationale
1 All departments and staff involved with the patient must be made aware of the diagnosis.	To allow them to make their own precautionary arrangements.
2 All request cards to be labelled appropriately.	To alert the receiving department of the diagnosis.
3 All specimens to be labelled appropriately and correctly bagged. (For further information on specimen collection see Chapter 38.)	To alert the receiving department of the diagnosis and prevent contamination of the environment.
4 If a patient who is bleeding has to be transported elsewhere, the porter involved should be provided with the following:	To prevent the contamination of the porter or other patients.
(a) Disposable gloves and aprons.	
(b) Disposable trolley sheets or chair covers.	
(c) Cleaning equipment for the trolley or chair before use by the next patient.	

Death of a patient with hepatitis B

Action	Rationale
1 There should be minimal handling of the body.	To reduce the risk of infecting the nursing staff.

2	Nurses should wear disposable plastic aprons and gloves when handling the body.	
3	The body should be totally enclosed in a plastic cadaver bag specifically designed for infected patients.	To reduce the risk of infecting the nursing staff.
4	The mortuary staff should be informed of the diagnosis.	To ensure that all staff are aware of the infection risk.
5	If the relatives want to view the body, they must be supervised.	To prevent contamination.

Discharging the patient

Action

Rationale

1	The majority of precautions can cease.	Discharge normally implies that the risk of cross-infection is no longer present.
2	The patient should be advised not to share razors, toothbrushes or similar personal property likely to be contaminated by blood.	To prevent cross-infection.
3	If bleeding occurs, the patient clears up the blood himself/herself and disposes safely of such items as contaminated tissues by burning, flushing down the toilet or sealing in a polythene bag for routine council rubbish collection. If regular persistent bloodstained waste is generated, the health authority must be requested to make special collections.	To prevent cross-infection.
4	If emergency treatment or dental care is required, the patient must inform the health care worker of the fact that he/she has a recent history of hepatitis B infection.	To allow the correct precautions to be taken.

NON-A NON-B HEPATITIS

Definition

Due to major advances in knowledge concerning hepatitis, hepatitis A, B, C, D and E have been distinguished. There remains the theoretical possibility of hepatitis F and beyond being reported. Until this time, the hepatitis virus non-A non-B (NANB) is the term given to all clinical hepatitis that does not fall into the above-mentioned categories (Editorial, 1990).

REFERENCE MATERIAL

There are no accepted serological tests for NANB. Diagnosis is achieved by excluding infections associated with NANB. (Main *et al.*, 1992). These include symptoms associated with hepatitis A, hepatitis B, cytomegalovirus, Epstein–Barr virus, toxic and drug-induced liver injury (including alcoholic liver disease), circulatory abnormalities, shock, sepsis, biliary tract disease and metabolic liver disease (Dienstag, 1983).

Non-A and non-B hepatitis has been shown to occur in patients who have received:

(1) Blood transfusions (Dienstag *et al.*, 1977).
(2) Clotting factors for coagulation disorders.
(3) Haemodialysis.
(4) Outbreaks of epidemics in tropical areas (Wong *et al.*, 1980).
(5) Sporadic cases with no identifiable cause.

Transmission appears to be similar to that of hepatitis B, i.e. principally through blood and blood products. There is an increased incidence in drug addicts due to the sharing of contaminated needles and syringes (Bamber &

Thomas, 1983). There is evidence, however, of sporadic cases with no obvious contributory factors (Farrow *et al.*, 1981).

The incubation period is estimated at 6–8 weeks followed by clinical features similar to hepatitis B, although as a rule acute illness tends to be less severe.

Despite its relatively mild, often asymptomatic and anicteric presentation during acute infection, approximately 20% of people infected with NANB will develop cirrhosis and may die from hepatic-related death such as hepatocellular carcinoma (Lefkowitch *et al.*, 1987). Assessment of treatment protocols for chronic NANB hepatitis has been hindered by the lack of viral markers (Ellis, 1990).

Recombinant interferon is showing promising results in the management of NANB hepatitis (Hoofnagle *et al.*, 1986). Generally, treatment involves responding to the signs and symptoms as they occur. Liver transplantation is the treatment of the future for patients with liver failure (Dusheiko, 1990).

It is essential that safe techniques are used at all times when in contact with blood and body fluids. Human immunoglobulin should be given prophylactically following a previous history of needlestick injuries.

References and further reading

Bamber, M. & Thomas, H. C. (1983) Acute type A, B and non-A non-B hepatitis in a hospital population in London clinical and epidemiological features. *Gut*, 24, 561–4.

Barlow, D. & Sherrard, J. (1992) Sexually transmitted diseases. *Public Health Laboratory Service Digest*, 9(3), 129–31.

Dienstag, J. L. (1983) Non-A non-B hepatitis recognition epidemiology and clinical features. *Gastroenterology*, 85, 439–62.

Dienstag, J. L. *et al.* (1977) Non-A non-B post transfusion hepatitis. *Lancet*, 1, 560–2.

Dusheiko, G. M. (1990) Hepatocellular carcinoma associated with chronic viral hepatitis. Aetiology, diagnosis and treatment. *British Medical Bulletin*, 46(2), 492–511.

Editorial (1990) The A to F of viral hepatitis. *Lancet*, 336, 1158–60.

Ellis, M. E. (1990) Non-A non-B hepatitis; quandaries in serological testing and treatment. *Journal of Infection*, 21, 235–40.

Farrow, L. J. *et al.* (1981) Non-A non-B hepatitis in West London. *Lancet*, 1, 982–4.

Hoofnagle, J. H. *et al.* (1986) Treatment of chronic non-A non-B hepatitis with recombinant human alpha interferon. *New England Journal of Medicine*, 315, 1575–8.

Inarson, S. *et al.* (1973) Multiple attacks of hepatitis in drug addicts. *Journal of Infectious Disease*, 12, 165–9.

Lefkowitch, J. H. *et al.* (1987) Liver cell dysplasia and hepatocellular carcinoma in non-A non-B hepatitis. *Arch. Path. Lab. Med.*, III, 170–73.

Main, J. *et al.* (1992) The diagnosis and management of viral hepatitis. *Communicable Disease Report*, 2(10), R117–R120.

Wong, O. C. *et al.* (1980) Epidemic and endemic hepatitis in India: evidence for a non-A non-B hepatitis virus aetiology. *Lancet*, 2, 876–8.

GUIDELINES: NON-A NON-B HEPATITIS

The procedure should be as for hepatitis B (see above).

HEPATITIS C VIRUS (HCV)

Definition
Hepatitis C is an acute infectious disease caused by hepatitis C virus (HCV).

REFERENCE MATERIAL
HCV is a single-stranded RNA virus, which was discovered in 1989. It is reported to be the cause of 90–95% of cases of transfusion related non-A and non-B hepatitis (Mims *et al.*, 1993). It is also associated with chronic liver disease (Weinstock *et al.*, 1993).

The prevalence of hepatitis C in the UK is estimated to be between 0.1% and 1% of the general population (Department of Health, 1995). Hepatitis C virus is transmitted primarily through contact with blood and blood products (Crowe, 1994). One important means of transmission is misuse of intravenous drugs and sharing of needles (Department of Health, 1995). Studies do not exclude sexual transmission as a mode of transmission, but indicate that it is not transmitted frequently by this route (Bresters *et al.*, 1993; Weinstock *et al.*, 1993). The possibility of intrafamilial transmission has been suggested on the basis of HCV antibody detection in a family of two persons (Kamitsukasa *et al.*, 1989).

The incubation period following infection varies from 6 to 8 weeks (Teo, 1992). The clinical manifestations of hepatitis C infection are non-specific and include fatigue, malaise and nausea, with only about 5% of patients developing acute jaundice (Girakar *et al.*, 1993). The disease may be mild and go unnoticed by the infected person (Griffiths-Jones, 1994), with patients recovering spontaneously and completely (Smith, 1993).

However, up to 50% of patients develop chronic active hepatitis and 20% progress to cirrhosis. Infection with hepatitis C also appears to be associated with cancer of the liver (Mims *et al.*, 1993).

Diagnosis of acute hepatitis C infection is established by the presence of antibodies to hepatitis C (anti-HCV IgG) in the blood. Results are confirmed by recombinant immunoblot assay (Department of Health, 1995).

Cases should be referred to a specialist in liver disease for evaluation, observation and care. This may involve liver biopsy and liver function tests. Patients considered to be at risk of progressive liver disease may be offered anti-viral interferon therapy, which reduces the incidence of serious long-term disease (Davis *et al.*, 1989). Although between 40% and 80% of patients show an initial response to interferon, the response is sustained in only about 50% of cases. Response rates depend on the patient's hepatitis C genotype (Department of Health, 1995).

Transfusion services in the UK began to screen for antibodies to HCV in September 1991 (Department of Health, 1995). The screening programme is likely to have a considerable positive effect on the prevention of post-transfusion HCV infection (Teo, 1992). It is estimated that 1 in 2000 blood donors in the UK may have been anti-HCV positive when screening was introduced (Communicable Disease Report, 1995). Recipients of blood or blood components from donors now known to be carriers of HVC are being traced with the view to providing counselling, testing and referral to a specialist, if appropriate.

Transmission of hepatitis C virus following percutaneous exposure to blood has been documented (Marranconi *et al.*, 1992). Follow-up care for health care workers who report accidents involving patients with hepatitis C includes anti-HCV testing 3 and 6 months after the exposure. Routine anti-HCV testing of patients whose HCV status is not known is not routinely recommended unless a significant percutaneous incident has occurred. The routine use of human immunoglobulin or hepatitis B immunoglobulin as prophylaxis for HCV infection is not recommended, as there is no published evidence to suggest that such prophylaxis is of value, and documented instances exist where it has failed to prevent the spread of HCV infection (Public Health Laboratory Service Hepatitis Sub-committee, 1993).

Nursing care for the patient infected with hepatitis C is the same as for patients with hepatitis B (see Guidelines: Hepatitis B, above).

References and further reading

Bresters, D. *et al.* (1993) Sexual transmission of hepatitis C. *Lancet*, 342, 210–11.

Communicable Disease Report (1995) Hepatitis C and blood transfusion. *Communicable Disease Report*, 5(3), 1. Public Health Laboratory Service Communicable Disease Surveillance Centre.

Crowe, H. M. (1994) Forum: a perspective on hepatitis. *Asepsis*, 16(2), 13–17.

Davis, G. L. *et al.* (1989) Treatment of chronic hepatitis C with recombinant interferon-alpha: a multicenter randomized, controlled trial. *New England Journal of Medicine*, 321, 1501–1506.

Department of Health (1995) *Hepatitis C and blood transfusion look back. PL CMO (95)1.* Department of Health, London.

Girakar, A. *et al.* (1993) Hepatitis C virus: when to suspect, how to detect. *Journal of Critical Illness*, 8, 1287–95.

Griffiths-Jones, A. (1994) Hepatitis revisited. *Nursing Times*, 90(46), *Journal of Infection Control Nursing*, S4–S8.

Kamitsukasa, H. *et al.* (1989) Intrafamilial transmission of hepatitis C virus. *Lancet* 1, 987.

Marranconi, F. *et al.* (1992) HCV infection after accidental needlestick injury in health care workers. *Infections*, 20, 111.

Mims, C. A. *et al.* (1993) *Medical Microbiology*, Mosby, London.

Public Health Laboratory Service Hepatitis Sub-committee (1993) Hepatitis C virus: guidance on the risks and current management of occupational exposure. *Communicable Disease Report Review*, 3(10), R135–R139.

Smith, J. P. (1993) Hepatitis C: a major public health problem. *Journal of Advanced Nursing*, 18(3), 503–506.

Teo, C. G. (1992) The virology and serology of hepatitis: an overview. *Communicable Disease Report*, 2(10), R109–R114.

Weinstock, H. S. *et al.* (1993) Hepatitis C virus infection among patients attending a clinic for sexually transmitted diseases. *Journal of the American Medical Association*, 269(3), 392–4.

HEPATITIS D

Definition

Hepatitis D virus (HDV), also referred to as Delta Virus (Mims *et al.*, 1993), is a new human pathogen which is always associated with hepatitis B virus (HBV) and causes both fulminane hepatitis and the accelerated progression of pre-existing HBV hepatitis (Monjardino *et al.*, 1990).

REFERENCE MATERIAL

Hepatitis D is uncommon in the UK and USA, but common in parts of South America and Africa. Worldwide it is present in about 5% of HBV carriers (Mims *et al.*, 1993).

HDV is a very small RNA virus which can only multiply in a cell which is infected with hepatitis B as it is dependent on HBV for its surface antigens (Barbara & Contreras, 1990). HDV is transmitted in the same way as HBV (Crowe, 1994).

HDV has a relatively short incubation period of 3–6 weeks (Teo, 1992). Infection with HBV or HDV results in a more severe and symptomatic illness than infection with HBV (Crowe, 1994). It has been suggested that high dose interferon-alpha may be beneficial in chronic HDV infection, although relapses can occur (Farci *et al.*, 1994).

Diagnosis relies on the detection of HDV antibody in serum (Centers for Disease Control, 1990). Prevention is based on vaccination (Mims *et al.*, 1993).

Presenting symptoms and nursing care are the same as for hepatitis B (see Hepatitis B, above).

References

Barbara, J. A. J. & Contreras, M. (1990) Infectious complica-

tions of blood transfusions. *British Medical Journal*, 300, 450–53.
Centers for Disease Control (1990) Protection against viral hepatitis. *Morbidity and Mortality Weekly Report*, 39(RR2), 1–26.
Crowe, H. M. (1994) Forum: perspective on hepatitis. *Asepsis*, 16(2), 13–17.
Farci, P. *et al.* (1994) Treatment for chronic hepatitis D with interferon alpha-2a. *New England Journal of Medicine*, 330, 88–94.
Mims, C. A. *et al.* (1993) *Medical Microbiology.* Mosby, London.
Monjardino, J. P. *et al.* (1990) Delta hepatitis. The disease and the virus, *British Medical Bulletin*, 46, 2, 399–407.
Teo, C. G. (1992) The virology and serology of hepatitis: an overview. *Communcable Disease Report*, 2(10), R109–R114.

HEPATITIS E

Definition
Hepatitis E is the term given for enterically transmitted non-A, non-B, hepatitis, producing a self-limiting disease resembling hepatitis A, although chronic liver disease and persistent viraemia has not been observed.

REFERENCE MATERIAL
Hepatitis E is an RNA virus, which has caused outbreaks of infection involving tens of thousands of cases in developing countries of the world, particularly China, India, Burma and Kyrgyzston (Bradley, 1992). Cases in Western countries are associated with foreign travel (Centers for Disease Control, 1993), with young to middle-aged people primarily affected. A distinguishing characteritic of this disease is a high mortality of about 20% in pregnant women (Crowe, 1994), with disseminated intravascular coagulation during the third trimester (Mims *et al.*, 1993).

Hepatitis E is transmitted by faecally contaminated drinking water or by contact with a faecally contaminated environment (Viswanathan, 1957), with a low secondary attack rate occurring among exposed household members. This indicates that person to person transmission is uncommon. The incubation period ranges between 2 and 9 weeks, with an average of 6 weeks (Teo,

1992). The virus is eliminated from the body on recovery, which prevents carriage of the virus (Mims *et al.*, 1993).

Diagnosis is made by detecting HEV antibody in serum (Tilton, 1994). Very little is known about the virus, but it is considered to be unstable, which may account for the difficulty in producing a clear profile of the virus (Bradley, 1990).

Barrier nursing is necessary for patients with hepatitis E infection.

References and further reading
Bradley, D. W. (1990) Enterically transmitted non-A non-B hepatitis. *British Medical Bulletin*, 46(2), 442–61.
Bradley, D. W. (1992) Hepatitis E: epidemiology, etiology and molecular biology. *Review of Medical Virology*, 2, 19.
Centers for Disease Control (1993) Hepatitis E among US travellers, 1989–1992. *Morbidity and Mortality Weekly Report*, 42, 1–4.
Crowe, H. M. (1994) Forum: a perspective on hepatitis. *Asepsis*, 16(2), 13–17.
Mims, C. A. *et al.* (1993) *Medical Microbiology.* Mosby, London.
Teo, C. G. (1992) The virology and serology of hepatitis: an overview. *Communicable Disease Report*, 2(10), R109–R114.
Tilton, R. C. (1994) Forum: a perspective on hepatitis. *Asepsis*, 16(2), 18–22.
Viswanathan, R. (1957) Infectious hepatitis in Delhi 1955–56. A critical study epidemiology. *Ind. J. Med. Res.* (supplement), 45, 1–30.

HEPATITIS F

Definition
Hepatitis F is the name given to a recently discovered hepatitis causing virus, thought to be a hepatitis B virus mutant (Uchida *et al.*, 1994a).

REFERENCE MATERIAL
The introduction of sensitive molecular biology techniques has revealed the existance of a non-A, non-B, non-C, non-D, non-E hepatitis, named hepatitis F (Fagan, 1994). It appears to cause acute and chronic liver disease (Uchida *et al.*, 1994b). Much remains to be learned about this virus. Nursing care is as for hepatitis B.

References

Fagan, E. A. (1994) Acute liver failure of unknown pathogenesis: the hidden agenda. *Hepatology*, 19(5), 1307–12.

Uchida, T. *et al.* (1994a) Silent hepatitis B virus mutants are responsible for non-A, non-B, non-C, non-D, non-E hepatitis. *Microbiology and Immunology*, 38(4), 281–5.

Uchida, T., Shimojima, M., Gotoh, K., Shikata, T. & Mima, S. (1994b) Pathology of livers infected with silent hepatitis B virus mutant. *Liver*, 14(5), 251–6.

THE HERPES VIRUSES

There are four human herpes viruses which cause infection. These are detected more frequently in immunocompromised people than in immunologically intact individuals (Kedzierski, 1991). The four types are:

(1) Cytomegalovirus (CMV).
(2) Epstein–Barr virus (EBV).
(3) Herpes simplex virus (HSV).
(4) Varicella zoster virus (VZV).

CYTOMEGALOVIRUS (CMV)

Definition

Cytomegalovirus (CMV) is a herpes virus which causes a transient infectious mononucleosis-like syndrome, often in childhood (Horowitz, 1986). Later in life, especially in the immunosuppressed person, the infection can reactivate, causing viraemia, fever and sometimes hepatitis and pneumonitis (Pomeroy & Englund, 1987).

REFERENCE MATERIAL

CMV is distributed widely throughout the world, mostly among those from the lower socioeconomic groups (Krech *et al.*, 1981), and homosexual males are known to have high rates of CMV seropositivity (Drew *et al.*, 1981). Increased rates of CMV infection can be found in children in group day care and institutions (Pass *et al.*, 1984).

There are many strains of CMV, with identical strains found in individuals connected with one another. Babies born with congenital CMV infection, for example, have the same strain as their mother (Griffiths, 1991). Reinfection can also occur (Ryan *et al.*, 1995), probably because of CMV's antigenic diversity (Alford & Britt, 1993).

CMV infection can be acquired by intrauterine, perinatal (Stagno *et al.*, 1986), intrafamilial and sexual transmission (Handfield *et al.*, 1985) as well as following blood transfusion (Hersman *et al.*, 1982) or transplantation (Peterson *et al.*, 1980). Approximately 50% of the population in the UK carry the antibody to CMV. Consequently, many people are capable of transmitting the infection through blood donation. Those most recently infected appear to be more likely to do so (Barbara, 1990).

During primary infection, the virus can be isolated from saliva, tears, urine, breast milk, blood, semen and cervical secretions (Pomeroy *et al.*, 1987). After initial infection, the virus establishes a latent infection thought to be in the lymphocytes. The latent infection may subsequently reactivate with production of infectious virions. Reactivation is generally controlled by the host's cell-mediated immune response. Hence, CMV infection is common in immunocompromised people (Meyers *et al.*, 1986), particularly patients with AIDS (Weller, 1993).

Approximately 1% of all babies have congenital CMV infection, and 90–95% of these infants are asymptomatic. Some infants with asymptomatic symptoms at birth may have sensorineural hearing loss (Stagno *et al.*, 1977) and others may have mild learning disabilities (Hanshaw *et al.*, 1976). CMV-associated morbidity has been seen in both full-term (Kumar *et al.*, 1984) and pre-term infants (Yeager *et al.*, 1983).

Patients with malignancies, or those receiving chemotherapeutic therapies, transplantation of kidney (Chou, 1986), heart (Hofflin *et al.*, 1987) or bone marrow (Meyers *et al.*, 1988), have a high risk of contracting CMV disease, including CMV pneumonia, hepatitis, pancreatitis, colitis, mononucleosis, retinitis and encephalitis (Rubin *et al.*, 1979). Diagnosis of CMV is by cell culture from lung, liver and kidney tissue, as well as from urine and blood. Alternatively tissue immunofluoresence, complement fixation and enzyme linked immunosorbent assay can be used to detect antibody to CMV (Pomeroy & Englund, 1987).

Treatment of active CMV infection using acyclovir, vidarabine, ganciclovir and alpha-interferon has been used as therapy in immunosuppressed patients. However, mortality remains high (Meyers *et al.*, 1988).

Prevention relies on decreasing the risk of virus acquisition and reactivation. Therefore, blood products used should either derive from CMV seronegative donors or be free from viable leucocytes, which can be achieved by irradiating or washing the blood product (Rubin *et al.*, 1979).

Transmission of CMV within the hospital setting from seropositive patients to seronegative patients (Spector, 1983), and staff (Lipscomb *et al.*, 1984) has been seen but is thought to be low (Adler, 1986; Adler *et al.*, 1986). Routine blood and body fluid precautions are essential to maintain these numbers at their low level.

Patients with CMV infection generally do not require barrier nursing as they feel ill and do not mix closely with other patients. Therefore, patient-to-patient transmission is unlikely.

References and further reading

Adler, S. P. (1986) Nosocomial transmission of cytomegalovirus. *Pediatric Infectious Disease*, 5(2), 239–46.

Adler, S. P. *et al.* (1986) Molecular epidemiology of cytomegalovirus in a nursery: lack of evidence for nosocomial transmission. *Journal of Pediatrics*, 108, 117–23.

Alford, C. A. & Britt, W. J. (1993) Cytomegalovirus. In: *The Herpes Viruses*, (eds B. Roizman, R. J. Whitley & C. Lopez). Raven Press, New York.

Barbara, J. (1990) Microbiology in the national blood transfusion service. *Public Health Laboratory Service Microbiology Digest*, 7(1), 4–7.

Chou, S. (1986) Acquisition of donor strains of cytomegalovirus by renal transplant recipients. *New England Journal of Medicine*, 314, 1418–23.

Drew, W. L. *et al.* (1981) Prevalence of cytomegalovirus infection in homosexual men. *Journal of Infectious Diseases*, 143, 188.

Griffiths, P. D. (1991) Advances in the prevention and treatment of cytomegalovirus infection in hospital patients. *Journal of Hospital Infection*, 18, Supplement A, 330–34.

Handfield, H. N. *et al.* (1985) Cytomegalovirus infection in sex partners – evidence for sexual transmission. *Journal of Infectious Diseases*, 151, 344–8.

Hanshaw, J. B. *et al.* (1976) School failure and deafness after silent congenital cytomegalovirus infection. *New England Journal of Medicine*, 295, 468–70.

Hersman, J. *et al.* (1982) The effect of granulocyte transfusion on the incidence of CMV infection after allogenic marrow transplantation. *Annals of International Medicine*, 96, 149–52.

Hofflin, J. M. *et al.* (1987) Infectious complications in heart transplant recipients receiving cyclosporine and corticosteroids. *Annals of International Medicine*, 106, 209–16.

Horowitz, C. A. *et al.* (1986) Clinical and laboratory evaluation of cytomegalovirus in previously healthy individuals. *Medicine*, 65, 124–33.

Kedzierski, M. (1991) Diseases of the herpes viruses. *Nursing Standard*, 5(31), 28–32.

Krech, U. *et al.* (1981) A collaborative study of cytomegalovirus antibodies in mothers and young children in 19 countries. *Bull. WHO*, 59, 605–10.

Kumar, M. L. *et al.* (1984) Postnatally acquired cytomegalovirus infection in infants of CMV-excreting mothers. *Journal of Paediatrics*, 104, 669.

Lipscomb, J. A. *et al.* (1984) Prevalence of cytomegalovirus antibody in nursing personnel. *Infection Control*, 5(11), 513–18.

Meyers, J. D. *et al.* (1986) Risk factors for cytomegalovirus infection after human marrow transplantation. *Journal of Infectious Diseases*, 153, 478–88.

Meyers, J. D. *et al.* (1988) Infection complicating bone marrow transplantation. In: *Clinial Approach to Infection in the Compromised Host*, (eds R. H. Rubin & L. S. Young), pp. 525–55. Plenum Medical Books, New York and London.

Pass, R. F. *et al.* (1984) Increased frequency of cytomegalovirus infection in children in group day care. *Paediatrics*, 74, 121–6.

Peterson, P. K. *et al.* (1980) Cytomegalovirus disease in renal allograft recipients: a prospective study of the clinical features, risk factors and impact on renal transplantation medicine. *Medicine*, 59, 283–300.

Pomeroy, C. & Englund, J. A. (1987) Cytomegalovirus epidemiology and infection control. *American Journal of Infection Control*, 15(3), 107–19.

Pomeroy, C. *et al.* (1987) Cytomegalovirus epidemiology and infection control. *American Journal of Infection Control*, 15, 107–19.

Rubin, R. H. *et al.* (1979) Summary of workshop on cytomegalovirus infection during organ transplantation. *Journal of Infectious Diseases*, 139, 728–34.

Ryan, M. *et al.* (1995) Cytomegalovirus infection in England and Wales, 1992 and 1993. *Communicable Disease Report*, 5(5), R74–R76.

Spector, S. A. (1983) Transmission of cytomegalovirus among infants in hospital documented by restriction-endonuclease-digestion analyses. *Lancet*, 2, 378–81.

Stagno, S. *et al.* (1977) Auditory and visual defects resulting from symptomatic and subclinical congenital cytomegalovirus and toxoplasma infections. *Paediatrics*, 59, 669–78.

Stagno, S. *et al.* (1986) Primary cytomegalovirus infection in pregnancy. *Journal of the American Medical Association*, 256, 1904–8.

Weller, I. V. D. (1993) Treatment and infections and antiviral agents. In: *ABC of AIDS*, (ed. M. W. Adler), 3rd edn. British Medical Journal Publishing Group, London.

Yeager, A. S. *et al.* (1983) Sequelae of maternally derived cytomegalovirus infection in premature infants. *Journal of Paediatrics*, 102, 918.

EPSTEIN–BARR VIRUS

Definition

Epstein–Barr virus (EBV) is a herpes virus which causes infectious mononucleosis.

REFERENCE MATERIAL

EBV primary infection in childhood is usually asymptomatic, although occasional cases have been seen to resemble chronic active hepatitis (Lloyd-Still *et al.*, 1986). In adolescence, approximately 50% of cases are accompanied by fever, malaise, pharyngitis and lymphadenopathy (Hoagland, 1960). In people over 40 years of age, infection can be accompanied by abdominal pain and fever (Horowitz *et al.*, 1983).

EBV can persist in the host and reactivate at a later time, particularly during immunosuppression (Crawford *et al.*, 1981), commonly following transplantation

(Strauch *et al.*, 1974) or in people with cancer or leukaemia (Lange *et al.*, 1978). Initially, EBV replication appears to take place in epithelial cells of the nasopharynx (Sixbey *et al.*, 1984) followed by infection of B lymphocytes. The incubation period between exposure and clinical manifestation in normal people varies from 30 to 50 days.

EBV is found in the saliva (Sixbey *et al.*, 1984) and on the cervix (Sixbey *et al.*, 1986), and can be transmitted by kissing and sexual contact, and rarely by blood transfusion (McMonigal *et al.*, 1983). Diagnosis relies on serological methods that detect the presence of IgG and IgM antibodies to EBV viral capsid antigen (Wielaard *et al.*, 1988).

EBV infection in healthy people is generally self-limiting with spontaneous recovery. Interferon, acyclovir and dihydroxy-2-propoxy-methyl guanine (DHPG) treatment for immunosuppressed patients is being investigated (Hirsch, 1988).

Barrier nursing is not necessary for EBV infection, but the patient should avoid kissing and sexual contact while symptoms persist. The patient's personal hygiene articles must not be shared.

References and further reading

Crawford, D. H. *et al.* (1981) Long-term T cell-mediated immunity to Epstein-Barr virus in renal allograft recipients receiving cyclosporin A. *Lancet*, 1, 10–13.

Hirsch, M. S. (1988) Herpes group virus infections in the compromised host. In: *Clinical Approach to Infection in the Compromised Host*, (eds R. H. Rubin & L. S. Young), pp. 347–66. Plenum Medical Books, New York and London.

Hoagland, R. J. (1960) The clinical manifestation of infectious mononucleosis. A report of 200 cases. *American Journal of Medical Science*, 240, 55–63.

Horowitz, C. A. *et al.* (1983) Infectious mononucleosis in older patients aged 40 to 72 years. Report of 27 cases including 3 without hyeterophile antibody response. *Medicine*, 62, 256–62.

Lange, B. *et al.* (1978) Longitudinal study of Epstein-Barr virus antibody titre and excretion in paediatric patients with Hodgkin's disease. *International Journal of Cancer*, 22, 521–7.

Lloyd-Still, J. D. *et al.* (1986) The spectrum of Epstein-Barr virus hepatitis in children. *Paediatric Pathololgy*, 5, 337–51.

McMonigal, K. *et al.* (1983) Post-perfusion syndrome due to Epstein-Barr virus. Report of 2 cases and review of the literature. *Transfusion*, 23, 331–5.

Sixbey, J. W. *et al.* (1984) Epstein-Barr virus replication in oropharyngeal epithelial cells. *New England Journal of Medicine*, 310, 1225–30.

Sixbey, J. W. *et al.* (1986) A second site for Epstein-Barr virus shedding the uterine cervix. *Lancet*, 2, 1122–4.

Strauch, J. W. *et al.* (1974) Oropharyngeal excretion of Epstein-Barr virus by renal transplant recipient and other patients treated with immunosuppressive drugs. *Lancet*, 1, 234–7.

Wielaard, F. *et al.* (1988) Development of an antibody-capture IgM enzyme-linked immunosorbent assay for diagnosis of acute Epstein-Barr virus infection. *J. Virol. Meth.*, 21, 105–15.

HERPES SIMPLEX VIRUS (HSV)

Definition

HSV causes a range of infections, from painful vesicular lesions (cold sores) to life-threatening illness in the immunocompromised patient (Goodall, 1992). It has an affinity for the skin and nervous system.

HSV has two presentations:

(1) HSV 1 infections (oral herpes or cold sores) tend to occur on the face or lips. However, primary infection can occur in the conjunctiva, where it causes conjunctivitis and keratitis; in the fingers, where it causes herpetic whitlow; and in the mouth where it causes herpes gingivomatitis (Arvin & Prober, 1991).
(2) HSV 2 infections (herpes genitalis or genital herpes) are usually limited to the genital region (Corey *et al.*, 1983). However, both types of herpes can be contracted either genitally or orally.

REFERENCE MATERIAL

Herpes simplex infections are world-wide in distribution. HSV 1 usually infects children between the ages of 2 and 10 years. Latent infection is then lifelong (Kedzierski, 1991). Transmission is primarily by contact with oral secretions. HSV 1 is chiefly responsible for perioral, ocular and encephalitic infections in adults. HSV 2 is spread by genital contact. Statistical information about HSV 2, and a number of other sexually transmitted diseases, is passed to the Department of Health by clinics specializing in these diseases (Barlow & Sherrard, 1992). HSV 2 is the major cause of penile vesicular lesions, cervicovaginitis and proctitis, as well as neonatal disseminated disease (Hirsch, 1988).

Recurrent infection occurs frequently, generally as a result of reactivation of the virus, since HSV 1 may become latent within the trigeminal sensory nerve ganglion, and HSV 2 within the corresponding sacral ganglion (Mims & White, 1984). Infection or reactivation in the normal host tends to be a mild, self-limiting disease (Kedzierski, 1991). The reactivated disease tends to be less severe than the primary infection (Williams, 1994). In most cases there are prodromal symptoms such as burning and tingling sensations before blisters appear (Goodall, 1992).

Individuals who are immunocompromised are susceptible to more severe presentations of HSV infections. Examples include: organ transplant recipients (Rubin, 1993); patients receiving cytotoxic chemotherapy for cancer (Muller *et al.*, 1972); people with congenital or acquired cellular immune defects (Seigal *et al.*, 1981); burns patients (Foley *et al.*, 1970); people with skin disorders (Wheeler *et al.*, 1966); and people with AIDS (Drew *et al.*, 1988). In an individual with no other cause of underlying immunodeficiency, but with laboratory evidence of the presence of HIV, chronic mucocutaneous HSV infection for longer than one month is diagnostic of AIDS (Centers for Disease Control, 1987).

HSV infection in immunosuppressed patients can produce large, chronic ulcerated lesions (Herpes phagenda). In addition, HSV 2 can cause severe perianal and rectal damage (although this is primarily found in homosexual men with AIDS) (Stine, 1993), diffused interstinal pneumonitis, oesophagitis. The liver, adrenals (Hirsch, 1988) gastrointestinal tract and central nervous system can be involved and may persist for some months to years (Hirsch, 1988).

Transmission of HSV is by direct contact with oral, genital or oro–genital secretions. One means of minimizing the risk of infection is to avoid contact with infected lesions. Gloves are essential for all health care staff in direct contact with lesions. The use of condoms is advisable to minimize the risk of transmission during sexual intercourse (Corey *et al.*, 1983b).

Caesarean section for women with clinically apparent cervical or genital infection prevents transmission of the infection to the infant (Corey *et al.*, 1983b), provided that sound infection control measures are adopted by the mother when handling the child. Caesarean section should be performed before the rupture of the membranes (Kedzierski, 1991).

Diagnosis
Mucocutaneous HSV infections are often easily recognizable. Visceral involvement is more difficult to identify. Confirmation of diagnosis is obtained by isolation of the virus in cell culture, and by an increase in antibody levels (Mims *et al.*, 1993).

Therapy
The majority of infections in normal hosts resolve spontaneously. For the immunocompromised patient, prompt treatment with antiviral chemotherapy reduces morbidity and the risk of serious complications. Oral, intravenous and topical preparations of acyclovir are available. The choice of route of administration, dose and duration of treatment depends on the nature and severity of the infection (Mims *et al.*, 1993).

Nursing care
Barrier nursing is essential in cases of extensive infection with herpes virus. Psychological support may be required (Williams, 1994). Studies have shown that 50%
of people with recurrent herpes infection experience depression, 15% have suicidal thoughts and 10% avoid sexual relationships (Chandiok, 1992). Goodall (1992) suggests that these effects may be a result of insufficient information and understanding of the true nature of HSV infection.

References and further reading
Arvin, A. M. & Prober, C. G. (1991) Herpes simplex viruses. In: *Manual of Clinical Microbiology*, (eds A. Balows *et al.*), 5th edn., pp. 822–8. American Society for Microbiology, Washington.

Barlow, D. & Sherrard, J. (1992) Sexually transmitted diseases. *Public Health Laboratory Service Microbiology Digest*, 9(3), 129–31.

Centers for Disease Control (1987) Revision of the CDC surveillance case definition for Acquired Immunodeficiency Syndrome. *Morbidity and Mortality Weekly Report*, 36, 15.

Corey, L. *et al.* (1983a) Genital herpes simplex virus infection. Clinical manifestations, cause and complications. *Annals of Internal Medicine*, 98, 958–72.

Corey, I. *et al.* (1983b) Genital herpes simplex virus infection. Current concepts in diagnosis, therapy and prevention. *Annals of Internal Medicine*, 98, 973–83.

Chandiok, S. (1992) The GP's role in the management of viral STDs. *Journal of Sexual Health*, 1(1), 32–3.

Drew, W. L. *et al.* (1988) Herpes virus infections. In: *The Management of AIDS*, (eds M. A. Sande & P. A. Volberding). W. B. Saunders, London.

Foley, F. D. *et al.* (1970) Herpes virus infection in burns patient. *New England Journal of Medicine*, 282, 652–6.

Goodall, B. (1992) A recurring problem. *Nursing* 5(5), 23–4.

Hirsch, M. S. (1988) Herpes group virus infection in the compromised host. In: *Clinical Approach to Infection in the Compromised Host*, (eds R. H. Rubin & L. S. Young), 2nd edn., pp. 347–66. Plenum Medical Books, New York and London.

Kedzierski, M. (1991) Diseases of the herpes viruses. *Nursing Standard*, 5(31), 28–32.

Mims, C. A. & White, D. O. (1984) *Viral Pathogenesis and Immunology*. Blackwell Scientific Publications, Oxford.

Mims, C. A. *et al.* (1993) *Medical Microbiology*, Mosby, London.

Muller, S. A. *et al.* (1972) Herpes simplex infections in hematologic malignancies. *American Journal of Medicine*, 52, 102–14.

Rubin, R. H. (1993) Infectious disease complications of renal transplantation. *Kidney International*, 44, 221–36.

Seigal, E. P. *et al.* (1981) Severe acquired immunodeficiency in male homosexuals, manifested by chronic perianal ulcerative herpes simplex lesions. *New England Journal of Medicine*, 305, 1439–44.

Stine, G. J. (1993) *AIDS Update 1993*. Prentice Hall, New Jersey.

Wheeler, C. E. *et al.* (1966) Eczema herpeticum: primary and recurrent. *Archives of Dermatology*, 93, 162–73.

Williams, K. (1994) Fact or fiction. *Nursing Times*, 90(3), 38–41.

VARICELLA ZOSTER VIRUS (VZV)

Definition

Initial infection with VZV causes varicella (chicken pox). Following clinical recovery, the virus persists in the latent form in the dorsal root ganglia of nerves; reactivation of the latent VZV causes zoster (shingles) (Mims *et al.*, 1993).

REFERENCE MATERIAL

The varicella incubation period is 11–21 days. The infected individual is infectious for two days before the rash appears and remains so until all the lesions have healed. Initial entry of VZV is unclear, although the respiratory tract, skin or conjunctiva are likely possibilities. Following local replication, the virus will be carried by the bloodstream to other sites. Recovery from varicella in a fit person is usually spontaneous and without sequelae (Mims *et al.*, 1993).

In the immunocompromised child, a much more serious presentation occurs. Visceral dissemination and death is not uncommon in children with cancer. When peripheral blood lymphocyte counts are below 500/mm³, the mortality rate is 7%–30% (Fieldman *et al.*, 1975). Varicella may be especially severe in transplant recipients, particularly among children who have received bone marrow grafts. In these patients the motality rate for untreated varicella is 35% (Atkinson *et al.*, 1979). In the immunocompromised patient visceral involvement involving the lung usually occurs three to seven days after the onset of skin lesions. Neurological complications occur less commonly and generally present 4–8 days after the onset of rash, and often indicate a poor prognosis. The liver is less commonly involved (Hirsch, 1989).

The diagnosis of chicken pox can usually be made from the characteristic pattern of vesicles. Treatment of varicella is normally only necessary for immunosuppressed patients, and involves the use of antiviral agents such as acyclovir, which reduces time of new lesion formation, fever and visceral complications.

Immunosuppressed children without a history of varicella and, in some cases, children with a history of varicella, but who are currently on high-dose chemotherapy, should receive varicella zoster immunoglobulin (VZIg) when exposed to varicella or zoster. To be effective, VZIg must be administered as soon after exposure as possible (Wisnes, 1978), which will give protection for approximately 4 weeks. Second cases of chicken pox in healthy people are extremely rare. However, among the immunosuppressed, second cases have been seen to occur and are often referred to as atypical disseminated zoster or varicelliform zoster. They do not have dermatomal distribution (Dolin *et al.*, 1978).

Every year, about four in every 1000 people suffer an attack of zoster (Milbourn, 1989). It is thought that zoster appears when cell-mediated immunity fails to curtail virus reactivation. This may happen as a result of age, the side-effects of drugs, or disease. The virus reactivates randomly in the nerve ganglion and spreads down the peripheral nerve producing vesicular skin lesions at the site supplied by the affected neurons (Mims *et al.*, 1993).

Cancer patients are particularly susceptible to zoster, which is more common during advance stage disease and develops more frequently at areas of regionalized tumour and/or localized radiotherapy. Most cases of zoster occur within the first year after diagnosis of cancer, although no single chemotherapeutic regimen or agent has been consistently implicated (Dolin *et al.*, 1978).

Patients with AIDS or AIDS-related complex (ARC) appear to be at increased risk of zoster; the incidence of zoster in an HIV antibody positive person appears to be a sign for the development of AIDS (Melbye *et al.*, 1987).

People who have not been infected with VZV can acquire varicella from individuals infected with varicella or zoster. However, there is little evidence to support the view that in healthy people, zoster can be contracted by exposure to zoster or varicella (Dolin *et al.*, 1978).

Neuralgia often proclaims the onset of zoster and can occur several days before skin signs occur. Erythematous patches are the first sign. They progress to macules then to papules and finally to vesicles. New outbreaks of vesicles continue in untreated persons for some time (Couillard-Getreuer, 1982). Fever, headaches and malaise can accompany the rash (Mims *et al.*, 1993). The vesicles generally correspond in distribution to one or more sensory nerves. Secondary bacterial infection of the lesions can develop (Hirsch, 1988). To minimize the risk of infection, care must be taken not to break the vesicles. Daily hygiene must be meticulous. Dissemination of zoster in an immunosuppressed patient generally occurs 6–10 days after the onset of localized lesions and is usually limited to cutaneous involvement, with occasional involvement of the central nervous system (CNS), lung, heart or gastrointestinal tract (Jemsek *et al.*, 1983).

Chicken pox during the first year of life predisposes to zoster infections in childhood. The incidence of childhood zoster is five times greater following infection with varicella at 0–2 months (Baba *et al.*, 1986). This is presumed to be a result of immunological immaturity (Craddock-Watson, 1990). A small number of cases of childhood zoster occur in children who themselves have no history of varicella, but whose mothers had the disease during the third to seventh months of pregnancy (Brunell Kotchmar, 1981). Maternal varicella immediately pre- and post-partum can lead to neonatal varicella, in most cases a mild clinical form of the disease (Craddok-Watson, 1990). More than 30 cases of infants with major abnormalities following varicella in the first 20 weeks of pregnancy have been described (Higa *et al.*, 1987).

The diagnosis of zoster can be made from the typical picture and distribution of the lesions. Confirmation can be obtained from virology culture of vesicle fluid. Treatment involves the use of antiviral agents such as acyclovir, which should begin within 72 hours of lesion formation. Adverse reactions to acyclovir and VZV resistance to acyclovir have been reported (Gnann & Whitley, 1991). Herpetic neuralgia and healing time will be shortened, although scarring may result in severe zoster (Balfour *et al.*, 1983). Prompt treatment of the eye if it is in any way involved is essential (Dolin *et al.*, 1978).

Nursing care

Only staff who have had varicella should have contact with patients with varicella or zoster. Barrier nursing is essential (see the beginning of this chapter). The door of the room must be kept closed to minimize airborne transmission of the virus (Josephson & Gombert, 1988).

References and further reading

Atkinson, M. K. *et al.* (1979) Analysis of late infections in 89 long-term survivors of bone marrow transplantation. *Blood*, 53, 720–31.

Baba, K. *et al.* (1986) Increased incidence of Herpes zoster in normal children infected with Varicella zoster during infancy. *Journal of Pediatrics*, 108, 372–7.

Balfour, H. H. *et al.* (1983) Acyclovir halts progression of herpes zoster in immune-compromised patients. *New England Journal of Medicine*, 308, 1448–53.

Brunel, I. P. A. & Kotchmar G. S. (1981) Zoster in infancy: failure to maintain virus latency following intrauterine infection. *Journal of Pediatrics*, 98, 71–3.

Couillard-Getreuer, D. L. (1982) Herpes zoster in the immunocompromised patient. *Cancer Nursing*, 10, 361–70.

Craodock-Watson, J. E. (1990) Chickenpox in pregnancy. *Public Health Laboratory Service Microbiology Digest*, 7(2), 40–45.

Dolin, R. *et al.* (1978) Herpes zoster varicella infections in immunosuppressed patients. *Annals of Internal Medicine*, 89, 374–88.

Fieldman, S. *et al.* (1975) Varicella in children with cancer. *Paediatrics*, 56, 388–97.

Gnann, J. W. & Whitley, R. J. (1991) Natural history and treatment of Varicella zoster in high-risk patients. *Journal of Hospital Infection*, 18, Supplement A, 317–29.

Higa, K. *et al.* (1987) Varicella zoster virus infection during pregnancy: hypothesis concerning the mechanism of congenital malformation. *Obstetrics and Gynecology*, 69, 214–22.

Hirsch, M. S. (1988) Herpes group virus infection in the compromised host. In: *Clinical Approach to Infection in the Compromised Host*, (eds R. H. Rubin & L. S. Young), 2nd edn, pp. 347–66. Plenum Medical Books, New York and London.

Jemsek, J. *et al.* (1983) Herpes zoster-associated encephalitis in immunosuppressed patients. *Annals of Internal Medicine*, 89, 375–88.

Josephson, A. & Gombert, M. E. (1988) Airborne transmission of nosocomial varicella from localized zoster. *Journal of Infectious Diseases*, 158(1), 238–41.

Melbye, M. *et al.* (1987) Risk of AIDS after herpes zoster. *Lancet*, 1, 728–31.

Milbourn, S. (1989) Caring for patients with herpes zoster ophthalmicus. *Professional Nurse*, January, 186–7.

Mims, C. A. *et al.* (1993) *Medical Microbiology*. Mosby, London.

Wisnes, R. (1978) Efficacy of zoster immunoglobulin in prophylaxis of varicella in high-risk patients. *Acta Paediatr. Scand.*, 67, 77–82.

LEGIONNAIRE'S DISEASE

Definition

Legionnaire's disease is an acute bacterial pneumonia caused by infection with *Legionella pneumophilia*.

REFERENCE MATERIAL

In the summer of 1976 an outbreak of pneumonia occurred among about 5000 people who had attended an American Legion convention in Philadelphia. There were 182 cases and 29 deaths. The epidemic aroused enormous public interest. Epidemiological investigations showed that the focus was the lobby of a famous hotel, but the cause remained unidentified for months until a small Gram-negative organism was found, which subsequently became known as *Legionella pneumophilia* (Fraser *et al.*, 1977).

Since 1976 at least 34 additional species, comprising 53 different serogroups, have been isolated from a range of environmental sites including lakes, rivers, soils and man-made water systems such as cooling towers and water distribution systems (Cooper, 1991). The latter two sites have been responsible for numerous outbreaks of legionnaire's disease, which have occurred mainly during June to October (Center for Disease Control, 1978). Since 1987 countries in Europe have collaborated in surveillance of legionnaires' disease. Over 50 clusters of travel related disease have been reported. Many cases are associated with Mediterranean countries, reflecting the large numbers of holidaymakers from across Europe who visit the area (Public Health Laboratory Service, 1994).

Up to 30% of sporadic cases of hospital acquired pneumonias are caused by legionnella (Hart & Makin, 1991). The pattern of infection is unique. The outbreaks are site specific and associated with factors which predispose to infection, including water systems contaminated with the organism. *Legionella pneumophilia* is a thermophile which flourishes at temperatures from 25 to 42°C and can survive a range of temperatures from 5 to 58°C. However, it is unusual for this organism to proliferate in temperatures of below 20°C (Health and Safety Executive, 1991). The most critical temperature is 36°C. Every effort should be made to avoid stagnant water conditions and to store and supply water outside this critical temperature (Harper, 1986).

Legionella is ubiquitous in surface water. It multiplies in warm water, particularly in 'dead ends' and loops in plumbing systems where sludge has formed. This predisposes to proliferation of the organism, providing ideal conditions and the opportunity for the organism to grow and cause infection (Health and Safety Executive, 1991).

Legionnaires' disease is not a notifiable disease, but since 1977 the Communicable Disease Surveillance Centre has maintained a surveillance programme of cases reported voluntarily by medical microbiologists. Between 1980 and 1990 an average of 188 cases were seen each year (Health and Safety Executive, 1992).

The major route of infection is by aerosal dispersion and inhalation of the bacteria from, for example, shower heads (Alderman, 1988), or more commonly by air conditioning systems where the organism may multiply in the water of cooling towers. When water from these sources evaporates, droplets containing *Legionella* may be drawn into the air intakes of the building or fall on people passing by.

Virulence is coupled to a susceptible host. The disease tends to affect males, by a factor of 2 or 3 to 1. Those who smoke or consume excess alcohol, people who are already immunocompromised and the elderly are all predisposed to infection (Stout, 1987).

The incubation period is about 2–10 days following first exposure. The signs and symptoms include malaise, general aches and headache, diarrhoea and vomiting, followed by high temperature, cough, rigors and respiratory distress. Some patients do not develop pneumonia but progress to profound septicaemia with confusion, symptoms of diplopia and mental confusion (Potterton, 1985).

Diagnosis relies on laboratory diagnosis by:

(1) Isolation of the causative organism.
(2) Demonstration of the presence of the organism, its antigen or its products in the patient's body fluids or tissues (Harrison, 1985).
(3) Demonstration of specific antibodies directed against the organism, its antigens or its products (Harrison, 1985).

Coupled to the clinical picture and chest X-ray findings, treatment includes the antibiotic erythromycin (Center for Disease Control, 1978) with supportive therapy for complications as they arise, which may include pulmonary failure, shock and acute renal failure. Person-to-person spread has never been demonstrated (Hart & Makin, 1991) and therefore barrier nursing is not required. However, careful disposal of sputum and encouraging patients to cover their mouth and nose when coughing are necessary precautions.

Prevention relies on regular inspection and maintenance of the water system, including planning, installation and commissioning (Finch, 1988). Each case of nosocomial legionnaires' disease must be investigated to ensure that the outbreak has been contained (Fallon, 1994).

References and further reading

Alderman, C. (1988) The cooler culprits. *Nursing Standard*, 2(33), 22.

Center for Disease Control (CDC) (1978) Legionnaire's disease, diagnosis and management. *Annals of Internal Medicine*, 88, 363–5.

Cooper, J. (1991) Positive discrimination. *Laboratory Practice*, 40(1), 16–17.

Fallon, R. J. (1994) How to prevent an outbreak of legionnaires' disease. *Journal of Hospital Infection*, 27, 247–56.

Finch, R. (1988) Minimizing the risk of Legionnaire's disease. *British Medical Journal*, 296, 1343–5.

Fraser, D. W. *et al.* (1977) Legionnaire's disease: description of an epidemic of pneumonia. *New England Journal of Medicine*, 297, 1189–97.

Harper, D. (1986) Legionnaire's disease: prevention better than cure. *Health and Safety at Work*, March, 41–6.

Harrison, T. G. (1985) A nasty family from Philadelphia. *Medical Laboratory World*, September, 19–23.

Hart, C. A. & Makin, T. (1991) Legionella in hospitals: a review. *Journal of Hospital Infection*, 18, Supplement A, 481–9.

Health and Safety Executive (1991) *The Control of Legionellosis including Legionnaires' Disease.* HMSO, London.

Health and Safety Executive (1992) *Joint Health and Safety Executive and Department of Health Working Group on Legionellosis.* HMSO, London.

Potterton, D. (1985) Mystery of the organism. *Nursing Times*, 82(22), 20–21.

Public Health Laboratory Service (1994) European surveillance of legionnaires' disease associated with travel. *Communicable Disease Report*, 4(6), 25.

Stout, J. E. (1987) Legionnaire's disease acquired within the homes of two patients. *Journal of the American Medical Association*, 257(9), 1215–17.

LISTERIOSIS

Definition

Listeriosis is an infectious disease caused by *Listeria monocytogenes*. Listeria is a Gram-positive bacterium with widespread distribution in the environment, including soil, dust and vegetation (Watkins *et al.*, 1981). It inhabits the gastrointestional tract of animals and humans, who remain symptomless (Botsen-Moller, 1972).

REFERENCE MATERIAL

The genus Listeria includes many types which are non-pathogenic to man. *Listeria monocytogenes* is recognized as being the cause of listeriosis in man (Lamont *et al.*, 1988).

Growth of this organism is optimal at 37°C but it will survive and multiply at a range of 26–42°C, and is not easily inactivated by environmental influences such as freezing, thawing and strong sunlight (Gray, 1963). Instances of human infection are increasing (McLauchlin, 1988), particularly among immunocompromised people.

The fetus and the newborn are especially prone to infection due to the immaturity of their immune systems. In the UK, there is about one incidence in every 9700 of perinatal listeriosis births (McLauchlin, 1987). Maternal symptoms are often absent, and neonatal listeriosis presents as meningitis or occasionally as septicaemia (Gill, 1988). Abortion and stillbirths due to listeriosis have been reported (MacNaughton, 1962). Infection in immunocompromised adults varies from a mild, chill-like illness to bacteraemia, septicaemia and meningitis.

Treatment

Ampicillin is usually regarded as the drug of choice (Trautman *et al.*, 1985), often in combination with gentamicin (Azimi *et al.*, 1979). However, even with prompt antibiotic therapy, mortality may be as high as 30% in patients with other serious underlying conditions.

The mode of transmission can be via sexual contact, following localization in both male and female genital tracts (Gray, 1960). However, contaminated food is becoming increasingly important as a vehicle of spread (McLaughlin & Gilbert, 1990). There are increasing reports of listeria found in raw meat, fruit and vegetables which predispose to contamination of, for example, coleslaw. An outbreak involving coleslaw prepared from contaminated cabbage involved seven adults and 34 newborn babies in Canada (Schlech *et al.*, 1983). Prepared mixed salads have a much higher rate of contamination than individual salad ingredients, probably because prepared salads are contaminated during the chopping, mixing and packaging process (Valani & Robert, 1990).

Prevention entails scrupulous preparation of cooked food for immunocompromised people and the avoidance of uncooked foods. Person-to-person transmission during normal contact is unlikely. However, careful disposal of blood fluids and thorough handwashing after contact with the patient is essential.

References and further reading

Azimi, P. H. *et al.* (1979) *Listeria monocytogenes*. Synergistic effects of ampicillin and gentamicin. *American Journal of Clinical Pathology*, 72, 974–7.

Botsen-Moller, J. (1972) Human listeriosis, Diagnostic epidemiological and clinical studies. *Acta. Pathol. Microbiol. Scand.* (Suppl.), 229, 1–57.

Gill, P. (1988) Is listeriosis often a food-borne illness? *Journal of Infection*, 17, 1–5.

Gray, M. L. (1960) Genital listeriosis as a cause of repeated abortions. *Lancet*, 2, 315–17.

Gray, M. L. (1963) Epidemiological aspects of listeriosis. *American Journal of Public Health*, 53, 554–63.

Lamont, R. J. *et al.* (1988) *Listeria monocytogenes* and its role in human infection. *Journal of Infection*, 17, 7–28.

MacNaughton, M. C. (1962) *Listeria monocytogenes* in abortion. *Lancet*, 11, 484.

McLauchlin, J. (1987) *Listeria monocytogenes*: recent advances in the taxonomy and epidemiology of listeriosis in humans. *J. Appt. Bacteriol.*, 63, 1–11.

McLauchlin, J. (1988) Listeriosis and food-borne transmission. *Lancet*, 1, 177–8.

McLaughlin, J. & Gilbert, R. J. (1990) Listeria in food. *Public Health Laboratory Service Microbiology Digest*, 7(3), 54–5.

Schlech, W. F. *et al.* (1983) Epidemic listeriosis. Evidence of a transmission by food. *New England Journal of Medicine*, 308, 203–6.

Trautman, M. *et al.* (1985) Listeria meningitis: report of 10 cases and review of current therapeutic recommendations. *Journal of Infection*, 10, 107–14.

Valani, S. & Robert, D. (1990) *Listeria monocytogenes* and other listeria spp. in pre-packed mixed salads and individual salad ingredients. *Public Health Laboratory Service Microbiology Digest*, 8(1), 21–2.

Watkins, J. *et al.* (1981) Isolation and enumeration of *Listeria monocytogenes* from sewage, sewage study and river water. *J. Appt. Bacteriol.*, 5, 1–9.

PNEUMOCYSTOSIS

Definition
Pneumocystosis is an infection caused by the organism *Pneumocystis carinii*.

REFERENCE MATERIAL
Pneumocystis carinii was first discovered in 1909 and was associated with outbreaks of pneumonia in people subjected to malnutrition and overcrowding (Radman, 1973). The organism has been recognized as being an important cause of pneumonia in the immunocompromised host for over 20 years. Three types of patients have been particularly affected:

(1) Patients of all ages receiving immunosuppressive agents for the treatment of cancer and during organ transplantation (Walzer *et al.*, 1973).
(2) Children and infants with primary immunodeficiency disorders, particularly severe combined immunodeficiency (SCID) (Gajdusek, 1957).
(3) Patients with acquired immune deficiency syndrome (AIDS), particularly in patients whose blood CD_4 T lymphocytes are below $200/mm^3$ of blood (Phair *et al.*, 1990). (CD_4 is an antigenic marker of helper T cells.)

Most epidemiological studies have focused on clusters of cases within hospitals, orphanages or private clinics. All have a common denominator of overcrowding, protein calorie malnutrition, prematurity or immunosuppressive disease, predisposing to *Pneumocystis carinii* pneumonia. These studies give the impression of outbreaks of infection, when no spread has actually occurred; rather the disease probably occurred from reactivation of latent infection triggered by immunosuppression (Dutz, 1970).

Watanable and colleagues (1965) reported a cluster of infection in a family of three. A healthy woman developed fatal *Pneumocystis carinii* pneumonia several days before her husband who had acute lymphatic leukaemia, and who also died. Their 7-year-old daughter had had a typical respiratory disease 2 months before her parents' illness. Although she recovered, she may have transmitted the disease to her non-immune parents, suggesting that person-to-person or airborne transmission is possible among immunologically naive subjects.

Pneumocystis carinii infections associated with deprivation in children are reported to be slow and insidious in onset, with initial non-specific signs of restlessness, lethargy, poor feeding over a period of weeks, resulting in tachypnoea, severe dyspnoea, use of accessory muscles for breathing, marked cyanosis and exhausting nonproductive cough (Perera *et al.*, 1970).

Children and adults with underlying disease such as neoplasm often experience an abrupt onset of illness, with high lever, tachypnoea and cough, which can progress to a fatal outcome even with treatment (Walzer, 1970).

Until recently, diagnosis has relied upon the demonstration of organisms in either open lung or transbronchial biopsy, although considerable controversy surrounds these invasive procedures because of the potential complications of haemorrhage and pneumothorax. Fibreoptic bronchoscopy or bronchial washings are now favoured because of the increase of *Pneumocystis carinii* infection among AIDS patients, where large numbers of organisms are generally present in bronchial secretions, sputum and transtrachial aspirations. Unfortunately, if such specimens yield negative results, open lung biopsy may have to be undertaken expeditiously, before the patient deteriorates further. Survival is related directly to the aggressiveness with which the diagnosis is pursued in the early stages of disease and with the early institution of appropriate therapy (Young, 1984).

Treatment is by pentamidine intramuscularly, daily for 14 days; although longer therapy may be necessary for more recalcitrant infections. Major side-effects can be experienced (Pearson *et al.*, 1985).

Other treatment includes the use of trimethoprim sulphamethoxazole given orally or intravenously. However, the cumulative toxicity from both individual components has made this drug the most toxic of all anti-pneumocystis treatments (Wharton *et al.*, 1986). Oral trimethoprim sulphamethoxazole is generally given prophylactically to severely immunocompromised patients when discharged from hospital. It is continued for the duration of their immunosuppression, and discontinued on improvement of immuological function and/or a decrease in therapeutic immunosuppression (Ruskin, 1989).

Aerosolized pentamidine prophylaxis has significantly improved prognosis for patients with AIDS (Miller *et al.*, 1989). However, a real concern has emerged that the use of aerosolized pentamidine has predisposed patients to disseminated disease, which has been reported with increased frequency; for example, *Pneumocystis carinii* thyroiditis (Galland, 1988), otitis media, mastoiditis (Gherman, 1988), choroidopathy (Friedberg *et al.*, 1990), gastrointestinal (Carter *et al.*, 1988), hepatic (Poblete *et al.*, 1989) and splenic disease (Pilon *et al.*, 1987). This indicates that the systemic absorption of aerosolized pentamidine is minimal, allowing *Pneumocystis carinii* to infect extrapulmonary sites. Therefore, patients receiving aerosolized prophylaxis must be monitored carefully for signs of disseminated disease (Dubé & Sattler, 1993).

Hospitalized patients who develop *Pneumocystis*

carinii pneumonia may well be cared for in areas where there are large concentrations of immunosuppressed patients. Due to the reports of clustering of this disease and the difficulty of distinguishing whether this represents person-to-person spread, patients with a productive cough should be placed in a single room until the cough improves. Precautions other than careful hand washing following patient contact are unnecessary.

References and further reading

Carter, T.-R. *et al.* (1988) *Pneumocystis carinii* infection of the small intestine in a patient with acquired immunodeficiency syndrome. *American Journal of Clinical Pathology*, 89, 679–83.

Dubé, M. & Sattler, F. R. (1993) Prevention and treatment of opportunistic infections. *Current Opinion in Infectious Disease*, 6, 230–36.

Dutz, W. (1970) *Pneumocystis carinii* pneumonia. *Path. Ann.*, 5, 309.

Friedberg, D.-N. *et al.* (1990) Asymptomatic dissemination *Pneumocystis carinii* infection detected by ophthalmoscopy. *Lancet*, 2, 1256–7.

Gajdusek, D. C. (1957) *Pneumocystis carinii* etiologic agent of interstitial plasma cell pneumonia of young and premature infants. *Paediatrics*, 19, 543.

Galland, J. E. (1988) *Pneumocystis carinii* thyroiditis. *American Journal of Medicine*, 84, 303–6.

Gherman, C. R. (1988) *Pneumocystis carinii* otitis media and mastoiditis as the initial manifestation of the acquired immunodeficiency syndrome. *American Journal of Medicine*, 85, 250–2.

Miller, R. F. *et al.* (1989) Nebulized pentamidine as treatment for *Pneumocystis carinii* pneumonia in the acquired immunodeficiency syndrome. *Thorax*, 44, 565–9.

Pearson, R. D. *et al.* (1985) Pentamidine for the treatment of *Pneumocystis carinii* pneumonia and other protozoan diseases. *Annals of Internal Medicine*, 103, 782–6.

Perera, D. R. *et al.* (1970) *Pneumocystis carinii* pneumonia in a hospital for children. *Journal of the American Medical Association*, 214, 1074–8.

Phair, J. *et al.* (1990) The risk of *Pneumocystis carinii* pneumonia among men infected with human immune deficiency virus type 1. *New England Journal of Medicine*, 322, 161–5.

Pilon, V. A. *et al.* (1987) *Pneumocystis carinii* infection in AIDS. *New England Journal of Medicine*, 316, 1410–11.

Poblete, R. B. *et al.* (1989) *Pneumocystis carinii* hepatitis in the acquired immunodeficiency syndrome. *American Journal of Internal Medicine*, 110, 737–8.

Radman, J. C. (1973) *Pneumocystis carinii* pneumonia in an adopted Vietnamese infant. *Journal of the American Medical Association*, 230, 1561–3.

Ruskin, J. (1989) Parasitic disease in the compromised host. In: *Clinical Approaches to Infection in the Compromised Host*, (eds R. H. Rubin & L. S. Young), 2nd edn. Plenum Medical Book Company, London.

Walzer, P. D. *et al.* (1973) *Pneumocystis carinii* pneumonia and primary immune deficiency disease in infancy and childhood. *Journal of Paediatrics*, 82, 416–22.

Walzer, P. D. (1970) *Pneumocystis carinii* infection. Review article. *Southern Medical Journal*, 70(11), 1330–33.

Watanable, J. M. *et al.* (1965) *Pneumocystis carinii* pneumonia in a family. *Journal of the American Medical Association*, 193, 113.

Wharton, M. *et al.* (1986) Trimethoprim sulphamethoxazole or pentamidine for *Pneumocystis carinii* pneumonia in the acquired immunodeficiency syndrome. *Annals of Internal Medicine*, 105, 37–44.

Young, L. S. (1984) Clinical aspects of pneumocystosis in man. In *Pneumocystis carinii Pneumonia*, (ed. L. S. Young), pp. 139–74. Marcel Dekker, New York.

TUBERCULOSIS

Definition

Tuberculosis is a destructive infectious disease caused by *Mycobacterium tuberculosis*. Other species of mycobacterium which cause infection are referred to as 'atypical' mycobacteria (Mims *et al.*, 1993).

REFERENCE MATERIAL

Mycobacterium tuberculosis is an acid-fast bacillus. It is acid-fast because of a waxy material in the cell wall, which resists simple laboratory staining techniques unless treated with hot carbol fuchsin, which allows impregnation by the dye. This is retained despite attempts to decolourize it with acid or alcohol (Mims *et al.*, 1993).

Mycobacteria are distributed widely throughout the world, and only a few species are pathogenic to man, such as *Mycobacterium tuberculosis*, whose main host is man, and *Mycobacterium bovis*, the bovine type of tubercle bacillus, which is pathogenic to man as well as to cattle. This causes characteristically chronic granulamatous lesions, mainly in the lungs, but the glands, bones, joints, brain and meninges and other internal organs may be affected (Alvarez *et al.*, 1984).

Studies have shown that the prevalence of mycobacteria infection is six times greater in patients with cancer than in patients who do not have cancer. Lung cancer was the most common neoplasm in patients with mycobacteria infection (Ortbals, 1978).

There are also three atypical mycobacteria associated with patients who are severely immunocompromised due to human immunodeficiency virus (HIV) infection. These are: *Mycobacterium avium intracellulare*, *M. xenopi* and *M. kansasii*. In the past, these types rarely caused disease in man, but now cause a disease which quickly disseminates to most organs in the body

(Young *et al.*, 1986), and they are highly resistant to treatment.

Atypical mycobacteria are not highly adapted to humans like *Mycobacteria tuberculosis* and are not transmitted from person to person. They survive in the environment and pass from there to human hosts. Infection occurs when the atypical organisms are inhaled from the air, ingested with milk or inoculated through the skin. Atypical mycobacteria do not respond as readily to established tuberculosis drugs (Chaisson, 1993).

Worldwide, tuberculosis is the leading cause of death due to infectious disease. An estimated 8 million new cases and 3 million deaths occur annually (Marwick, 1993). Ninety-five per cent of all new cases occur in developing countries where the disease is frequently associated with infection with HIV (Joly *et al.*, 1993). The year on year decline in reported cases of tuberculosis in the UK ended in the late 1980s. Since then there has been a small annual rise in incidence (Watson, 1993). Factors which may have contributed to the observed increase in numbers of cases is improved reporting and the increased proportion of tuberculosis among Asian people (Hayward & Watson, 1995). Numbers may also have increased as a result of the association of tuberculosis with HIV (Drobniewski *et al.*, 1994). Approximately 5% of patients with AIDS develop tuberculosis (Watson, 1993).

Certain conditions predispose to the development of tuberculosis, including general physical debilitation and lowered resistance due to disease, immunosuppressive drugs and alcoholism. In addition, poor economic status and population groups such as Asians and those with little immunity, such as the very young and elderly are also susceptible (Drobniewski *et al.*, 1994). The mode of spread for tuberculosis is occasionally by ingestion, for example, by drinking infected milk, but principally by inhalation of small droplets produced by coughing. These droplets are probably the most effective vehicle of spread since they dry rapidly in the air to yield droplet nuclei of less than 5 nm in diameter which, when inhaled, can reach the alveoli. The organism can survive in moist or dried sputum for up to six weeks, but is killed by a few hours' exposure to direct sunlight (Loudon *et al.*, 1969).

Special attention must be given to equipment contaminated with mycobacterium species. Thorough cleaning followed by autoclaving is the sterilization method of choice. As certain equipment such as endoscopes can be damaged by autoclaving, disinfection must be used. A greater resistance by the organism to glutaraldehyde solution has been seen, and so thoroughly pre-cleaned equipment must be totally immersed for 60 minutes in a freshly prepared glutaraldehyde solution (Department of Health and Social Security, 1986).

Diagnosis

A provisional diagnosis can be based on microscopical findings of acid-fast bacilli in sputum, tissue, urine or cerebrospinal fluid, for example. This is termed smear positive. Confirmation and species identification by culture may take several weeks and is termed culture positive (Orobniewski *et al.*, 1994).

Patients with smear-positive pulmonary disease are infectious, those with smear-negative or non-pulmonary disease are not. Once appropriate combination chemotherapy has commenced (Skinner *et al.*, 1995), smear-positive people are considered non-infectious after two weeks of treatment (Subcommittee of the Joint Tuberculosis Committee of the British Thoracic Society, 1990).

Treatment

Treatment until the 1960s included bed rest and attention to diet but chemotherapy is now the preferred treatment. It involves the use of combination drugs designed to reduce viable bacteria as rapidly as possible in order to minimize the risk of ineffective treatment in those patients infected by drug-resistant bacteria (Cooke, 1985).

In the UK resistance to certain tuberculosis drugs is increasing. In New York, multi-drug-resistant tuberculosis is found in 20% of cases. This is thought to be due to the use of inappropriate combinations of drugs and the failure of some patients to complete their full course of treatment (Goldsmith, 1993). In the USA cases have been reported of transmission of *Mycobacterium tuberculosis* to patients and staff, including multi-drug-resistant strains (Pitchenik *et al.*, 1990; Centers for Disease Control, 1990). Outbreaks of hospital acquired multi-drug-resistant tuberculosis have been associated with mortality rates of 72–89% (Beck-Sage *et al.*, 1992). Deaths have occurred among health care staff in the USA who are believed to have contracted tuberculosis at work (Di Perri *et al.*, 1992).

Tuberculosis continues to be a notifiable disease under the revised Public Health Act, 1985. It is the responsibility of the Medical Officer for Environmental Health to follow up all contacts of infected people. This has proved to be a valuable and worthwhile procedure (British Thoracic and Tuberculosis Association, 1978). Generally, hospital staff are followed up by the hospital infection control officer in liaison with the hospital occupational health unit (Thornbury, 1985). The World Health Organization and the International Union Against Tuberculosis and Lung Disease have published two joint statements, one on the prevention of tuberculosis in people infected with HIV, and one on the prevention of the transmission of tuberculosis in health care settings in developing countries (WHO 1993a, b). Guidance in these statements reflects advice published by the British Thoracic Society in 1990 and 1992.

The priorities for tuberculosis control are early detection of cases, examination of contacts, barrier nursing if appropriate and immunization of tuberclenegative people with Bacillus Calmette-Guérin vaccine (BCG). It is recommended that BCG vaccination should be offered routinely in schools to children aged 10–14 years. This programme has been shown to be effective in preventing tuberculosis (Sutherland, 1987; Colditz et al., 1994).

Certain professions, for example, those working in hospitals, prisons, old people's homes and schools, should be screened on employment. This may include a tuberculin test and chest radiography (Jachuck, 1988) for staff who have not received BCG vaccination in the past. It is extremely uncommon for hospital staff in the UK to acquire tuberculosis from patients (Capewells et al., 1986). Staff in contact with untreated, smear-positive patients for a week or more should be reported to the occupational health department, and a chest X-ray arranged for 6 months' time. However, if the employee develops suspicious symptoms such as an unexplained cough lasting longer than 3 weeks, persistent fever or weight loss, then a full examination must be undertaken.

Nursing care
Patients who are smear positive must be barrier nursed until they have been taking combination drug therapy for at least 2 weeks. A longer period is necessary if drug resistant tuberculosis is suspected (Skinner et al., 1995).

Patients must be taught to cover their mouths when coughing to prevent droplet spread, and to wash their hands after coughing. Patients must expectorate into sputum pots with tight fitting lids. Pots must be changed, frequently.

In the USA, where drug-resistant tuberculosis is more common and health care staff are not routinely given BCG vaccine, the use of high efficiency particulate respirators when attending patients with suspected or confirmed tuberculosis is being discussed (Wilcox, 1995).

References and further reading

Alvarez, S. et al. (1984) Extrapulmonary tuberculosis revisited. A review of experience at Boston City and other hospitals. Medicine (Baltimore), 63, 25.

Ayliffe, G. A. J. et al. (1984) Chemical Disinfection in Hospital, p. 3. Public Health Laboratory Service, London.

Beck-Sage, C. et al. (1992) Hospital outbreak of multidrug resistant Mycobacterium tuberculosis infection: factors in transmission to staff and HIV-infected patients. Journal of the American Medical Association., 268, 1280–86.

British Thoracic and Tuberculosis Association (1975) Tuberculosis among immigrants related to length of residence in England and Wales. British Medical Journal, 3, 698–9.

British Thoracic and Tuberculosis Association (1978) A study of standardized contact procedure in tuberculosis. Tubercle, 59, 245–59.

Capewells, S. et al. (1986) Tuberculosis in the NHS – is it a problem? Thorax, 41, 708.

Centers for Disease Control (1990) Guidelines for preventing the transmission of tuberculosis in health care settings with special focus on HIV-related issues. Morbidity and Mortality Weekly Report, 39, Supplement RR-17, 1–29.

Centers for Disease Control (1993) Estimates of future global tuberculosis morbidity and mortality. Morbidity and Mortality Weekley Report, 42, 961–4.

Chaisson, R. (1993) Mycobacterial infections and AIDS. Current Opinion in Infectious Diseases, 6, 237–43.

Colditz, G. A. et al. (1994) Efficacy of BCG vaccine in the prevention of tuberculosis. Journal of the American Medical Association, 271, 698–702.

Cooke, N. J. (1985) Treatment of tuberculosis. British Medical Journal, 291, 497–8.

Department of Health and Social Security (1986) Safety Information Bulletin 28. DHSS, London.

Di Perri, G. et al. (1992) Transmission of HIV associated tuberculosis of health care workers. Lancet, 340(8820), 682.

Drobniewski, F. A. et al. (1994) Molecular biology in the diagnosis and epidemiology of tuberculosis. Journal of Hospital Infection, 28, 249–63.

Goldsmith, M. F. (1993) New reports make recommendations, ask for resources to stem TB epidemic. Journal of the American Medical Association, 269(2), 187–8, 191.

Hayward, A. C. & Watson, J. M. (1995) Tuberculosis in England and Wales 1982–1993; notification exceeded predictions. Communicable Disease Report Review, 5(3), R29–R32.

Jachuck, S. J. (1988) Is a pre-employment chest radiograph necessary for NHS employees? British Medical Journal, 296, 1187–8.

Joint Tuberculosis Committee of the British Thoracic Society (1990) Control and prevention of tuberculosis in Britain: an updated code of practice. British Medical Journal, 300, 995–9.

Joint Tuberculosis Committee of the British Thoracic Society (1992) Guidelines on the management of tuberculosis and HIV infection in the United Kingdom. British Medical Journal, 304, 1231–3.

Joly, V. et al. (1993) Mycobacterium tuberculosis infection. Current Science, 6, 171–8.

Loudon, R. G. et al. (1969) Cough frequency and infectivity in patient with pulmonary tuberculosis. American Review of Respiratory Disease, 99, 109–111.

Marwick, C. (1993) Resurgence of tuberculosis prompts US search for effective drugs, expanded research effort. Journal of the American Medical Association, 269(2), 191–5.

Mims, C. A. et al. (1993) Medical Microbiology. Mosby, London.

Ortbals, D. W. (1978) A comparative study of tuberculosis and mycobacterial infection and their associations with malignancy. *American Review of Respiratory Disease*, 117, 39.

Pitchenik, A. E. *et al.* (1990) Outbreaks of drug-resistant tuberculosis to health care workers and HIV infected patients in urban hospitals. *Morbidity and Mortality Weekly Report*, 39, 718–22.

Skinner, C. *et al.* (1995) *Control and Prevention of Tuberculosis in the United Kingdom: Code of Practice 1994.* Joint Tuberculosis Committee of the British Thoracic Society.

Subcommittee of the Joint Tuberculosis Committee of the British Thoracic Society (1990) Control and prevention of tuberculosis in Britain. An updated code of practice. *British Medical Journal*, 300, 995–9.

Sutherland, I. *et al.* (1987) Effectiveness of BCG vaccination in England and Wales in 1983. *Tubercle*, 68, 81–92.

Thornbury, G. (1985) TB or not TB. *Nursing Times*, 81(32), 43–4.

Watson, J. M. (1993) Tuberculosis in Britain today. *British Medical Journal*, 306, 221–2.

WHO (1993a) Tuberculosis preventive therapy in HIV-infected individuals. A joint statement of the World Health Organization Tuberculosis Programme and the Global Programme on AIDS, and the International Union Against Tuberculosis and Lung Disease. *Weekly Epidemiology Record*, 68(49), 361–4.

WHO (1993b) Control of tuberculosis transmission in health care settings. A joint statement of the World Health Organization Tuberculosis Programme and the International Union Against Tuberculosis and Lung Disease. *Weekly Epidemiology Record*, 68(50), 369–71.

Wilcox, M. H. (1995) Protection against hospital acquired tuberculosis. *Journal of Hospital Infection*, 29, 165–8.

Young, L. S. *et al.* (1986) Mycobacterial infection in AIDS patients with the emphasis on the *Mycobacterium* complex. *Review of Infectious Diseases*, 8, 1024–33.

CHAPTER 6
Bladder Lavage and Irrigation

Definitions

Lavage
Bladder lavage is the washing out of the bladder with sterile fluid.

Irrigation
Bladder irrigation is the continuous washing out of the bladder with sterile fluid.

Indications
Bladder lavage or irrigation is indicated for the following reasons:

Lavage
(1) To clear an obstructed catheter.
(2) To remove the potential souces of obstruction, e.g. blood clots or sediment from infection.

Irrigation
(1) To prevent the formation and retention of blood clots, e.g. following prostatic surgery.
(2) On rare occasions to remove heavily contaminated material from a diseased urinary bladder.

REFERENCE MATERIAL

Solutions used for lavage and irrigation
A number of solutions are available for cleansing the bladder and the selection of a particular solution will depend on its therapeutic properties in relation to the patient's needs.

0.9% sodium chloride is the agent most commonly recommended for lavage and irrigation and should be used in every case unless an alternative solution is prescribed. It is isotonic so it does not affect the body's fluid or electrolyte levels, therefore large volumes may be used as necessary. Three litre bags of saline are available for irrigation purposes.

Studies of water and saline (Harper & Matz, 1975,

1976) showed them to be the least erosive irrigating solutions when tested in rat bladders. Ferrie *et al.* (1979) and Blannin and Hobden (1980) recommended the use of tap water as a purely mechanical means of flushing out the catheter for patients at home. The use of large volumes of sterile water is not recommended, however, as its absorption through the bladder wall may increase the blood volume to unacceptable levels.

Bladder wash outs using antiseptic solutions in order to prevent, reduce or treat urinary tract infections have commonly been used but these have been found to be ineffective. The use of regular chlorhexidine bladder wash outs has been found to lead to the development and selection of resistant organisms (Walker & Lowes, 1985; Baillie, 1987). Davies *et al.* (1987) found the chlorhexidine lacked bactericidal effect in long-term catheterized patients and it can also cause haematuria and bladder erosion (Harper, 1981). Antiseptic solutions do not prevent or eradicate urinary infections in catheterized patients (Slade & Gillespie 1985; Kunin 1987). Therefore their use in long-term catheterized patients is not advocated (Stickler & Chawla, 1987; Stickler, 1990).

The use of bladder lavage to reduce or prevent catheter obstruction may be beneficial with certain patients (Brocklehurst & Brocklehurst, 1978; Ferrie *et al.*, 1979; Blannin & Hobden, 1980). Getliffe's (1994a) study attempted to identify characteristics of patients who were at greater risk of obstructing their catheters. Patients who 'blocked' their catheters were found to have high urinary pH and ammonia concentrations. High ammonia concentration and alkaline urine are found when urine is infected with urease producing micro-organisms, such as *Proteus mirabilis*. Significantly more females were classed as 'blockers', this may be due to the greater risks females have of developing catheter associated urinary infections (Kennedy *et al.*, 1983), as the shorter female urethra may allow more rapid colonization. 'Blockers' were also found to be significantly less mobile than 'non-blockers'. There was no significant relationship noted between non-blockers and high average daily fluid intake; this study therefore does not support the advice conventionally given to 'drink plenty' to reduce mineral precipitation.

Catheter encrustations

Catheter encrustations commonly consist of magnesium ammonium phosphate and calcium phosphate (Bruce *et al.*, 1974; Cox *et al.*, 1987) which precipitate from urine when it becomes alkaline during infection from urease secreting micro-organisms (Griffith & Musher, 1976).

A number of different solutions have been used to prevent or reduce instances of catheter blockage by encrustation of the catheter lumen:

- mandelic acid (1%) is used to prevent the growth of urease-producing bacteria by acidifying the urine;
- 6% citric acid solution is used to dissolve persistent crystallization in the bladder or catheter; and
- citric acid (3.23%) and magnesium oxide solution prevent and dissolve crystallization in the catheter or bladder (Waghorn *et al.*, 1988).

A study carried out by Kennedy *et al.* (1992) showed that citric acid solution with (Suby G) and without

magnesion oxide (solution R) administered twice weekly for 3 weeks did not have a demonstrable effect in preventing crystal formation. Getliffe's (1994b) *in vitro* study suggested that mandelic acid solution may be particularly effective in reducing encrustation. However, both researchers identify the need for further studies to be carried out in this area.

Potential damage to the bladder endothelium from bladder wash out reagents or from the physical effects of irrigation has been identified (Elliott *et al.*, 1989; Kennedy *et al.*, 1992). Reassessment of bladder irrigation methods and the indication for their use is therefore called for.

Cytotoxic agents given intravesically

For details on the administration of cytotoxic agents, see Chapter 13, Cytotoxic Drugs, section entitled Guidelines: Intravesical instillation of cytotoxic drugs.

Catheters used for irrigation

A three-way urinary catheter must be used for irrigation in order that fluid may simultaneously be run into, and drained out from, the bladder. This catheter is commonly passed in theatre when irrigation is required, e.g.

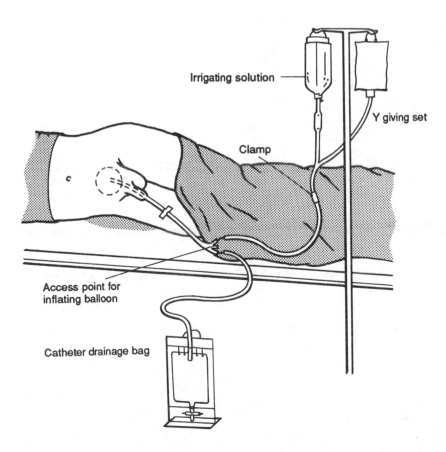

Irrigating solution

Y giving set

Clamp

Access point for inflating balloon

Catheter drainage bag

Figure 6.1 Closed urinary drainage system with provision for intermittent or continuous irrigation.

after prostatectomy (Maxfield *et al.*, 1994). Occasionally if a patient is admitted with a heavily contaminated bladder, e.g. blood clots, bladder irrigation may be started on the ward. If the patient has a two-way catheter, this must be replaced with a three-way type (Fig. 6.1).

It is recommended that a three-way catheter is passed if frequent intravesical installations of drugs or antiseptic solutions are prescribed and the risk of catheter obstruction is not considered to be very great. In such cases the most important factor is minimizing the risk of introducing infection and maintaining a closed urinary drainage system, for which the three-way catheter allows.

References and further reading

Baillie, L. (1987) Chlorhexadine resistance among bacteria isolated from urine of catheterised patients. *Journal of Hospital Infection*, 10, 83–6.

Blannin, J. & Hobden, J. (1980) The catheter of choice. *Nursing Times*, 76, 2092–3.

Brocklehurst, J. C. & Brocklehurst, S. (1978) Management of indwelling catheters. *British Journal of Urology*, 50, 102–5.

Bruce, A. W. *et* al. (1974) The problem of catheter encrustation. *Canadian Medical Association Journal*, 111, 238–41.

Cox, A. J. *et al.* (1987) Calcium phosphate in catheter encrustation. *British Journal of Urology*, 59, 159–63.

Datta, P. K. (1981) The post-prostatectomy patient. *Nursing Times*, 77, 1759–61.

Davies, A. J. *et al.* (1987) Does instillation of chlorhexidine into the bladder of catheterised geriatric patients help reduce bacteriuria? *Journal of Hospital Infection*, 9, 72–5.

Dudley, M. N. & Barriere, S. L. (1981) Antimicrobial irrigations in the prevention and treatment of catheter-related urinary tract infections. *American Journal of Hospital Pharmacy*, 38, 59–65.

Elliott, T. (1990) Disadvantages of bladder irrigation (in catheterized patients. Brief research report). *Nursing Times*, 86, 52.

Elliott, T. S. *et al.* (1989) Bladder irrigation on irritation? *British Journal of Urology*, 64, 391–4.

Ferrie, B. G. *et al.* (1979) Long-term urethral catheter drainage. *British Medical Journal*, 279, 1046–7.

Getliffe, K. A. (1994a) The characteristics and management of patients with recurrent blockage of long-term urinary catheters. *Journal of Advanced Nursing*, 20, 140–49.

Getliffe, K. A. (1994b) The use of bladder wash-outs to reduce urinary catheter encrustation. *British Journal of Urology*, 73, 696–700.

Gilbert, V. & Gobbi, M. (1989) Bladder irrigation (Principles and methods). *Nursing Times & Nursing Mirror*, 85, 40–2.

Gopal, R. G. & Elliott, T. S. (1988) Bladder irrigation. *Age and Ageing*, 17(6), 373–8.

Griffith, D. P. & Musher, O. N. (1976) Urease: the primary cause of infection induced urinary stones. *Investigative Urology*, 13(5), 346–82.

Harper, W. (1981) An appraisal of 12 solutions used for bladder irrigation or installation. *British Journal of Urology*, 53, 433–8.

Harper, W. & Matz, L. (1975) The effect of chlorhexidine irrigation of the bladder in the rat. *British Journal of Urology*, 47, 539–43.

Harper, W. & Matz, L. (1976) Further studies on effects of irrigating solutions on rat bladders. *British Journal of Urology*, 48, 463–7.

Kennedy, A. (1984) Trial of new bladder washout system. *Nursing Times*, 80, 48–51.

Kennedy, A. P. *et al.* (1983) Factors relating to the problems of long-term catheterization. *Journal of Advanced Nursing*, 8, 207–12.

Kennedy, A. P. *et al.* (1992) Assessment of the use of bladder washouts/instillations in patients with long term indwelling catheters. *British Journal of Urology*, 70, 610–15.

Kunin, C. M. (1987) *Detection, Prevention and Management of Urinary Tract Infections*, 4th edn. Lea and Febiger, Philadelphia.

Lowthian, P. (1991) Using bladder syringes sparingly. *Nursing Times*, 87(10), 61–4.

Macaulay, D. (1994) Urinary drainage systems. In: *Urological Nursing*, (ed. C. Laker). Scutari Press, Harrow.

Martindale, W. (1982) *The Extra Pharmacopoeia*, 28th edn. The Pharmaceutical Press, London.

Maxfield, J. *et al.* (1994) Prostatic problems. In: *Urological Nursing*, (ed. C. Laker). Scutari Press, Harrow.

Roe, B. H. (1989) Use of bladder washouts: a study of nurses' recommendations. *Journal of Advanced Nursing*, 14(6), 494–500.

Roe, B. (1990) The basis for sound practice. *Nursing Standard*, 4, 25–7.

Slade, N. & Gillespie, W. A. (1985) *The Urinary Tract and the Catheter – Infection and Other Problems*. John Wiley, Chichester.

Stickler, D. J. (1990) The role of antiseptics in the management of patients undergoing short term indwelling bladder catheterisation. *Journal of Hospital Infection*, 16, 89–108.

Stickler, D. J. & Chawla, J. C. (1987) The role of antiseptics in the management of patients with long term indwelling bladder catheters. *Journal of Hospital Infection*, 10, 219–28.

Stickler, D. J. *et al.* (1981) Some observations on the activity of three antiseptics used as bladder irrigants in the treatment of UTI in patients with indwelling catheters. *Paraplegia*, 19, 325–33.

Waghorn, D. J. *et al.* (1988) Urinary catheters. *British Medical Journal*, 296, 1250.

Walker, E. M. & Lowes, J. A. (1985) An investigation into in vitro methods for the detection of chlorhexadine resistance. *Journal of Hospital Infection* 6, 389–97.

Warren, J. *et al.* (1978) Antibiotic irrigation and catheter-associated urinary tract infection. *New England Journal of Medicine*, 299, 570–3.

GUIDELINES: BLADDER LAVAGE

EQUIPMENT

1 Sterile dressing pack.
2 Sterile bladder syringe, 60 ml.
3 Sterile jug.
4 Antiseptic solution.
5 Bactericidal alcohol hand rub.
6 Clamp.
7 New catheter bag (for balloon two-way catheter) or sterile spigot (for three-way catheter).
8 Sterile receiver.
9 Sterile solution for lavage.

PROCEDURE

Action	Rationale
1 Explain and discuss the procedure with the patient.	To ensure that the patient understands the procedure and gives his/her valid consent.
2 Screen the bed. Ensure that the patient is in a comfortable position allowing access to the catheter.	For the patient's privacy and to reduce the risk of cross-infection. Curtains are drawn at this stage so that dust and airborne organisms disturbed by the curtains do not settle on the sterile field.
3 Perform the procedure using an aseptic technique.	To prevent infection. (For further information on aseptic technique see Chapter 4.)
4 If necessary, draw up solutions using a 60 ml syringe, preferably with needle adapter. Cap the syringe and place it in a sterile receiver.	It is easier to draw up solutions from vials in the clinical area than at the bedside.
5 Take the trolley to the bedside, disturbing the screens as little as possible. Open the outer wrappings of packs and put them on the top shelf of the trolley.	To minimize airborne contamination. To begin to prepare equipment for procedure.
6 Prepare the sterile field. Pour the lavage solution into the sterile jug.	To prepare equipment for procedure.
7 Wash hands with a bactericidal alcohol hand rub.	To minimize the risk of infection.
8 Clamp the catheter. Place a sterile paper towel under the junction of the catheter and the tubing of the drainage bag and disconnect them.	To prevent leakage when the catheter is disconnected. To create a sterile field and reduce the risk of cross-infection. When the patient has a three-way catheter the drainage bag will not need disconnecting as the washout fluid is injected through the side-arm of the catheter. This should be spigoted off after use and the fluid remaining in the bladder will drain into the catheter bag.
9 Clean gloved hands with a bactericidal alcohol hand rub. Clean around the end of the catheter with sterile low-linting gauze and an antiseptic solution.	To remove surface organisms from gloves and catheter and thus reduce the risk of introducing infection into the catheter.

Guidelines: Bladder lavage (cont'd)

Action	Rationale
10 Draw up the irrigating fluid into the bladder syringe and insert the nozzle into the end of the catheter.	To prepare syringe for lavage.
11 Release the clamp on the catheter and gently inject the contents of the syringe into the bladder, trying not to inject air.	Rapid injection of fluid could be uncomfortable for the patient. Large volumes of air in the bladder cause distension and discomfort.
12 Remove the syringe and allow the bladder contents to drain by gravity into a receiver placed on a sterile towel.	To allow catheter to drain gently. To reduce risk of cross-infection.
13 Repeat steps 11 and 12 of the procedure until the washout is complete or the returning fluid is clear.	To ensure bladder is free of contaminants.
14 If the fluid does not return naturally, aspirate gently with the syringe.	Gentle suction is sometimes required to remove obstructive material from the catheter. If suction is applied too forcefully the urethelium may be sucked into the eyes of the catheter, preventing drainage and causing pain and trauma which may predispose to infection (Lowthian, 1991; Macauly, 1994).
15 Connect a new catheter bag or sterile spigot if a three-way catheter is in place, and allow the remaining fluid to drain out.	A closed drainage system must be re-established as soon as possible to reduce the risk of bacterial invasion through the catheter.
16 If the solution is to remain in the bladder, the catheter should be clamped when all the fluid has been injected and the clamp released after the desired period.	To allow solution to act on bladder mucosa/catheter.
17 Measure the volume of washout fluid returned and compare it with the volume of fluid injected. Record any discrepancies of volume in the appropriate documents.	To keep an accurate record of urinary output and to observe for catheter obstruction.
18 Make the patient comfortable, remove equipment, clean the trolley, and wash hands.	To reduce the risk of cross-infection.

As an alternative to the use of bladder syringe and irrigating solution, a pre-packed filled reservoir with sterile catheter adaptor called Uro-tainer is now available. Kennedy (1984) found that the use of Uro-tainer compared with traditional saline washout procedure produced a reduced incidence of urinary tract infection.

GUIDELINES: CONTINUOUS BLADDER IRRIGATION

EQUIPMENT

1 Sterile dressing pack.
2 Antiseptic solution.
3 Bactericidal alcohol hand rub.

4 Clamp.
5 Sterile irrigation fluid.
6 Disposable irrigation set.
7 Infusion stand.
8 Sterile jug.

PROCEDURE

Commencing bladder irrigation

Action	Rationale
1 Explain and discuss the procedure with the patient.	To ensure that the patient understands the procedure and gives his/her valid consent.
2 Screen the patient and ensure that he or she is in a comfortable position allowing access to the catheter.	For the patient's privacy and to reduce the risk of cross-infection. Curtains are drawn at this stage so that dust and airborne organisms disturbed by the curtains do not settle on the sterile trolley.
3 Perform the procedure using an aseptic technique.	To prevent infection. (For further information on aseptic technique, see Chapter 4.)
4 Open the outer wrappings of the pack and put it on the top shelf of the trolley.	To prepare equipment.
5 Insert the end of the irrigation giving set into the fluid bag and hang the bag on the infusion stand. Allow fluid to run through the tubing so that air is expelled.	To prime the irrigation set so that it is ready for use. Air is expelled in order to prevent discomfort from air in the patient's bladder.
6 Clamp the catheter.	To prevent leakage of urine through irrigation arm when spigot is removed.
7 Clean hands with a bactericidal alcohol hand rub. Put on gloves.	To minimize the risk of cross-infection.
8 Place a sterile paper towel under the irrigation inlet of the catheter and remove the spigot.	To create sterile field. To prepare catheter for connection to irrigation set.
9 Discard the spigot.	To prevent re-use.
10 Clean gloved hands with a bactericidal alcohol hand rub. Clean around the end of the irrigation arm with sterile low linting gauze and an antiseptic solution.	To remove surface organisms from gloves and catheter and to reduce the risk of introducing infection into the catheter.
11 Attach the irrigation giving set to the irrigation arm of the catheter. Keep the clamp of the irrigation giving set closed.	To prevent over-distension of the bladder, which can occur if fluid is run into the bladder before the drainage tube has been unclamped.
12 Release the clamp on the catheter tube and allow any accumulated urine to drain into the catheter bag. Empty the urine from the catheter bag into a sterile jug.	Urine drainage should be measured before commencing irrigation so that the fluid balance may be monitored more accurately.
13 Discard the gloves.	These will be contaminated, having handled the catheter bag.
14 Set irrigation at the required rate and ensure that fluid is draining into the catheter bag.	To check that the drainage system is patent and to prevent fluid accumulating in the bladder.

Guidelines: Bladder lavage (cont'd)

Action	Rationale
15 Make the patient comfortable, remove unnecessary equipment and clean the trolley.	
16 Wash hands.	To reduce the risk of cross-infection.

Care of the patient during irrigation

Action	Rationale
1 Adjust the rate of infusion according to the degree of haematuria. This will be greatest in the first 12 hours following surgery (average fluid input is 6–9 litres during the first 12 hours, falling to 3–6 litres during the next 12 hours). The aim is to obtain a drainage fluid which is rosè in colour.	To remove blood from the bladder before it clots and to minimize the risk of catheter obstruction and clot retention.
2 Check the volume in the drainage bag frequently when infusion is in progress, e.g. half-hourly or hourly, or more frequently as required.	To ensure that fluid is draining from the bladder and to detect blockages as soon as possible, also to prevent over-distension of the bladder and patient discomfort. Frequent checking means, in addition, that full catheter bags are noticed and can be emptied before they reach capacity.
3 Using rubber-tipped 'milking' tongs, 'milk' the catheter and drainage tube regularly, as required.	To remove unseen clots from within the drainage system and to maintain an efficient outlet.
4 Record the fluid balance chart accurately. The fluid balance of all patients having bladder irrigation must be monitored.	So that urine output is known and any related problems, e.g. renal dysfunction, may be detected quickly and easily.

BLADDER IRRIGATION RECORDING CHART

The bladder irrigation recording chart (Fig. 6.2) is designed to provide an accurate record of the patient's urinary output during the period of irrigation.

Procedure for the use of the chart

Record the time (column A) and the fluid volume in each bag of irrigating solution (column B) as it is put up.

When the irrigating fluid has all run from the first bag into the bladder, record the original volume in the bag in column C. Record the corresponding time in column A. Do not attempt to estimate the fluid volume run in while a bag is in progress as this will be inaccurate. If, however, a bag is discontinued, the volume run in can be calculated by measuring the volume left in the bag and deducting this from the original volume. This should be recorded in column C.

The catheter bag should be emptied as often as is necessary, the volume being recorded in column D and the corresponding time in column A. The catheter bag must also be emptied whenever the bag of irrigating fluid is empty, and the volume recorded in column D.

When each bag of fluid has run through, add up the total volume drained by the catheter in column D, and write this in red. Subtract from this the total volume run in (column C) to find the urine output (D − C = E). Write this in column E. Draw a line across the page to indicate that this calculation is complete and continue underneath for the next bag.

Patient name: Hospital no:

(A) Date and time	(B) Volume put up	(C) Volume run in	(D) Total volume out	(E) Urine	(F) Urine running total
10/7/96 10.00	2000				
10.30			700		
11.10			850		
11.40		2000	600		
			2150	150	150
11.45	2000				
12.30			500		
13.15			700		
14.20		2000	800		
			2400	400	550
14.25	2000				
15.30			850		
17.00	Irrigation stopped	1200	800		
			1650	450	1000

Figure 6.2 Bladder irrigation recording chart.

NURSING CARE PLAN

Problem	Cause	Suggested action
Fluid retained in the bladder when the catheter is in position.	Fault in drainage apparatus, e.g.	
	Blocked catheter.	'Milk' the tubing. Wash out the bladder with 0.9% sodium chloride.
	Kinked tubing.	Straighten the tubing.
	Overfull drainage bag.	Empty the drainage bag.
	Catheter clamped off.	Unclamp the catheter.
Distended abdomen related to an overful bladder during the irrigation procedure.	Irrigation fluid is infused at too rapid a rate.	Slow down the infusion rate.
	Fault in drainage apparatus.	Check the patency of the drainage apparatus.
Leakage of fluid from around the catheter.	Catheter slipping out of the bladder.	Insert the catheter further in. Decompress balloon fully to assess the amount of water necessary. Refill balloon until it remains *in situ*, taking care not to over fill beyond safe level (see manufacturer's instructions).

Nursing care plan (cont'd)

Problem	Cause	Suggested action
	Catheter too large or unsuitable for the patient's anatomy.	If leakage is profuse or catheter is uncomfortable for the patient, replace the catheter with one of smaller size.
Patient experiences pain during the lavage or irrigation procedure.	Volume of fluid in the bladder is too great for comfort.	Reduce the fluid volume within the bladder.
	Solution is painful to raw areas in the bladder.	Inform the doctor. Administer analgesia as prescribed.
Retention of fluid with or without distended abdomen, with or without pain.	Perforated bladder.	Stop irrigation. Maintain in recovery position. Call medical assistance. Monitor vital signs. Monitor patient for pain, tense abdomen.

For further details, see Chapter 45, Nursing care plan with the catheter in place.

CHAPTER 7

Bone Marrow Procedures

Definition

Bone marrow procedures involve the removal of haemopoietic tissue from the iliac crest, sternum and spinal processes using a special needle. In children aged less than 2 years the upper end of the tibia may be used (Dacie & Lewis, 1991).

Bone marrow procedures include the following:

(1) *Aspiration* Withdrawal of the bone marrow fluid. Tests performed on this sample include observation of haemopoiesis, cytology of cells and infiltrates, assessment of iron stores, cytochemistry and immunotyping (MIMS, 1994).
(2) *Trephine biopsy* Removal of a core of the bone including marrow. Tests performed on this sample include histological examination and assessment of marrow cellularity, classification of marrow infiltrates, diagnostic information where the aspirate is unsatisfactory and imprint preparations for cytology (MIMS, 1994).
(3) *Harvest* Withdrawal of bone marrow including stem cells for autologous and allogenic bone marrow transplantation or for cryopreservation.

Indications

Tests on the bone marrow are performed for haematological conditions where there is a decrease or increase in a blood element, e.g. anaemia, leukaemia and for diagnosis of diseases not primarily affecting the blood system, e.g. malignancies, infections and hereditary conditions (Monteil, 1987). The study of bone marrow in haematological diseases was first introduced by Arinkin in 1929.

REFERENCE MATERIAL

Anatomy and physiology

In early gestation the yolk sac is the primary area for haemopoiesis. From 6 to 7 months of fetal life through to adulthood the bone marrow is the only source of haemopoiesis (Monteil, 1987). The bone marrow is spe-cialized soft tissue filling the spaces in cancellous bone of the epiphyses (Mosby, 1994). It is one of the largest organs in the body representing 3.4–4.6% of the total body weight (Monteil, 1987).

Haemopoietic stem cells give rise to all haemopoietic cell lines. Stromal cells, fat cells and a microvascular network provide a suitable network for stem cell growth and development (Hoffbrand & Pettit, 1985). There are two types of bone marrow:

(1) Red bone marrow, which is responsible for haemopoeisis. It is found in the proximal epiphyses of the humerus and femur and in the sternum, ribs and vertebral bodies of adults (Mosby, 1994).
(2) Yellow bone marrow. This consists of fat cells, blood vessels, reticulum cells and fibres. Some of the fatty bone marrow is capable of reversion to haemopoeisis (Hoffbrand & Pettit, 1985).

The most common sites for obtaining bone marrow tissue are posterior iliac crest, sternum, anterior superior iliac crest and spinal processes (Monteil, 1987) (Fig. 7.1).

Aspiration and trephine biopsy

Patients may be anxious about the procedure and a mild sedative may be indicated. The procedure is performed under local anaesthetic, although due to the nature of the pain (often described as a dragging sensation) the actual aspiration may remain painful. The iliac crests are often used for patients requiring frequent marrow procedures as the use of the right and left crests can be alternated, both anterior and posterior surfaces may be used and there are no vital organs nearby that may be punctured by the procedure. The posterior iliac crest is often preferred as the procedure can then be performed outside the patient's field of vision.

Bone marrow harvest

Bone marrow harvests are performed under a general anaesthetic. This is done because:

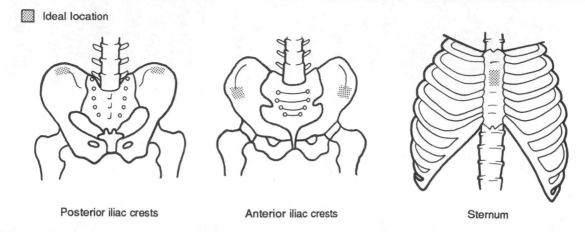

Ideal location

Posterior iliac crests   Anterior iliac crests   Sternum

Figure 7.1 Common sites for bone marrow examination, arranged in order of preference. Normally, only aspirations and not biopsies are done on the sternum because of its small size and proximity to vital organs.

(1) The procedure may last approximately 1 hour compared with the 5–15 minutes for an aspiration and biopsy.
(2) Multiple puncture sites are used and the patient may be approached from both sides.
(3) The procedure can be very painful.

A volume of 1 litre or more (dependent on the harvest cell count in relation to the recipient's body weight) is aspirated from multiple puncture sites. If large volumes of marrow are harvested the patient may require a blood transfusion. The marrow may be harvested for immediate use or may be cryopreserved for the future.

Contraindications
Bone marrow aspirate and trephine biopsy are contraindicated in those patients who are unable to co-operate or have a coagulation defect such as increased clotting time, unless this is correctable. Patients in extreme pain may not be able to adopt the lateral position for posterior iliac crest sampling. In this case the anterior iliac crest or, if biopsy is not needed, the sternum can be used (MIMS, 1994).

Complications
Complications are extremely rare but include the following:

(1) Cardiac tamponade. This is compression of the heart produced by the accumulation of blood or fluid in the pericardial sac. It can be caused by the rupture of a blood vessel in the myocardium caused by the aspirate or trephine needle. The actual risks associated with a sternal puncture are extremely small (Dacie & Lewis, 1991), especially with the use of a guarded needle.

(2) Haemorrhage. This occurs almost exclusively in those patients with thrombocytopenia. It may be avoided by applying adequate pressure to the puncture site for a few minutes following the procedure and by the administration of platelet transfusions where indicated.
(3) Infection, particularly in the neutropenic patient.
(4) Bone fractures, particularly in small children.

References and further reading
Abrahams, P. & Webb, P. (1975) *Clinical Anatomy of Practical Procedures.* Pitman Medical, London.
Arinkin, M. J. (1929) Intravitale Untersuchungsmethodik der Knochenmarks. *Folia Haematol (Leipz)*, 38, 233.
Ayliffe, G., Lowbury, E., Geddes, A. & Williams, J. (1992) *Control of Hospital Infection: A Practical Handbook*, 3rd edn. Chapman & Hall, London.
Bevan, J. (1978) *A Pictorial Handbook of Anatomy and Physiotherapy.* Mitchell Beazley, London.
Booth, J. A. (1983) *Handbook of Investigations.* Harper & Row, London.
Brunner, L. S. & Suddarth, D. S. (1982) *The Lippincott Manual of Medical-Surgical Nursing*, Vol. 2. Harper & Row, London.
Dacie, J. & Lewis, S. M. (1991) *Practical Haematology*, 7th edn. Churchill Livingstone, Edinburgh.
Frazer, I. & Gough, K. R. (1968) Bone marrow biopsy. In: *Biopsy Procedures in Clinical Medicine*, (ed. A. E. Read). John Wright, Bristol.
Henke, Y. C. (1990) Physiology of normal bone marrow. *Seminars in Oncology Nursing – Adult Leukaemia*, 6(1), 3–8.
Hoffbrand, A. & Pettit, J. (1985) *Essential Haematology*, 2nd edn. Blackwell Scientific Publications, Oxford.
Keele, C., Neil, E. & Joels, N. (1983) *Samson Wrights Applied Physiology*, 13th edn. Oxford University Press, Oxford.
Markus, S. (1981) Taking the fear out of bone marrow examinations. *Nursing* (US), 11(4), 64–7.

MIMS (1994) *Handbook of Haematology*. Haymarket Medical Imprint, London.

Monteil, M. M. (1987) Bone marrow. In: *Clinical Hematology and Fundamentals of Hemostasis*, (eds D. Harmening Pittiglio & R. A. Sacher). F. A. Davies, Philadelphia.

Mosby (1994) *Mosby's Medical, Nursing and Allied Health Dictionary*, 4th edn. Mosby, London.

Navarett, D. (1981) Assisting with bone marrow aspiration. In: *Mosby's Manual of Clinical Nursing Procedures*, (eds J. Hirsch & J. Hancock). C. V. Mosby, St Louis.

Pagnana, K. D. & Pagnana, T. J. (1986) *Diagnostic Testing and Nursing Implications*, 2nd edn. C. V. Mosby, St Louis.

Skydell, B. & Crowder, A. (1975) *Diagnostic Procedures – A Reference for Health Practitioners and a Guide for Patient Counselling*. Little, Brown, Boston.

GUIDELINES: BONE MARROW ASPIRATION AND TREPHINE BIOSPY

EQUIPMENT

1 Antiseptic skin cleansing agent (chlorhexidine in isopropyl alcohol 70%).
2 Sterile dressing pack.
3 Selection of syringes and needles for administration of local anaesthetic.
4 Local anaesthetic.
5 Marrow aspiration needle and guard, e.g. Salah needle.
6 Microscope slides and coverslips.
7 Specimen bottles (plain and with heparin).
8 Polyurethane semi-permeable dressing or spray.

PROCEDURE

Action	Rationale
1 Explain and discuss the procedure with the patient.	To ensure that the patient understands the procedure and gives his/her valid consent.
2 Give medication, such as sedation, as ordered, allowing sufficient time for it to have effect.	Usually this is only necessary for very anxious patients.
3 Help the patient into the correct position: (a) Supine. (b) Prone or on side.	For sternal puncture. For anterior or posterior iliac crest puncture.
4 Continue to observe the patient throughout the procedure. Assist the doctor as required. Reassure the conscious patient. Follow the appropriate procedure if the patient is anaesthetized.	To detect signs of discomfort or pain and to minimize anxiety.
5 Procedure is performed by a doctor: (a) Skin is cleansed with antiseptic solution.	To maintain asepsis throughout the procedure and thus minimize the risk of infection.
(b) Local anaesthetic is injected intradermally and through the various layers until the periosteum is infiltrated.	To minimize pain during the procedure. Transitory pain will be felt both as the periosteum is punctured and when the marrow is aspirated.
(c) Once the local anaesthetic has taken effect the doctor inserts the marrow needle with the guard on, into the anaesthetized area.	The needle guard ensures the correct positioning of the needle in the marrow cavity and diminishes the risk, particularly in the sternal puncture, of inadvertently puncturing vital organs.
(d) If the patient has not been anaesthetized, the doctor warns the patient he/she will	To allay anxiety and to ensure the patient's maximum cooperation.

Guidelines: Bone marrow aspiration and trephine biospy (cont'd)

Action	Rationale
feel a brief episode of sharp pain as the marrow is withdrawn. The needle is advanced into the bone marrow and the required amount of marrow is withdrawn.	
(e) The needle is removed from the puncture site.	
6 Once the doctor has removed the needle, apply pressure over the puncture site using a sterile topical swab until the bleeding stops.	To minimize bruising and to prevent haematoma formation. Prolonged pressure, 5–10 minutes, is required if the patient has a low platelet count (thrombocytopenia).
7 Once the bleeding stops, cover the site with plaster or a plastic dressing. Ask the patient not to bathe or wash the area for 24 hours.	To provide an airtight seal over the puncture site and to prevent the entry of bacteria.
8 Make the patient comfortable. He/she may be mobile, as desired, depending on the level of sedation.	Some patients will have this procedure performed in the outpatient department and will be asked to wait in the clinic for a further 30 minutes to ensure that no further bleeding occurs.
9 Ensure equipment is removed and disposed of safely.	To prevent spread of infection.
10 Record necessary information in the appropriate documents and ensure that specimens are sent to the appropriate laboratory department, correctly labelled and with the necessary forms.	

NURSING CARE PLAN

Problem	Cause	Suggested action
Pain experienced over the puncture site for 1–2 days following the procedure.	Bruising of the tissues at the time of puncture or haematoma formation due to inadequate pressure on the puncture site following the procedure.	Administer a mild analgesic as prescribed by the doctor.
Haemorrhage from the puncture site following the procedure.	Low platelet count or inadequate pressure on the puncture site following the procedure.	Ensure that pressure is applied for a minimum of 5 minutes on the puncture site. Report excessive or uncontrollable bleeding to the appropriate personnel.
Haematoma formation over the puncture site.	Haemorrhage following the procedure.	Administer analgesics as prescribed. If the haematoma is severe, report this to the doctor as aspiration may be required.

GUIDELINES: BONE MARROW HARVEST

EQUIPMENT

1 Sterile syringes: $1 \times 2\,ml$, $1 \times 5\,ml$.
2 Transfer pack 600 ml – collect from Haematology.
3 Small sterile dressing.
4 FBC Haematology forms.
5 Sterile sampling coupling spike – collect from Haematology.
6 Sterile gown pack.
7 Sterile gloves.
8 Swab saturated with 70% isopropyl alcohol.
9 64 ml of CPD (citrate phosphate dextrose) per transfer pack if marrow to be infused fresh – collect from Haematology.
10 Chlorhexidine 0.5% in 70% isopropyl alcohol.
11 500 ml bag of 0.9% sodium chloride.
12 5 ml ampoules of heparin, 1000 units per ml (preservative free).
13 Aspiration needles (short sternal needles) of appropriate size.
14 Bone marrow needles (e.g. Islam) of appropriate size.
15 Sterile pack containing 5 inch bowl, Gallipot, gauze swabs, two sponge holders, five towel clips, drapes.

PROCEDURE

Follow pre-, intra- and post-operative guidelines for general care during bone marrow harvest procedure.

Action	Rationale
1 Prepare the area (iliac crests or sternum) cleaning with 0.5% Chlorhexidine in 70% isopropyl alcohol.	To reduce risk of wound contamination (Ayliffe *et al.*, 1992).
2 Drape the area with sterile towels. Secure the towels with towel clips.	To provide and maintain a sterile field around the operation site.
3 Place two swabs on the towels.	To be available to remove blood exudate from the puncture site.
4 Flush syringe and aspiration needles with heparinized saline solution prepared on sterile trolley.	To reduce clotting risk in the aspiration needle and syringe.
5 Using the appropriate size aspiration needle make a small hole in the skin over the posterior iliac crest.	To facilitate smooth introduction of the bone marrow needle.
6 Introduce the bone marrow aspiration needle into the bone with firm controlled pressure. Initially it should enter the bone to a depth of approximately 1 cm.	The posterior iliac crest is 5–7 cm thick and there are no structures in the surrounding area which can be damaged by the introduction of a needle.
7 Firmly site the bone marrow needle.	To prevent slippage.
8 Remove the trocar.	To enable aspiration of the bone marrow.

Guidelines: Bone marrow harvest (cont'd)

Action	Rationale
9 Place a 20 ml syringe which has been heparinized on the end of the aspiration needle taking a volume of 10–25 ml.	To draw marrow into syringe for collection.
10 Pass the syringe containing marrow to the circulating nurse who injects the bone marrow into the heparinized transfer pack.	To maintain the sterility of the operating personnel. The transfer pack is not sterile on the outer surface.
11 After two aspirations from the same site, replace trocar and move the position of the bone marrow needle to another place in the bone approximately 2 cm from the first entry site.	To reduce risk of wound infection and excessive cell depletion. No further skin puncture is necessary due to the elasticity of the skin. If more than two aspirates are taken from one site the cells become depleted.
12 Move the bone marrow needle around over an area 2.5–5 cm from the entry site in the skin and introduce the needle every 2 cm until 400–500 ml of marrow have been removed in total.	The required amount of bone marrow can be harvested using the original hole in skin. It is normally possible to obtain sufficient bone marrow from the patient's iliac crests, if any more is required the sternum is used.
Place bone marrow in the transfer pack.	The number of cells required for re-engraftment is calculated using the recipient's body weight. Generally 2×10^8 per/kg body weight of cells are required, although more can be obtained if desired.
13 Take sample of aspirate from transfer pack and place in full blood count specimen container and send to the laboratory.	To establish the white cell count of the bone marrow aspirate and the number of stem cells present in each pack.
14 Seal the transfer pack with sterile plug.	To maintain sterility and prevent spillage.
15 Record amount in ml of bone marrow aspirate on outside of the transfer bag.	To establish total amount of bone marrow in each bag.
16 If the bone marrow is to be used fresh add 64 ml citrate phosphate dextrose (CPD) to the bone marrow in the transfer pack.	To prolong the life of the bone marrow and maintain its liquid form for up to 24 hours.
17 Withdraw needle and place gauze swab over site; apply digital pressure for 5 minutes, or longer if required.	To stop leakage and formation of haematoma.
18 Inspect puncture site for bleeding. Apply opsite spray and small sterile dressing.	To prevent wound infection. To seal wound.
19 Take fresh bone marrow to designated fridge in Haematology laboratories.	To ensure constant temperature and viability of stem cells.

CHAPTER 8
Bowel Care

GENERAL INTRODUCTION
It should be borne in mind that many patients are too embarrassed to talk about bowel function and will often delay reporting the problem until it has been present for a few days. Generally, complaints will be either that the patient has diarrhoea or is constipated. Both diarrhoea and constipation should be seen as symptoms of some underlying disease or malfunction, and managed accordingly.

The nurse's priority in either case is immediate resolution of the problem and re-education of the patient to avoid such problems in the future. However, it is necessary to assess what the patient means by the terms diarrhoea and constipation as well as to assess the cause.

REFERENCE MATERIAL

Anatomy and physiology
From the ileocaecal sphincter to the anus the colon is approximately 1.5 m in length. Its main function is to eliminate the waste products of digestion by the propulsion of faeces towards the anus. In addition, it produces mucus to lubricate the faecal mass, thus aiding its expulsion. Other functions include the absorption of fluid and electrolytes, the storage of faeces and the synthesis of vitamins B and K by bacterial flora.

Faeces consist of the unabsorbed end products of digestion, bile pigments, cellulose, bacteria, epithelial cells, mucus and some inorganic material. They are normally semi-solid in consistency and contain about 70% water.

The movement of faeces through the colon towards the anus is by peristaltic action. The colon absorbs about 2 litres of water in 24 hours. If faeces are not expelled they will, therefore, gradually become hard due to dehydration and will be difficult to expel. If there is insufficient roughage (fibre) in the faeces, colonic stasis occurs. This leads to continued water absorption and the faeces will harden still further.

Faeces normally remain in the sigmoid colon until the stimulus to defaecate occurs. This stimulus varies in individuals according to habit. The stimulus can be controlled by conscious effort. After a few minutes the stimulus disappears and does not return for several hours. If these natural reflexes are inhibited on a regular basis they are eventually suppressed and reflex defaecation is inhibited. The result is that the individual becomes severely constipated. In response to the stimulus faeces move into the rectum.

The rectum is very sensitive to rises in pressure, even of 2–3 mm Hg, and distension will cause a perineal sensation with a consequent desire to defaecate. A co-ordinated reflex empties the bowel from mid-transverse colon to the anus. During this phase the diaphragm, abdominal and levator ani muscles contract and the glottis closes. Waves of peristalsis occur in the distal colon and the anal sphincter relaxes, allowing the evacuation of faeces.

Diarrhoea
Diarrhoea has been defined as an

'abnormal increase in the quantity, frequency and fluid content of stool and associated with urgency, perianal discomfort and incontinence' (Basch, 1987).

The cause of diarrhoea needs to be ascertained. Roberts (1987) suggests that *acute* causes of diarrhoea include, for example, the following:

(1) Infective agents.
(2) Food poisoning.
(3) Unwise eating (spices, excessive fruit).
(4) Allergy to food constituents.

Chronic causes include:

(1) Drugs (e.g. broad-spectrum antibiotics).
(2) Gastrectomy.
(3) Malabsorption.
(4) Systemic illnesses.

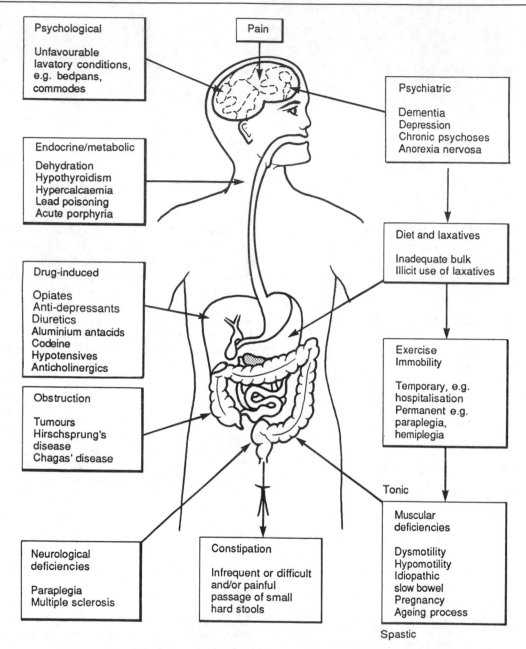

Figure 8.1   Classification of constipation – combined sources.

(5) Diseases of the large colon, including carcinoma, diverticular disease and inflammatory bowel disease, which can affect the small intestine as well.

(6) Radiation enteritis.

It must also be remembered that faecal impaction can cause diarrhoea overflow concealing an impacted colon. Continuing episodes of diarrhoea need to be investigated to rule out inflammatory bowel disease or infection. Mild or severe diarrhoea before or after breakfast can be an indication of irritable bowel disease. In the management of diarrhoea, the nurse can ensure that the patient's diet is altered. Foods having a high fibre content can be avoided and fluid intake can be increased. Such measures as the provision of soft toilet paper, easy access to toilet facilities and a suitable barrier cream to prevent anal excoriation can be implemented and will be much appreciated by the patient. Constipation, however, demands the use of more elaborate nursing skills.

Constipation

Constipation is a symptom. Its management depends on its cause. Definitions and classifications differ but for most patients it means irregular, infrequent defaecation associated with the passage of hard faeces (see Fig. 8.1). The patient usually complains of difficulty in defaecating with accompanying discomfort or pain.

Traditionally, the treatment of constipation has been left to the nurse (Milton-Thompson, 1971). As the patient often presents in hospital with an acute problem of constipation, nurses will need to formulate a short-term plan to evacuate the bowel as completely and as quickly as possible. For this reason enemas, suppositories and laxatives have remained the treatments of choice. Very often little thought is given either to the cause of the problem or to a more long-term plan. Duffin *et al.* (1981) have shown that a total of 3428 enemas were given on the geriatric wards of a district general hospital over a 6-month period. There were 1120 admissions in this period, which gave an overall average of three enemas per patient. The same study found that although enemas frequently produced a good bowel evacuation, they also embarrassed the patient and produced symptoms ranging from nausea and abdominal pain to faecal incontinence. Hurst (1970) felt that enemas were probably only of use where there was a mechanical delay between the splenic flexure and anus. Dorgu (1971) felt that the main benefit of enemas was that they acted within minutes of their administration and were useful in acute conditions of impaction before drug therapy could be effective.

Assessment of the problem

The myth of daily bowel evacuation being essential to healthy living has persisted through the centuries. This myth has resulted in laxative abuse becoming one of the commonest type of drug abuse in the Western world.

On the use and abuse of purgatives, Hurst (1970) showed that £10 million was expended in 1921 on patent medicines, the majority of which contained purgatives. In the 1960s, a survey of Londoners showed that over 30% were treating themselves with laxatives (Rutter & Maxwell, 1976).

However, the indications for the use of laxatives are fairly limited. The nurse should always stress the importance of diet and exercise to the patient before recommending other ways of evacuating the bowel.

Defining constipation is undoubtedly a problem while the notion of essential daily evacuations persists. The first objective should be for the nurse to assess what is 'normal' for an individual patient. A bowel action every third day may be quite adequate for some people; for others 3 times a day will be the norm. This does not mean that the first person is constipated or that the second has diarrhoea.

Many factors may affect normal bowel functioning. Among those pertinent to hospital admission are the following:

(1) Change in diet.
(2) Lack of exercise.
(3) X-ray investigation of the bowel involving the use of barium.
(4) The use of drugs, particularly analgesics.

Laxatives are often required to overcome these effects (Table 8.1).

Weller (1989) defines laxatives as medicine that loosens bowel contents and encourages evacuation. A laxative with a mild or gentle effect is also known as an aperient and one with a strong effect is referred to as a cathartic or a purgative. Purgatives should be used only in exceptional circumstances, i.e. where all other interventions have failed, or when they are prescribed for a specific purpose. Wherever possible the most natural means of bowel evacuation should be employed.

Table 8.1 Types of laxatives.

Type of laxative	Example	Brand names and sources
Bulk producers	Dietary fibre Mucilaginous polysaccharides Methylcellulose	Bran, wholemeal bread, Fybogel, Celevac
Stool softeners	Synthetic surface active agents, liquid paraffin	Agarol, Dioctyl Petrolager, Milpar
Osmotic agents	Sodium, potassium and magnesium salts	Magnesium sulphate, milk of magnesia, lactulose
Chemical stimulants	Sodium picosulphate, glycerin	Senna, Senokot, bisacodyl, Dulcolax, co-danthrusate, Picolax, glycerol

Laxatives alter the natural functioning of the alimentary tract. Often a period of no bowel evacuations follows their use and this usually causes the patient to take more laxatives; thus a cycle of dependence ensues (Mortimer, 1970).

The nurse should always make a rectal examination to establish whether the patient is constipated and to what degree. Wilson & Muir (1975) in their trial on geriatric faecal incontinence found that there was little correlation between a nurse's subjective assessment of whether a patient was constipated and the actual evidence gained from a rectal examination.

The use of the bedpan should always be avoided if possible. If the patient can get out of bed, a commode is preferable as the amount of energy expended is considerably less than that required for balancing on a bedpan. Lewin (1976) quoted from research by an American team investigating the straining forces of bowel evacuation by objective methods. They showed that straining was increased 3–6 times when a patient uses the bedpan and that its use requires a 50% greater consumption of oxygen than a commode by the bedside.

Manual evacuation of the rectum should be avoided if possible. It is a distressing, often painful and potentially dangerous procedure for the patient. If the procedure proves to be unavoidable, it may be necessary to sedate the patient before carrying it out. It is recommended by Pirrie (1980) that the procedure should be performed only by medical staff.

Laxatives

The many different types of laxatives available may be grouped into four types according to the action they have (Table 8.1).

Stool softeners

These act by lowering the surface tension of faeces which allows water to penetrate and soften the stool. They may also have a weak stimulatory effect (Barrett, 1992), but drugs of this type are often given in combination with a chemical stimulant. Softening agents take 24–48 hours to work (Martindale, 1993).

Liquid paraffin acts as a lubricant as well as a stool softener by coating the faeces and allowing easier passage. However, its use should be avoided as there are a number of problems associated with this preparation. The repetitive use of liquid paraffin may increase the risks of alimentary tract malignancies (Janes, 1979) and it also interferes with the absorption of fat-soluble vitamins. Accidental inhalation of droplets of liquid paraffin may result in lipoid pneumonia (Milton-Thompson, 1971; Barrett, 1992).

Osmotic agents

These may be divided into two sub-groups: lactulose and magnesium preparations. Lactulose is a synthetic disaccharide which exerts an osmotic effect in the small bowel. Colonic bacteria metabolize lactulose into short chain organic salt which is then absorbed, therefore the osmotic effect does not continue throughout the colon (Barrett, 1992). Faecal weight, volume and water are significantly increased by lactulose, which acts within 2 days (Bass & Dennis, 1981). Flatulence, cramps and abdominal discomfort are associated with high dosages. Magnesium preparations also exert an osmotic effect on the gut; they have a rapid effect, working within 2–6 hours. Fluid intake is important with these preparations as patients may easily become dehydrated (Martindale, 1993). These preparations should be avoided in patients with renal impairment as magnesium ions may be absorbed (Portenoy, 1987).

Stimulant laxatives

These stimulate the nerve plexuses in the gut wall causing irritation and increased peristalsis in the small and large bowel (Roe, 1992). Abdominal cramping may be increased if the stool is hard and a stool softener may be used in combination with this group of drugs (Martindale, 1993). Long-term use of these laxatives should be avoided, except for patients on long-term opiates, as they may lead to impaired bowel function such as atonic non-functioning colon (Martindale, 1993).

Preparations containing Danthron are restricted to certain groups of patients, i.e. the elderly, the terminally ill and some cardiac patients, as some rodent studies have indicated a potential carcinogenic risk (Martindale, 1993). Danthron preparations should not be used for incontinent patients especially those with limited mobility as prolonged skin contact will colour the skin pink or red and superficial sloughing of the discoloured skin will occur (Marindale, 1993).

Bulking agents

These work by retaining water and promoting microbial growth in the colon. This increases faecal mass production which stimulates peristalsis. These agents need plenty of fluid in order to work; they take a few days to exert their effect so are not suitable to relieve acute constipation. They are not suitable for use in patients who have bowel obstruction or reduced muscle tone. Increasing the bulk may worsen impaction, it may lead to increased colonic faecal loading (Donald et al., 1985) and may also increase the risk of faecal incontinence (Ardron & Main, 1990).

Recently, more favour has been shown towards the bulk laxatives which can be incorporated into the diet, e.g. whole-grain cereals and high-fibre bread. Bulk laxatives work by increasing the mass of the faeces. They do this by attracting water. This in turn promotes peristalsis and reduces the time taken by the faeces to move through the colon. An increased fluid intake is required when bulk laxatives are used, particularly in the elderly, to prevent intestinal obstruction occurring. Another problem initially is that bulk laxatives tend to distend the abdomen, often making the patient feel full and uncomfortable. Sometimes this leads to temporary anorexia. Harris (1980) discussed fully the merits of introducing bran into the diet, especially of the elderly, and the consequent drastic reduction in the number of enemas administered. She also showed that the cost of using bran compared with other laxatives, even other bulk laxatives, was very much lower.

However, more care now needs to be taken in the use of supplementary bran; unprocessed wheat bran, commonly used to increase the fibre in a diet, contains high levels of phytates, which can combine with minerals essential to a healthy diet, such as calcium, iron, copper and zinc. This can lead to a deficit in those people at risk from an inadequate diet, especially the elderly. More use should be made of normal foods which are rich in 'high-fibre' content, e.g. cereals, vegetables, especially root vegetables and broad beans, and fruit.

There is evidence indicating that 'dietary fibre' can reduce the postprandial levels of glucose and insulin (Haber et al., 1977; Jenkins et al., 1981). However, the value of this relationship to diabetic patients is unclear. Studies have now shown that there are a number of types and components of 'dietary fibre', which makes this too imprecise a term for health care professionals to use: its closest, more exact description is now 'non-starch polysaccharides'. A more detailed discussion of this area can be found in *Dietary Reference Values for Food Energy and Nutrients for the United Kingdom* (Department of Health, 1991).

ENEMAS

Definition
An enema is the introduction into the rectum or lower colon of a stream of fluid for the purpose of producing a bowel action or instilling medication.

Indications
Enemas may be prescribed for the following reasons:

(1) To clean the lower bowel before surgery; X-ray examination of the bowel using contrast medium; before endoscopy examination or in cases of severe constipation.

(2) To introduce medication into the system.
(3) To soothe and treat irritated bowel mucosa.
(4) To decrease body temperature (due to contact with the proximal vascular system).
(5) To stop local haemorrhage.
(6) To reduce hyperkalaemia (calcium resonium).
(7) To reduce portal systemic encephalopathy (phosphate enema).

Contraindications
Enemas are contraindicated under the following circumstances:

(1) In paralytic ileus.
(2) In colonic obstruction.
(3) Where the administration of tap water or soap and water enemas may cause circulatory overload, water intoxication, mucosal damage and necrosis, hyperkalaemia and cardiac arrhythmias.
(4) Where the administration of large amounts of fluid high into the colon may cause perforation and haemorrhage.
(5) Following gastrointestinal or gynaecological surgery, where suture lines may be ruptured (unless medical consent has been given).
(6) The use of micro-enemas and hypertonic saline enemas in patients with inflammatory or ulcerative conditions of the large colon.

REFERENCE MATERIAL

Types of enemas

Evacuant enemas
An evacuant enema is a solution introduced into the rectum or lower colon with the intention of its being expelled, along with faecal matter and flatus, within a few minutes. The following solutions are used:

(1) Phosphate enemas with standard or long rectal tubes in single-does disposable packs.
(2) Dioctyl sodium sulphosuccinate 0.1%, sorbitol 25% in single-dose disposable packs.
(3) Sodium citrate 450 mg, sodium alkysulphoacetate 45 mg, sorbic acid 5 mg in single-dose disposable packs.
(4) Oxyphenisatin in powder for reconstitution.
(5) Tap water.

Enemas containing dioctyl sodium sulphosuccinate lubricate and soften impacted faeces. Phosphate enemas are useful in bowel clearance before X-ray examination and surgery.

Tap water may be dangerous when administered as an enema to a child or to those with poor cardiac function, as excessive absorption could lead to circulatory overload (Milton-Thompson, 1971).

Green soap was formerly very popular as an evacuant enema, especially before childbirth. However, its use has now fallen into disfavour due to numerous adverse reports of mucosal damage, necrosis, extensive sloughing of mucosa, severe haemorrhage, anaphylactic shock and death (Edgell & Johnson, 1973; Lewis, 1965; Pike *et al.*, 1971; Smith, 1967). The limiting factors in soap are alkalis, potash and phenol. In Hirschsprung's disease, deaths following soap enema have occurred when a potassium-based soap was used. Hyperkalaemia resulted, causing cardiac arrhythmias (Lewin, 1976). Soap is probably a simple irritant; the higher the concentration, the greater the mucosal inflammation that results.

Retention enemas

A retention enema is a solution introduced into the rectum or lower colon with the intention of being retained for a specified period of time. Three types of retention enema are in common use:

(1) Arachis oil (may be obtained in a single-dose disposable pack).
(2) Olive oil.
(3) Prednisolone.

Enemas containing olive oil will soften and lubricate impacted faeces. Retention enemas given to administer medications will be prescribed by the doctor. The product must be checked with the prescription before its administration.

SUPPOSITORIES

Definition
A suppository is a solid or semi-solid pellet introduced into the anal canal for medicinal purposes.

Indications
The use of suppositories is indicated under the following circumstances:

(1) To empty the bowel before certain types of surgery.
(2) To empty the bowel to relieve acute constipation or when other treatments for constipation have failed.
(3) To empty the bowel before endoscopic examination.
(4) To introduce medication into the system.
(5) To soothe and treat haemorrhoids or anal puritus.

Contraindications
The use of suppositories is contraindicated when one or more of the following pertain:

(1) Chronic constipation, which would require repetitive use.
(2) Paralytic ileus.
(3) Colonic obstruction.
(4) Following gastrointestinal or gynaecological operations, unless on the specific instructions of the doctor.

REFERENCE MATERIAL
Many elderly people find repeated enemas both unpleasant and uncomfortable, and in cases of severe stasis and impaction, whole gut irrigation or colonic lavage may be preferable (Currie, 1979). Hunt (1974) states that the advantages of colonic lavage are that it clears the colon more effectively when visual observation of the interior of the colon is necessary and in cases of disordered action with constipation. However, the disadvantages include the risk of bowel perforation and the inadvertent washing away of the protective mucus which the bowel secretes. Its use is contraindicated in cases of diverticular disease and colitis.

Suppositories may be favoured as they are both easier to adminster and generally cause the patient less discomfort.

Administration of suppositories
The use of suppositories dates back to about 460 BC. Hippocrates recommended the use of cylindrical suppositories of honey smeared with ox gall (Hurst, 1970). Several types are now commonly available.

Lubricant suppositories, e.g. glycerine, should be inserted directly into the faeces and allowed to dissolve to enable softening of the faecal mass. However, stimulant types, such as bisacodyl, must come into contact with the mucus membrane of the rectum if they are to be effective. Other types, such as sodium bicarbonate and anhydrous sodium acid phosphate, exert their influence by releasing carbon dioxide, causing rectal distension when they contact water or mucous membrane.

RECTAL LAVAGE

Definition
Rectal lavage is the washing out of the rectum using large volumes of non-sterile fluid.

Indications
Rectal lavage is performed for the following purposes:

(1) To clear the lower bowel before investigation by barium enema and thus enable good images to be obtained.
(2) To assist in clearing the lower bowel before major

abdominal surgery and thus decreasing the risk of infection and aiding satisfactory healing.

(3) To clear the lower bowel of residual faecal matter following previous surgery, e.g. formation of colostomy.

Contraindications

Rectal lavage is contraindicated in patients who have a history of any one of the following:

(1) Severe or prolapsed haemorrhoids.
(2) Anal fissure.
(3) Inflammatory bowel disease.
(4) Large tumour in the rectum or sigmoid colon.
(5) Post-radiation proctitis.
(6) Internal fistulae.
(7) Previous extensive deep X-ray therapy to the pelvis.
(8) Recent bowel surgery.
(9) Congestive cardiac failure.
(10) Impaired renal function.

In points 1 to 8 of the contraindications listed above, the reason for employing caution is because of the damage that could be inflicted by the mechanical aspects of rectal lavage. When the bowel has already been traumatized there is a greater potential risk of causing irritation or, in extreme cases, perforation while inserting the catheter and running large volumes of fluid in and out of the rectum.

With the last two contraindications the potential risk lies with the possibility of large amounts of fluid and/or electrolytes becoming absorbed through the bowel. (Generally speaking, with the amounts and type of fluid used and the relatively short time that it stays in the bowel, this should not present a major problem.)

REFERENCE MATERIAL

Choice of fluid
Several solutions can be used to clear the bowel.

Hypertonic solutions
Hypertonic solutions, e.g. sodium phosphate and sodium acid phosphate in solution, act by drawing water from the intestinal cells by osmosis. This increases the fluid in the faecal mass, causing first distension then contraction and defaecation.

For patients who have a large amount of faecal matter to evacuate, small volumes of these solutions are very effective. Hypertonic solutions should not be given to patients whose capacity to utilize sodium is affected, as some sodium may be absorbed. These solutions are available as commercially prepared enemas but are not suitable for administration in large volumes.

Tap water
Rectal lavage is a procedure that is normally used in combination with other methods of clearing the bowel, e.g. oral aperients and dietary restrictions. In this situation, it can be anticipated that there will be very little residue remaining in the lower bowel. What is needed, therefore, is a simple, non-sterile solution that can be used with relative safety in large volumes to wash out the residual faecal matter. The solution which fulfils these criteria ideally is tap water.

Rectal lavage using tap water is not without risk as large volumes of this hypotonic solution can upset the patient's electrolyte balance. Water is drawn by osmosis into the intestinal cells and water intoxication can result, with symptoms of weakness, sweating, pallor, vomiting, coughing and dizziness. However, this is a relatively rare complication and generally tap water is very well tolerated.

The other advantages of tap water are as follows:

(1) It is cheap and easily available.
(2) It can be easily warmed to the correct temperature.
(3) It is non-irritant to the bowel mucosa.
(4) It does not cause excessive peristalsis with resulting cramps and colic.

Caution should be exercised when giving tap water lavage to infants or patients with altered kidneys or cardiac reserve, but otherwise tap water is the solution of choice.

Isotonic saline
An isotonic saline solution can be substituted for patients with compromised electrolyte status. This is prepared by adding 2 level teaspoons of salt to 1 litre of plain water. Its effect on the bowel is similar to that of water in that it stimulates peristaltic action by distending the intestinal walls. With isotonic saline, however, there is less danger of electrolyte imbalance.

Choice of catheter
Several manufacturers produce rectal catheters. The criteria for selection should be as follows:

(1) The catheter should be of an adequate length. Most are approximately 30 cm long.
(2) The lumen should be large enough to allow the free drainage of particulate matter, i.e. a minimum Charrière gauge of 24.
(3) The tip of the catheter should be open ended or have large opposed eyelets to minimize the possibility of blockage.
(4) The catheter should be made from a soft flexible material; rubber or plastic is suitable.

References and further reading

Ardron, M. E. & Main, A. N. H. (1990) Management of constipation. *British Medical Journal*, 300, 1400.

Barrett, J. A. (1992) Faecal incontinence. In: *Clinial Nursing Practice. The Promotion and Management of Continence*, (ed. B. Roe). Prentice Hall, New York.

Basch, A. (1987) Symptom distress changes in elimination. *Seminars in Oncology Nursing*, 3(4), 287–92.

Bass, P. & Dennis, S. (1981) The laxative effects of lactulose in normal and constipated subjects. *Journal of Clinical Gastro-enterology*, 3 (Supplement 1), 23–8.

Booth, S. & Booth, B. (1986) Aperients can be deceptive. *Nursing Times*, 24 September, 82(39), 38–9.

British Medical Association/Pharmaceutical Society of Great Britain (1988) *British National Formulary*. BMA, London.

Clarke, B. (1988) Making sense of enemas. *Nursing Times*, 84(30), 40–4.

Cooper, P. (1976) The treatment of constipation. *Midwife, Health Visitor and Community Nurse* 12, 165.

Corman, M. *et al.* (1975) Cathartics. *American Journal of Nursing*, 75, 237–9.

Currie, J. E. J. (1979) Whole gut irrigation. *Nursing Times*, 75, 1570–1.

Department of Health (1991) *Report on Health and Social Subjects 41, Dietary Reference Values for Food Energy and Nutrients for the United Kingdom* pp. 61–71. HMSO, London.

Donald, I. P. *et al.* (1985) A study of constipation in the elderly living at home. *Gerontology*, 31, 112–18.

Dorgu, R. E. O. (1971) *Bowel Function – Disorders and Management*. Butterworths, London.

Duffin, H. M. *et al.* (1981) Are enemas necessary? *Nursing Times*, 77(45), 1940–1.

Edgell, R. W. & Johnson, W. D. (1973) Postpartum hypotension and erythema: an adverse reaction to soap enema. *American Journal of Obsterics and Gynecology*, 117, 1146–7.

Greenwood, J. (1955) Treatment with dignity. *Nursing Times*, 91(17), 65–7.

Haber, G. B. *et al.* (1977) Depletion and disruption of dietary fibre. *Lancet*, 2, 679–82.

Hanham, S. (1990) Management of constipation. *Nursing*, 4(17), 28–31.

Harris, W. (1980) Bran or aperients? *Nursing Times*, 76, 81–3.

Hunt, T. (1974) Colonic irrigation. *Nursing Mirror*, 139(1), 76–7.

Hurst, Sir A. (1970) *Selected Writings of Sir Arthur Hurst* (1989–1944). Spottiswode, Ballantyne.

Janes, E. (1979) Constipation: keeping a true perspective. *Nursing Mirror*, 149(13), Supplement, p. x.

Jenkins, D. J. A. *et al.* (1981) Glycaemic index of foods: a physiological basis for carbohydrate exchange. *American Journal of Clinical Nutrition*, 34, 362–6.

Lewin, D. (1976) Care of the constipated patient. *Nursing Times*, 72, 444–6.

Lewis, A. E. (1965) Dangers inherent in soap enemas. *Pacific Medicine and Surgery*, 73, 131–3.

Martindale, W. (1993) *The Extra Pharmacopia*, 30th edn., (ed. J. E. F. Reynolds). The Pharmaceutical Press, London.

Milton-Thompson, G. J. (1971) Constipation. *Nursing Mirror*, 132, 30–3.

Mortimer, P. M. (1970) A worrying problem – constipation. *Health Visitor*, 43, 47–8.

Pike, B. F. *et al.* (1971) Soap colitis. *New England Journal of Medicine*, 285(4), 217–18.

Pirrie, J. (1980) Constipation in the elderly. *Nursing*, 1(17), 753–4.

Portenoy, R. K. (1987) Constipation in the cancer patient: causes and management. *Medical Clinics of North America*, 71(2), 303–11.

Roberts, A. (1987) Systems of life, No. 146. *Nursing Times*, 83(5), 47–8.

Roberts, M. F. (1993) Diarrhoea: a symptom. *Holistic Nurse Practioner*, 7(2), 73–80.

Rutter, K. & Maxwell, D. (1976) Constipation and laxative abuse. *British Medical Journal*, 2, 997–1000.

Sadler, C. (1988) The power of purgatives. *Community Outlook*, June, 11–12.

Smith, D. (1967) Severe anaphylactic reaction after a soap enema. *British Medical Journal*, 215(4), 215.

Smith, S. (1987) Drugs and the gastrointestinal tract. *Nursing Times*, 83(26), 50–2.

Stilwell, B. (1992) Skills update: assessing the adult with constipation. *Community Outlook*, 2(9), 26–7.

Thompson, M. & Bottomley, H. (1980) Normal and abnormal bowel function. *Nursing*, 1(17), 721–2.

Walker, R. (1982) Suppository insertion. *World Medicine*, 18, 58.

Weller, B. (1989). *Encyclopaedic Dictionary of Nursing and Health Care*, Baillière Tindall, Eastbourne.

White, T. (1995) Dealing with constipation in terminal illness. *Nursing Times*, 91(14), 57–8.

Wieck, L. *et al.* (1986) *Illustrated Manual of Nursing Techniques*, 3rd edn. J. B. Lippincott, Philadelphia.

Wilson, A. & Muir, T. (1975) Geriatric faecal incontinence. *Nursing Mirror*, 140(16), 50–2.

GUIDELINES: ADMINISTRATION OF ENEMAS

EQUIPMENT

1 Disposable incontinence pad.
2 Disposable gloves.

3 Topical swabs.
4 Lubricating jelly.
5 Rectal tube and funnel (if not using a commercially prepared pack).
6 Solution required or commercially prepared enema.
7 Bath thermometer.

PROCEDURE

Action	Rationale
1 Explain and discuss the procedure with the patient.	To ensure that the patient understands the procedure and gives his/her valid consent.
2 Ensure privacy.	To avoid unnecessary embarrassment to the patient.
3 Allow patient to empty bladder first if necessary.	A full bladder may cause discomfort during procedure.
4 Ensure that a bedpan, commode or toilet is readily available.	In case the patient feels the need to expel the enema before the procedure is completed.
5 Warm the enema to the required temperature by immersing in a jug of hot water, testing with a bath thermometer. A temperature of 40.5–43.3°C is recommended for adults. Oil retention enemas should be warmed to 37.8°C.	Heat is an effective stimulant of the nerve plexi in the intestinal mucosa. An enema temperature of body temperature or just above will not damage the intestinal mucosa. The temperature of the environment, the rate of fluid administration and the length of the tubing will all have an effect on the temperature of the fluid in the rectum.
6 Assist the patient to lie in the required position, i.e. on the left side, with knees well flexed, the upper higher than the lower one, and with the buttocks near the edge of the bed.	This allows ease of passage into the rectum by following the natural anatomy of the colon. In this position gravity will aid the flow of the solution into the colon. Flexing the knees ensures a more comfortable passage of the enema nozzle or rectal tube.
7 Place a disposable incontinence pad beneath the patient's hips and buttocks.	To reduce potential infection caused by soiled linen. To avoid embarrassing the patient if the fluid is ejected prematurely following administration.
8 Wash hands with bactericidal soap and water or bactericidal alcohol hand rub, and put on disposable gloves.	To reduce cross-infection.
9 Place some lubricating jelly on a topical swab and lubricate the nozzle of the enema or the rectal tube.	To prevent trauma to the anal and rectal mucosa by reducing surface friction.
10 Expel excessive air and introduce the nozzle or tube slowly into the anal canal while separating the buttocks. (A small amount of air may be introduced if bowel evacuation is desired.)	The introduction of air into the colon causes distention of its walls, resulting in unnecessary discomfort to the patient and increases peristalsis. The slow introduction of the lubricated tube will minimize spasm of the intestinal wall. (Evacuation will be more effectively induced due to the increased peristalsis.)
11 Slowly introduce the tube or nozzle to a depth of 10–12.5cm.	This will bypass the anal canal (2.5–4cm in length) and ensure that the tube or nozzle is in the rectum.

Guidelines: Administration of enemas (cont'd)

Action	Rationale
12 If a retention enema is used, introduce the fluid slowly and leave the patient in bed with the foot of the bed elevated by 45° for as long as prescribed.	To avoid increasing peristalsis. The slower the rate at which the fluid is introduced the less pressure is exerted on the intestinal wall. Elevating the foot of the bed aids in retention of the enema by force of gravity.
13 If an evacuant enema is used, introduce the fluid slowly by rolling the pack from the bottom to the top to prevent backflow, until the pack is empty or the solution is completely finished.	The faster the rate of flow of the fluid the greater the pressure on the rectal walls. Distention and irritation of the bowel wall will produce strong peristalsis which is sufficient to empty the lower bowel.
14 If using a funnel and rectal tube, adjust the height of the funnel according to the rate of flow desired.	The forces of gravity will cause the solution to flow from the funnel into the rectum. The greater the elevation of the funnel, the faster the flow of fluid.
15 Clamp the tubing before all the fluid has run in.	To avoid air entering the rectum and causing further discomfort.
16 Slowly withdraw the tube or nozzle.	To avoid reflex emptying of the rectum.
17 Dry the patient's perineal area with a gauze swab.	To promote patient comfort and avoid excoriation and infection.
18 Ask the patient to retain the enema for 10–15 minutes before evacuating the bowel.	To enhance the evacuant effect.
19 Ensure that the patient has access to the nurse call system, is near to the bedpan, commode or toilet, and has adequate toilet paper.	
20 Remove and dispose of equipment.	To avoid infection.
21 Wash hands.	To reduce risk of cross-infection.
22 Record in the appropriate documents that the enema has been given, its effects on the patient and its results (colour, consistency, content and amount of faeces produced).	To monitor the patient's bowel function.

NURSING CARE PLAN

Problem	Cause	Suggested action
Unable to insert the nozzle of enema pack or rectal tube into the anal canal.	Tube not adequately lubricated.	Apply more lubricating jelly.
	Patient in an incorrect position.	Ask the patient to draw knees up further towards the chest.

	Patient apprehensive and embarrassed about the situation.	Ensure adequate privacy and give frequent explanations to the patient about the procedure.
	Patient unable to relax anal sphincter.	Ask the patient to take deep breaths and 'bear down' as if defaecating.
Unable to advance the tube or nozzle into the anal canal.	Spasm of the canal walls.	Insert the tube or nozzle more slowly, thus minimizing spasm.
Unable to advance the tube or nozzle into the rectum.	Blockage by faeces.	Allow a little solution to flow and then insert the tube further.
	Blockage by tumour.	If resistance is still met, stop the procedure and inform a doctor.
Patient complains of cramping or the desire to evacuate the enema before the end of the procedure.	Distension and irritation of the intestinal wall, which produce a stong peristalsis sufficient to empty the lower bowel.	Temporarily stop the insertion of fluid by clamping the tubing or lowering the funnel until the patient says the feeling has subsided.
Patient unable to open bowels after an evacuant enema and the fluid has not returned.	Reduced neuromuscular response in the bowel wall.	Insert a rectal tube and try to siphon the fluid off. Measure and record the amount. If this is not successful, perform rectal lavage. (For further information, see Rectal lavage, above.) Measure and record the amount returned.

GUIDELINES: ADMINISTRATION OF SUPPOSITORIES

EQUIPMENT

1 Disposable incontinence pad.
2 Disposable gloves.
3 Topical swabs or tissues.
4 Lubricating jelly.
5 Suppository(ies) as required (check the prescription before administering a medicinal suppository, e.g. aminophylline).

PROCEDURE

Action	Rationale
1 Explain and discuss the procedure with the patient. If you are administering a medicated suppository, it is best to do so after the patient has emptied his/her bowels.	To ensure that the patient understands the procedure and gives his/her valid consent. To ensure that the active ingredients are not impeded from being absorbed by the rectal mucosa or that the suppository is not expelled before its active ingredients have been released.
2 Ensure privacy.	To avoid unnecessary embarrassment to the patient.

Guidelines: Administration of suppositories (cont'd)

Action	Rationale
3 Ensure that a bedpan, commode or the toilet is readily available.	In case of premature ejection of the suppositories or rapid bowel evacuation following their administration.
4 Assist the patient to lie in the required position, i.e. on the left side, with the knees flexed, the upper higher than the lower one, with the buttocks near the edge of the bed.	This allows ease of passage of the suppository into the rectum by following the natural anatomy of the colon. Flexing the knees will reduce discomfort as the suppository is passed through the anal sphincter.
5 Place a disposable incontinence pad beneath the patient's hips and buttocks.	To avoid unnecessary soiling of linen, leading to potential infection and embarrassment to the patient if the suppositories are ejected prematurely or there is rapid bowel evacuation following their administration.
6 Wash hands with bactericidal soap and water or bactericidal alcohol hand rub, and put on gloves.	To reduce the risk of cross-infection.
7 Place some lubricating jelly on the topical swab and lubricate the blunt end of the suppository if it is being used to obtain systemic action. Separate the patient's buttocks and insert the suppository blunt end first, advancing it for about 2–4 cm. Repeat this procedure if a second suppository is to be inserted.	Lubricating reduces surface friction and thus eases insertion of the suppository and avoids anal mucosal trauma. Research has shown that the suppository is more readily retained if inserted blunt end first. (For further information see Suppositories, above.) The anal canal is approximately 2–4 cm long. Inserting the suppository beyond this ensures that it will be retained.
8 Once suppository(ies) has been inserted, clean any excess lubricating jelly from the patient's perineal area.	To ensure the patient's comfort and avoid anal excoriation that may then lead to infection.
9 Ask the patient to retain the suppository(ies) if it is of an evacuant type. If it is medicated, ask the patient to retain the suppository for 20 minutes, or until he/she is no longer able to do so.	This will allow the suppository to melt and release the active ingredients.
10 Remove and dispose of equipment. Wash hands.	To reduce risk of infection.
11 Record that the suppository(ies) have been given, the effect on the patient and the result (amount, colour, consistency and content) in the appropriate documents.	To monitor the patient's bowel function.

GUIDELINES: ADMINISTRATION OF RECTAL LAVAGE

EQUIPMENT

1 Rectal lavage pack containing a large funnel, rubber tubing, a straight connector, a one-litre jug and a rectal catheter (Charrière gauge 24). (Commercial packs are also available.)

2 Non-sterile topical swabs.
3 Lubricating jelly.
4 Disposable gloves.
5 Disposable incontinence pad.
6 Plastic sheet and draw sheet.
7 Large non-sterile jug.
8 Bucket.
9 Gate clip or clamp.
10 Toilet paper or tissues.
11 Disposable plastic apron.
12 Large disposable bag.
13 Measured volume of warm tap water (37–40°C).

PROCEDURE

Action

1 Explain and discuss the procedure with the patient.

2 Prepare the area where the lavage is to be performed, i.e. the patient's bed or a couch in the room where rectal lavage is to take place. Protect the bed or couch with plastic sheet and draw sheet. Place a disposable incontinence pad on the floor.

3 Wash hands with bactericidal soap and water or bactericidal alcohol hand rub, and dry hands, clean the trolley and prepare the equipment for the procedure by opening the pack and laying out the contents on the top of the shelf.

4 Attach a large disposable bag to the trolley.

5 Fill a large non-sterile jug with a measured volume of warm (37–40°C) tap water. Check the temperature with a lotion thermometer. Place the filled jug on the lower shelf of the trolley. Put a bucket for receiving effluent by the side of the bed or couch.

6 Assist the patient to lie in the required position, i.e. on the left side, with the knees well flexed, the upper higher than the lower one, and with the buttocks near the edge of the bed. Tilt the foot of the bed slightly upwards if possible.

7 Check that the patient's clothing is tucked out of the way and that both the patient and the bed are adequately protected. Ensure that the patient is as comfortable as possible before continuing with the procedure.

Rationale

To ensure that the patient understands the procedure and gives his/her valid consent.

To prevent non-disposable equipment becoming contaminated with faecal matter, thus minimizing the risk of cross-infection.

Although this is not an aseptic procedure, care must be taken to avoid unnecessary contamination.

To provide a suitable receptacle for safe disposal of potentially large amounts of contaminated waste.

As the bowel is not sterile, there is no need to use sterile fluid. A large volume needs to be available for use, up to a maximum of six litres, although the total amount used will vary with each patient and may be much less. If the solution is too warm, the intestinal mucosa may be damaged; if too cold, unnecessary cramping may occur.

This position allows ease of access for insertion of the catheter into the rectum, follows the natural anatomy of the colon and aids gravity in promoting the flow of fluid into the sigmoid and descending colon. Tilting the bed also aids the flow.

As the procedure can be lengthy and is potentially messy, the patient needs to be as relaxed and well protected as possible to aid successful completion.

Guidelines: Administration of rectal lavage (cont'd)

Action	Rationale
8 Wash hands with bactericidal soap and water or bactericidal alcohol hand rub, and put on disposable gloves and a disposable plastic apron.	To reduce the risk of cross-infection and for nurse's protection.
9 Connect up the funnel, tubing and rectal catheter, using a straight connector between the latter two items. Fix a gate clamp or clip in position approximately 15 cm from the end of the rectal catheter.	To allow the tubing and the catheter to be primed and filled with fluid, thus preventing the entry of air into the rectum and discomfort to the patient.
10 Using non-sterile topical swab lubricate the last 15 cm of the rectal catheter with a generous amount of lubricating jelly.	To aid insertion and minimize patient discomfort and trauma to the rectal mucosa.
11 Fill a small jug with one litre from the measured volume of warm tap water.	A small jug is more manageable and allows measurement of the amount of fluid used each time.
12 Prime the catheter and the tubing.	To prepare equipment.
13 Gently insert 7.5–10 cm of the catheter into the rectum.	The rectum is approximately 12.5 cm long and the anal canal 2.5 cm. Inserting the catheter 7.5–10 cm ensures that the rectum will be adequately filled with the minimum trauma to the patient.
14 Encourage the patient to take deep breaths.	Deep breathing relaxes the anal sphincter.
15 Check that the patient is comfortable.	
16 Fill the funnel with approximately 400 ml of fluid from the jug.	The rectum will hold 200–400 ml without causing trauma.
17 Hold the funnel about 30 cm above the rectum, release the clamp and allow the fluid to run into the rectum, holding the catheter in position.	Aqueous solution exerts pressure of 0.225 kg for every 30 cm of elevation. The pressure should not exceed 0.45 kg as this may cause cramping or even rupture of the intestinal wall.
18 Ask the patient to rock gently from side to side.	To ensure efficient lavage of the bowel lumen.
19 Before the funnel is completely empty, invert it over the bucket to allow the lavage fluid and faecal matter to drain out.	To prevent unnecessary amounts of air entering the rectum and causing the patient discomfort.
20 Refill the funnel with another measure of fluid, keeping the tubing pinched or clamped and the funnel at patient level until it is filled.	To prevent entry of air into rectum and discomfort to the patient.
21 Repeat the last two procedures until: (a) The effluent runs clear. (b) A maximum volume of 6 litres has been used.	If the bowel is not clear after this volume, other methods need to be employed.
22 Note how much fluid was used during the procedure.	To ensure that not more than 6 litres are used to reduce the risk of circulatory fluid overload.

23 At the end of the procedure:
(a) Measure the amount of effluent obtained and compare it with the volume run in.

To ensure that the patient has not absorbed fluid in such a quantity that will carry the risk of fluid overload.
To reduce risk of infection.

(b) Clear away and dispose of equipment.
(c) Ensure that the patient is clean and tidy.

24 Settle the patient into bed, on an incontinence pad and with a bedpan or commode at hand.

To reduce risk of infection caused by soiled linen.

NURSING CARE PLAN

Problem	Cause	Suggested action
Fluid will not run in freely.	Catheter is pressed against the bowel wall. Catheter is blocked with faecal material. Insufficient gravity flow.	Gently manoeuvre the catheter around in the rectum. Remove the catheter and unblock. Reinsert and recommence procedure. Raise the funnel slightly.
Leakage of fluid around the catheter.	Poor positioning of the catheter or displacement following insertion. Poor tone of the anal sphincer muscles.	Check that the catheter is 7–10 cm into the rectum. Hold it gently in position. Ask the patient to try and tighten muscles as fluid is run in. Elevate the foot of the bed to aid flow.
Discomfort and/or cramping when the fluid is run in.	Fluid is too cold. Pressure of the fluid entering the rectum is too high. Extreme tension and anxiety. Perforation of the rectum.	Check the temperature of the fluid and warm it if necessary. Lower the funnel to stop fluid from running until the spasm passes, but leave the catheter in to relieve distension. When the spasm has passed, gradually raise the funnel and allow fluid to enter very slowly. Encourage deep breathing through the mouth to relax the abdominal muscles and decrease colonic pressures. Stop the procedure immediately. Inform a doctor.
Severe pain accompanied by perspiration, pallor and tachycardia.	Perforation of the gut around the site of a large tumour due to increased peristalsis.	Check the patient's vital signs. Inform a doctor. Do not allow the patient to eat or drink until seen by a doctor.
Blood is returned in the effluent.	Insertion of the catheter has caused internal haemorrhoids to bleed.	Stop the procedure and inform a doctor. Record the appropriate amount of blood that has been

Nursing care plan (cont'd)

Problem	Cause	Suggested action
		passed and observe further bowel motions.
	Trauma to rectal mucosa.	
Large discrepancy between amount of fluid run in and the effluent obtained.	Excessive leakage on to pads during the procedure.	Try to estimate the amount of fluid on pads, etc.
	Patient has retained a certain amount of fluid that may be passed later.	Measure carefully all subsequent bowel actions.
	Patient has absorbed the excess fluid.	Check the patient's vital signs. Record further intake and output carefully. Inform a doctor.
Sudden onset of pallor, perspiration, vomiting, coughing and dizziness.	Water intoxication due to absorption of water from the rectum.	Stop the procedure immediately. Inform a doctor. Check the patient's vital signs.

CHAPTER 9
Breast Aspiration

Definition

Breast aspiration is the insertion of a needle into the breast to obtain cells for cytological examination or to remove fluid to drain a cyst. It is usually carried out using a fine needle and so is often referred to as fine needle aspiration or FNA.

REFERENCE MATERIAL

Anatomy and physiology

The breast is a glandular organ designed to produce milk (Fig. 9.1). It contains 15–20 lobes and each lobe branches into lobules. The lobules end in tiny sacs called alveoli where milk is actually produced. The lobules are connected to the nipple by ducts. The entire breast is enclosed by a membrane called the fascia. Superficially this lies between the breast and the skin, the deep fascia separates the breast tissue from the muscle of the chest wall. Beneath the breast are two muscles: the pectoralis major and pectoralis minor. The breasts are situated on the chest wall between the third and sixth or seventh rib (Gray, 1977). Most of the normal breast is composed of fat and less than 5% is made up of duct epithelial cells. It is in these cells that cancers arise (Case, 1984).

The cells of the breast are sensitive to hormonal changes and the ducts and alveoli increase in size under the influence of oestrogen and decrease under the influence of progesterone. As this happens every month under the influence of the menstrual cycle the breasts are subject to constant change which may result in the development of nodularity. This nodularity or lumpiness is more pronounced in some women and is sometimes classed as benign breast disease. Where a lump is found in the breast it is necessary to perform aspiration or surgical biopsy in order to eliminate the possibility of cancer. It is often difficult to differentiate between generalized lumpiness and a discrete lump so mammography or ultrasound can help to guide the insertion of the needle (Case, 1984).

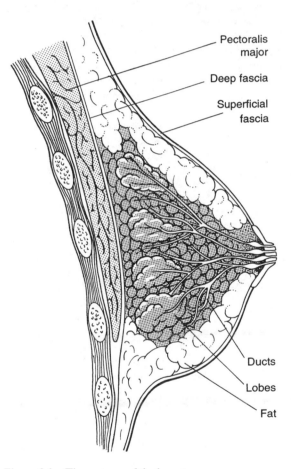

Figure 9.1   The anatomy of the breast.

Breast cancer

Breast cancer is a disease that affects 26 000 women in the UK every year (Cancer Research Campaign, 1991). Experience suggests that a vast majority of breast cancers arise in the ducts of the breast. Those that arise in the lobules only account for a small minority. The remainder are made up of rare tumours such as Paget's disease, inflammatory carcinoma and sarcoma of the breast. Most breast cancers are invasive, i.e. the cells have begun to spread through the linings of the ducts into surrounding tissue, but a few may be non-invasive or *in situ*. *In situ* cancers are the earliest changes that can be identified as malignant.

Many more women find a lump in their breast that turns out to be benign, such as a cyst or fibroadenoma. When lumps are biopsied, only two in ten turn out to be cancer (Case, 1984). Consequently large numbers of women are undergoing investigations to exclude malignancy. It is therefore important to find a simple, non-invasive test that can determine malignancy within given resources at minimal inconvenience to the patient.

Diagnostic methods

Historically, where breast cancer was suspected diagnosis was made by surgical excision of a tumour (known as excision biopsy) under general anaesthetic and then examination of the tumour by a histopathologist. The patient was given the results and subsequently, if positive, needed further excision requiring a second anaesthetic. Alternatively, histopathological examination was carried out rapidly using a frozen section of the tumour while the patient was anaesthetized. Where the tumour was shown to be malignant, further excision or even mastectomy was carried out at the time. While this had the advantage of giving the patient only one anaesthetic, the disadvantage was that patients frequently went to theatre not knowing whether they had cancer or indeed whether they would undergo a mastectomy. Fine needle aspiration and cytological examination normally help to overcome this problem as the patient knows the diagnosis prior to surgery and the extent of surgery required can be discussed with them.

Another alternative to excision biopsy is trucut biopsy. This is where an incision is made in the breast under local anaesthetic and a wide bore needle used to take a core of breast tissue. This also gives the patient the diagnosis before surgery but is more invasive and more painful than a fine needle aspiration. It also causes more trauma to the breast and may make subsequent surgery more difficult. However, unlike FNA, it can distinguish between invasive or non-invasive tumours.

Many other prognostic markers can now be measured from fine needle aspirations. In conjunction with immunocytochemistry it is possible to measure oestrogen receptor, progesterone receptor and other markers such as the p53 enzyme (Trott, 1991).

Accuracy

Although aspiration cytodiagnosis has been possible since the 19th century, the first report of its widespread use (3479 patients) was in 1968 in Scandinavia (Franzen & Zajicek, 1968). It has been slow to be widely accepted because of concerns about its accuracy. The problems arise because only small amounts of aspirate are obtained and in inexperienced hands there are often not enough cells to make a diagnosis. Even where cells are obtained it is possible to miss the cancer cells and so achieve a false negative result. It is also essential to have an experienced cytologist who is able to make diagnoses on small amounts of material. If the practitioner and cytologist are not experienced the accuracy can fall to 50%. This would result in the test being too unreliable to use for diagnostic purposes. It is therefore essential that any individual who is to undertake this procedure should undergo specific training, have excellent manual dexterity and have their competence assessed before proceeding to breast aspiration routinely (Koss, 1993). To achieve consistent results the technique needs to be practised at least several times a week (Ljung *et al.*, 1994). However, it is possible to reach very high accuracy. In the series conducted by Franzen & Zajicek (1968) there was 92.1% agreement between FNA and subsequent histology. Currently most centres are reporting false positive rates (i.e. mistaken diagnosis of cancer) generally under 0.5% and false negative rates of about 5% (Layfield *et al.*, 1993).

Preparation of the sample

Once obtained the aspirate is expressed onto two microscope slides and sent to the Cytology Department. Two main staining techniques are used for the visualization of the slides. The Papanicolaou stain requires fixing in spirit (95% ethanol) before it dries so is suitable for a thick smear of cells. The Romanovsky technique using the May–Grunwald Giemsa stain requires the cells to dry almost instantaneously in order to achieve good staining and therefore is better when the smear is scanty. Ideally both stains should be made for each specimen as different lesions are more easily identifiable using the different techniques (Trott, 1991). The cytologist will also find it useful to be given a description of what is felt in the breast when the needle is inserted. Cancers often feel more gritty and benign lesions feel more rubbery (Kline *et al.*, 1979).

If the lump turns out to be a cyst then the fluid will drain out on aspiration and the lump disappear. Clear fluid aspirated from breast cysts need not have cytologic examination unless the lump has not disappeared. Discoloured or cloudy fluid, either blood-stained or green, should be sent to the laboratory for examination as carcinoma can be associated with a cyst (Trott, 1991).

Patient anxiety

Many patients undergoing this procedure will be very anxious due to concern over the possible diagnosis of cancer. Anxiety may increase the perceived pain of the procedure and if the patient is restless due to anxiety they may move when the needle is inserted. If the patient moves then the FNA may not be accurate and the chances of haematoma and pneumothorax are increased. It is of the utmost importance, therefore, that a full explanation is given and the procedure carried out in a sensitive manner to minimize the distress of the patient.

Problems

It is possible to pierce the lung and cause pneumothorax so care should be taken when performing aspiration in those areas of the breast where there is little breast tissue. However, there is no report of any serious complication from this (Trott, 1991). In a small breast or where aspiration is carried out in a thin layer of breast tissue it is wise to use a 23 g (blue) needle to minimize this risk.

Tumours are often vascular so there is a risk of haematoma formation if care is not taken. This can be reduced by using a small (23 g) needle and by applying pressure directly to the puncture site after withdrawal of the needle (Kline et al., 1979). Experience has indicated this should be for at least 5 minutes. Because of the possibility of haematoma it is not usually advisable to do mammography for at least one week after FNA. Haematoma or the trauma of the needle may cause distortion of the mammogram and therefore be difficult to interpret.

The process can be uncomfortable or even painful for some. Local anaesthetic is not normally used because this may distort the area to be needled and decrease the accuracy. From general experience most people find the administration of the local anaesthetic to be as painful as the FNA itself.

There is no evidence that tumour cells can be disseminated along the needle tract (Zajicek et al., 1970).

Conclusion

In conclusion, fine needle aspirate is cost effective and accurate (Koss, 1993) and causes less discomfort and emotional distress than open biopsy (Layfield et al., 1993). With the proviso that the procedure and examination of cells are undertaken by experienced personnel, for many centres this is now the preferred method of diagnosis in breast cancer.

References

Cancer Research Campaign (1991) *Factsheet 6. Breast Cancer*. Cancer Research Campaign, London.

Case, C. (1984) *The Breast Cancer Digest*, 2nd edn. US Department of Health and Human Services, National Cancer Institute, Maryland.

Franzen, S. & Zajicek, J. (1968) Aspiration biopsy in diagnosis of palpable lesions of the breast: critical review of 3479 consecutive biopsies. *Acta Radiologica*, 7, 241–62.

Gray, H. (1977) *Gray's Anatomy*. Bounty Books (American edition), New York.

Kline, T. et al. (1979) Fine needle aspiration of the breast: diagnosis and pitfalls *Cancer*, 44, 1458–64.

Koss, L. (1993) The palpable breast nodule: a cost-effectiveness analysis of alternate diagnostic approaches. *Cancer*, 72(5), 1499–1502.

Layfield, L. et al. (1993) The palpable breast nodule: a cost-effectiveness analysis of alternate diagnostic approaches. *Cancer*, 72(5), 1642–51.

Ljung, B.-M. et al. (1994) Fine needle aspiration techniques for the characterization of breast cancers. *Cancer*, 74, 1000–1005.

Trott, P. (1991) Aspiration cytodiagnosis of the breast. *Diagnostic Oncology*, 1, 79–87.

Zajicek, J. et al. (1970) Cytologic diagnosis of mammary tumors from aspiration biopsy smears. Comparison of cytologic and histologic findings in 2111 lesions and diagnostic use of cytophotometry. *Acta. Cytology*, 14, 370–76.

GUIDELINES: BREAST ASPIRATION

EQUIPMENT

1 70% isopropyl alcohol swabs.
2 Sterile syringes (10 ml).
3 Sterile needles 21 g or 23 g.
4 Microscope slides.
5 Universal container.
6 Slide tray.
7 Fixative (ethanol).
8 Low-linting gauze,
9 Plaster/surgical tape.
10 Sharps container.
11 Cytology request form.
12 Microscope slide holders.

Guidelines: Breast aspiration (cont'd)

PROCEDURE

Action

Rationale

1 Explain and discuss the procedure with the patient.

To ensure that the patient understands the procedure and gives his/her valid consent.

2 Place slides on a tray.

In preparation for breast aspirate.

3 Prepare syringe by introducing 2 ml of air into the barrel.

To prevent aspirated material being sucked into the syringe.

4 Choose appropriate size needle and attach to the syringe.

Usually 23 g, but for a large breast or deep lesion 21 g may be necessary.

5 Clean area of patient's skin with single use sterile swab saturated with 70% isopropyl alcohol.

To reduce the risk of infection.

6 Firmly fix breast lump or area of clinical interest between the fingers of one hand.

To stabilize the area before introducing the needle to ensure the correct area sampled.

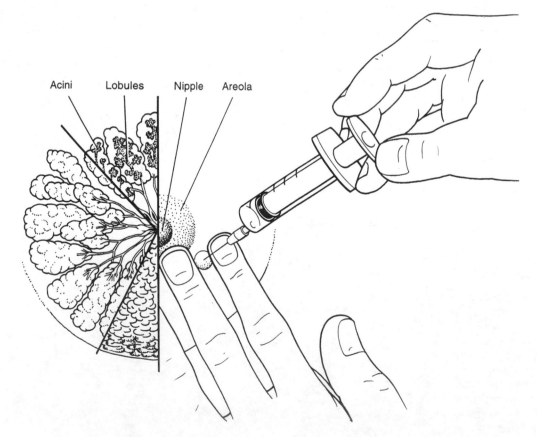

Acini   Lobules   Nipple   Areola

Figure 9.2 Performing fine needle aspiration of the breast.

7	Warn the patient that a needle is about to be inserted.	To prevent the patient moving.
8	Push the needle tip into the centre of the lump or area of clinical interest. Note consistency. (Fig. 9.2).	To obtain specimen from appropriate area. Consistency can be a diagnostic indicator, i.e. gritty (malignant) or rubbery (benign). This information is of use to the cytologist.
9	If the lump is thought to be cystic be careful not to move the needle whilst withdrawing fluid. Withdraw the needle when no further fluid appears in the syringe. If the fluid is discoloured send for cytology.	The needle must be kept in place in the cyst sack whilst withdrawing fluid to enable complete drainage of the cyst and reduce chances of it refilling. Clear fluid is indicative of a cyst only. Anything else should be sent to the laboratory to exclude malignancy.
10	Aspirate a solid lesion or area of clinical interest using the maximum amount of suction moving the tip of the needle back and forth and in different directions without withdrawing the needle through the skin.	To enable sampling of different areas and to obtain an adequate sample for transferring to the slide.
11	After aspiration, allow the barrel of the syringe to return to 2 ml before withdrawing the needle to eliminate any negative pressure in the syringe.	To avoid the contents of the needle being sucked into the syringe.
12	After withdrawal of the needle from the breast, express the aspirate on to two slides. If the aspirate is thick then four slides will be required. Smear the cells evenly on the slides, usually with a second slide.	To prepare the cells for cytodiagnosis. A monolayer is required because if the smear is blood stained or there is too much material on the slide staining can be a problem and the cytologist cannot make a diagnosis.
13	Low linting swab should be placed over the puncture site and pressure applied for at least one minute or until bleeding has stopped.	To prevent haematoma.
14	Leave one slide to dry in the air and add fixative to the other as required by the cytologist. Label appropriately.	When such a small amount of material is available the cytologist will require different staining techniques for accurate diagnosis.
15	If the aspirate is lost into the barrel of the needle 5 ml of 0.9% sodium chloride should be drawn into the syringe through the same needle and the resultant suspension placed in a universal container.	So that the sample can be recovered by centrifugation and then stained as normal. A large percentage of the cells will still be lost.
16	Dispose of needle and syringe in sharps container.	To reduce risk of injury and infection to staff.
17	Label slides with name, number and which breast.	To ensure correct identification of specimen.
18	Apply a plaster or non-allergenic dressing to puncture site.	To protect clothing.
19	Complete cytology forms with full details.	To ensure correct identification and most accurate information for diagnosis.
20	Place slides in slide holder. Slide holder and cytology forms to be placed in plastic specimen bag.	To ensure safe transfer to laboratory.

CHAPTER 10
Cardiopulmonary Resuscitation

Definition
Cardiac arrest can be defined as the abrupt cessation of cardiac function which is potentially reversible. Respiratory and cardiac arrest may produce similar signs but there is one important difference: cardiac arrest – no arterial pulse; respiratory arrest – arterial pulse is present.

The three arrhythmias which cause cardiac arrest are:

(1) Asystole.
(2) Ventricular fibrillation.
(3) Electromechanical dissociation.

Indications
Indications of cardiac arrest are as follows:

(1) The patient rapidly loses consciousness, becoming pale and cyanosed with absent pulses in major vessels (carotid and femoral arteries).
(2) Respiration is slow and stertorous or absent.
(3) The pupils become dilated and unresponsive to light.

REFERENCE MATERIAL

Principles
The primary objective of cardiopulmonary resuscitation is to prevent irreversible cerebral damage due to anoxia by restoring effective circulation within four minutes.

Resuscitation is the emergency treatment of any condition in which the brain fails to receive enough oxygen. The basic technique involves a rapid simple assessment of the patient followed by the ABC of resuscitation (Colqhhoun *et al.*, 1995) (Fig. 10.1a–d).

A Assessment and airway control
There are two stages of assessment:

(1) An immediate assessment by the first-aider to ensure that cardiopulmonary resuscitation may safely proceed (i.e. checking there is no immediate hazard to the patient or others from electrical equipment, for example).
(2) Assessment by the first-aider of any injury sustained by the patient, particularly injury to the cervical spine.

Check the patient's level of consciousness by shaking him/her gently gently and asking, 'Are you alright?'. If there is no response, establish and maintain a clear airway.

B Breathing
If the patient is not breathing, commence and maintain artificial ventilation either by expired air method, i.e. mouth to mouth, or use of an airway plus Ambu-bag and face mask. The patient should initially be given two slow expired breaths of air, each sufficient to cause the chest to rise (ERC Guidelines, 1994).

C Circulation
If the patient does not have a pulse in a major artery, i.e. carotid or femoral, then circulation must be established by external cardiac massage (Fig. 10.2a,b) (ERC Guidelines, 1994).

The first intervention should be the pre-cordial thump. This is delivered from about 20 cm above the chest, sharply on the junction between the lower and middle third of the sternum. The pre-cordial thump is of most value in asystole or ventricular tachycardia. A thump can also be effective on rare occasions within a few seconds of the onset of ventricular fibrillation. It carries little risk and takes only a few seconds (Colqhhoun *et al.*, 1995).

Causes
(1) *Cardiac*: cardiac causes are due to coronary occlusion, cardiac tamponade, cardiomyopathy and electrocution.
(2) *Respiratory*: respiratory causes are due to airway obstruction, i.e. foreign bodies, pulmonary embolism, pneumothorax and drowning.

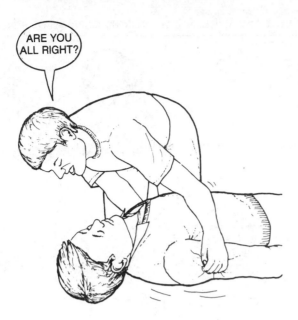

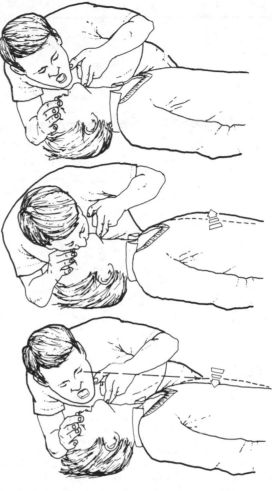

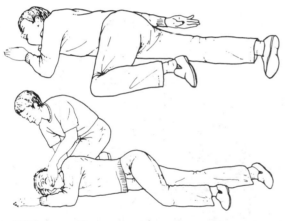

Recovery position

Figure 10.1 (a) The ABC of resuscitation, Rapid, simple assessment of patient, and placement in the recovery position.

Expired air resuscitation

Figure 10.1 (b) If the patient is not breathing, expired air respiration must be started immediately.

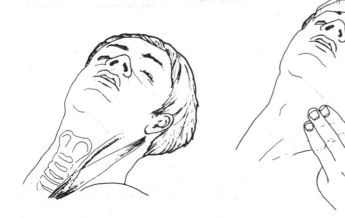

Figure 10.1 (c) If the patient does not have a pulse in a major artery (carotid), or if there is a neck injury, the femoral artery may be felt. Circulation must then be established with compression.

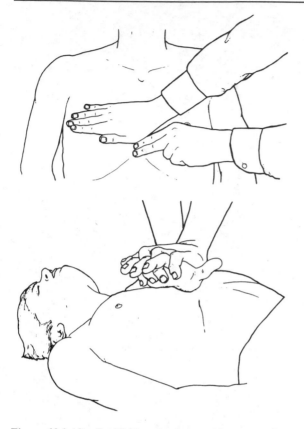

Figure 10.1 (d) Establishing circulation with compression. Note fingers are clear of chest wall. (Courtesy of Colqhhoun, M., Handley, A.J. & Evans, T.R. (1995) *ABC of Resuscitation*, 3rd edn. BMJ Publishing Group).

(3) *Cerebral*: cerebral causes are due to depression of respiratory centre due to:
    (a) Head injury with increased intracranial pressure.
    (b) Overdose of depressant drugs.
    (c) Hypothermia.
    (d) Hypertension.
    (e) Lesions of the central nervous system.
(4) Metabolic disruption of the normal acid–base balance and/or electrolyte profile, i.e. hypo/hyperkalaemia, acidosis, hypovolaemia, severe sepsis (Oh, 1995).

Treatment

Treatment of cardiac arrest is carried out in three stages:

(1) Restoration of breathing and circulation.
(2) Correction of acid–base balance.
(3) Assessment and correction of fluid and electrolyte imbalance.

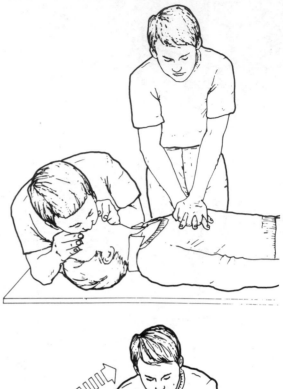

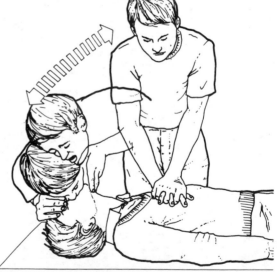

Figure 10.2 Establishing circulation by external cardiac massage. (a) When only one rescuer is present, the compression to ventilation ratio is 15:2. (b) When two rescuers are present, the compression to ventilation ratio is 5:1. (Courtesy of Colqhhoun, M., Handley, A.J. & Evans, T.R. (1995) *ABC of Resuscitation*, 3rd edn. BMJ Publishing Group).

Drugs

The drugs used in the treatment of cardiac arrest are:

(1) Adrenaline 1 mg (10 ml of a 1 : 10 000 solution) given intravenously. The main purpose of adrenaline is to utilize its inotropic effect to maintain coronary and

cerebral perfusion during a prolonged resuscitation attempt.

(2) Atropine 3 mg given intravenously. Reduces cardiac vagal tone, increases the rate of discharge of the sinoatrial node and increases the speed of conduction through the atrioventricular node. It is advisable to give atropine for asystole following administration of adrenaline because it blocks all parasympathetic activity (Tinker & Zapol, 1991).

(3) Calcium chloride (10 ml of 10%) is used for the treatment of electromechanical dissociation when the cause is hyperkalaemia, hypocalcaemia, or when calcium antagonist toxicity is present. Calcium has no proven efficacy in asystolic cardiac arrest (Tinker & Zapol, 1991).

(4) Sodium bicarbonate 8.4% is only used in prolonged cardiac arrest or according to blood gas analyses. Potential adverse effects of excessive sodium bicarbonate administration include hypokalaemia, exacerbation of respiratory acidosis and increased affinity of haemoglobin for oxygen. The high concentration of sodium is also contraindicated by cerebral oedema. Other adverse effects are increased cardiac irritability and impaired myocardial performance. The usual dose of sodium bicarbonate is aliquots of 10–20 mmol repeated as necessary (Oh, 1995).

The Resuscitation Council of the United Kingdom has issued new guidelines for drug administration and defibrillation sequence (ERC Guidelines, 1994). Cardiopulmonary resuscitation should not be interrupted for more than 10 seconds, and should be continued for up to 2 minutes after each drug is administered. If an intravenous line cannot be established, then double doses of adrenaline or lignocaine may be given via the endotracheal tube, but drug absorption is unpredictable using this method. When intravenous access is problematic, the intra-osseus route may be utilized. The intra-osseus route is sometimes used in accident and emergency departments when venous access is difficult, especially in children (ERC Guidelines, 1994).

Defibrillation

Defibrillation causes a simultaneous depolarization of the myocardium and aims to restore normal rhythm to the heart. This is the immediate treatment for ventricular fibrillation and ventricular tachycardia. Defibrillation can be used for a patient who has had a cardiac arrest even if a monitor is not available.

The carrying out of defibrillation by nurses in special units, i.e. coronary care and intensive care, is becoming an accepted practice, provided nurses have received proper training. This also depends on guidelines laid down in hospital policies.

Please see Fig. 10.3 for the European Resuscitation Council algorithm of electromechanical dissociation, ventricular fibrillation and asystole.

The resuscitation team

Most hospitals now have a designated cardiac arrest team. It is essential that the team works in an efficient and effective manner, with one member acting as co-ordinator. There are usually four or five team members (Colqhhoun et al., 1995):

(1) A duty medical registrar.
(2) An anaesthetic registrar.
(3) Senior house officer.
(4) A porter (and trolley).
(5) A nurse skilled in resuscitation.

The team will require bleeps, with a speech channel so that the operator can give the exact location of the emergency.

Statistics

Sudden cardiac death most frequently occurs in the first 1–2 hours after the onset of symptoms due to fatal arrhythmias, usually ventricular fibrillation (Tinker & Zapol, 1991).

Cozart Rosequist (1987) suggests that if cardiopulmonary resuscitation is initiated quickly and promptly by well-trained lay people or emergency medical personnel, then between 40 and 80% of patients with documented ventricular fibrillation can be resuscitated successfully.

In the UK, community resuscitation has been slower to improve (Evans, 1990). However, with the advent of a nationwide programme of extended training of ambulance staff in resuscitation, and the introduction of a training programme aimed at the general public by a few hospitals (Ferguson, 1990), this situation can only improve.

Of equal importance is the fact that hospital staff often do not possess the necessary skills. Wynn (1987) has shown the poor performance by nursing staff in resuscitation. This indicates an obvious need for more training, and a revision of skills. The UKCC has indicated that in the near future nurses will require a certificate of competence to perform cardiopulmonary resuscitation in order to renew registration.

Ethics

The increase in skills, knowledge, technology and pharmacological support have proved very effective in prolonging quality of life. However, the assessment of patients suitable for resuscitation is controversial. There are many important factors which need to be considered in deciding whether to resuscitate a patient or not:

ADVANCED CARDIAC LIFE SUPPORT

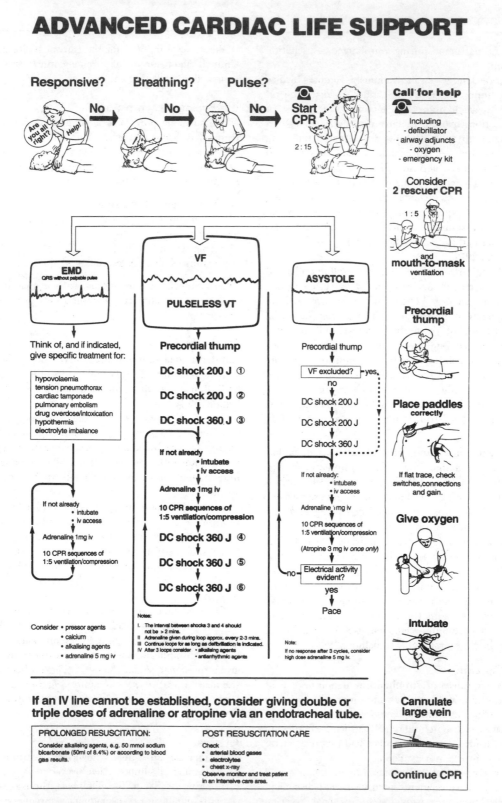

Figure 10.3 The European Resuscitation Council algorithm. (Courtesy of the European Resuscitation Council guidelines for Advanced Life Support, endorsed by Resuscitation Council (UK).)

(1) The patient's disease and prognosis.

(2) Events leading to cardiopulmonary arrest.

(3) The patient's wishes and the wishes of the family or friends.

(4) The quality of life of the patient and expected quality after discharge.

The decision on whether or not to resuscitate should involve all personnel in the clinical team. Ideally, this decision should be made before the event. However or whenever these decisions are made, the problems must be discussed openly and freely, so that the medical profession is not accused of prolonging misery because personnel are afraid to make the decision.

Dangers associated with resuscitation

Diseases such as auto-immune deficiency syndrome (AIDS) and hepatitis B and C have now come into focus with regard to mouth-to-mouth resuscitation. Research into the human immunodeficiency virus (HIV) virus being transmitted during resuscitation is still in its infancy although there is no evidence to date that HIV is transmitted by saliva, and there are airway adjuncts which can be used. Pocket face masks and mouth shields are available commercially, but such devices must not hinder airflow.

References and further reading

Andreoti, K. G. *et al.* (1975) *Comprehensive Cardiac Care*, 3rd edn. C. V. Mosby, St Louis.

Bridges, W. & MacLeod Clark, J. (1981) *Communication in Nursing*. I HM & M Publishers, London.

Cavanagh, S. J. (1990) Education aspects of cardiopulmonary resuscitation (CPR) training. *Intensive Care Nursing*, 6(1), 38–40.

Cozart Rosequist, C. (1987) Current standards and guidelines for cardiopulmonary resuscitation and emergency cardiac care. *Heart and Lung Journal of Critical Care (Heart Lung)*, 16(4), 408–18.

ERC Guidelines (1994). Laerdal Medical, London.

Colqhhoun, M. *et al.*, (1995) *ABC of Resuscitation*, 3rd edn. BMJ Publishing Group, London.

Ferguson, A. (1990) Cardiopulmonary resuscitation . . . a teaching guide. *Nurse Education Today*, 10(1), 50–3.

Lawrence, J. A. (1982) The nurse should consider: critical care ethical issues. *Journal of Advanced Nursing*, 7(3), 223–9.

McPhail, A. *et al.* (1981) One hospital's experience with a 'do not resuscitate' policy. *Canadian Medical Association Journal*, 125, 830–6.

Neatherlin, J. S. & Brillhart, B. (1988) Glasgow Coma Scores in the patient: post-cardiopulmonary resuscitation. *Journal of Neuroscience Nursing*, 20(2), 104–9.

Oh, T. E. (1995) *Intensive Care Manual*. Butterworths, Sydney, Australia.

Sloman, M. (1988) Paediatric cardiopulmonary resuscitation. *Nursing Times*, 84(43), 50–2.

Stirba, C. (1988) Cardiopulmonary resuscitation in patients with acquired immunodeficiency syndrome (letter). *Archives of Internal Medicine*, 149(10), 2380.

Tinker, J. & Zapol, W. (1991) *Care of the Critically Ill Patient*. Springer-Verlag, London.

Voladez, L. & Garcia, R. M. (1987) Resusci annie proves safe. *Journal of Continuing Education in Nursing*, 18(5), 160–2.

Wynn, G. (1987) Inability of trained nurses to perform basic life support. *British Medical Journal*, 294(6581), 1198.

GUIDELINES: CARDIOPULMONARY RESUSCITATION

EQUIPMENT

All hospital wards and appropriate departments, i.e. computerized axial tomography (CT) scanning departments, should have a cardiac arrest trolley or box. A list of the items should be drawn up and checked weekly or immediately after use, by ward staff or designated personnel.

1 Airways (different sizes).

2 Mouth to face resuscitation mask.

3 Ambu-bag with valve and mask.

4 Oxygen tubing.

5 Suction apparatus.

6 Oropharyngeal suction catheters.

7 Laryngoscope with spare bulbs and batteries.

8 Magill's forceps.

9 Pre-prepared endotracheal tubes (different sizes according to patient populations), and introducer.

10 Gauze swabs.

11 Lubricating jelly.

12 10ml syringe for use with endotracheal tube.

Guidelines: Cardiopulmonary resuscitation (cont'd)

13 Artery forceps.
14 Endotracheal suction catheter.
15 Bandage or tracheostomy tape.
16 Scissors.
17 Catheter mount with swivel connector.
18 Emergency cardiac drugs (prefilled syringes).
19 Intravenous infusion giving sets including large bore central lines.
20 Selection of intravenous cannulae – including large bore central lines.
21 Strapping.
22 Syringes and needles (various sizes).
23 70% isopropyl alcohol swabs.
24 Intravenous infusion stand.
25 ECG monitor plus adhesive electrodes.
26 Defibrillator with conductive gel pads for defibrillation.

PROCEDURE

Action

1 Note time of arrest, if witnessed.

2 Give patient pre-cordial thump.

3 Summon help. If a second nurse is available, he/she can call for the cardiac arrest team, bring emergency equipment and screen off the area.

4 Lie patient flat on firm surface. A King's Fund bed now provides such a surface; failing this, a board may be placed under the mattress, or the patient may be placed on the floor.

5 If patient is in bed, remove bed head, and ensure adequate space between back of bed and wall.

6 Ensure a clear airway. If cervical spine injury is excluded, extend, not hyperextend, the neck (thus lifting the tongue off the posterior wall of the pharynx). This is best achieved by lifting the chin forwards with the finger and thumb of one hand while pressing the forehead backwards with the heel of the other hand. If this fails to establish on airway, there may be obstruction by a foreign body. Try to remove the obstruction if possible.

Do not remove well-fitted dentures.

7 Insert airway, and place mask over patient's mouth and nose, making sure a seal is created.

Rationale

Lack of cerebral perfusion for approximately 3–4 minutes can lead to irreversible brain damage.

This may restore cardiac rhythm, which will give a cardiac output.

Cardiopulmonary resuscitation is more effective with two rescuers. One is responsible for inflating the lungs, and the other for chest compressions. Continue until medical help arrives.

Effective external cardiac massage can be performed only on a hard surface.

To allow easy access to patients' head in order to facilitate intubation.

To establish and maintain airway, thus facilitating ventilation.

They help to create a mouth seal during ventilation.

To ventilate lungs, and avoid escape of air around face mask. It avoids contact with patient's mouth, thus minimizing risk of disease transmission.

8 Locate the base of the sternum, then place one hand the width of two fingers above this point over the lower third of the sternum, midline. Ensure that only the heel of the dominant hand is touching the sternum.

Place the other hand on top, straighten the elbows and make sure shoulders are directly over the patient's chest.
The sternum should be depressed sharply by 2–4cm. The cardiac compressions should be forceful, and sustained at a rate of 60–80 per minute.

To ensure accuracy of external cardiac compression.

Pressure on the lower half of the sternum of sufficient weight will compress the sternum and force blood out of the ventricles and improve blood flow (Oh, 1995).

9 Compress the Ambu-bag in a rhythmical fashion: the bag should be attached to an oxygen source. In order to deliver 100% oxygen, a reservoir may be attached to the Ambu-bag. If, however, oxygen is not immediately available, the Ambu-bag will deliver ambient air.

To ensure a constant and steady supply of oxygen. The brain and heart have a very low tolerance to hypoxia, and any increase in the blood oxygen content will improve the chances of survival of these organs. Room air contains only 21% oxygen (Oh, 1995).

10 Maintain cardiac compression and ventilation at a ratio of 15:2 for one-rescuer resuscitation, and 5:1 for two-rescuer resuscitation (Fig. 10.2a,b). This rate can be achieved effectively by counting out loud 'one and two' etc. There should be a slight pause to ensure that the delivered breath is sufficient to cause the patient's chest to rise. This must continue until cardiac output returns and the patient has a palpable blood pressure.

Counting aloud will ensure coordination of ventilation and compression ratio. To maintain circulation and oxygenation, thus reducing risk of damage to vital organs.

11 When the cardiac arrest team arrives, it will assume responsibility for the arrest in liaison with the ward staff.

To ensure an effective expert team coordinates the resuscitation.

12 Attach patient to ECG monitor using three electrodes or defibrillation patches/paddles.

To obtain adequate ECG signal. Accurate recording of cardiac rhythm will determine the appropriate treatment to be initiated.

Intubation

Action

Rationale

13 Continue to ventilate and oxygenate the patient before intubation.

The risks of cardiac arrhythmias due to hypoxia are decreased.

14 Equipment for intubation should be checked before handing to appropriate medical staff:
   (a) Suction equipment is operational.
   (b) The cuff of the endotracheal tube inflates and deflates.
   (c) The endotracheal tube is well lubricated.
   (d) That catheter mount with swivel connector is ready for use.

Guidelines: Cardiopulmonary resuscitation (cont'd)

Action	Rationale
15 During intubation, the anaesthetist may request cricoid pressure. This involves compressing the oesophegus between the cricoid ring and the sixth cervical vertebra to prevent regurgitation.	Aspiration of stomach contents during intubation can cause a chemical pneumonitis with an increased mortality (Oh, 1995).
16 Recommence ventilation and oxygenation once intubation is completed.	Intubation should interrupt resuscitation only for a few seconds to prevent the occurrence of cerebral anoxia.

Intravenous lines

Action	Rationale
17 Venous access must be established through a large vein as soon as possible.	To administer emergency cardiac drugs and fluid replacement.
18 Asepsis should be maintained throughout.	To prevent local and/or systemic infection.
19 The correct rate of infusion is required.	To ensure maximum drug and/or solution effectiveness.
20 Accurate recording of the administration of solutions infused and drugs added is essential.	For reference in the event of any queries.

Defibrillation

Used to terminate ventricular fibrillation or ventricular tachycardia.

Post-resuscitation care

Complete recovery from cardiac arrest does not happen immediately. The patient may require 24 hours of mechanical ventilation after cardiac arrest.

1 Check the patient by assessing breathing, circulation, blood pressure and urine output.
2 Check arterial blood gases and electrolytes.
3 Monitor patient's cardiac rhythm.
4 Chest X-ray should be taken.
5 Continue respiratory therapy.
6 Assess patient's level of consciousness. This can be done by use of the Glasgow Coma Scale. Although this is intended primarily for head injury, it is clinically relevant. It contains five levels of consciousness:
   (a) Conscious and alert.
   (b) Drowsy but responsive to verbal commands.
   (c) Unconscious but responsive to minimal painful stimuli.
   (d) Unconscious and responsive to deep painful stimuli.
   (e) Unconscious and unresponsive.
7 The patient should be made comfortable and nursed in the appropriate position, i.e. upright or the recovery position. Careful explanation and reassurance is vital at all times, particularly if the patient is conscious and aware.

The patient should be transferred to a special unit, i.e. coronary care or intensive care.

NURSING CARE PLAN

Problem	Cause	Suggested action
Only one nurse immediately available.	Colleagues in other areas of ward. If an emergency occurs during the night, the second nurse may be having rest break.	Use emergency buzzer to summon help, or shout. Commence resuscitative measures immediately using airway, breathing and circulation (ABC) technique.
Breathing is absent.	Obstructed airway due to the tongue falling onto the posterior pharyngeal wall. Airway obstruction can occasionally be caused by foreign bodies, e.g. food, dentures, etc.	Establish and maintain a clear airway: extend (*not* hyperextend) the neck and lift the chin forward with the finger and thumb of one hand, and press down on the forehead with the other. Check for foreign bodies. If this does not relieve obstruction and patient is still not breathing, commence expired air respiration immediately either by mouth-to-mouth resuscitation or by using an airway or Ambu-bag and mask. For effective ventilation, ensure the mask covers the nose and mouth correctly in order to create an airtight seal.
Patient has a radioactive source implanted.		See the procedures for sealed and unsealed sources.

CHAPTER 11
Central Venous Catheterization

Definition

Placement of an indwelling catheter within the superior or inferior vena cava or right atrium, or a large vein leading to these vessels.

Indications

This procedure is indicated in the following circumstances:

(1) To monitor central venous pressure in seriously ill patients.
(2) For the administration of large amounts of intravenous fluid or blood, e.g. in cases of shock or major surgery.
(3) To provide long-term access for:
    (a) Hydration or electrolyte maintenance.
    (b) Repeated administration of drugs, such as cytotoxic and antibiotic therapy.
    (c) Repeated transfusion of blood or blood products.
    (d) Repeated specimen collection.
(4) For total parenteral nutrition (Bjeletich & Hickman, 1980).

REFERENCE MATERIAL

The catheter

In the past decade there have been numerous developments in both catheter design and materials, resulting in a greater range of devices. This has had a beneficial effect on patient care due to improvements in insertion techniques and nursing management.

Table 11.1 lists examples of available catheters. This is not intended to be a comprehensive list as recent progress has been rapid, with many new products entering clinical use. Double and triple lumen catheters have provided solutions to the problems of multiple access and the inclusion of the extra features such as 'on/off' switches and non-return valves have simplified nursing practice. Impregnated coatings have reduced the risk of infection.

Insertion of the catheter

The catheter may be inserted at any of the sites shown in Fig. 11.1. If the site chosen is the antecubital fossa, a 'long line' will be used as the catheter has to pass a substantial distance through the venous system.

The catheter may be inserted directly into the vein or it may be tunnelled subcutaneously for a short distance prior to entry (see Fig. 11.1). Skin tunnelling is usually performed if the catheter is intended to provide long-term access over a number of months, during which the patient may be discharged and readmitted. The purpose of the tunnel is to remove the entry site into the vein from the exit site on the skin, so providing a barrier to infection. Catheters specifically designed for skin tunnelling frequently have a Dacron cuff which should be sited at least 5 cm from the entry site (Stacey *et al.*, 1991). The catheter currently used at The Royal Marsden NHS Trust has a Dacron cuff which is situated 22 cm from the top of the bifurcation on a dual lumen catheter (Fig. 11.2). This measurement may assist the practitioner in locating the cuff during removal of the catheter. However, this may vary according to the type of catheter. The cuff is positioned in the subcutaneous tunnel and tissue granulates around it, so reinforcing the barrier to invading organisms and providing security. Local site infection can be observed and treated, the incidence of septicaemia is reduced and removal of the catheter due to contamination is not always necessary. An example of this type of catheter is the Hickman.

A recent development also aimed at reducing complications due to infections is an implantable drug delivery system, consisting of a portal attached to a silicone catheter (Fig. 11.3). It is usually inserted under general anaesthetic. Among the advantages of this system over conventional central or skin tunnelled catheters are less frequent heparinization and a more aesthetically pleasing effect. Claims have been made that the risk of sepsis is reduced and there is evidence of this in a number of studies reviewed by Richard Alexander (1994).

Table 11.1 Central venous catheters: materials and features.

Catheter type	Material	Features	Common insertion site	Recommended indwelling life and common uses
Short-term percutaneous	Polyurethane Silicone	Multiple lumen Antimicrobial collagen cuff Heparin, antibiotic and antiseptic coatings	Jugular Subclavian	Intended for days to several weeks of intravenous access
Peripherally inserted central catheter (PICC)	Silastic Polyurethane Aquavene	Double lumen Groshong valve	Antecubital fossa	Used primarily for patients requiring several weeks or months of intravenous access. Also for patients with chest injuries, radical neck dissection, radiotherapy to the chest, unstable for surgical procedure
Tunnelled catheters	Silastic Polyurethane	Groshong valve Antimicrobial collagen cuff Multiple lumen	Cephalic Axillary Subclavian Antecubital fossa	Indefinite. Used for long-term intermittent, continuous or daily intravenous access. May be appropriate for short-term use if reliable access needed
Implanted venous access ports	*Catheter* Silastic *Port* Titanium Stainless steel Plastic	Dual ports Peripheral ports Dual lumen Groshong valve	Antecubital fossa Subclavian	Indefinite. Used for long-term intermittent, continuous or daily intravenous access

External jugular vein

Internal jugular vein

Subclavian vein

Axillary vein

Incision

Cephalic vein

Basilic vein

Skin insertion (exit site)

Figure 11.1 The ideal position and site for a long-term indwelling catheter.

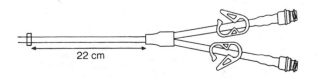

22 cm

Figure 11.2 Distance from cuff to bifurcation of skin tunnelled catheter.

However, sample groups have not been matched and so the comparisons made should be approached with caution. The portal system can be used for bolus injections, infusions of drugs, blood products, total parenteral nutrition and blood sampling (Speechley & Davidson, 1989).

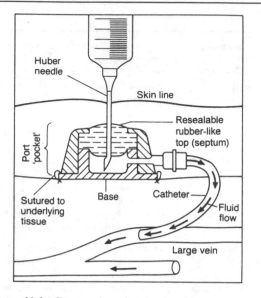

Figure 11.3 Cross-section of an implantable port, accessed with Huber point needle.

Table 11.2 Hazards of catheter insertion (Speer, 1990).

Sepsis	Air embolism	Pneumothorax
Hydrothorax	Haemorrhage	Haemothorax
Brachial plexus injury	Thoracic duct trauma	Misdirection or kinking
Catheter embolism	Thrombosis	Cardiac tamponade
		Cardiac arrhythmias

important to check the manufacturer's recommendations (Rasor, 1991).

The hazards associated with the insertion of a central venous catheter are substantial (Table 11.2). For that reason the procedure should be performed in a controlled environment, and the operating theatre or anaesthetic room is preferred to reduce the risk of complications and have access to an experienced team (Stacey *et al.*, 1991). When this is not possible, a quiet environment with a minimum of activity is recommended, in order to control for potential contamination.

A general anaesthetic may be necessary for some insertions but now the procedure is frequently performed under heavy sedation using local anaesthesia (Stacey *et al.*, 1991). The doctor inserts the catheter with the nurse assisting. The nurse's responsibilities are:

(1) To ensure the patient has been given a full explanation of the procedure and to teach the patient techniques which may be required during insertion; for example the Valsalva manoeuvre (see below).
(2) To ensure that any specific preoperative instructions have been carried out.
(3) To explain the post-operative procedures and the appearance and function of the catheter or device.
(4) To assemble the equipment requested.
(5) To prepare fluids with which to test the patency of the catheter.
(6) To prepare local anaesthesia and dressing materials.
(7) To ensure the correct positioning of the patient during insertion, that is, in the supine or Trendelenburg position, with the head down and a roll of towel along the spinal column.
(8) To attend to the physical and psychological comfort of the patient during and immediately following the procedure.
(9) To ensure that no fluid or medication is infused before the correct position of the catheter is confirmed on X-ray by medical staff.

Reducing the likelihood of the above complications and preventing distress to the patient may be achieved by careful insertion techniques, strict asepsis, correct positioning and radiological confirmation of the catheter

The portal is placed under the skin and sutured to the chest wall. The catheter is tunnelled as previously described and the tip rests in a major vein. The reformation of the skin barrier prevents the entry of micro-organisms, and aseptic technique should result in a minimal contamination rate.

A variety of catheters and portals are available, the choice of which is dependent on a number of factors. For example, whether the patient is a child or an adult, amount of access necessary, etc. The portal is accessed using a special Huber point needle when therapy is required and this may remain in place for up to one week (see Guidelines: Care of Implantable Ports, below).

The midline catheter offers an alternative to peripheral and central venous access. Where patients present with poor peripheral venous access and when use of a central venous catheter is contraindicated, the midline catheter provides venous accessibility along with easy, less hazardous insertion at the antecubital fossa. X-ray verification is not required. The insertion is performed using either an over-the-needle or Seldinger technique. Benefits to the patient include less frequent resiting of the catheter and a reduction in associated venous trauma. However, mechanical phlebitis is a common side-effect and close observation and appropriate management is indicated. Once *in situ*, the catheter should be managed exactly as a central venous catheter, although the list of drugs that can be administered via a midline catheter does not always include vesicant cytotoxics because of the risk of extravasation damage. Therefore it is

placement. The catheter should be heparinized or 0.9% sodium chloride infused slowly, 10–20ml/h, until X-ray results confirm the correct placement of the catheter (Stacey *et al.*, 1991).

The Valsalva manoeuvre

This may be performed by conscious patients to aid the insertion of the catheter. The patient is placed in the supine or Trendlenburg position which increases venous filling. He/she is asked to breathe in and then try to force the air out with the mouth and nose closed (i.e. against a closed glottis). This increases the intrathoracic pressure so that the return of blood to the heart is reduced momentarily and the veins in the neck region become engorged. A distension of the vein up to 2.5cm can be achieved in this way (Ostrow, 1981).

Principles of catheter care

Prevention of infection

Strict aseptic technique and compliance with recommendations for equipment and dressing changes are essential if microbial contamination is to be prevented. (See Chapter 4, Aseptic Technique.)

Whenever the insertion site is exposed or the closed system is broken, aseptic technique should be practised. As blood or body fluids may be present, gloves should be worn to comply with safe technique and practice. The insertion site should be checked regularly post-operatively and the dressing renewed if there is haemoserous discharge. There may be local swelling and drainage from the tunnel when a skin-tunnelled catheter has been inserted. A pressure dressing or application of an ice pack may reduce the severity of these problems. Complaints of soreness, unexpected pyrexia and damaged, wet or soiled dressing are reasons for immediate inspection and renewal. (For further details, see Guidelines: Changing the dressing on a central venous catheter insertion site, page 165.

When the dressing is changed the site should be inspected for inflammation and/or discharge, and the condition of the skin noted. A dry sterile low-linting dressing secured with the minimum of (hypoallergenic) tape is most suitable for patients with delicate skin. The dressing should be changed daily. A central venous catheter dressing should: provide an effective barrier to bacteria; allow the catheter to be securely fixed; be sterile and easy to apply and remove; and be comfortable for the patient (Royal College of Nursing and Infection Control Nurses' Association, 1992). Transparent dressings have the added advantage of allowing inspection of the inser-

tion site, and are waterproof (Baranowski, 1993; Keenleyside, 1993).

Recent research has investigated the infection risks and frequency of dressing changes of both sterile gauze and transparent dressings. Whilst some studies indicate that there is no significant difference between the two types of dressings in these respects (Petrosino *et al.*, 1988), others describe slightly higher levels of bacterial colonization with transparent dressings (Hoffman *et al.*, 1992). No agreement has been reached about exactly what level of colonization represents an infection risk. Consequently choice of dressing depends on which is most suitable for a particular catheter site or type of skin, and on information emerging from ongoing research.

Chlorhexidine in 70% alcohol has been shown to be the most effective agent for skin cleansing around the catheter exit site prior to insertion and between dressing changes (Maki *et al.*, 1991). Following healing of the skin tunnel, which takes approximately 7 days, sutures at the entry site may be removed. Sutures at the exit site of a skin tunnelled catheter should be removed after 21 days. Thereafter no dressing is usually required unless the patient requests one.

Maintenance of a closed system

If equipment becomes disconnected, air embolism or profuse blood loss may occur, depending on the condition and position of the patient at the time (Ostrow, 1981). Luer locks provide a more secure connection and all equipment should have these fittings, i.e. giving sets, extension sets, injection caps and syringes. Care should be taken to clamp the catheter firmly when changing equipment, and the switch provided on some catheters must be used. Connections must be double checked and precautions taken to prevent the introduction of air into the system when making additions to, or taking blood from, the central catheter.

Maintenance of a patent catheter

It is important at all times for the patency of the catheter to be maintained. Blockage predisposes to catheter damage, infection, inconvenience to patients and disruption to protocols. Occlusion of the catheter is usually the result of clot formation due to:

(1) An administration set or mechanical aid being turned off accidentally and left for a prolonged period.
(2) Insufficient or incorrect flushing of the catheter when not in use.
(3) Precipitate formation due to inadequate flushing between incompatible medications.

Patency of the catheter may also be impaired by kinking of the catheter. Meticulous intravenous technique will prevent the majority of these problems.

When used for intermittent therapy, the catheter should be flushed after each use with the appropriate flushing solution. (Guidelines for volumes, concentrations and frequency of flushing are commonly established within individual institutions.) The lack of consensus nationally, and even within regions, causes concern and confusion among health care professionals and patients (Gilles & Rogers, 1985; Clarke & Cox, 1988; Ridley, 1990; Kelly *et al.*, 1992). Heparinized saline is the accepted solution for maintaining the patency of devices for intermittent use. Use of 0.9% sodium chloride alone is not yet widespread and remains controversial. Flushing regimes ranging from once daily to once weekly have been found to be effective. However, irrespective of the amount used and the frequency, it is important to use the push – pause method to create turbulent flow (administer solution 1 ml at a time) and complete the procedure using a positive pressure technique. This is thought to minimize reflux of blood into the catheter tip and to prevent clotting and blockage (Baranowski, 1993).

If occlusion does occur, gentle aspiration may dislodge the clot and a flush with 0.9% sodium chloride may be all that is required to restore patency. Gentle pressure and suction may need to be repeated if the catheter has been left for a long time and a larger thrombus has formed. Silicone catheters expand on pressure and allow fluid around a clot facilitating its dislodgement. Use of heparin solution may also be tried (Stokes *et al.*, 1989; Haire *et al.*, 1990).

The enzymes urokinase and streptokinase have both been used to dissolve thrombi and restore catheter patency. Although effective, these are potentially dangerous substances and their use must be approved by the medical staff and prescribed accordingly (Wachs, 1990; Wickham *et al.*, 1992; Richard Alexander, 1994).

When using implanted drug delivery systems, the manufacturer's literature should be consulted with reference to heparinization. The most widely stated recommendation is a flush with 500 units of heparin monthly.

Preventing damage of the catheter and performing a repair

Silicone catheters are prone to cracking or splitting if handled incorrectly but fortunately both temporary and permanent repairs can be performed. However, prevention of this occurrence is preferred.

Artery forceps, scissors or sharp-edged clamps should not be used on or near the catheter. A smooth clamp should be placed on the reinforced section of the catheter provided for this purpose. If this is not present, one can be created by placing a tape tab over part of the catheter. A second alternative is to move the clamp up or down the catheter at regular intervals.

Accidents do occur, however, and the nurse must be familiar with the action to be taken. Immediate clamping of the catheter proximal to the fracture or split is essential to prevent blood loss or air embolism. The split area should be covered with an alcohol swab and emergency repair equipment collected, together with sterile gloves to ensure that all manipulations are aseptic.

A permanent repair should be performed as soon as possible using the specific kit provided by the manufacturer. This should be done by a member of the medical staff or other designated personnel (Bjeletich, 1982; McMenamin, 1993).

Pyrexia of unknown origin

In the event of the patient developing a persistent pyrexia or tachycardia, contamination of the catheter should be suspected. However, the catheter should not be removed until infection has been confirmed, unless the clinical condition dictates otherwise. The doctor should be informed and the following investigations performed:

(1) Blood cultures:
    (a) From the catheter.
    (b) From a peripheral vein.
    (c) Swab from entry site.
(2) A full blood count.
(3) Midstream specimen of urine for microscopy, culture and sensitivity.
(4) Chest X-ray.
(5) Other tests, e.g. wound swabs, throat swabs, to eliminate other sources of infection, as appropriate.

Indications for catheter removal

(1) Blood cultures from the catheter when tested indicate the presence of micro-organisms.
(2) A positive wound swab from the entry site.
(3) Generalized septicaemia.
(4) A leaking or damaged catheter.
(5) Blockage.
(6) Termination of therapy.

Catheters should not be removed without consultation with medical staff. The device should be removed carefully using aseptic technique. The tip of the catheter should be sent for bacteriological examination only if the catheter is infected, or there are signs of infection that lead the medical staff to suspect the catheter as the source of infection.

Reading central venous pressure

Central venous pressure (CVP) is the pressure within the superior vena cava or the right atrium. Measure-

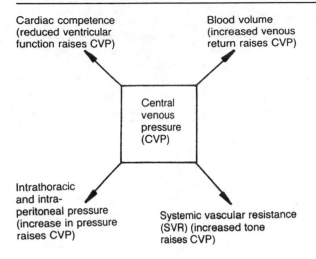

Cardiac competence
(reduced ventricular
function raises CVP)

Blood volume
(increased venous
return raises CVP)

Central venous pressure (CVP)

Intrathoracic
and intra-
peritoneal pressure
(increase in pressure
raises CVP)

Systemic vascular resistance
(SVR) (increased tone
raises CVP)

Figure 11.4 Determinants of central venous pressure.

ments of CVP reflect the relationship between the circulating blood volume (Fig. 11.4), the competence of the heart as a pump and the vascular resistance.

Purpose of CVP readings

(1) To serve as a guide to fluid balance in critically ill patients.
(2) To estimate the circulating blood volume.
(3) To assist in monitoring circulatory failure.

Measuring CVP

The CVP measurement should be taken from a site in line with the right atrium. Either of the sites indicated in Fig. 11.5 may be used, remembering that the sternal angle should be used only with the patient in the supine position, whereas the mid-axilla can be used when the patient is in a variety of other positions. It should be established at the outset which point is to be used, as

there is a difference in pressure of about 5 cm of water between them. It is useful to mark the chosen site for future readings and note both the site and the patient's position on the CVP recording chart and also in the patient's care plan. The normal values for CVP readings are: 0–5 cm of water at the sternal angle, and 5–10 cm of water at the mid-axilla.

Where patients are critically ill, the CVP is transduced electronically via a central monitoring system.

Discharging patients with a central venous catheter *in situ*

Patients with skin-tunnelled catheters or implanted devices may be discharged home with their catheter *in situ*. No special instructions are required for implanted ports as the catheter will be heparinized and the needle removed before the patient leaves hospital. Reheparinization is necessary once a month.

Patients with skin-tunnelled catheters must be instructed and supervised in the care of their catheters before discharge. Aspects to be covered with the patient, relatives and/or friends include:

(1) Care of the exit site.
(2) Heparinization techniques.
(3) The amount and type of activity permitted.

The sutures should only be removed once the catheter has become well established and the Dacron cuff is covered with fibrous tissue. This usually takes 2–3 weeks. Once the sutures are removed, there is usually no longer any need for a dressing unless the patient requests it. Sterile, low-linting swabs and hypoallergenic tape may initially be supplied. While sutures remain in place, patients should change the dressing after their daily shower, having dried the area with clean cotton wool and wiped the exit site with a chlorhexidine soaked swab. When in the bath, water should not come into contact with the exit site: this should be cleaned separately using

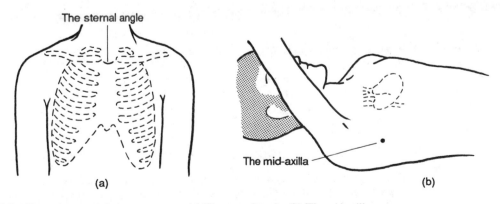

The sternal angle

The mid-axilla

(a)   (b)

Figure 11.5 Measuring central venous pressure. (a) The sternal angle. (b) The mid-axilla.

fresh water and low-linting swabs to clean and dry. The only other time that a dressing is required is when patients go swimming or take part in water sports. In this instance the whole catheter and exit site should be covered completely with an occlusive dressing one hour before entering the water. The dressing is removed immediately afterwards.

Before discharge the patient should observe the heparinization technique and perform it with and without supervision. Relatives and friends may be involved in this procedure. Sufficient equipment must be supplied to enable the patient to care for the catheter from the time of discharge until the next outpatient appointment or admission. A kit should be assembled containing the following:

(1) Spare Luer lock caps with an injection site.
(2) A spare, smooth-edged clamp.
(3) A supply of heparinized saline, 50 iu in 5 ml 0.9% sodium chloride.
(4) Chlorhexidine in 70% alcohol/swab saturated with isopropyl alcohol to clean the injection site on the cap.
(5) A supply of sterile 5 ml syringes.
(6) 23 g needles (blue) to draw up the heparinized saline.
(7) 25 g needles (orange) to inject through the intermittent injection cap.
(8) Instruction booklet to provide the patient with a point of reference if in doubt about procedures when at home.
(9) A designated sharps container.

The patient's technique and confidence when caring for the catheter should be assessed as safe before discharge and the importance of asepsis during all handling procedures stressed. If a patient is discharged before sutures are removed, the site should be dressed before discharge, and arrangements made for the dressing to be removed when necessary.

There are few restrictions with reference to activity. Modifications of dressing technique to allow the patient to engage in water sports are mentioned above. The psychological impact of an indwelling catheter on body image should not be overlooked, especially when patients are sexually active. Additionally, normal activities may be affected, for example, driving may become uncomfortable due to pressure from a seat belt on the catheter or clamp (Thompson *et al.*, 1989).

Removal of the catheter

Non-skin tunnelled catheters
If a catheter is not tunnelled through the skin it may be removed by nursing staff. The nurse must be familiar with the procedure and confident about performing it.

Aseptic technique must be adhered to and the site cleaned with chlorhexidine soaked swabs before removal to prevent a false-positive result when the catheter tip is sent for bacteriological examination. Major vessels usually heal quickly but direct pressure must be applied to the site until cessation of bleeding confirms this. A sterile dressing is applied and should remain in place for at least 24 hours.

Skin-tunnelled catheters
Removal techniques for skin-tunnelled catheters vary. Removal should only be performed by specially trained nurses or doctors. It is recommended that the patient is placed supine and that aseptic technique is used throughout. There are two methods for removal.

Surgical excision
This method involves locating the Dacron cuff and performing a minor surgical excision under local anaesthetic. A small incision is made over the site of the cuff and, using blunt dissection, the cuff and the catheter are freed from the surrounding fibrous tissue, and then the catheter is cut in order to remove the distal and proximal ends separately. Once the catheter has been removed, the wound is sutured using interrupted sutures, which can be removed after 7 days.

Traction method
This method involves using traction and therefore there is a greater risk of the catheter breaking, which could result in a catheter embolism. The catheter is gripped firmly and constant traction applied. It may take a few minutes for the catheter and cuff to become loose before sliding free. Constant steady pressure will remove the complete catheter, however the catheter should be checked on removal to ensure it is complete. The catheter and cuff may be pulled through; however, the cuff may remain attached to tissue. This is of no significance and may be left in place. Difficulty with removal or a break in the catheter will require surgical intervention.

Since the vein closes after the catheter is removed, no bleeding occurs at the insertion site but there may be slight bleeding at the exit site immediately after removal of the catheter because of the passage of the cuff (Bjeletich & Hickman, 1980).

Following either removal method, pressure should be applied to the site and a dressing may be required for up to 24 hours (Weinstein, 1993). The patient should be encouraged to rest for at least an hour.

If the tip is required for microbiological examination, care should be taken to clean the exit/incision site with chlorhexidine in 70% alcohol, prior to removal, to prevent a false positive tip culture. The tip should be placed into a sterile container immediately upon removal.

Total parenteral nutrition

Total parenteral nutrition (TPN) is the direct infusion, into a vein, of solutions containing the essential nutrients in quantities sufficient to meet all the daily needs of the patient.

The decision to administer TPN should be an elective one and should be used only if alternative enteral methods are considered inappropriate or unsatisfactory. Total parenteral nutrition is indicated in any disease or circumstances when the digestive and absorptive functions of the small intestine are seriously impaired. See Chapter 29, Nutritional Support.

TPN solutions

The basic components of a TPN regime are provided by solutions of:

(1) Amino acids (nitrogen source).
(2) Glucose (carbohydrate energy source).
(3) Fat emulsion (non-carbohydrate energy source).
(4) Electrolytes and trace elements.

TPN is usually administered from a single infusion container in which all the requirements for a 24-hour feed are pre-mixed. Such infusions are prepared either by the hospital pharmacy or are purchased. It may be necessary sometimes to exclude fat emulsion from the mixture and to administer it concurrently from separate containers. See Chapter 29, Nutritional Support.

To allow for the possible need to vary the constituents of the infusion in response to changes in the patient's nutritional status, TPN solutions should be ordered daily, except on weekends and public holidays, when it is usually necessary to order and prepare them in advance on Fridays or the last working day before the holiday.

Delivery of TPN and recommendations for intravenous management

The major hazard associated with delivery of TPN is infection and the following detailed recommendations are designed to prevent this. They reflect the current policy of The Royal Marsden NHS Trust that was compiled by a multidisciplinary team:

(1) Catheter insertion should take place in theatre where possible, using aseptic technique.
(2) A skin-tunnelled silicone catheter is the catheter of choice for long-term nutrition.
(3) A separate peripheral cannula may be required for insulin infusion via a syringe pump.
(4) Peripheral venous access should be assessed before catheter placement; if the veins available are consid-

ered inadequate to support the patient for the duration of therapy, a double- or triple-lumen central venous catheter should be inserted.
(5) Only in the event of peripheral access deteriorating during the course of parenteral nutrition, should an adaptor for dual access to the nutrition catheter be used. The adaptor should be streamlined and possess Luer lock fittings.

Dressing of the insertion site

A sterile semi-occlusive transparent dressing will be applied to the insertion site while the patient is in theatre. This should not be touched but the site should be inspected daily. Exceptions to this are:

(1) If the site is inflamed, sore or if there is haemoserous discharge.
(2) If the dressing is not adequately secured, or torn, it should be changed in order to maintain an adequate barrier to infection.

The dressing must be performed in accordance with hospital procedure for the dressing of central venous catheters. The entry site is cleaned with 0.4% chlorhexidine in 70% spirit (Maki *et al.*, 1991), then an appropriate dressing applied. If the site is inflamed, a swab must be sent to the bacteriology department for culture and sensitivity, and the medical staff notified.

Administration sets

Administration sets must be changed every 24 hours, as directed by hospital policy, always using an aseptic technique. Administration sets must have a Luer lock fitting. Infusion containers will be prepared under aseptic conditions in the pharmacy and may be delivered to the ward with administration sets attached. In this instance, the nurse is required to prime the tubing and connect it to the catheter. Before changing the line, the connections should be cleaned thoroughly with a chlorhexidine in 70% spirit soaked swab. The line should then be disconnected and the new one attached. Existing injection sites on the administration set should never be used for the giving of additional medications, as TPN is incompatible with numerous medications.

Administration of medications

No additional medications or blood products should be given by means of a parenteral nutrition catheter. It should not be used for central venous pressure (CVP) measurements. The procedure detailed under catheter insertion should be followed, i.e. a peripheral line should be established.

Control of the rate of infusion

A volumetric infusion pump should be used to ensure accurate delivery of TPN and to provide a means of closely monitoring the infusion. No bag should be used for longer than 24 hours. No adjustment greater than four drops per minute every 15 minutes should be made to an infusion rate. Never attempt to 'catch up' rapidly if fluid is running slowly. In the event of the patient developing septicaemia or a pyrexia of unknown origin, the principles outlined above apply.

Clinical conditions dictating removal of the catheter

Elective
See 'Indications for catheter removal', above.

Termination of therapy
Total parenteral nutrition should only be terminated following discussion with the medical and surgical staff and dietician. At the end of parenteral nutrition, the catheter need not be removed immediately as it may continue to be used for access or hydration. (See Chapter 29, Nutritional Support.) When the catheter is removed, aseptic technique must be used. A sterile airtight dressing should be placed on the exit site and left in place for at least 24 hours to prevent air embolism.

Heparinization
Occasionally certain investigations, e.g. computerized tomography, may require the infusion to be discontinued and the catheter heparinized. Simultaneous insulin infusions must also be discontinued. Partly-used infusion containers should never be used again but must be discarded and a fresh one requested from the pharmacy. Problems should be referred to the appropriate member of medical, anaesthetic, pharmacy or nursing staff.

References and further reading
Anderson, M. A. *et al.* (1982) The double-lumen Hickman catheter. *American Journal of Nursing*, 82(2), 272–7.

Baranowski, L. (1993) Central venous access devices – current technologies, uses and management strategies. *Journal of Intravenous Nursing*, 16(3), 167–94.

Bjeletich, J. (1982) Repairing the Hickman catheter. *American Journal of Nursing*, 82(2), 274.

Bjeletich, J. & Hickman, R. O. (1980) The Hickman indwelling catheter. *American Journal of Nursing*, 80(1), 62–5.

Brunner, L. S. & Suddarth, D. S. (1986) *The Lippincott Manual of Nursing Practice*, 4th edn. J. B. Lippincott, Philadelphia.

Clarke, J. & Cox, E. (1988) Heparinisation of Hickman catheters. *Nursing Times*, 84(15), 51–3.

Davies, J. *et al.* (1978) Disinfection of the skin of the abdomen. *British Journal of Surgery*, 65, 855–8.

Finnegan, S. & Oldfield, K. (1989) When eating is impossible: TPN in maintaining nutritional status. *Professional Nurse*, March, 4(6), 271–5.

Flannigan, M. (1982) Intravenous feeding. *Nursing Mirror*, 156(16), 44–6; 154(17), 48–52.

Ford, R. (1986) History and organisation of the Seattle-area Hickman catheter committee. *Journal of the Canadian Intravenous Nurses Association*, 2(2), 4–13.

Gilles, H. & Rogers, H. J. (1985) Is repeated flushing of Hickman catheters necessary? *British Medical Journal*, 290, 1708.

Goodman, M. S. & Wickham, R. (1984) Venous access devices: an overview. *Oncology Nurses Forum*, 11(5), 16–23.

Gyves, J. *et al.* (1982) Totally implanted system for intravenous chemotherapy in patients with cancer. *American Jorunal of Medicine*, 73, 841–5.

Haire, W. D. *et al.* (1990) Hickman catheter induced thoracic vein thrombosis. *Cancer*, 66, 900–908.

Hinds, C. T. (1988) *Intensive Care*, pp. 32–9. Baillière Tindall, Eastbourne.

Hoffman, K. K. *et al.* (1992) Transparent polyurethane film as an intravenous catheter dressing. *JAMA*, 267(15), 2072–6.

Hollingsworth, S. (1987) Getting on line. *Nursing Times*, 83(29), 61–2.

Hurtibise, M. R. *et al.* (1980) Restoring patency of occluded central venous catheters. *Archives of Surgery*, 115, 212–13.

Keenleyside, D. (1993) Avoiding an unnecessary outcome. A comparative trial between IV 3000 and a conventional film dressing to assess rates of catheter related sepsis. *Professional Nurse*, February, 288–91.

Kelly, C. *et al.* (1992) A change in flushing protocol of CVC. *Oncology Nursing Forum*, 19(4), 599–605.

Keohane, P. P. *et al.* (1983) Effects of catheter tunnelling and a nutrition nurse on catheter sepsis during parenteral nutrition. *Lancet*, 2(17), 1388–90.

Lawson, M. *et al.* (1982) The use of urokinase to restore the patency of occluded central venous catheters. *American Journal of IV Therapy and Clinical Nutrition*, 9(9), 29–32.

Maki, D. R. *et al.* (1991) Prospective randomized trial of povidone iodine, alcohol and chlorhexidene for prevention of infection associated with CVC and arterial catheters. *Lancet*, 338, 339–43.

McMenamin, E. M. (1993) Catheter fracture: a complication in venous access devices. *Cancer Nursing*, 16(6), 464–7.

Mehtar, S. & Taylor, P. (1982) Bacteriological survey of patients undergoing TPN and an IV policy's effects. *British Journal of Intravenous Therapy*, 3(8), 3–11.

Mughal, D. L. (1991) Infected feeding lines. *Care of the Critically Ill*, 6(6), November, 228–32.

Ostrow, L. S. (1981) Air embolism and central venous lines. *American Journal of Nursing*, 81(21), 40–2.

Petrosino, B. *et al.* (1988) Infection rates in CVC dressings. *Oncology Nursing Forum*, 15(6), 709–17.

Plumer, A. L. (1987) *Principles and Practices of Intravenous Therapy*, 4th edn. Little, Brown & Co., Boston.

Rasor, J. J. (1991) Review of catheter related infection rates: comparison of conventional catheter materials with aquavene. *Journal of Vascular Access Network*, 1(3), 8–16.

Richard Alexander, H. (1994) Thrombotic and occlusive complications in long-term venous access. In: *Vascular Access in the Cancer Patient*, Chapter 6. J. B. Lippincott, Philadelphia.

Ridley, R. A. (1990) The use of unpreserved 0.9% sodium chloride injection for the maintenance of multilumen subclavian catheters. *Canadian Intravenous Nurses Association*, 6(1), 5–9.

Royal College of Nursing and Infection Control Nurses' Association (1992) *Intravenous Line Dressings – Principles of Infection Control*. Smith & Nephew Medical Ltd.

Sellu, D. (1985) Long-term intravenous therapy. *Nursing Times*, 81(21), 40–2.

Speechley, V. & Davidson, T. (1989) Managing an implantable drug delivery system. *Professional Nurse*, March, 4(6), 284–8.

Speer, E. W. (1990) CVC issues associated with the use of single and multiple lumen catheters. *Journal of Intravenous Nursing*, 13(1), 30–39.

Stacey, R. G. W. *et al.* (1991) Percutaneous insertion of Hickman type catheters. *British Journal of Hospital Medicine*,

46, 396–8.

Stokes, D. C. *et al.* (1989) Early detection: a simplified management of obstructed Hickman and Broviac catheters. *Journal of Paediatric Surgery*, 24(3), 257–62.

Thompson, A. *et al.* (1989) Long-term central venous access: the patient's view. *Intensive Therapy and Clinical Monitoring*, May, 10(5), 142–5.

Viall, C. (1990) Daily access of implanted venous port. *Journal of Intravenous Nursing*, 13(5), 294–6.

Wachs, T. (1990) Urokinase administration in paediatric patients with occluded central venous catheters. *Journal of Intravenous Nursing*, 13(2), 100–2.

Weinstein, S. M. (1993) *Plumer's Principles and Practice of Intravenous Therapy*, 5th edn. J. B. Lippincott, Philadelphia.

Wickham, R. *et al.* (1992) Long-term CVs issues for care. *Seminars in Oncology Nursing*, 8(2), 133–47.

Woods, S. (1982) Parenteral nutrition. *Nursing*, 2(4), 105–7.

GUIDELINES: READING CENTRAL VENOUS PRESSURE

EQUIPMENT

1 Spirit level.
2 Manometer.
3 Central venous pressure (CVP) monitoring intravenous administration set.

PROCEDURE

Action	Rationale
1 Explain and discuss the procedure with the patient.	To ensure that the patient understands the procedure and gives his/her valid consent.
2 Ascertain the point of CVP reading, i.e. sternal angle or mid-axilla. If the patient agrees, this point should be marked on the patient and noted in the care plan chart for future reference.	CVP must always be read from the same point because the sternal angle reading is about 5 cm of water higher than the mid-axilla reading. To show an accurate trend the figure should be 0.
3 Assist the patient to get into a recumbent or semi-recumbent position to a maximum angle of 45°.	The position of the patient must allow the baseline of the manometer to be level with the patient's right atrium. If the patient is upright or is lying on his/her side, the right atrium will not be in line with the sternal angle or the mid-axilla. However, if it is impossible for the patient to be in any other position, the CVP reading may be recorded with the patient sitting up at a 90° angle, but this must be recorded on the observation chart.
4 Position the manometer so that the baseline is level with the right atrium.	To obtain an accurate CVP reading, the baseline and the right atrium must be level.
5 Loosen the securing screw and slide the scale up or down until the baseline figure lies next	

Guidelines: Reading central venous pressure (cont'd)

Action	Rationale

to the arm of the spirit level (Fig. 11.6a) This figure should be 0.

6 Check that the baseline and right atrium are level by extending the arm of the spirit level to the sternal angle or to the mid-axilla. Move the manometer until the bubble is between the parallel lines of the spirit level (Fig. 11.6b).

7 Care should be taken when flushing the line regarding the volume and type of fluid.

To ensure the patency of the line and to check for leaks, kinks, blockages, etc.

8 Turn off the three-way tap to the patient (Fig. 11.7). Allow the manometer to fill slowly.

To allow the intravenous fluid to run into the manometer. To avoid:
- bubbles, which cause inaccurate readings;
- overfilling of, and spillage from, the manometer that would put the patient at risk from infection.

9 Turn off the three-way tap to the intravenous fluid (Fig. 11.8).

To allow fluid from the manometer to enter the patient's right atrium.

10 The column of water should fall rapidly.

Indicating patency of the line, resulting in an accurate CVP reading.

11 When the level of fluid in the manometer ceases to drop, and oscillates with the pateint's respirations, this is the CVP reading.

The pressure of the column of water in the manometer now equals the pressure in the right atrium.

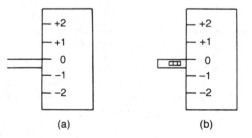

(a)   (b)

Figure 11.6 (a) Setting the baseline. (b) Checking the baseline.

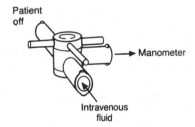

Figure 11.7 Turn off the three–way tap to the patient.

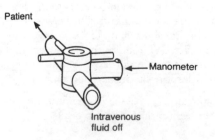

Figure 11.8 Turn off the three–way tap to intravenous fluid.

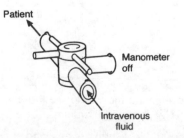

Figure 11.9 Turn off the three-way tap to manometer.

12	Turn off the three-way tap to the manometer (Fig. 11.9).	To restore the intravenous line.
13	Readjust the infusion rate.	
14	Record the CVP measurement on the appropriate chart. Compare this measurement with the patient's acceptable CVP limits as stated by the medical team.	Acceptable CVP values vary with the patient observations and his/her overall condition. Deviations from these limits may require urgent medical intervention.

GUIDELINES: CHANGING THE DRESSING ON A CENTRAL VENOUS CATHETER INSERTION SITE

Before commencing the procedure it is important to check whether there is a variation to standard technique for individual patients, e.g. those receiving TPN, children.

EQUIPMENT

1 Sterile dressing pack.
2 Clamp for the catheter, if necessary.
3 Alcohol-based hand scrub.
4 Alcohol-based skin cleansing preparation, e.g. chlorhexidine in 70% alcohol.
5 Intravenous administration set and extension set or intermittent injection cap.
6 Sterile low-linting dressing.
7 Hypoallergenic tape.
8 Bacteriological swab.

PROCEDURE

Action

Rationale

1	Explain and discuss the procedure with the patient.	To ensure that the patient understands the procedure and gives his/her valid consent.
2	Perform the dressing using an aseptic technique.	To prevent infection. (For further information on asepsis, see Chapter 4, Aseptic Technique.)
3	Screen the bed. Assist the patient into supine position, if possible.	To allow dust and airborne organisms to settle before the wound and the sterile field are exposed. To help prevent embolus.
4	Wash hands with bactericidal soap and water or bactericidal alcohol hand rub. Place all equipment required for the dressing on the bottom shelf of a clean dressing trolley.	To prevent cross-infection.
5	Prime the giving set, keeping the Luer lock sterile.	So that the infusion is ready for use when the current giving set is discontinued.
6	Take the trolley to the patient's bedside, disturbing the screens as little as possible.	To minimize airborne contamination.
7	Attach a yellow clinical waste bag to the side of the trolley below the level of the top shelf.	

Guidelines: Changing the dressing on a central venous catheter insertion site (cont'd)

Action	Rationale
8 Open the outer cover of the sterile dressing pack and slide the contents onto the top shelf of the trolley.	So that areas of potential contamination are kept to a minimum.
9 Open the sterile field using the corners of the paper only. Using the forceps in the pack, arrange the sterile field with the handles of the instruments in one corner.	So that contaminated material is below the level of the sterile field.
10 Open the other sterile packs, tipping their contents gently onto the centre of the sterile field. Pour lotions into gallipots or an indented plastic tray.	To reduce risk of contamination of contents.
11 Wash hands with bactericidal alcohol hand rub.	Hands may have become contaminated by handling the outer packs, etc.
12 Loosen the old dressing gently, touching only the tape, etc securing it.	So that the dressing can be lifted off easily with the forceps.
13 Put on clean gloves.	To protect the nurse from any contact with patient's blood.
14 Using gloved hands or forceps, remove the old dressing and discard it, together with the forceps into the yellow clinical waste bag.	
15 If the site is red or discharging, take a swab for bacteriogical investigation.	For identification of pathogens. To predict colonization of the site.
16 Clean gloved hands with bactericidal alcohol hand rub.	To minimize the risk of introducing infection.
17 Clean the wound with chlorhexidine in 70% isopropyl alcohol as necessary, working from the inside to the outside of the area and dealing with the cleanest parts of the wound first.	To minimize the risk of infection spread from a 'dirty' to a 'clean' area.
18 Apply appropriate dressing, moulding it into place so that there are no folds or creases.	
19 Remove gloves and wash hands with bactericidal soap and water or bactericidal alcohol hand rub.	
20 Discontinue the infusion in progress. Clamp the catheter using the clamp supplied or a smooth clamp if the catheter is of silicone, or artery forceps over sterile topical swabs if it is of plastic.	To prevent entry of air or leakage of blood when the catheter is disconnected. Swabs prevent cracking of a plastic catheter by artery forceps.
21 Either (a) put on gloves or (b) clean hands with bactericidal alcohol hand rub.	Where potential spillage of patient's blood or certain drugs may occur, e.g. cytotoxics; to minimize the risk of introducing infection into the catheter after handling unsterile parts of the system.
22 Clean connections thoroughly with chlorhexidine in 70% spirit before disconnection.	To minimize infection risk at connection site.

23 Disconnect the catheter from the old giving set and connect the prepared new set. Check that no air bubbles are present in the system. Unclamp the catheter and continue infusion. Where no clamping of the line is possible, the Valsalva manouvre should be used.	To reduce the risk of air embolism.
24 Tape the giving set into a position comfortable for the patient, and attend to his/her general comfort.	To ensure the patient's comfort and to minimize the risk of accidentally dislodging the catheter.
25 Ensure that the drip rate is satisfactory.	
26 Alternatively, attach a Luer lock intermittent injection cap and heparinize the catheter, if continuous infusion is not required (see Heparinization, below).	To maintain a patent catheter for intermittent use.
27 Fold up the sterile field, place it in the yellow clinical waste bag and seal it before moving the trolley. Draw back the curtains. Dispose of waste in appropriate containers.	To prevent environmental contamination.

GUIDELINES: HEPARINIZATION OF A CENTRAL VENOUS CATHETER

This is a simple procedure which may be performed after each use or once weekly (or less frequently in some circumstances) when no therapy is necessary.

EQUIPMENT

1 Flushing solution ready prepared in a syringe, with 25g (orange) needle attached, in clinically clean container.
2 Chlorhexidine in 70% alcohol/swab saturated with 70% isopropyl alcohol.

PROCEDURE

Action	Rationale
1 Explain and discuss the procedure with the patient.	To ensure that the patient understands the procedure and gives his/her valid consent.
2 Wash hands thoroughly or use an alcohol-based hand scrub.	To avoid microbiological contamination.
3 Swab the injection cap with chlorhexidine in 70% spirit/swab saturated with 70% isopropyl alcohol and allow to dry.	To avoid microbiological contamination.
4 Insert the needle, unclamp the catheter and inject contents of the syringe.	To flush the catheter thoroughly.
5 Clamp the catheter while injecting the final 0.5 ml of solution.	To maintain positive pressure and prevent back-flow of blood into the catheter, and possible clot formation.
6 Remove needle from cap and dispose of equipment safely.	To prevent injury.

Guidelines: Heparinization of a central venous catheter (cont'd)

Action	Rationale
7 Demonstrate the procedure clearly and methodically.	To ensure the patient is aware of each step, and the need for good hand washing/drying techniques, etc. as he/she may be performing this procedure on discharge.

GUIDELINES: TAKING BLOOD SAMPLES FROM A CENTRAL VENOUS CATHETER

EQUIPMENT

1 Sterile dressing pack.
2 Clamp for catheter, if necessary.
3 Alcohol-based hand wash solution.
4 Extra 10 ml blood bottle without heparin or sterile 10 ml syringe.
5 Vacuum system container holder (shell).
  Vacuum system adaptor.
  Appropriate vacuumed blood bottles.
  or
  Sterile syringe of appropriate size for sample required.
6 Intermittent injection cap.
7 10 ml syringe of 0.9% sodium chloride.
8 Flushing solution, as per policy.

PROCEDURE

Action	Rationale
1 Explain and discuss the procedure with the patient.	To ensure that the patient understands the procedure and gives his/her valid consent.
2 Perform procedure using an aseptic technique.	To prevent infection. (For further information on asepsis see Chapter 4, Aseptic Technique).
3 Wash hands with bactericidal soap and water or bactericidal alcohol hand rub.	
4 Prepare a tray or trolley and take it to the bedside. Cleanse hands as above. Open sterile pack and prepare equipment.	
5 If intravenous fluid infusion is in progress, switch it off.	
6 Clamp the catheter with the clamp supplied or a smooth clamp if the catheter is of silicone or with artery forceps over sterile topical swabs if it is of plastic, or move catheter 'on/off' switch to 'off'.	To prevent entry of air or leakage of blood via the catheter. Swabs prevent the artery forceps from cracking a plastic catheter.
7 Wash hands with a bactericidal alcohol hand rub. Put on gloves. Clean hub thoroughly with chlorhexidine.	To minimize the risk of introducing infection into the catheter, and prevent contamination of practitioner's hands with blood.

8 Disconnect the giving set from the catheter and cover the end of the set with the syringe cover or remove the injection cap and discard.

To reduce the risk of contaminating the end of the giving set.

9 For vacuum sampling:
(a) Attach vacuum container holder and release clamp. Attach extra sample bottle: fill and discard.

To remove blood, heparin and intravenous fluids from the 'dead space' of the catheter. Samples from this 'dead space' are likely to cause inaccuracies in blood tests.

(b) Attach required sample bottles for requested specimens.

To obtain sample. It is not necessary to clamp the catheter when changing collection bottles, as the system is not broken.

(c) Re-clamp catheter and detach vacuum container holder.

To prevent blood loss or air embolism.

10 For syringe sampling:
(a) Attach a 10 ml syringe to the catheter. Release the clamp and withdraw 5–10 ml of blood.
(b) Re-clamp the catheter and discard the sample and syringe.

To remove blood, heparin and intravenous fluids from the 'dead space' of the catheter. Samples from this 'dead space' are likely to cause inaccuracies in blood tests.

(c) Attach a new syringe of appropriate size. Release the clamp and withdraw the required amount of blood.

To obtain the sample.

(d) Re-clamp the catheter and detach the syringe.

To prevent blood loss or air embolism.

11 Flush with 10 ml 0.9% sodium chloride.

To ensure removal of all blood in catheter and prevent occlusion.

12 Reconnect the giving set, unclamp the catheter and recommence infusion or attach new intermittent injection cap, release clamp and flush catheter through injection cap using positive pressure technique.

To prevent the catheter clotting in between uses. To continue therapy.

13 Ensure that blood samples have been placed in the correct containers and agitated as necessary to prevent clotting. Label them with patient's name, number, etc. and send them to the laboratory with the appropriate forms.

To make certain that the specimens, correctly presented and identified, are delivered to the laboratory, enabling the requested tests to be performed and the results returned to the correct patient's records.

Double- or triple-lumen catheters are now inserted routinely. Where these catheters have different-sized lumens, the largest should be reserved where possible for blood products and blood sampling only.

Difficulty may be encountered when taking blood samples. This is particularly true when the central catheter is made of silicone and has been in place for a period of time. The main cause is that the tip of the soft catheter lays against the wall of the vessel and the suction required to draw blood brings this into close contact, so leading to temporary occlusion.

Measures to try to dislodge the tip include asking the patient to:

1 Cough and breathe deeply.
2 Roll from side to side.
3 Raise his/her arms.

Guidelines: Taking blood samples from a central venous catheter (cont'd)

4 Perform the Valsalva manoeuvre, if possible.
5 Increase general activity, e.g. walk up and down stairs.

If these are unsuccessful, irrigation of the catheter with 0.9% sodium chloride or a dilute solution of heparin may be helpful. However, it may be necessary to take blood from a peripheral vein (see Chapter 46, Venepuncture).

GUIDELINES: CARE OF IMPLANTABLE PORTS

Placement of a Huber point needle into the implantable port is to be performed by a doctor or by nurses who have been taught and assessed as being competent. The needle will be connected to an extension set and a Luer-lock injection cap placed at the end of this. The needle and extension set remain in position for seven days and will then be changed, if required, after that time. For general procedures please refer to relevant Guidelines for Intravenous Management, Chapter 23.

EQUIPMENT

As for Guidelines: Administration of drugs by direct injection, bolus or push (items 1–13, Chapter 23, Intravenous Management), together with the following:

14 Non-sterile gloves.

PROCEDURE

To give a bolus injection

Action	Rationale
1 Explain and discuss the procedure with the patient.	To ensure that the patient understands the procedure and gives his/her valid consent.
2 Perform the procedure using aseptic technique.	To prevent infection.
3 Screen the bed, assist patient into the supine position.	To allow dust and airborne organisms to settle before the sterile field is exposed.
4 Wash hands with bactericidal soap and water or bactericidal alcohol hand rub.	
5 Remove the dressing.	To inspect for any obvious signs of sepsis, inflammation, haematoma, accumulation of serous fluid or movement of needle.
6 Put on gloves.	
7 Using a 10 ml Luer lock syringe, flush the catheter with 0.9% sodium chloride and/or draw back blood (you may not always succeed in drawing back blood). However, if any pressure is experienced when flushing the catheter, advice should be sought.	Syringes smaller than 10 ml exert too great a pressure on the catheter. To confirm the patency of the catheter.
8 Inject the drugs as per hospital procedure.	

Flush with 10 ml 0.9% sodium chloride and heparinize the port using 500 iu heparin in 5 ml 0.9% sodium chloride.	To maintain patency of catheter.
Remove the needle.	

To use for intermittent single injections or infusions

1–8 as for bolus injections.	
9 Flush with 10 ml 0.9% sodium chloride. Heparinize the catheter with 50 iu heparin in 5 ml 0.9% sodium chloride after each use. If the catheter is not to be used in the next 24 hours, it should be flushed with 500 iu heparin in 5 ml 0.9% sodium chloride (Plumer, 1993), using the push – pause method and positive pressure technique.	To maintain patency.

To commence an infusion or to change giving set

1–4 as for bolus injections.	
5 Prime a Luer lock giving set.	So infusion is ready to attach.
6 Remove dressing and inspect insertion site as previously described.	To observe for any abnormalities.
7 Put on gloves.	
8 Inject at least 10 ml 0.9% sodium chloride and draw blood as previously described.	To confirm patency.
9 Clamp extension set with clamp or artery forceps protected with low-linting swab.	To prevent entry of air or leakage of blood when catheter is disconnected; swabs prevent cracking of plastic catheter by forceps.
10 Remove intermittent injection cap or giving set and attach primed giving set.	To commence infusion or change giving set in accordance with hospital policy (24-hour set changes).
11 Unclamp forceps and commence infusion, regulate infusion accordingly.	

Discontinuation of infusion

1–4 as for bolus injections.	
5 Clamp extension set.	To prevent entry of air or leakage of blood when giving set is disconnected.
6 Disconnect giving set and replace with intermittent injection cap.	
7 Unclamp extension set.	

Guidelines: Care of implantable ports (cont'd)

Action	Rationale
8 Flush with 10 ml 0.9% sodium chloride and heparinize using 500 iu heparin in at least 5 ml 0.9% sodium chloride.	To maintain patency.

Heparinization of implantable port

It must be heparinized after each use and at monthly intervals between treatments.

Removal of the needle

The needle should be removed if no further treatment is anticipated or before discharge.

Action	Rationale
1–6 as for bolus injections.	
7 Flush with at least 10 ml 0.9% sodium chloride.	To flush the device thoroughly.
8 Heparinize the port using heparin 500 iu in 5 ml 0.9% sodium chloride.	To maintain patency.
9 Clamp extension set while still maintaining positive pressure (i.e. keep thumb on syringe plunger).	To prevent back-flow of blood and possible clot formation.
10 Press down on portal of implantable port with two fingers.	To support portal.
11 Withdraw the needle using steady traction.	To prevent trauma to the skin.
12 No dressing is required.	

GUIDELINES: REMOVAL OF A NON-SKIN TUNNELLED CENTRAL VENOUS CATHETER

EQUIPMENT

As for Guidelines: Changing the dressing on a central venous catheter insertion site (items 1–9, above) plus:

10 Sterile scissors.
11 Small sterile specimen container.
12 Stitch cutter.
13 Additional sterile low-linting gauze swab (a new administration set, etc. is not required).

PROCEDURE

Proceed as for a dressing procedure, steps 1–15 (above) then continue as follows:

Action	Rationale
16 Clean the insertion site.	To prevent contamination of the catheter on removal, and a false-positive culture result.

| 17 | Discontinue the infusion, if in progress. Clamp the catheter as previously described or move the catheter 'on/off' switch to 'off'. | To prevent entry of air or leakage of blood when the catheter is disconnected. |

| 18 | Clean gloved hands with a bactericidal alcohol hand rub. | To minimize the risk of infection after handling unsterile parts of the system. |

| 19 | Cut and remove any skin suture securing the catheter. | To facilitate removal. |

| 20 | Disconnect the catheter from the remainder of the infusion system. | To ease handling and removal. |

| 21 | Ask the patient to perform the Valsalva manoeuvre. | To reduce the risk of air embolus. |

| 22 | Cover the insertion site with a thick pad of several sterile topical swabs. | Swabs are used to discourage the entry of organisms into the insertion site and to absorb any leakage of blood. |

| 23 | Hold the catheter with one hand near the point of insertion and pull firmly and gently. As the catheter begins to move, press firmly down on the site with the swabs. | Pressure is applied to prevent haemorrhage and to encourage resealing of the vein wall. It also prevents the entry of air into the vein. |

Maintain pressure on the swabs for about five minutes after the catheter has been removed.

Continued pressure is necessary to allow time for the puncture in the vein to close.

| 24 | When bleeding has stopped (approximately 5 minutes), swab site for bacteriological examination and cover with padded dressing. | To detect any infection at exit site. |

| 25 | If the catheter is removed because of infection, carefully cut off the tip (approximately 5 cm) of the catheter using sterile scissors and place it in a sterile container for microbiological investigation. | To detect any infection related to the catheter, and thus provide necessary treatment. |

| 26 | Fold up the sterile field, place it in the yellow clinical waste bag and seal it before moving the trolley. Dispose of the equipment in the appropriate containers. | To prevent environment contamination. |

| 27 | Make the patient comfortable. | |

This procedure may be adapted for removal of a skin-tunnelled catheter.

GUIDELINES: SURGICAL REMOVAL OF A SKIN TUNNELLED CENTRAL VENOUS CATHETER

EQUIPMENT

1 Plastic apron.
2 Sterile gloves.
3 Minor operations set.
4 10 ml Luer lock syringe.
5 25 g needle.
6 21 g needle.

Guidelines: Surgical removal of a skin tunnelled central venous catheter (cont'd)

7 10 ml plain lignocaine 2%.
8 10 cm × 10 cm low-linting gauze swabs ×5.
9 3/0 mersilk suture on a curved needle.
10 2 cm micropore tape.
11 Chlorhexidine in 70% alcohol.
12 Steristrips (to be used if necessary).

PROCEDURE

Action	Rationale
1 Check the patient's full blood count and clotting profile for that day.	To ensure that the patient is not at risk of bleeding or infection from this invasive procedure. The platelets should be above 150×10^9/litre, the white blood count >2 and the international normalized ratio (INR) <1.3.
2 Explain and discuss the procedure with the patient.	To ensures that the patient understands the procedure and gives his/her valid consent.
3 Ask patient to remove clothing down to the waist.	To ensure ease of access to the patient's chest.
4 Ask patient to lie as flat as possible with their arms by their sides.	To minimize the risk of bleeding from gravitational pressure and to dissuade the patient from touching the sterile field.
5 Palpate and identify the position of the cuff in the patient.	To locate the area for the incision.
6 If the cuff cannot easily be felt measure 22 cm up from the bifurcation at the end of the catheter distal to the patient (see Fig. 11.2) then palpate again. If it still cannot be felt ask for help.	To locate the probable site of the cuff. To guard against malplaced incisions.
7 Open the outer bag of the minor operation pack. Put on plastic apron and wash hands, then dry hands on sterile towel provided in the pack.	To reduce risk of infection.
8 Accept and put on sterile gloves from assistant and assemble all necessary equipment on the sterile pack.	To maintain asepsis and to prepare for the procedure and maximize efficiency.
9 Advise the patient that you will explain each step of the procedure as you go along.	This should take into account the patient's individual wish for information.
10 Clean the area directly over the cuff with swabs soaked in chlorhexidine in 70% alcohol. Use a circular motion working out from the centre directly over the cuff.	To reduce the risk of infection.
11 Position the two sterile green towels – one horizontally across the waist and the other longitudinally down the side of the patient between yourself and the patient.	To create a sterile field to operate within and therefore reduce the risk of infection.

12 Inform the patient that you are about to administer the local anaesthetic and that this will cause a stinging sensation.	The first injection can be painful and does cause a stinging sensation.
13 With a 25 g needle administer the first ml of local anaesthetic subcutaneously directly over the cuff site causing a raised bleb.	To commence the numbing of the area to be incised. To provide a raised area for the next injection and identification of the site.
14 Give further 1 ml of local anaesthetic subcutaneously using the bleb as the area for the insertion of the needle, but directing the area out around the cuff site area.	To reduce pain for the patient with repeated injections. To ensure all the incision area is numb.
15 Attach the 21 g needle and with the last remaining 4 ml of local anaesthetic give two deeper injections to either side of the cuff area.	To ensure anaesthesia at a deeper level during the blunt dissection around the cuff.
16 Test the area above the cuff for numbness and then make the incision over the cuff site. This should be about two cms in length. Ensure that the incision is through the epidermis and dermis.	To ensure that the patient will not experience any pain. To facilitate identification and removal of the cuff. To allow access to the cuff which is situated below the dermis.
17 With one of the artery forceps commence blunt dissection of tissue from around the cuff. At intervals place your finger into the site and feel the cuff.	To free the cuff from the surrounding fibrous tissue. To assess the mobility of the cuff.
18 Continue with blunt dissection around and under the cuff until it feels mobile.	To facilitate the loosening of the cuff.
19 With one artery forcep clamp onto the cuff and lift it up out of the incision whilst looking down the incision to identify the catheter below the cuff.	To identify the catheter to allow the lower portion to be severed.
20 Once the catheter is clearly visible, maintaining your grip on the cuff with the forceps cut through the full thickness with the blade. Then pull the portion of the catheter below the cuff out through the exit site.	To remove the lower half of the catheter below the cuff.
21 Still maintaining your grip on the cuff gently dissect away the fibrous tissue from around the cuff and the first 5 mm of the catheter immediately above the catheter.	To free the cuff in readiness for removal of the top portion of the catheter.
22 Once the cuff is free still maintaining your grip on the cuff gently and carefully peel away the thin straw-coloured tissue from the catheter with the blade.	To free the catheter from the anchoring fibrous bands to enable removal.
23 As the last bands are divided you should feel the catheter becoming free and you should be able to see the whiteness of the catheter.	To ensure that you have completely freed the catheter for removal.
24 Whilst holding a low linting swab to the incision site gently pull out the catheter.	To remove the catheter and be prepared for any bleeding.

Guidelines: Surgical removal of a skin tunnelled central venous catheter (cont'd)

Action	Rationale
25 Close the incision with three or four sutures. Commence the first suture in the middle of the incision.	To close the incision efficiently. To ensure that the skin edges are brought together in alignment.
26 If there continues to be any bleeding Steristrips can be applied across the incision over the sutures.	To minimize blood loss.
27 Apply a dry dressing and advise the patient that there might be some oozing and to reapply a dry dressing. Advise the patient that the sutures should be removed in 7 days.	To absorb any slight bleed and to maintain a clean site. To ensure that the incision has fully closed and healed.
28 Ask the patient to rest on the bed for the next 30 minutes to an hour, or longer if required.	To reduce the risk of a bleed as the patient sits or gets up.
29 Liaise with the nursing team and document the removal and findings in the nursing and medical notes.	To ensure there is good communication between all teams and a written record of the procedure.

NURSING CARE PLAN

Problem	Cause	Suggested action
Dyspnoea, chest pain or cyanosis (may be slow in onset).	Hydrothorax, pneumothorax or haemothorax due to insertion technique.	Inform a doctor. Arrange for a chest X-ray. Assist with any immediate treatment and with chest drainage if necessary.
Change in pulse rate and rhythm after insertion of catheter.	Cardiac irritability.	Inform a doctor.
Dyspnoea, chest pain, tachypnoea, disorientation, cyanosis, raised CVP, coma, cardiac arrest.	Air embolism due to air entering circulation during the insertion procedure or via the catheter.	Monitor the patient. If signs or symptoms develop, clamp the catheter to prevent further air entry. Lay the patient on the left side in Trendelenburg position. Inform a doctor. Give oxygen or external cardiac compression in the event of cardiac arrest.
Change in pulse rate, rhythm, dyspnoea, cyanosis, cardiac arrest.	Ventricular rupture due to insertion.	Observe patient closely. Inform doctor immediately. Prepare to commence cardiac massage.
Tingling in fingers, shooting pain down arm, paralysis.	Injury to brachial plexus during insertion.	Inform a doctor. Treatment is symptomatic. Physiotherapy may be necessary.
Oedma of the arm on the side of the catheter insertion, may be	Thoracic duct injury at insertion, resulting in alterations in lymph	Inform a doctor. Removal of the catheter is usually necessary.

Problem	Cause	Suggested action
associated with pain or limb discolouration.	flow. Thrombosis in major vessel due to irritation by foreign body (catheter).	
Pyrexia, tachycardia, rigors indicating systemic infection.	Infection due to poor aseptic technique. Careless use and handling of equipment, e.g. stopcocks, over-flooding of manometer.	Culture of the patient's blood is required. Take a swab of the infusion site, employing strict asepsis and minimum handling of the equipment. Administer antimicrobials as prescribed. Observe the patient closely. Removal of line is sometimes indicated.
Unable to draw back blood.	Catheter tip occluded by the vein wall. Tip of catheter covered by fibrin sheath	Encourage the patient to move arms, or position on the side where catheter is inserted, and ask patient to perform the Valsalva manoeuvre.
	Catheter blocked by blood clots due to: (1) infusion being too slow or switched off; (2) heparinization not having been carried out previously.	Attempt to flush using 5 or 10 ml syringe of 0.9% sodium chloride. If unsuccessful, instil 50 iu heparin in 5 ml 0.9% sodium chloride using a 'to and fro' motion (Wickham, 1992) over a few minutes. Attempt to aspirate clots and then flush with heparinized saline. Repeat if necessary or use other solution, e.g. urokinase. 5000 iu in 2–5 ml 0.9% sodium chloride. Inject slowly and clamp catheter Leave for one hour and then attempt to aspirate.
Leakage of fluid onto the dressing.	Loose connection in the system. Cracking of catheter or hub.	Check and tighten connections. Report to the intravenous nursing staff and/or medical staff.
Catheter required for many functions, e.g. blood sampling and extra drug	Limited routes of access available to satisfy the patient's requirements.	Consider multi-lumen catheter before insertion. Simple regimes and methods of administration. Use extension sets and administration sets available for this purpose.
Fluid overload resulting in dyspnoea, oedema, raised pulse rate and blood pressure.	Infusion is too fast. Inaccurate fluid monitoring.	Revise the patient's fluid intake regimen. Use flow control devices. Keep accurate records of the patient's fluid balance and weight. Inform a doctor.

Nursing care plan (cont'd)

Problem	Cause	Suggested action
Inaccurate CVP readings.	Patient in a position different from that in which the initial reading was taken.	Position should be documented in the patient's records.
	Reference point on the patient not observed.	Zero of the manometer must be level with the patient's right atrium at the point marked on the patient, i.e. mid-axilla or sternal angle.
	Faulty pressure reading technique.	If the CVP reading is outside the limits deemed acceptable for that patient and it is considered to be an accurate reading, recheck it after 15 or 30 minutes and inform a doctor if unchanged.
Elevated CVP.	Increased intrathoracic pressure caused by coughing, increased movement or pain.	Encourage coughing before taking the reading. Ensure that the patient is comfortable and pain free.
	Lower extremities elevated.	Position the patient so that he/she is lying in a supine position.
	Patient having intermittent positive-pressure ventilation.	Read the CVP at the end expiratory level (lowest point of fluctuation). This will always be higher that the 'normal' reading.
	Anxiety and/or restlessness..	Verify the cause of the anxiety or restlessness and take action to reassure patient.
	Blood in progress via the CVP line.	Flush the catheter well with 0.9% sodium chloride and read again.
	Shivering and/or muscular spasm, e.g. post-anaesthetic reaction (see Chapter 32, Peri-operative Care).	Assess the patient's general condition, e.g. pulse, blood pressure, temperature. Check that the patient is warm enough. Inform a doctor.
Low CVP reading.	Leak in the system or equipment adjusted inaccurately.	Check and readjust the system.
	Changing of the patient's position from recumbent to semi-recumbent.	Re-read with the patient in the original position.
Potential pulmonary embolus due to catheter tip embolus. Symptoms include chest pain, cool clammy skin, haemoptysis, tochycardia, hypotension.	Occasionally occurs after the removal of the catheter, especially the skin-tunnelled type.	All skin-tunnelled catheters must be removed by medical staff or trained nursing staff. Notify a doctor immediately if the patient develops any of the related symptoms.

Problem	Cause	Suggested action
Bleeding at the insertion site following removal of the catheter.	Opening in the vein wall.	Apply pressure over the site with sterile topical swabs, until bleeding has stopped. Patients prescribed warfarin or heparin will require a longer period of pressure to compensate for the prolonged clotting time. Apply sterile dressing. If bleeding persists, the doctor must be informed.

In addition, the care plan associated with intravenous management (Chapter 15, Drug Administration) may contain useful and relevant information.

CHAPTER 12
Continent Urinary Diversions

Definition

A urinary diversion is a surgical procedure to create an alternative method of removing urine from the body when either the bladder or urethra is no longer viable.

The urine leaves the body through an opening on the abdomen created during the operation. This opening is termed a stoma. There are two types of urinary diversion: an ileal conduit urinary diversion (incontinent) and a continent urinary diversion.

The formation of an ileal conduit urinary diversion is an operation involving the construction of a tube of ileum with one end formed into a protruding spout on to the abdomen (called a stoma) and the ureters implanted into the other, as described by Woodhouse (1991). It continually leaks urine (an incontinent stoma) necessitating the wearing of an appliance. (See procedure on stoma care, Chapter 39.)

A continent urinary diversion (Fig. 12.1) is an operation involving either the preservation of the patient's bladder or the formation of a new bladder called a urinary reservoir, into which the patient's ureters have been implanted. The bladder or urinary reservoir is then connected to the abdomen by a continent urinary stoma created from the appendix, ureter, fallopian tube or small bowel (Fig. 12.1). The continent urinary stoma does not leak urine. Instead of wearing an appliance, patients self-catheterize into the continent urinary stoma every 3–4 hours to empty the urine. These operative techniques were devised by Mitrofanoff (1980) and Kock *et al.* (1987).

Indications for the formation of a continent urinary diversion

(1) To expel urine from the body if the ureter, bladder or urethra are no longer viable due to disease (Horn, 1990).
(2) So that urine does not leak continuously (Horn, 1990), therefore:
   (a) It prevents skin excoriation.
   (b) It improves the individual's body image since it is not necessary to wear an appliance.

(Boyd *et al.*, 1987.)

REFERENCE MATERIAL

Principles of a continent urinary diversion

Following the formation of an ileal conduit (see Chapter 39, Stoma Care), the patients' perception of their body image and sexuality may be altered, which may affect their ability to form and maintain social and sexual relationships (Delvin & Plant, 1979; Jeffrey *et al.*, 1988; Jones *et al.*, 1981).

The formation of a continent urinary diversion is an alternative to the formation of an ileal conduit. The opening on the abdomen (stoma), compared with the ileal conduit stoma, is small and flush with the skin. The continent urinary stoma is tunnelled through the muscle of the bladder or reservoir. This prevents urine leaking through the stoma. The size of the continent urinary stoma depends upon the type of material used to create it. The ureter is the smallest (approximately 3.9 mm in diameter), while the small intestine is the largest at 9–10 mm in diameter.

The continent urinary diversion involves the patient having two admissions into hospital. The first is to form the continent urinary diversion. Following the operation, a sterile fine-bore tube is left in the continent urinary stoma to keep it patent and allow the urine to drain into a catheter bag. After recovering from the operation, patients are taught how to take care of the tubing, leg bags and night drainage systems. Patients are then discharged home to be readmitted 6 weeks after the operation to be taught self-catheterization. This admission lasts between 24 and 48 hours. During this time, patients are taught self-catheterization and encouraged to practise the technique. Nursing staff are available to detect and rectify any problems. This allows patients time to gain confidence in self-catheterization before they return home.

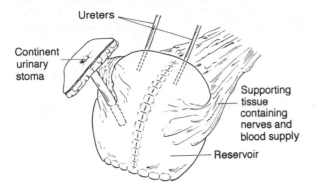

Figure 12.1 Continent urinary diversion.

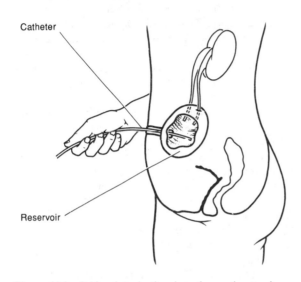

Figure 12.2 Self-catheterization into the continent urinary stoma.

Urine drains into the urinary reservoir or bladder through the ureters. Patients self-catheterize into the continent urinary stoma every 3–4 hours to empty the urine reservoir (Fig. 12.2). They go into a toilet, adjust any restrictive clothing and insert a special tube into the continent urinary stoma, pointing the other end into the toilet. The urine drains out. The tube is then removed, washed with water and replaced in its container (usually a plastic bag, spectacle case or cosmetic bag).

Before each discharge, patients are given verbal and written advice (Horn, 1990), and can contact the hospital 24 hours a day.

Types of continent urinary diversions

There are a number of types of continent urinary diversions. Essentially the principles and the nursing care are the same, with only minor modifications. Two examples

are the Mitrofanoff and Kock's pouch (Figs. 12.1 and 12.2).

The Mitrofanoff pouch was devised in the late 1970s/ early 1980s by Paul Mitrofanoff (1980) in France. Initially, it was devised for patients with bladder neck obstruction or incompetence. The bladder was preserved and the appendix was used as the continent urinary stoma. The operation was later modified so that in the absence of an appendix, a piece of ureter or fallopian tube could be used. If the bladder is unviable, the sigmoid colon can be resected and created into a urinary reservoir. Further modifications have been made by Duckett & Snyder (1985, 1986).

The Kock pouch was devised by Kock et al. (1987), in Sweden, initially as a continent ileostomy; in the early 1980s it was adapted into a continent urinary diversion. A section of the small bowel is resected and used to create both the reservoir and the continent urinary stoma. The Kock pouch continent urinary stoma is larger then the Mitrofanoff stoma which uses the smaller appendix, ureter or fallopian tube. Skinner & Boyd (1984) have made further modifications to refine the surgical technique. The decision about which technique to use is made according to the availability of an appendix, fallopian tube, ureter or small bowel for the continent urinary stoma. If the bladder can be preserved, a Mitrofanoff procedure is performed. If not, either a Mitrofanoff or a Kock's procedure may be carried out (Cummings et al., 1987; Woodhouse, 1989). Whilst there is little published evidence to suggest that one procedure is superior to the other, Galister & Woodhouse (1991) express a preference for the Mitrofanoff procedure over the Kock's pouch.

Indications for the surgical formation of a continent urinary diversion

The indications for the formation of a continent urinary diversion and an ileal conduit are similar. (See Chapter 39, Stoma Care.) However, an ileal conduit can be converted into a continent urinary diversion and vice versa.

(1) Cancer of the bladder, ureters or urethra.
(2) Invasive cancer of the cervix or ovary requiring a pelvic exenteration. This is an operation involving a cystectomy, hysterectomy and colectomy.
(3) An unviable bladder or urethra following radiotherapy.
(4) Congenital urinary tract deformities.
(5) Bladder neck obstructions or incompetence.
(6) Neuropathic bladder. A condition where the nerve impulses do not reach the bladder.
(7) Trauma to the bladder, ureters or urethra.
(8) An ileal conduit or ureterostomy can be converted into a continent urinary diversion.

Table 12.1   Advantages and disadvantages of an ileal conduit (from Horn, 1990).

Advantages	Disadvantages
(1) Tried and tested technique, in use since 1950 (Bricker & Eisenman, 1950, cited in Boyd & Lieskovsky, 1988).	(1) Continual urine leakage necessitating the wearing of an appliance.
(2) Surgery is not as extensive as with a continent urinary diversion.	(2) Potential problem of skin excoriation.
(3) The skills to care for an ileal conduit are relatively easy to learn.	(3) Potential problem of altered body image to patients and others.
(4) Lower incidence of post-operative problems.	(4) Fear of maintaining or creating new relationships.

(Mitrofanoff, 1980; Skinner & Boyd, 1984; Duckett & Snyder, 1985; Kock *et al.*, 1987; Woodhouse, 1989, 1991; Horn, 1990.)

Patient selection

Patients are selected carefully for this type of surgery. Horn (1990) describes how potential patients should have good renal function and a suitable continent urinary stoma. They must be motivated towards self–catheterization and be dexterous. Patients should be physically and psychologically able to undergo major surgery. If they have cancer it should be either curable or controllable and without metastases. The operation is a lengthy one, further treatment may be required, and there is an increased risk of surgical complications (Galister & Woodhouse, 1991).

Specific pre-operative preparation

Patients undergo the usual preparation for anaesthesia (see Chapter 32, Peri-operative Care). Only the specific preparation is discussed here although physical preparation may vary according to the individual surgeon's preference.

Pre-operative counselling

Once patients have been selected as suitable candidates, psychological preparation should begin as soon as possible. Boore (1978), Hayward (1978), Zeimer (1983), Morris *et al.* (1989), Raleigh *et al.* (1990) and Roberts (1991) have illustrated the importance of pre-operative information and explanation in reducing postoperative physical and psychological stress to the individual following the formation of a stoma (ileal conduit or colostomy). Their research is also applicable to patients receiving continent urinary diversion stomas. This is discussed in Chapter 39, Stoma Care.

Patients should receive a full explanation of the operation and its effects. The amount and type of information should be adapted to the individual's requirements.

When circumstances permit, patients have the opportunity to choose between an ileal conduit and a continent urinary diversion. This usually takes place in an outpatients clinic, and is reiterated when the patient has been admitted to the ward. The formation of an ileal conduit as well as a continent urinary diversion is discussed with the patient in case the latter is not a viable option. The advantages and disadvantages of both operations should be fully discussed with the patients and their family and friends (Tables 12.1 and 12.2). They should be shown pictures of the continent urinary diversion and ileal conduit stomas, and are encouraged to familiarize themselves with the equipment: pouches, wafers, catheterization tubes and bladder syringes.

Useful aids
(1) Information booklets.
(2) Samples of equipment.
(3) Diagrams.
(4) Being visited by patients who have had a continent urinary diversion and an ileal conduit formed (ideally, of similar age, sex and background to the patient).

The effect on diet and bowel movements
Horn (1991) describes in a patient information booklet the effect of evacuating the patient's bowels and intestinal manipulation during the operation, and how the patient can adjust to temporary effects such as diarrhoea (e.g. by replacing fluids orally). Patients should be warned about the necessity to evacuate their bowels of faeces before the operation. The procedure to do this and the surgical manipulation of the bowel during the operation results in the bowel not working for several days after the surgery. When their bowels do start to work again, patients may experience loose, watery stools which will become firmer as the appetite returns (Horn, 1991).

Horn (1991) describes how the slow return of both a normal appetite and bowel function is a common feature

Table 12.2 Advantages and disadvantages of a continent urinary diversion (from Horn, 1990; Galister & Woodhouse, 1991).

Advantages	Disadvantages
(1) No need to wear an appliance.	(1) Patient must be enthusiastic and motivated towards self-catheterization.
(2) Small stoma, 0.5–1 cm in diameter.	(2) There are problems with the operation technique, which is being refined to improve stoma continence.
(3) No urine leakage.	
(4) Improves or maintains body image.	(3) Operation still involves a laparotomy and drain-site scars, which do fade but may cause an altered body image.
(5) No skin excoriation.	(4) Consider whether patient will have the physical ability to be able to self-catheterize in 5–10 years' time.
	(5) It is a long operation with a high risk of post-operative problems, and requires two hospitalizations.
	(6) Lack of familiarity in outside specialist centres.
	(7) Long-term problems are unknown.
	(8) Surgical and nursing care techniques are modified regularly.
	(9) Patients may fear they are being used to test the operation.

following this type of operation and it can give much anxiety. The patient should be advised to take small, light meals supplemented with nutritious drinks. It may take 2–3 months before patients return to a completely normal appetite. Once recovered, the patient can eat and drink a normal diet.

Patients are reassured that the new urine reservoir and stoma are completely separate from their normal bowel action. Stools will not pass through the continent urinary stoma (Horn, 1991).

Bowel preparation

Patients are admitted 3 days before surgery to commence a regime to evacuate all faecal matter from the intestine. The regime used depends on the surgeon's preference.

Alexander Williams (1980) explains why it is necessary to remove all faecal matter:

(1) To prevent hard faecal masses from impacting proximal to an anastomosis.
(2) To prevent faeces spilling from the cut ends of the bowel during the operation.
(3) To reduce bacterial contamination when the bowel is opened.

However, it is important to know that this faeces removing procedure can cause the patient to suffer hypovolaemia and electrolyte imbalance. Therefore, it is important that the fluid loss is replaced orally or intravenously (Skinner & Lieskovsky, 1988; Woodhouse, 1989).

Sexual dysfunction

Following the formation of a continent urinary diversion possible sexual impairment for both men and women may occur. This is the same as for other stoma patients and is discussed in Chapter 39, Stoma Care.

Pre- and post-operative counselling is given to each patient and partner. Each person's potential sexual dysfunction is discussed and treated on an individual basis.

Specific post-operative care

Horn (1990) describes the post-operative nursing care given to patients following the formation of a continent urinary diversion. The surgery involves intestinal manipulation, which causes a paralytic ileus. Manipulation of the ureters in a highly vascular area results in a risk of haemorrhage and local oedema, leading to uteric obstruction. This may prevent the urine draining into the urinary reservoir (Woodhouse, 1989; Horn, 1990; Galister & Woodhouse, 1991; Woodhouse, 1994).

Apart from the routine immediate postoperative care (see Chapter 32, Peri-operative Care), nursing care is based on early detection of these problems. Due to the paralytic ileus, patients are unable to eat or drink, and receive total parental nutrition through a cannula in the internal jugular or subclavian vein (see Chapter 29, Nutritional Support). A gastrostomy or nasogastric tube drains any gastric fluid that collects due to gastric stasis. The nasogastric and gastrostomy tubes are removed and parental nutrition is discontinued when the ileus has resolved. A wound drain is inserted into the wound

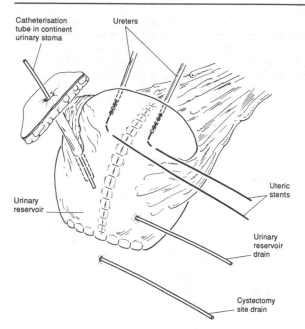

Catheterisation tube in continent urinary stoma

Ureters

Urinary reservoir

Uteric stents

Urinary reservoir drain

Cystectomy site drain

Figure 12.3 Siting of wound drains to prevent haematoma and abscess formation.

site to prevent haematoma and abscess formation (Fig. 12.3).

Ureteric obstruction can be avoided by inserting a small, hollow, plastic tube called a stent into each ureter, which is then passed through the urinary reservoir and onto the abdomen, and connected to a urine-measuring apparatus. This allows the urine to drain out and is usually removed 10 days post-operatively when local oedema has reduced. A fine-bore nasogastric tube is inserted into the continent urinary stoma to prevent occlusion due to surgical trauma and to allow urine to drain into a measuring device. This remains in position for 6 weeks (Woodhouse, 1989).

If the urinary reservoir is allowed to fill before the anastomosis can heal it may rupture, and therefore a bladder drain is inserted to drain the urine. It is removed aseptically within 7–10 days. The main post-operative problems are the collection of post-surgery debris and, if a urinary reservoir has been created, the mucus produced by the intestinal lining of the urine reservoir (Mitrofanoff, 1980; Skinner & Boyd, 1984; Woodhouse, 1989, 1991). These can collect and block the bladder drain and continent urinary stoma, which may lead to increased pressure on the anastomosis. Horn (1990) describes how to remove the debris by irrigating the reservoir drain and continent urinary stoma tubing with sterile 0.9% sodium chloride twice a day.

Although the debris is eventually removed, the mucus

secretion may cause obstruction (Woodhouse, 1989; Horn, 1990). Therefore, patients are taught how to flush the reservoir twice a day. At home tap water can be used to flush the continent urinary stoma (Lapides, 1971, 1974; Diokno et al., 1983; Lindehall et al., 1994). This is described in more detail in Guidelines: Self-catheterization, below.

Patient education before first discharge

The stoma therapist visits the patients on the ward to continue the relationship established before the operation, to check on post-operative recovery and to act as a resource for the nursing staff. As patients recover from the operation they should be taught the care of the urine drainage systems by the stoma therapist and experienced ward nurses. The care of the urine drainage system then gradually becomes the patient's responsibility rather than the ward nurses'. Before discharge, patients should be taught how to flush the continent urinary stoma tubing using tap water (Lapides, 1971), secure the tube in place and attach drainage bags. They are taught how to recognize a urinary tract infection and advised to drink at least 2–3 litres of fluid daily to prevent it happening. They are also advised to wear a medical aid bracelet, so that if they are found unconscious at any time a doctor or nurse will know how to empty the urine drainage system.

When patients are well enough to be discharged, they are allowed to go home for a few weeks before being readmitted to be taught self-catheterization. Patients are seen by the stoma therapist before discharge and a community nurse is requested to visit the patients after discharge. An explanatory letter and the relevant literature is supplied. Patients are encouraged to seek advice from the ward staff at any time.

Second admission

Patients are readmitted 6 weeks after the operation to be taught intermittent self-catheterization by the stoma therapist and experienced ward staff, as described by Horn (1990). Before such teaching, a pouchogram may be performed. A radio-opaque dye is poured into the urinary reservoir to ascertain the amount of fluid the bladder or urinary reservoir can hold, and to ensure all the anastomoses have healed. The patient is then taught intermittent self-catheterization. See 'Teaching intermittent self-catheterization', below.

Second discharge advice

Once proficient with intermittent self-catheterization, patients are discharged home with a 2–4 week outpatient clinic appointment to see the surgeon and stoma therapist. The advice now extends to include the following:

(1) Emptying the bladder or reservoir every 3–4 hours, to prevent overdistension of the reservoir.

(2) To ensure an undisturbed sleep by reducing the amount of fluid the patient drinks 3 hours before going to sleep. The patient should catheterize before going to sleep and on waking.

(3) To keep a tube available at all times (in suit, car, handbag, at work and at home), in case patient needs to empty the urine.

(4) A small amount of mucus may leak from the continent urinary stoma and a piece of gauze can be worn to protect clothing.

(5) On discharge, patients are given a supply of low friction self-catheterization catheters. These are normally used for urethral self-catheterization to reduce trauma during catheterization. Suction catheters should not be used. Various makes of low friction catheter are available on prescription. The hospital will tell the patient how to obtain further supplies.

(6) Once the tubing has been taken out of its original sterile packet, it can be used repeatedly for up to 7 days providing it is rinsed with tap water between uses and stored in its own container (a plastic bag, cosmetic bag, spectacle case).

(7) If the patient finds it difficult to insert the catheter into the stoma, he or she is advised to pause and rest for 10 minutes before attempting to insert the catheter again. This is to allow any swelling around the stoma to subside (Horn 1990, 1991). If it is still difficult, then a warm bath sometimes dilates the stoma. The patient should then try again, with a size smaller tube. If it is still difficult, the hospital should be contacted.

(8) If there is trauma during catheterization, such as some spotting of blood, the patient should wait 10 minutes and then try again. Trauma may be caused by rough catheterization technique, using the wrong size of catheter or by a problem with the continent urinary stoma which requires further investigation. A doctor should be consulted if the bleeding continues or increases.

(9) Patients should be told that it can take a while to become confident with this procedure. However, they can contact the hospital at any time for advice and reassurance.

Long- and short-term problems

Horn (1990) summarized the following problems which were encountered by the surgeons who had performed this technique:

- Septicaemia (due to urine leaking during the operation).

- Breakdown of the anastomosis.
- Perforation or stenosis of the continent urinary stoma.
- Calculi forming on the clips in the anastomosis.
- Swelling due to trauma, which may block the stoma.
- Urine leaking from the stoma which necessitates further surgery.

(Mitrofanoff, 1980; Skinner & Boyd, 1984; Duckett & Snyder, 1985, 1986; Kock, 1987; Woodhouse, 1989, 1991). McCahill et al. (1992) describe toxic shock in one patient, caused by poor hygiene during catheterization. Fistulae in the reservoir and stoma necrosis and prolapse have also been reported (Arai et al., 1993). As the formation of a continent urinary diversion is a relatively new surgical technique, it is not known if there are any other short- or long-term problems.

Long-term psychological effects

Several surveys have been undertaken to compare ileal conduits with Mitrofanoff/Kock's continent urinary diversions in terms of social and sexual effects, and to assess the effect on the patient of converting an ileal conduit to a continent urinary diversion (Boyd et al., 1987; Mansson et al., 1988, 1991; Oishi et al., 1993). Each examined the effect of cystectomy and investigated issues such as depression, adjustment to the new skills required for self-catheterization or use of stoma appliances, and changes in social, sports and sexual activity. The evidence suggests that patients are able to learn the manual skills required of them, but that all experience some degree of depression and altered body image. Patients with ileal conduits reported a more negative body image and a higher incidence of depression compared with the other two groups. Patients with a primary continent urinary diversion also exhibited depression and altered body image. Patients whose ileal conduit was converted to a continent urinary diversion experienced less depression and fewer negative changes in body image. It is conjectured that this is because these patients perceive a definite improvement in their situation when the conversion is carried out (Boyd et al., 1987; Mansson et al., 1988, 1991; Oishi et al., 1993).

These studies did not investigate altered body image or psychological morbidity in patients whose ileal conduits or continent urinary diversions were performed for non-malignant disease. Kennedy et al. (1993), however, describe the experiences of four women who had successful pregnancies following continent urinary diversions for non-malignant disease.

The importance of the role of stoma therapists and nursing staff in providing information tailored for the individual and in teaching new skills is recognized by patients, and it is suggested that these functions play a part in adjustment to changes brought about by surgery

(Boyd *et al.*, 1987; Mansson *et al.*, 1988, 1991; Oishi *et al.*, 1993).

Useful addresses

The Urostomy Association
Central Office
'Buckland'
Beaumont Park
Danbury
Essex
CM3 4DE
Tel.: 01245 224294

Impotence Information Centre
PO Box 1130
London
WC1X 9JN

The Royal Marsden NHS Trust
Fulham Road
London
SW3 6JJ
Tel.: 0171 352 8171

Medic-Alert Foundation
17 Bridge Wharf
156 Caledonian Road
London
N1 9UU
Tel.: 0171 833 3034

References and further reading

Alexander Williams, J. (1980) Cleaning the gut for colonic surgery. *World Medicine*, 15(10), 18–19.

Arai, Y. *et al.* (1993) Long-term follow-up of the Kock and Indiana pouch procedures. *Journal of Urology*, 150(1), 51–5.

Blannin, J. P. & Hobden, J. (1980) The catheter of choice. *Nursing Times*, 76, 2092–3.

Boore, J. R. P. (1978) *A Prescription for Recovery: the Effects of Pre-operative Preparation of Surgical Patients on Post-operative Stress, Recovery and Infection.* Royal College of Nursing, London.

Boyd, S. D. & Lieskovsky, D. (1988) Creation of the continent Kock ileal reservoir as an alternative to cutaneous urinary diversion. In: *Diagnosis and Management of Genitourinary Cancer*, (eds D. Skinner & D. Lieskovsky), Chapter 46. W. B. Saunders, Philadelphia.

Boyd, S. D. *et al.* (1987) Quality of life survey of urinary diversion patients: comparison of ileal conduits versus continent urinary reservoirs. *Journal of Urology*, 138, 1386–9.

Brocklehurst, J. C. & Brocklehurst, S. (1978) Management of indwelling catheters. *British Journal of Urology*, 50(2), 102–5.

Cummings, J. *et al.* (1987) The choice of suprapubic continent catheterisable urinary stoma. *British Journal of Urology*, 60, 227–30.

Delvin, H. B. & Plant, J. (1979) Sexual function – an aspect of stoma care. *British Journal of Sexual Medicine*, 1, pp. 2, 6, 22, 26, 33–4, 37.

Diokno, A. C. *et al.* (1983) Fate of patients started on clean intermittent self-catheterisation therapy ten years ago. *Journal of Urology*, 3(2), 191–3.

Duckett, J. W. & Snyder, H. M. (1985) Use of the Mitrofanoff principal in urinary reconstruction. *World Journal of Urology*, 3, 191–3.

Duckett, J. W. & Snyder, H. M. (1986) Continent urinary diversion – the Mitrofanoff principal. *Journal of Urology*, 136, 58–62.

Galister, J. S. & Woodhouse, C. R. (1991) Role of continent suprapubic diversion in pelvic cancer. *British Journal of Urology*, 68(4), 376–9.

Hayward, J. (1978) *Information – A Prescription Against Pain.* Royal College of Nursing, London.

Horn, S. A. (1990) Nursing patients with a continent urinary diversion. *Nursing Standard*, 4(21), 24–6.

Horn, S. A. (1991) *Continent Urinary Diversions – Your Questions Answered. Patients' Information Booklet.* The Royal Marsden Hospital, London.

Jeffrey, L. *et al.* (1988) The Mitrofanoff principal: an alternative form of continent urinary diversion. *Journal of Urology*, 140, 1529–31.

Jones, M. A. *et al.* (1981) Life with an ileal conduit: results of a questionnaire – surveys of patients and urological surgeons. *British Journal of Urology*, 52, 21–5.

Kennedy, W. A. *et al.* (1993) Pregnancy after orthotopic continent urinary diversion. *Surgery, Gynaecology and Obstetrics*, 177(4), 405–9.

Kock, N. G. *et al.* (1987) Appliance-free sphincter controlled bladder substitute. *Journal of Urology*, 138, 1150–4.

Lapides, S. (1971) Clean intermittent self-catheterization in the treatment of urinary tract disease. *Trans-American Association of Genitourinary Surgery*, 63, 92.

Lapides, J. *et al.* (1974) Follow-up on unsterile intermittent self-catheterisation. *Journal of Urology*, 11(1), 184.

Lawson, A. (undated) *Understanding Urostomy.* Squibb Surgicare.

Lindenhall, B. *et al.* (1994) Long-term intermittent catheterisation: the experience of teenagers and young adults with myelomeningocele. *Journal of Urology*, 152(1), 187–9.

Mansson, A. *et al.* (1988) Quality of life after cystectomy. *British Journal of Urology*, 62(4), 240–45.

Mansson, A. *et al.* (1991) Psychological adjustment to cystectomy for bladder carcinoma and effects on interpersonal relationships. *Scandinavian Journal of Caring Sciences*, 5(3), 129–34.

McCahill, P. D. *et al.* (1992) Toxic shock syndrome: a complication of continent urinary diversion. *Journal of Urology*, 147(3), 681–7.

Mitrofanoff, P. (1980) Cystomie continente trans appendiclaire dans le traitement des vessies neurologiques. *Chirurgie Pediatrique*, 21, 297–305.

Morris, J. *et al.* (1989) *The Benefits of Providing Information to*

Patients. The Centre for Health Economics, University of York.

Oishi, K. *et al.* (1993) Quality of life of patients with a continent urinary reservoir. *Hinyokika-kiyo*, 39(1), 7–14.

Raleigh, E. H. *et al.* (1990) Significant others benefit from preoperative information. *Journal of Advanced Nursing*, 15(8), 941–5.

Roberts, S. (1991) Theatre nursing operation reassurance, preoperative visiting. *Nursing Times*, 87(41), 70–71.

Skinner, D. G. & Boyd (1984) Techniques of creation of a continent urinary ileal reservoir (Kock pouch) for urinary diversion. *Urological Clinics of North America*, 11(4), 741–9.

Skinner, D. G. & Lieskovsky, D. (1988) Technique of radical cystectomy. In: *Diagnosis and Management of Genitourinary Cancer*, (eds D. G. Skinner & D. Lieskovsky). W. B. Saunders, Philadelphia.

Whitfield, H. N. & Hendry, W. F. (eds) (1985) *Textbook of Genito-Urinary Surgery*, Chapter 101, Pathophysiology of erection and ejaculation (G. S. Brindley); Chapter 102, Investigations and treatment of impotence (J. P. Pryor); Chapter 121, Bladder surgery (W. F. Hendry & H. N. Whitfield). Churchill Livingstone, Edinburgh.

Woodhouse, C. R. J. (1989) The Mitrofanoff principal for continent urinary diversions. *British Journal of Urology*, 63(1), 53–7.

Woodhouse, C. R. J. (1991) *Longterm Paediatric Urology*. Blackwell Scientific, Oxford.

Woodhouse, C. R. J. (1994) The Mitrofanoff pouch for urethral failure. *British Journal of Urology*, 73(1), 55–60.

Zeimer, M. M. (1983) Effects of information on post-surgical coping. *Nursing Research*, 32(5), 282–7.

TEACHING INTERMITTENT SELF-CATHETERIZATION OF A CONTINENT URINARY DIVERSION STOMA

Definition

Intermittent self-catheterization is when patients insert a self-catheterization catheter into the urinary reservoir via the continent urinary stoma using a clean technique. It is performed to evacuate or instill fluids, after which the tube is removed.

Indications

Intermittent self-catheterization may be carried out for the following reasons:

(1) To empty the contents of the urinary reservoir every 3–4 hours. If the reservoir is left too long between emptying it can become overstretched and lose its elasticity.

(2) To allow irrigation of the urinary reservoir for the removal of mucus which may occlude the continent urinary stoma.

REFERENCE MATERIAL

The following research has been gathered from urethral self-catheterization. However, the same principles would apply to a continent urinary stoma.

Intermittent self-catheterization is intended to make life easier and not more complicated. It is associated with a lower incidence of urinary tract infection than long-term indwelling catheters (Lapides, 1971, 1974; Diokno *et al.*, 1983; Lindenhall *et al.*, 1994).

Types of tubing used for intermittent self-catheterization

Blannin & Hobden (1980) suggest that the tubing used for intermittent self-catheterization should be: smooth-surfaced and flexible to prevent trauma; sterile so that it will not introduce infection; relatively resistant to the urine's acidity which can cause some materials to disintegrate or become inflexible, resulting in trauma; easily cleaned and stored for repeated use up to 7 days. Horn (1990) describes how fine-bore nasogastric tubes and low friction catheters may be used. The choice of tubing depends upon the size of the continent urinary stoma: that formed from ureter and fallopian tube may need a size 6–10 French gauge low friction catheter, while that formed from the appendix and small bowel may need size 10 French gauge upwards of a low friction catheter (1 French gauge = 0.66 mm).

Teaching self-catheterization

Intermittent self-catheterization should be taught in a place that offers privacy, with a good clear light and a full-length mirror (bathroom, toilet or at the patient's bedside) (Horn, 1990). It is a clean and not a sterile procedure. Patients can learn self-catheterization with the aid of a mirror or by touch, and are observed and assisted by a nurse until they are proficient (see Procedure, Guidelines: Self-catheterization, below).

During the day patients are encouraged to drink at least 2 litres of fluid to prevent any urinary tract infection and to catheterize every 3 or 4 hours to prevent the reservoir becoming distended and losing its elasticity. However, patients can reduce their fluid intake during the evening so that they need catheterize only before they go to sleep and again when they get up in the morning. The patient may feel bloated when the urine reservoir is full. Patients whose own bladder has been preserved may get a normal sensation of wanting to pass urine (Duckett & Snyder, 1986.

If a urinary reservoir has been created it may ooze mucus from its intestinal lining. This is normal, although it may stain the patient's clothing so a small protective dressing is advisable.

GUIDELINES: SELF-CATHETERIZATION

EQUIPMENT

1 Tubes for catheterization depending upon the size of the stoma.
2 Catheter-tipped syringe.
3 Tissues.
4 Clean jug or bowl.
5 Non-adherent dressing and non-allergenic skin protective tape to cover stoma if it oozes mucus.

PROCEDURE

Action	Rationale
1 Following explanation and discussion of self-catheterization the nurse should ensure the patient has all the equipment necessary for the procedure.	To ensure that the patient understands the procedure and gives his/her valid consent. To ensure all the equipment required is easily available.
2 Take the equipment to the toilet, bathroom or screened bed area.	To ensure the patient's privacy.
Ensure there is a good light and a full-length mirror.	To ensure the patient can see the stoma clearly.
3 The equipment should be arranged on a clean surface and within easy reach for the procedure.	To reduce the risk of contamination by surface bacteria. So that equipment is easily available.
4 The patient needs to remove any inhibiting clothing.	To ensure the patient can examine the stoma.
5 The patient should wash the hands with soap and water then dry them.	To ensure the hands are clean.
6 The patient should look at the stoma, if necessary with the aid of a hand or full-length mirror.	To look for mucus and swelling around the stoma.
7 The patient should wipe away any mucus with a tissue soaked in warm water and gently pat dry.	To ensure the opening of the stoma is clear and mucus does not block the catheter during insertion into stoma.
8 Remove the plastic tube from its container. Moisten the tip to be inserted with warm, running water or water-soluble lubricant.	To act as a lubricant to allow the tube to enter the urinary reservoir without causing internal trauma.
9 Ensure the untipped end of the tube is in a receiver, i.e. jug, bowl or toilet.	To ensure the urine goes into a bowl and not onto the patient.
10 The patient can use either a mirror to guide the tube into the opening of the stoma or feel the opening with two fingers slightly apart with the stoma between.	To act as a guide to pass the tube into the continent urinary stoma.
11 Insert the tube gently into the stoma following the pathway inside (usually towards the middle of the abdomen) until urine starts to flow, then insert tube a further 4–6 cm.	The direction of insertion and the diameter of catheter inserted depends on the type, size and shape of continent urinary stoma.

12 When all the urine has stopped flowing gently remove the tubing. If urine starts to flow again wait until it stops before removing the tube any further.

To ensure complete emptying of the urinary reservoir.

13 Remove the tube. Hold one end up then the other end.

To allow complete drainage of the tube.

14 Rinse tubing through with lukewarm tap water.

To rinse out any urine.

15 Replace the tube in its plastic container.

To keep the tubing clean.

16 Cover the stoma with a non-adherent dressing and secure with skin-protective tape.

To prevent mucus staining the patient's clothing.

17 The patient should wash the hands with soap and water, and then dry them.

To remove any urine on the hands.

18 The patient can then dress, collect equipment and dispose of any soiled dressings.

To prevent cross-infection.

NURSING CARE PLAN

Problem	Cause	Suggested action
Cannot insert the tube into the stoma.	Using too large a tube. Unable to locate opening. Opening occluded, e.g. due to swelling.	Try a smaller sized tube. Use a magnifying mirror to find opening. Rest for 10 minutes to let stoma relax and then reinsert. Have a warm bath which sometimes helps to dilate the opening. If still unable to catheterize, then patient should contact the hospital. Doctor may give subcutaneous injection of steroid to reduce swelling. If the opening remains occluded, a suprapubic catheter may be inserted to allow the swelling to subside and drain the urine from the reservoir. The stoma may need to be dilated by a doctor.
Partial insertion only of tubing is possible.	Tubing kinked. Stricture in the stoma.	Remove tubing and try with fresh tubing of the same size. Or try with a size smaller tubing. If unable to catheterize, contact the hospital.
Patient has not catheterized for 4 hours and feels distended, is easily catheterized but no urine is passed.	Tubing not inserted into reservoir. Tubing kinked.	Insert tubing further. Do not use force. If there is resistance then stop. Contact the hospital.

Nursing care plan (cont'd)

Problem	Cause	Suggested action
	Tube blocked with mucus.	Cough. The increased intra-abdominal pressure may dislodge the plug of mucus. While the tube is inserted, flush it with tap water. Remove tubing, examine for mucus and reinsert once it is clear. Flush the urinary reservoir.
Stoma leaks urine between catheterizations.	Reservoir not emptied regularly. Mucus plug blocking tubing, preventing complete drainage. Stoma failure.	Catheterise every 3–4 hours. If the patient has drunk large amounts, or alcohol (a diuretic), or is taking diuretic medication, it may be necessary to catheterize more frequently. Flush reservoir at least twice a day. If still leaking inform the hospital. Surgical fashioning of the stoma may be necessary.
Staining of blood during catheterization.	Trauma due to rough technique. Using wrong type of self-catheterization catheter.	Lubricate the tube well with water and insert gently into stoma. Use lubricating jelly. If blood staining continues or increases in amount then inform the hospital. Use low friction self-catheterization catheter.

CHAPTER 13

Cytotoxic Drugs: Handling and Administration

Definition
The term cytotoxic literally translated means 'toxic to cells'. Hence these drugs are those which kill cells (malignant or non-malignant).

REFERENCE MATERIAL
In recent years there has been increasing concern about the occupational hazards associated with the handling of cancer chemotherapeutic agents. On the basis of the evidence available at present, risks to personnel involved in the reconstitution and administration of cytotoxic drugs fall into two categories:

(1) The proven local effects caused by direct contact with the skin, eyes and mucous membranes. These include the following:
   (a) Dermatitis.
   (b) Inflammation of mucous membranes.
   (c) Excessive lacrimation.
   (d) Pigmentation.
   (e) Blistering, associated with mustine.
   (f) Other, miscellaneous, allergic reaction (Speechley, 1984).

   These hazards have been recognized for a number of years. Protection using non-absorbent armlets, plastic aprons and gloves and masks (in certain circumstances) for reconstitution, and gloves and aprons for administration are required. A number of different protective glove materials, including latex, rubber and PVC, have been recommended (Wright, 1993). The key points to consider when selecting gloves are thickness and integrity (Laidlaw et al., 1984). Gloves should always be discarded immediately if they become contaminated or punctured (Gibbs, 1991). Goggles should fully cover the eyes to protect the handler, and meet BS2092C requirements (Gibbs, 1991; Allwood & Wright, 1993).

(2) Cytotoxic drugs may also have harmful short- or long-term systemic effects if inhaled or ingested during preparation. Many have been shown to be mutagenic, and several are suspected of being teratogenic and/or carcinogenic when given at therapeutic levels to animals and humans (Waksvik et al., 1987; Bingham, 1985). With the majority of the compounds there is little or no absorption through intact skin (the exceptions are those which are lipid soluble). Systemic complaints from handlers include:
   (a) Lightheadedness.
   (b) Dizziness.
   (c) Nausea.
   (d) Headache.
   (e) Alopecia.
   (f) Coughing.
   (g) Pruritus.
   (h) General malaise.

The working conditions in which these complaints were experienced were not desirable, i.e. a small, unventilated medicine closet (Speechley, 1984; Carter, 1986; Reymann, 1993). No formal collection of data was performed and the author readily admits to gathering information on an anecdotal basis, but the data are supported by the literature (*Drug Intelligence and Clinical Pharmacy*, 1983).

A number of experimental studies have suggested that serious long-term effects may result from exposure to cytotoxic drugs. Effects include chromosomal abnormalities (Waksvik et al., 1987), reproductive function disorders (Selevan et al., 1985). Mutagenic substances have been found in the urine of cytotoxic drug handlers, including nurses (Ames et al., 1975; Falck et al., 1979; Vennit et al., 1984).

Although alterations in cell structure have been detected in many of the published works, they appear to be transient and of a low level. It has yet to be demonstrated whether these changes in cell structure are harmful and if this level of mutagenesis can be equated with more serious consequences. Inconclusive or contradictory data, and doubts about the validity of the test, have yet to be quantified.

In summary, localized toxicity due to accidental contact with cytotoxic drugs is well documented and it is therefore only sensible to take precautions to minimize the risks. While long-term hazards remain largely undefined, the suggestion that some compounds may carry the insidious risk of teratogenicity or carcinogenicity is sufficiently strong that the only responsible course of action is that which minimizes exposure. This is best achieved through locally agreed policies based on the available national guidelines. In 1989 *The Control of Substances Hazardous to Health* (COSHH) regulations were introduced. Under these regulations employers are obliged to identify substances which are a hazard to staff. In hospitals where cytotoxic drugs are used frequently, the most effective means of minimizing the hazard is to arrange for all doses to be prepared on a named patient basis by trained pharmacy staff in a specially equipped area (Royal College of Nursing, 1989; Allwood & Wright, 1993).

Whatever the situation, written guidelines should be available to cover:

(1) Preparation of compounds – environment, staff training, staff protection, techniques, equipment.
(2) Administration of drugs – staff training, staff protection, technique, equipment.
(3) Disposal – of drugs, equipment, waste and excreta.
(4) Accidents – spillage and contamination of nurse, doctor or patient.
(5) A system for monitoring and recording any effects on hospital staff.

Note: Qualified nursing staff are increasingly given responsibility for the administration of intravenous medication, including cytotoxic drugs. For further information regarding these procedures see Chapter 23, Intravenous Management.

References and further reading

Allwood, M. & Wright, P. (eds) (1993) *The Cytotoxic Handbook*, 2nd edn. Radcliffe Medical Press, Oxford.

Ames, B. N. *et al.* (1975) Methods for detecting carcinogens and mutagens with the salmonella/mammalian microsome mutagenicity test. *Mutation Research*, 31, 347–64.

Anderson, M. *et al.* (1983) Development and operation of a pharmacy-based intravenous cytotoxic reconstitution service. *British Medical Journal*, 286, 32–6.

Anderson, R. *et al.* (1982) Risk of handling injectable antineoplastic agents. *American Journal of Hospital Pharmacy*, 39, 1881–7.

Bauman, B. & Duvall, E. (1980) An unusual accident during the administration of chemotherapy. *Cancer Nursing*, 3(4), 305–6.

Bingham, E. (1985) Hazards to health care professionals from antineoplastic drugs. *New England Journal of Medicine*, 313, 1120–2.

Calvert, A. H. (1981) The long-term sequelae of cytotoxic therapy. *Cancer Topics*, 3(7), 77–9.

Colls, B. M. (1985) Safety of handling cytotoxic agents: a cause for concern by pharmaceutical companies. *British Medical Journal*, 291, 318–19.

Cooke, J. *et al.* (1987) Environmental monitoring of personnel who handle cytotoxic drugs. *Pharmaceutical Journal*, 239(6452 suppl. R2).

Crudi, C. B. (1980) A compounding dilemma: I've kept the drug sterile but have I contaminated myself? *National Intravenous Therapy Association*, 3, 77–8.

Darbyshire, P (1986) Handle with care. *Nursing Times*, 82(40), 37–8.

Drug Intelligence and Clinical Pharmacy (1983) 17, 532–7.

Falck, K. *et al.* (1979) Mutagenicity in urine of nurses handling cytotoxic agents. *Lancet*, 1, 1250.

Gibbs, J. (1991) Handling cytotoxic drugs. *Nursing Times*, 87(11), 54–5.

Harris, J. & Dodds, L. (1985) Handling waste from patients receiving cytotoxic drugs. *Pharmaceutical Journal*, 235(6345), 289–91.

Health and Safety Executive (1983) *Precautions for the Safe Handling of Cytotoxic Drugs, Medical Series.* HMSO, London.

Health and Safety Executive (1988) *The Control of Substances Hazardous to Health Regulations.* HMSO, London.

HPG Welsh Office (1988) *Policy for the Safe Handling of Cytotoxic Drugs.*

Knowles, R. S. & Virden, J. E. (1980) Handling of injectable antineoplastic agents. *British Medical Journal*, 2, 589–91

Laidlaw, J. L. *et al.* (1984) Permeability of latex and polyvinyl chloride gloves to 20 antineoplastic drugs. *American Journal of Hospital Pharmacy*, 41, 2018–23.

Lee, L. (1993) The risks of handling cytotoxic therapy. *Nursing Standard*, 7(49), 25–8.

Nguyen, T. V. *et al.* (1982) Exposure of pharmacy personnel to mutagenic antineoplastic drugs. *Cancer Research*, 42, 4792–6.

Oakley, P. & Reeves, E. (1984) Setting up a reconstitution service. *Pharmaceutical Journal*, 232(6282), 739–40.

Oldcorne, M. A. *et al.* (1987) Letters to the editor. Handling cytotoxic drugs. *Pharmaceutical Journal*, 18 April, 238, 488.

Reymann, P. E. (1993) *Chemotherapy: Principles of Administration in Cancer Nursing*, (eds S. L. Groenwald *et al.*), 3rd edn, Chapter 15. Jones & Bartlett Publishers, Boston.

Richardson, M. L. & Bowron, J. M. (1985) The fate of pharmaceutical chemicals in the aquatic environment. *Journal of Pharmaceutical Pharmacology*, 37, 1–12.

Royal College of Nursing Oncology Nursing Society (1989) *Safe Practices with Cytotoxics.* Scutari Projects, Middlesex.

Selevan, S. G. (1986) Letter. *New England Journal of Medicine*, 16, 1048–51.

Selevan, S. G. *et al.* (1985) A study of occupational exposure to antineoplastic drugs and fetal loss in nurses *New England Journal of Medicine*, 19, 1173–8.

Speechley, V. (1982) Better safe than sorry. *Nursing Mirror*, 154(15), 11.

Speechley, V. (1984) Administration of cytotoxic drugs. *Nursing Mirror*, 158(2), 22–5.

Stokes, M. *et al.* (1987) Permeability of latex and polyvinyl chloride gloves to fluorouracil and methotrexate. *American Journal of Hospital Pharmacy*, 44, 1341–6.

Stuart, M. (1981) Sequence of administering vesicant cytotoxic drugs; Part A. *Oncology Nursing Forum*, 9(1), 53–4.

Thomas, P. H. & Fenton-May, V. (1987) Protection offered by various gloves to carmustine exposure. *Pharmaceutical Journal*, 20 June, 238, 775–7.

Vennit, S. *et al.* (1984) Monitoring exposure of nursing and pharmacy personnel to cytotoxic drugs: urinary mutation assays and urinary platinum as markers of absorption. *Lancet*, 1, 74–6.

Waksvik, H. *et al.* (1987) Chromosome analysis of nurses handling cytostatic agents. *Cancer Treatment Reports*, 65, 607–10.

Working Party of the Pharmaceutical Society of Great Britain on the Handling of Cytotoxic Drugs (1983) Guidelines for the handling of cytotoxic drugs. *Pharmaceutical Journal*, 230(6215), 230–1.

Wright, M. P. (1993) Protective clothing. In: *The Cytotoxic Handbook*, (eds M. Allwood & P. Wright), 2nd edn. Radcliffe Medical Press, Oxford..

GUIDELINES: PROTECTION OF THE ENVIRONMENT

EQUIPMENT

1 Two plastic overshoes.
2 Two disposable armlets.
3 Two clinical waste bags.
4 Two pairs of disposable non-sterile gloves.
5 Goggles (non-disposable).
6 Surgical masks.
7 Plastic apron.
8 Paper towels.
9 Plastic bucket.
10 Copy of spillage procedure.

Management of spillage

Action	Rationale
1 Act immediately.	Any spillage may become a health hazard.
2 Collect spillage kit.	It contains all necessary equipment.
3 Put on thick latex or PVC gloves and disposable plastic apron or tabard.	To provide personal protection.
4 If there is visible powder spill, put on a good-quality surgical face mask.	To prevent inhalation of powder.
5 If spillage is on hard floor, put on overshoes.	For protection and to minimize the spread of contamination.
6 Wipe up powder spillage quickly with well dampened paper towels and dispose of them as 'high-risk' waste.	To prevent dispersal of powder. To protect others and ensure safe disposal by incineration.
7 Mop up liquids which have been spilled on a hard surface with paper towels and dispose of them as 'high risk' waste.	To protect others and ensure safe disposal by incineration.
8 Wash hard surfaces well with copious amounts of cold, soapy water and dry with paper towels.	To remove residual contamination.

Guidelines: Protection of the environment (cont'd)

Action	Rationale
9 If spillage is on clothing, remove it as soon as possible and treat as 'soiled linen'.	To decontaminate clothing without hazard to laundry staff.
10 If spillage has penetrated clothing, wash contaminated skin liberally with soap and cold water.	To decontaminate skin and prevent drug absorption.
11 If spillage is on bed linen, change it immediately and treat as 'soiled linen'.	To protect the patient. To protect the laundry staff.
12 Any accident or spillage involving direct skin contact with a cytotoxic drug must be reported to the occupational health department (see Guideline: Protection of nursing staff when handling cytotoxic drugs, below).	To ensure that details of accidental contact are entered in the nurse's health record, and appropriate follow-up initiated.

Disposal of waste

Action	Rationale
1 'Sharps' should be placed in the special container provided.	To ensure incineration and to prevent laceration and/or inoculation during transit and disposal.
2 Dry waste, intravenous administration sets and other contaminated material should be placed in 'high-risk' waste disposal bags.	To ensure careful handling and disposal by incineration.
3 A small amount (a part dose) of drug solution may be flushed down the main drainage system, using copious amounts of cold water, only if no alternative means of safe disposal is available.	Many water authorities prohibit drug waste disposal in the drainage system. This route of disposal must be used *only* if the waste cannot be safely transported elsewhere for disposal.
4 Re-usable trays and other equipment should be washed with copious amounts of water followed by the usual procedure for disinfection.	To prevent cross-contamination and cross-infection.
5 Unused doses of cytotoxics should be returned, unopened, to the pharmacy.	To enable them to be relabelled and re-issued, stability permitting, or to be destroyed safely.

Disposal of excreta from patients receiving cytotoxic drugs

Few cytotoxic agents are excreted as unchanged drug or active metabolites in urine or faeces. In order to comply with safe technique and practice, gloves should now always be worn, thus minimizing risks to the nursing staff.

GUIDELINES: PROTECTION OF NURSING STAFF WHEN HANDLING CYTOTOXIC DRUGS

Nursing staff should not be involved in routine reconstitution of cytotoxic drugs, as this is the function of the pharmacy unit. However, there may be emergency situations when the nurse is requested to prepare chemotherapy and it is essential that this is performed safely. The following procedure should be used for guidance.

Action	Rationale
1 Reconstitution of cytotoxic drugs should take place in a well-ventilated room. Doors and windows should be closed to prevent draughts.	To prevent any unnecessary airborne exposure from possible powder or droplet aerosol released.
2 While reconstitution is in progress no other activities should be carried out within the area. Movement in and out of that area should be restricted.	As above.
3 The area should contain a sink and running water.	To clean surfaces and/or skin if spillage or contamination occurs.
4 The work surface should be smooth and impermeable.	To enable cleaning of surfaces to be undertaken easily and quickly.
5 Reconstitution should take place in a plastic tray or equivalent.	To enable containment of spillage and ease of cleaning.
6 Nursing staff should receive instruction in the techniques of reconstitution and the reasons for these recommendations.	To ensure staff are safe to practise and are aware of the risks involved.
7 Direct contact with drug solution can be entirely avoided by good technique and the use of thick latex/PVC gloves.	To minimize exposure to handler.
8 All cuts and scratches should be covered.	To prevent infiltration of the skin if damage to gloves occurs.
9 Use protective goggles or glasses.	To prevent contact between drugs and the eyes. If the nurse wears glasses these should provide protection.
10 Wash protective goggles with soap and water after use.	To prevent cross-contamination and/or cross-infection.
11 Use a good quality surgical face mask when reconstituting dry powder, especially if presented in an ampoule, e.g. bleomycin.	To prevent inhalation of any powder released during reconstitution.
12 Put on a disposable plastic apron or tabard.	To provide a barrier between the drug and the handler.
13 Ampoules should be held away from the face and covered with a sterile gauze swab when breaking them.	To prevent contamination of the gloves and skin. To prevent formation of aerosols or liberation of powder.
14 Luer-locking syringes should be used.	To reduce the incidence of accidental disconnection and spillage of drug.
15 A filtered air venting needle is recommended.	To prevent the development of pressure differentials between syringe and vial.
The alternative 'no airway' technique involves a 'push-pull' use of the syringe to add cyclically small quantities of diluent to, and remove air from, the closed vial. This technique is not recommended (see Chapter 15, Drug Administration, under the heading Guidelines: Administration of injections).	In inexperienced hands, the 'no airway' technique results in the danger of contamination. In extreme circumstances the vial and closure may separate, the syringe/needle junction may leak (especially if Luer slip syringes are used) or the vial may explode.

Guidelines: Protection of nursing staff when handling cytotoxic drugs (cont'd)

Action	Rationale
16 The diluent should be introduced slowly down the inside wall of the vial or ampoule.	To ensure that the powder is thoroughly wet before agitation, and is not released into the atmosphere.
17 Needles should be capped before the expulsion of air, or the tip should be covered with a sterile swab or the air should be expelled into the vial or ampoule.	To prevent aerosol formation.
18 Gloves and apron/tabard should continue to be worn during administration as the nurse is still handling the drugs and may become contaminated.	To prevent contamination at a later stage in the procedure.
19 Contamination of the skin, mucous membranes and eyes should be treated promptly. All areas should be washed with copious amounts of tap water or 0.9% sodium chloride. Eye wash may be available.	To prevent any local damage to tissue.
20 Accidental infiltration of the skin with a vesicant drug should be treated as an extravasation and the appropriate procedure followed (see Management of extravasation of vesicant drugs, below).	To prevent any local damage to tissue.
21 If erythema and/or other local reaction occurs in any circumstances, contact the occupational health unit or a member of the medical staff so that appropriate treatment may be advised.	To prevent further damage and/or complications.
22 It is essential after any accident involving direct contact with a cytotoxic drug, or if any local or systemic symptoms occur after handling such a drug, that the occupational health unit should be contacted.	To assist with recording and monitoring of staff exposure.
23 If pregnancy is suspected or intended, the occupational health unit should be contacted.	To discuss future work patterns and any anxiety that may be felt.

GUIDELINES: INTRAVENOUS ADMINISTRATION OF CYTOTOXIC DRUGS

The most frequently used route for administration of cytotoxic drugs is intravenously. This ensures rapid, reliable delivery of agents to the patients and the tumour site. In addition, many drugs have to be administered into a vein where rapid dilution by the blood can occur, as they are irritant to soft tissue and capable of causing necrosis. These drugs are called *vesicant agents*. The aim of the procedure for administration of chemotherapy intravenously is to protect both nurse and patient from contamination and also to prevent extravasation of drugs which could result in local tissue damage. An infusion of a cytotoxic vesicant drug may be administered into a verified central venous catheter, either with the aid of a mechanical device or by gravity. It is not recommended to administer infusions of vesicants via a peripheral device, due to the risk of possible extravasation. An infusion is acceptable only providing that the cannula is observed at all times. The large majority of cytotoxic agents will be delivered to the ward/unit individually packaged for delivery to a named patient, by injection or infusion. If this is not so, specific guidelines should be followed (see Guidelines: Protection of nursing staff when handling cytotoxic drugs, above).

Action	Rationale
1 Explain and discuss the procedure with the patient. Evaluate the patient's knowledge of cytotoxic therapy. If this knowledge appears to be faulty or incorrect, offer an explanation of the use, action, dose and potential side-effects of the drug or drugs involved.	To ensure that the patient understands the procedure and gives his/her valid consent. A patient has a right to information.
2 Put on gloves and an apron before commencing the procedure.	To protect the nurse from local contamination of skin or clothing Note: with careful handling technique, this risk is minimal but splashes can occur when changing syringes or infusion containers.
3 Prepare necessary equipment for an aseptic administration procedure, and ensure that this is followed carefully. (For further information on intravenous management, see Chapter 23.)	To prevent local and/or systemic infection. Patients are frequently immunosuppressed and at greater risk.
4 Check that all details on the syringe or infusion container are correct when compared with the patient's prescription, before opening the sterile packaging.	To ensure the patient is given the correct drug which has been dispensed for him/her. To prevent wastage.
5 Take the medication and the prescription chart to the patient. Check the patient's identity and the dose to be given.	To prevent error.
6 Inspect the infusion or injection site, and consult the patient about sensation around the device insertion site.	To detect any phenomena, e.g. phlebitis, which would render the vein unusable.
7 Establish the patency of the vein using 0.9% sodium chloride.	To determine whether the vein will accommodate the extra fluid flow and irritant drugs and remain patent.
8 Ensure the correct administration rate.	To prevent speed shock. To prevent extra pressure and irritation within the vein.
9 Be aware of the immediate effects of the drug.	To know what to observe during administration. To be prepared to manage any side-effects which occur.
10 Administer drugs in the correct order, i.e. vesicants first.	To ensure that those agents likely to cause tissue damage are given when venous integrity is greatest, i.e. at the beginning. Note: because of their irritant nature (approximately pH3 to 3.5) anti-emetics should be given half an hour before chemotherapy administration or at the end of the sequence.
11 Observe the vein throughout.	To detect any problems at the earliest moment.

Guidelines: Intravenous administration of cytotoxic drugs (cont'd)

Action	Rationale
12 Observe for signs of extravasation, e.g. swelling or leakage at the site of injection. Note the patient's comments about sensation at the site, e.g. pain.	To prevent any unnecessary damage to soft tissue, and to enable the remainder of the drug(s) to be given correctly at another site. To enable prompt treatment to be given, thus minimizing local damage, and possibly preserving venous access for future treatment. (For further information see Management of extravasation of vesicant drugs, below.)
13 Flush the device with 0.9% sodium chloride between drugs and after administration.	To prevent drug interaction. To prevent leakage of drug along the path of the cannula or from the puncture site.
14 Be aware of the patient's comfort throughout the procedure.	To minimize trauma to the patient. To involve the patient in treatment and detect any side-effects and/or problems that may then be avoided at the next treatment.
15 Record details of the administration in the appropriate documents.	To prevent any duplication of treatment and to provide a point of reference in the event of queries.
16 Protect the patient from contact with the drugs by:	
(a) Inserting the needle carefully into the injection site of the giving set, extension set or cannula injection cap.	To prevent exiting on the other side and contaminating or inoculating the patient.
(b) Careful removal of the blind hub and changing of needles/syringes, plus care when inserting the administration set into the infusion container or changing bags.	To avoid leakage or splashes and contamination of the nurse or patient.
(c) Securing a good bond between needle and syringe, always use Luer lock syringes.	To prevent leakage or separation, which may occur due to pressure during administration, resulting in spray and contamination.
(d) Checking the injection site or injection cap at the end of the procedure.	To ensure that there is no leakage.
(e) Acting promptly if any contamination is noted and washing the area with cold water or saline.	To prevent any local reaction on skin, mucous membranes, etc.

MANAGEMENT OF EXTRAVASATION OF VESICANT DRUGS

REFERENCE MATERIAL

The treatment of extravasations of chemotherapeutic agents is controversial. No treatments have well documented efficacy: controlled clinical trials are lacking and it is often difficult to ascertain whether an infiltration has actually occurred (Plumer, 1993). The use of warm or cold compresses is also controversial. Heat causes vasodilation and increases distribution and absorption of the drug, and may lead to further cellular damage (Plumer, 1993). Cold compresses promote localization of the drug by causing vasoconstriction and can alleviate local irritation and discomfort. They may also inactivate the locally destructive effects of some cytotoxic agents (Beason, 1990; Hastings–Tolsma *et al.*, 1993). A variety of antidotes are available, but again there is a lack of scientific evidence to demonstrate their value. Many are based on personal opinion and merely attempt to neutralize the drug (Rudolph & Larson, 1987).

Even when practitioners have many years of experience, extravasation of vesicant agents can occur and is an extremely stressful event. Early detection and treatment of extravasation is crucial: it is prevention, however, that remains the most effective strategy for managing this hazard to patients. The use of extravasation kits has been recommended (Beason, 1990). Kits should be assembled according to the particular needs of individual institutions. The procedure detailed here represents the policy of The Royal Marsden NHS Trust for the management by nursing staff of extravasation injury, drawn up with the assistance of pharmacy and medical colleagues.

Before administration of cytotoxic drugs the nurse should know which agents are capable of producing tissue necrosis. The following is a list of those in common use:

carmustine (concentrated solution)	mithramycin
dacarbazine (concentrated solution)	mitomycin C
dactinomycin	mustine
daunorubicin	streptozocin
doxorubicin	vinblastine
epirubicin	vincristine
idarubicin	vindesine

If in any doubt, the drug data sheet should be consulted or reference made to a trial protocol. Drugs should not be reconstituted to give solutions that are higher than the manufacturers' recommended concentration, and the method of administration should be checked, e.g. infusion, injection.

A variety of non-cytotoxic agents in frequent use are also capable of causing severe tissue damage if extravasated. They include:

amphotericin
acyclovir
ganciclovir
phenytoin
potassium chloride (if greater than 40 mmols/l)
hypertonic solutions of sodium bicarbonate (greater than 5%)
vancomycin

This potential hazard should always be remembered. The actions listed in this procedure may not be appropriate in all these instances. Drug data sheets should always be checked and the pharmacy departments should be consulted if the information is insufficient.

Extravasation should be suspected if:

(1) The patient complains of burning, stinging pain or any other acute change at the injection site. This should be distinguished from a feeling of cold which may occur with some drugs.

(2) Induration, swelling or leakage at the injection site is observed. It is important that this is distinguished from a 'flare' reaction: a redness or 'blistering' with doxorubicin and other red coloured drugs. It is similar in appearance to a nettle rash and is a local reaction to the dye (Beason, 1990; Wood & Gullo, 1993).

(3) No blood return is obtained. (If found in isolation this should not be regarded as an indication of a non-patent vein.)

(4) A resistance is felt on the plunger of the syringe if drugs are given by bolus.

(5) There is absence of free flow when administration is by infusion (Reymann, 1993).

Note: One or more of the above may be present. If extravasation is suspected or confirmed, action must be taken immediately.

The consequences of an untreated or poorly managed extravasation include:

• Pain from necrotic areas.
• Possible physical defect.
• The cost of hospitalization and possible plastic surgery.
• Treatment of disease may be delayed.
• Psychological distress (Plumer, 1993)

References and further reading

Allwood, M. & Wright, P. (1993) *The Cytotoxic Handbook*, 2nd edn, Chapter 9. Radcliffe Medical Press, Oxford.

Beason, R. (1990) Antineoplastic vesicant extravasation. *Journal of Intravenous Nursing*, March/April, 111–14.

Hastings-Tolsma, M. T. *et al.* (1993) Effect of warm and cold applications on the resolution of IV infiltrations. *Research in Nursing and Health*, 16, 171–8.

Oncology Nursing Society (1984) *Cancer Chemotherapy Guidelines and Recommendations for Nursing Education and Practice*. Oncology Nursing Society, Pittsburgh, USA.

Reymann, P. E. (1993) *Chemotherapy: Principles of Administration in Cancer Nursing. Principles and Practice*, (eds. S. L. Groenwald, M. Goodman, M. H. Frogge & C. H. Yarbro), 3rd edn, Chapter 15. Jones & Bartlett Publishers, Boston.

Rudolph, R. & Larson, D. L. (1987) Etiology and treatment of chemotherapeutic agent extravasation injuries: A review. *Journal of Clinical Oncology*, 5(7), 1116–26.

Smith, R. (1985a) Extravasation of intravenous fluids. *British Journal of Parenteral Therapy*, 6(2), 30–5/42.

Smith, R. (1985b) Prevention and treatment of extravasation. *British Journal of Parenteral Therapy*, 6(5), 114–20.

Weinstein, S. M. (1993) *Plumer's Principles and Practice of Intravenous Therapy*, 5th edn. J. B. Lippincott, Philadelphia.

Wood, L. S. & Gullo, S. M. (1993) IV vesicants: how to avoid extravasation. *American Journal of Nursing*, April, 42–50.

GUIDELINES: MANAGEMENT OF EXTRAVASATION

EQUIPMENT

To assist the nurse, an extravasation kit should be assembled and should be readily available in each ward/unit. It contains:

1 Instant cold pack ×1/instant hot pack ×1.
2 Dexamethasone injection 8 mg in 2 ml ×1/hyaluronidase 1500 units.
3 Hydrocortisone cream 1% 15 g tube ×1.
4 2-ml syringes ×1.
5 25 g needles ×2.
6 Alcohol swabs.
7 Documentation slips ×2.
8 Copy of extravasation management procedure.

PROCEDURE

Action	Rationale
1 Explain and discuss the procedure with the patient.	To ensure that the patient understands the procedure and gives his/her valid consent.
2 Stop injection *immediately*, leaving the cannula or winged infusion device in place.	To minimize local injury. To allow aspiration of the drug to be attempted.
3 Aspirate any residual drug and blood from the device and suspected extravasation site.	To minimize local injury by removing as much drug as possible. Subsequent damage is related to the volume of the extravasation, in addition to other factors.
4 Remove the cannula or winged infusion device.	To prevent the site from being used as an intravenous route.
5 Collect the extravasation pack and take it to the patient.	It contains all the equipment necessary for managing extravasation.
6 If vinca alkaloids: Draw up hyaluronidase 1500 units in 1 ml water for injection and inject volumes of 0.1–0.2 ml subcutaneously at points of the compass around the circumference of the area of extravasation. Apply warm pack.	This is the antidote for vinca alkaloids. The warm pack speeds up absorption of the drug by the tissues.
All other vesicants: Apply cold pack or ice instantly.	To localize the area of extravasation, slow cell metabolism and decrease the area of tissue destruction. To reduce local pain.
Draw up a dexamethasone injection 4–8 mg and inject 0.1 to 0.2 ml subcutaneously at each point of the compass around the circumference of the area of extravasation. Ensure the whole area is infiltrated.	To reduce local inflammation and improve the survival of tissues, especially those marginally injured.
7 Where possible elevate the extremity and/or encourage movement.	To minimize swelling and to prevent adhesion of damaged area to underlying tissue, which could result in restriction of movement.
8 Inform a member of the medical staff at the earliest opportunity.	To enable actions differing from agreed policy to be taken if considered in the best interests of the patient. To notify the doctor of the need to prescribe drugs.

9	Apply hydrocortisone cream 1% twice daily, and instruct the patient how to do this. Continue as long as erythema persists.	To reduce local inflammation and promote patient comfort.
10	Re-apply a long lasting cold pack of ice for 24 hours if vesicant is *other* than vinca alkaloids.	To localize the steroid effect in the area of extravasation. To reduce local pain and promote patient comfort.
11	Provide analgesia as required.	To promote patient comfort. To encourage movement of the limb as advised.
12	Document the following details, in duplicate, on the form provided: (a) Patient's name/number (b) Ward/unit (c) Date, time (d) Signs and symptoms. (e) Venepuncture site (on diagram). (f) Drug sequence. (g) Drug administration technique, i.e. 'bolus', infusion. (h) Approximate amount of the drug extravasated. (i) Diameter, length and width of extravasation area. (j) Appearance of the area. (k) Nursing management/action taken/ medical officer notified. (l) Patient's complaints, comments, statements (m) Signature of the nurse,	To provide an immediate full record of all details of the incident, which may be referred to if necessary. To provide a baseline for future observation and monitoring of patient's condition.
13	Explain to the patient that the site may remain sore for several days.	To reduce anxiety and ensure continued co-operation.
14	Observe the area regularly for erythema, induration, blistering or necrosis. *Inpatients*: monitor daily.	To detect any changes at the earliest possible moment.
15	Request outpatients to observe the area daily and to report immediately any increased discomfort, peeling or blistering of the skin.	To detect any changes as early as possible, and allow for a review of future management. This may include referral to a plastic surgeon.
16	If blistering or tissue breakdown occurs, begin sterile dressing techniques.	To prevent a superimposed infection.
17	If a shallow, clean ulcer develops, consider attempting to heal it using a starch-hydrogel type dressing.	To promote healing and avoid unnecessary surgery. This type of dressing has been observed to have a beneficial effect in some instances.
18	Consider referral for plastic surgery if no healing occurs and the patient's condition permits.	To prevent further pain or other complications as chemically induced ulcers rarely heal spontaneously.

ADMINISTRATION OF CYTOTOXIC DRUGS BY OTHER ROUTES

ORAL ADMINISTRATION

Nurses dispensing tablets or capsules should use a non-touch technique. If tablets have to be counted, this should be done using a triangle, which should be washed and dried after use.

Many tablets are coated and this protects the drug in its inner core. There is no handling risk if these coatings are not broken.

A small number of tablets are compressed powders, but there is no risk where there is no free powder visible. It is important that these tablets are not crushed.

Capsules are free from risk if they have not been opened or have not been either broken or leaked. They should not be crushed or opened.

Any visible spillage should be dealt with as previously directed (see Guidelines: Protection of the environment, above).

INTRAMUSCULAR AND SUBCUTANEOUS INJECTION

The local tissue toxicity of many cytotoxic drugs limits the use of this route. Drugs administered in this way are:

(1) Methotrexate.
(2) Bleomycin.
(3) Cytosine arabinoside.
(4) L-asparaginase.

Intramuscular and subcutaneous injections are often used for patient convenience, if regular administration is required and journeys to the hospital are impractical. Community nurses are responsible for administration and must be supplied with adequate information when the patient is discharged.

Although the volume of drug and diluent handled is less than for the intravenous route, preparation and re-constitution of the agents should be in line with the information listed under Guidelines: Protection of nursing staff when handling cytotoxic drugs, above. The nurse should continue to wear gloves during administration. Spillage and disposal of equipment should be dealt with as previously directed (see Guidelines: Protection of the environment, above) and systems of work modified to ensure this is possible.

Recommendations about administration should be followed carefully, e.g. deep intramuscular injection using a Z-track technique to prevent leakage onto the skin; rotation of sites to prevent local irritation developing.

INTRAPLEURAL INSTILLATION

Definition
Introduction of cytotoxic drugs, or other substances, into the pleural cavity following drainage of an effusion to prevent or delay a recurrence.

REFERENCE MATERIAL
Pleural effusion is a common complication of malignant disease and may pose a considerable management problem. The most common neoplasms associated with the development of malignant pleural effusions are those of the:

(1) Breast.
(2) Lung.

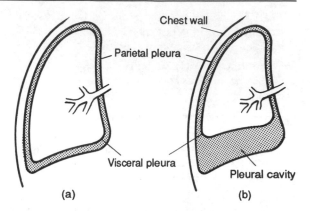

Figure 13.1   Lung anatomy. (a) Normal lung anatomy showing pleura. (b) Lung demonstrating presence of pleural effusion.

(3) Gastrointestinal tract.
(4) Prostate.
(5) Ovary.

The incidence varies, but may be as high as 50% in patients with primary lung or breast carcinoma. Such effusions can be very distressing to the patient, causing progressive discomfort, dyspnoea and death from respiratory insufficiency.

The alteration in normal anatomy due to the pressure of an effusion is illustrated in Fig. 13.1. In health less than 5 ml of transudate fluid are present between the visceral and parietal pleurae. This fluid acts as a lubricant and hydraulic seal. Infections and malignancies disrupt this mechanism, often repeatedly. Patients may survive for months or years; therefore, effective palliation is important in maintaining or improving their quality of life.

Several methods have been used to treat pleural effusions, including surgical techniques, such as ablation of the pleural space, radiotherapy and systemic chemotherapy and more recently the instillation of a pleural shunt (Tsang et al., 1990) and the insertion of a small bore catheter placement (Parker et al., 1989). In addition, instillation of sclerosing agents into the pleural space has been used for 30 years. These agents have included talc, radioactive phosphorus, thiotepa, tetracycline and, more recently, cytotoxic drugs. The drug most frequently instilled is bleomycin (Reymann, 1993).

Cytology may show the presence of tumour cells in effusion fluid but even when these are absent, instillation of drugs may be effective in preventing recurrence due to the inflammatory reaction which obliterates the pleural space.

Improvements in equipment used, for example flexible cannulae or catheters, and lengthening of both the initial drainage period and that following instillation of the drug, have contributed to increased patient comfort and greater effectiveness.

All studies recommend that the patient should be turned regularly following instillation of the drug to ensure its complete distribution over the pleural surfaces. The recommended timing varies and only one paper (Wood, 1981) provides a detailed procedure. The rationale for such turning is based on clinical observation and there is a lack of work comparing patients who were turned with those who were not.

Adequate analgesia and nursing measures must be provided to ensure patient comfort (Reymann, 1993).

References and further reading

Anderson, C. *et al.* (1972) The treatment of malignant pleural effusions. *Cancer*, 33, 916–22.

Paladine, W. *et al.* (1976) Intracavity bleomycin in the management of malignant effusions. *Cancer*, 38, 1903–8.

Parker, L. A. *et al.* (1989) Small bore catheter drainage and sclerotherapy for malignant pleural effusions. *Cancer*, 64, 1218–21.

Reymann, P. E. (1993) *Chemotherapy: Principles of Administration in Cancer Nursing. Principles and Practice,* (eds S. L. Groenwald, M. Goodman, M. H. Frogge & C. H. Yarbro), 3rd edn, Chapter 15. Jones & Bartlett Publishers, Boston.

Taylor, L. (1962) A catheter technique for intrapleural adminstration of alkylating agents: a report of ten cases. *American, Journal of the Medical Sciences*, 244(6), 706–16.

Tsang, V. *et al.* (1990) Pleuroperitoneal shunt for recurrent malignant pleural effusion. *Thorax*, 45, 369–72.

Wallach, H. (1975) Intrapleural tetracycline for malignant pleural effusions. *Chest*, 68, 510–12.

Wood, H. (1981) Developments in the support of patients with malignant pleural effusion. In: *Cancer Nursing Update*, (ed. R. Tiffany), pp. 69–76. Baillière Tindall, London.

GUIDELINES: ADMINISTRATION OF INTRAPLEURAL DRUGS

The procedure and nursing care plans related to intrapleural drainage (see Chapter 22) should be consulted for all aspects of thoracic drainage. The following information covers specific points regarding drug instillation.

PROCEDURE
Instillation of drug

Action	Rationale
1 Explain and discuss the procedure with the patient.	To ensure that the patient understands the procedure and gives his/her valid consent.
2 Administer premedication to the patient, if prescribed.	To relax the patient.
3 Prepare the required equipment (see Chapter 15, Drug Administration, under the heading Guidelines: Administration of injections) and cytotoxic drug with protective wear as necessary.	To ensure the procedure goes smoothly without interruption.
4 Assist the doctor with the installation and provide support for the patient.	To increase the efficiency of the procedure and reduce discomfort for the patient.
5 At the end of the procedure clamp the drainage tube and leave for the desired period.	To prevent back-flow of the drug.

Rotation of the patient

Action	Rationale
1 Assess the clinical status of the patient and ability to tolerate the desired rotation.	To prevent undue discomfort the patient may feel and to ensure that the doctor is informed of the patient's inability to comply.

Guidelines: Administration of intrapleural drugs (cont'd)

Action	Rationale
2 Turn the patient in the following rotation: (a) Left side. (b) Supine. (c) Right side. (d) Prone.	To ensure that the drug coats and washes the pleural cavity completely
3 Carry out the rotations as instructed. Examples are as follows: (a) Five minutes in each position, repeated once, equals 40 minutes. (b) Thirty minutes in each position, repeated once, equals 4 hours. (c) One hour in each position equals 4 hours.	As above.
4 Observe regularly for patient comfort. Administer analgesic as required.	To keep the patient comfortable and free from pain.
5 Record the patient's respirations and colour every 15 minutes for one hour, then every hour until stable, then 4-hourly, or as frequently as the patient's condition dictates. Record temperature 4-hourly.	To ensure there is no change in respiratory function following the procedure. To observe for pyrexia, a common side-effect that may indicate a developing infection or a reaction to chemotherapy.

Drainage of thoracotomy tube

Action	Rationale
1 Ensure the patient is in a comfortable position, and is aware of any limitations about movement.	To prevent discomfort or dislodgement of the drainage tube.
2 Unclamp the chest tube.	To allow drainage of the drug instilled.
3 Maintain the underwater seal until a volume of less than 50 ml is drained during 24 hours for 2 consecutive days or for a maximum of 7 days, or in consultation with medical staff.	To allow complete drainage of the drug instilled, and any additional fluid.
4 Record the colour and amount of fluid drained on the appropriate documents.	To monitor the immediate effectiveness of therapy.

NURSING CARE PLAN

Problem	Cause	Suggested action
Local or systemic effects associated with specific cytotoxic drugs, e.g. rigors due to bleomycin.	Absorption of the drug into circulation in sufficient quantities to cause toxicity.	Be aware that this can occur. Initiate preventive action, e.g. corticosteroid cover to prevent rigors, or observe for a reaction and treat symptomatically.

INTRAVESICAL INSTILLATION

Definition
The instillation of chemotherapeutic agents directly into the bladder, via a urinary catheter.

Indications
This therapy has been shown to be effective in the treatment of superficial papillary carcinoma of the bladder.

REFERENCE MATERIAL
Systemic chemotherapy has repeatedly produced disappointing results in bladder carcinoma although some recent combined modality studies have produced improved response rates. However, instillation of cytotoxic agents into the bladder via a urinary catheter has been used for many years in selected cases and has proven to be an effective and simple method of controlling superficial bladder cancer (Reymann, 1993).

A high concentration of drug bathes the endothelium. Local toxicity is not a major problem, being mainly confined to burning on urination, and there are minimal general side-effects.

The use of this method of therapy is limited to two clinical situations:

(1) Small, multiple, superficial, well differentiated, non-invasive papillomatous carcinomas.
(2) Prophylaxis, to minimize recurrence in patients with a history of multiple tumours known readily to seed locally.

Treatment protocols vary. Contact time with the bladder endothelium is 1 hour and therapy may be repeated on alternating days for three doses or weekly for varying lengths of time.

In measurable disease, however, response rates are similar with an average of 60% effectiveness. Approximately 30% of patients experience a complete response .

Cytotoxic drugs used are:

(1) Thiotepa.
(2) Mitomycin C.
(3) Doxorubicin.

A paper (Garnick *et al.*, 1987) has questioned the criteria on which efficacy of treatment is based and has suggested that the primary measure of success should be the development or not of invasive bladder carcinoma.

References and further reading
Carter, S. K. & Wasserman, T. H. (1975) The chemotherapy of urologic cancer. *Cancer*, 36, 729–47.

Dorr, R. T. & Fritz, W. L. (1980) *Cancer Chemotherapy Handbook*. Kimpton, London.

Garnick, M. B. *et al.* (1987) A determination of appropriate endpoints in assessing efficacy of intravesical therapies in superficial bladder cancer. In: *Proceedings of the American Society of Clinical Oncology*, Abstract No 412.

Manual of Cancer Chemotherapy (1981) *UICC Technical Reports* 56, pp. 223–4.

Reymann, P. E. (1993) *Chemotherapy: Principles of Administration in Cancer Nursing. Principles and Practice*, (eds S. L. Groenwald, M. Goodman, M. H. Frogge & C. H. Yarbro), 3rd edn, Chapter 15. Jones & Bartlett Publishers, Boston.

Swittes, D. D., Soares, S. E. & White, R. W. (1992) Nursing care of the patient receiving intravesical chemotherapy. *Urological Nurse*, 12(4), 136–9.

GUIDELINES: INTRAVESICAL INSTILLATION OF CYTOTOXIC DRUGS

Other relevant procedures are urinary catheterization (see Chapter 45) and bladder lavage and irrigation (see Chapter 6). Details of required procedure and problems which may be encountered are given in these chapters. The following guidelines and care plan deal with specific aspects of chemotherapy administration.

EQUIPMENT

1 Urotainer containing prescribed drug in clinically clean tray (delivered from pharmacy reconstitution unit).
2 Sterile, latex gloves.
3 Disposable apron and eye protection.
4 Gate clip or equivalent clamp for catheter.
5 Catheter drainage bag, if catheter is to remain in position.
6 10 or 20 ml sterile syringe.
7 Small dressing pack, containing sterile field.

Guidelines: Intravesical instillation of cytotoxic drugs (cont'd)

PROCEDURE

Action	Rationale
1 Explain and discuss the procedure with the patient.	To ensure that the patient understands the procedure and gives his/her valid consent.
2 Check the patient's full blood count, as instructed by the medical staff, and inform them of any deficit before administration.	Absorption of the drug through the bladder wall may cause some myelosuppression. However, there are differing opinions as to whether regular checks are necessary.
3 Check all the details on the container of cytotoxic drug against the patient's prescription chart.	To minimize the risk of error and comply with legal requirements.
4 Assemble all necessary equipment, including the cytotoxic drug container, and proceed to the patient.	To ensure that the instillation proceeds smoothly and without interruption.
5 Screen the patient's bed/couch.	To ensure privacy during the procedure.
6 Check that the patient's identity matches the patient's details on the prescription chart.	To ensure that the correct patient has been identified. To reduce the risk of error.
7 Ask the patient to empty bladder.	To enable the instillation of the drug.
8 Ensure the bladder is empty of urine.	To prevent dilution of the drug.
9 Put on an apron/eye protection.	To protect the nurse from contact with the cytotoxic drugs. With correct technique the risk of contamination is minimal, but splashes can occur.
10 If the catheter is already in place, using aseptic technique and sterile latex gloves, proceed to place sterile towel under the end of the catheter, clamp the catheter and disconnect the drainage bag.	To protect the patient from infection. To protect the nurse from drug spillage. To gain access to the catheter. To prevent urine from soiling the bed.
11 Remove the cover from the urotainer, connect to the catheter and release the clamp.	To facilitate drug instillation.
12 Gently squeeze the urotainer to administer the cytotoxic agent. Do not use force.	Rapid instillation would be uncomfortable for the patient, especially if the bladder is small or scarred from previous treatment or disease.
13 When the correct volume has been instilled, clamp the catheter	To prevent drainage of drug from the bladder.
14 (a) If the catheter is to stay in position, connect the catheter to a new drainage bag but do not unclamp it. (b) If the catheter is to be removed, withdraw the water from the catheter balloon using the sterile syringe and remove the catheter using gentle traction. Dispose of equipment into yellow clinical waste bag and seal.	To create a closed system, reducing the risk of bacterial contamination, and to retain the drug in the bladder. The catheter may not be required for continued urinary drainage, and may have been inserted to facilitate drug administration, particularly in the outpatient department. The risk of infection is greater if the catheter remains *in situ*.

| 15 | Make the patient comfortable and instruct him/her about changes of position required during the time the drug is *in situ*. | Frequent changes in position ensure the drug bathes all of the bladder mucosa. |

15 Make the patient comfortable and instruct him/her about changes of position required during the time the drug is *in situ*.

Frequent changes in position ensure the drug bathes all of the bladder mucosa.

16 If the patient is unable to turn himself/herself, nursing assistance must be provided.

As above.

17 Provide outpatients with information about the amount of movement required.

Following outpatient instillation, the journey home is usually sufficient to coat the bladder mucosa.

18 When the drug has been in the bladder for one hour, request the patient to micturate

or

release the clamp on the catheter to allow the drug and urine to drain into the bag.

One hour is the usual time specified for intravesical drugs to ensure the maximum therapeutic effect with minimum toxicity.

19 Advise the patient on fluid intake, suggesting ways in which he or she may increase it in the following 24-hour period. Patients should be aware that their urine may be cloudy.

To provide a good fluid output, washing out the bladder and reducing the likelihood of local irritation or difficulty in urination due to débris from the tumour.

20 Instruct the patient to report any discomfort or inability to pass urine immediately to ward staff or general practitioner/district nurse, or to telephone the hospital if anxious.

To detect any problems at the earliest moment. To reduce anxiety experienced by the patient.

NURSING CARE PLAN

Problem	Cause	Suggested action
No drainage of urine when the catheter is inserted.	Bladder is empty or the catheter is in the wrong place, e.g. in the urethra or in a false track. False tracks may develop after repeated cystoscopy or bladder surgery.	Do not inflate the balloon but tape the catheter to the skin to keep it in position. Check when the patient last micturated. Encourage the patient to drink a few glasses of fluid. Do not give the drug until urine flow is seen or correct positioning of the catheter is established. Inform a doctor if no urine has drained during the next 30 minutes.
Haematuria.	Trauma of catheterization or loosening of blood clots following cystoscopy by fluid injected into the bladder.	Inform a doctor. Observe the patient for signs of clot retention, shock, haemorrhage or fluid retention. Encourage the patient to drink fluids.
Leakage from around the catheter following administration of the drug.	Catheter slipping out of the bladder or bladder spasm caused by the drug.	Check the position of the catheter. Inform a doctor if leakage persists. Protect the patient's skin by wrapping sterile topical swabs around the catheter. Estimate the volume lost by leakage. Wash contaminated skin thoroughly.

Nursing care plan (cont'd)

Problem	Cause	Suggested action
Patient unable to retain the requisite drug volume in the bladder for the time required.	Low bladder capacity; weak sphincter muscles; unstable detrusor muscle causing uncontrolled bladder contractions.	Note actual duration of the drug in the bladder and inform a doctor.
Patient has pain during instillation of the drug or while the drug is in the bladder.	Following resection of mucosa, the bladder can become acutely sensitive to irritants, thus causing painful spasm resulting in possible expelling of the cytotoxic agent.	Allow the drug to drain out and/or stop instillation if the pain is severe. Inform a doctor. Administer Entonox if appropriate (see Chapter 17, Entonox Administration) and have analgesics prescribed for subsequent administration.
Patient unable to pass urine after the drug has been *in situ* for the required length of time.	Anxiety; poor bladder tone; prostatism.	Reassure the patient. Encourage the patient to drink fluids.
Urine does not drain from the catheter when the clamp is released.	Catheter wrongly placed. Catheter blocked with clots and/or debris.	Check the position of the catheter. Perform bladder lavage.

INTRA-ARTERIAL CHEMOTHERAPY

Definition

Delivery of a high concentration of cytotoxic drug to the tumour site by catheterization of the artery providing the blood supply to the affected organ.

Drugs may be administered by slow push injection or infusion, the latter being most common. Frequency of administration is determined by the doctor.

REFERENCE MATERIAL

Indications

Intra-arterial chemotherapy has been used to treat a variety of malignancies at a number of different sites during the past 20 years. These include:

- Head and neck lesions.
- Liver metastases from colorectal cancer.
- Sarcomas/melanomas of upper and lower limb (including isolated limb perfusion).
- Carcinoma of the stomach.
- Carcinoma of the breast.
- Carcinoma of the cervix.

Intra-arterial chemotherapy is possible when the regional artery can be easily isolated and catheterized.

Confirmation that the artery supplies the desired area can be achieved by installation of yellow fluorescence dye if the tumour site is visible, or contrast medium if an internal organ such as the liver is the target area.

Once the catheter is in place and secured, cytotoxic drugs may be administered by:

(1) Injection, using a syringe.
(2) Small volume infusion using a syringe pump.
(3) Large volume infusion using a volumetric pump.

Other variations on the delivery system include the implantable drug delivery system.

All delivery systems must be under pressure to combat arterial pressure, i.e. 300 mmHg. The majority of infusion pumps meet this requirement (Plumer, 1993).

The cytotoxic drugs used vary with the histology and site of the tumour. The following have all been used for intra-arterial administration:

actinomycin D	5-FUDR (floxuridine)
BCNU (carmustine)	methotrexate
bleomycin	melphalan
cisplatin	mitomycin C
doxorubicin	vincristine
5-FU (5-fluorouracil)	

A high concentration of drug can be delivered to the primary or secondary tumour mass. A reduction in systemic circulating levels of drugs has been shown to occur in many circumstances resulting in a corresponding reduction in side-effects to the patient, although this is difficult to predict (Reymann, 1993).

Principles of nursing care

Insertion is an operative procedure and consent must be obtained. Adequate explanation to the patient is essential, especially what to expect on return to the ward.

The area: to be shaved or otherwise prepared and the period of fasting should be checked with the anaesthetist.

The catheter is inserted in theatre or in the X-ray department and its position checked at that time. The catheter will be secured and an occlusive dressing applied. This should *not* be touched as it is essential that the catheter is *not* displaced.

A three- or one-way tap is connected to the catheter and it is at this point that all manipulations take place. An extension set should be connected to this at the time of insertion or on return to the ward to prevent unnecessary handling near the skin exit site.

The system will consist of: catheter/tap/extension set/administration set or infusion device.

Certain general rules apply:

(1) The dressing must not be touched but should be observed regularly for signs of bleeding. This should be reported immediately to the medical staff, including the radiologist.
(2) All procedures or manipulations associated with the pathway must use aseptic technique.
(3) All connections must be Luer locking to prevent exsanguination/air embolism or disconnection under pressure.
(4) The line must be clamped securely or switched off using the tap *in situ* before any equipment changes.
(5) Positive pressure, greater than arterial pressure, must be maintained at all times.
(6) When chemotherapy is not being infused, the flushing solution must be used to maintain patency. This should be via a syringe/syringe pump during transfer between wards or departments, or via a syringe pump/infusion pump in the ward. A nurse escort may be necessary for transfers. It should be delivered at the minimum rate sufficient to combat arterial pressure and maintain patency, approximately 3–5 ml per hour or 10 drops per minute, dependent on the device used (Plumer, 1993). If a special delivery system is used, then manufacturers' instructions should be followed.
(7) The patient must be instructed on the amount of mobility allowed. This may vary depending on the site of the catheter. Assistance may be needed to maintain personal hygiene and relieve pressure.

Aids may be required to prevent the development of pressure ulcers on all points of contact.

(8) The position of the catheter may be checked daily by X-ray, which will be performed on the ward. Fluoroscopy and installation of dye are other methods of confirming position.
(9) At the end of treatment, the patency of the arterial line should be maintained using an appropriate flushing solution until a decision has been made about removal. Instructions for this and the amount of heparin to be used should be prescribed in advance to enable the nurse to initiate the procedure when appropriate.
(10) Before removal, the tap may be switched off and the catheter allowed to clot. The catheter should be removed by a doctor and firm pressure applied for at least five minutes or until all bleeding has ceased. A dressing should be applied to the site. Pressure dressings are not indicated if bleeding has ceased and can obscure the formation of a haematoma.

Any problems should be referred to the medical staff (Consertino, 1987).

Conclusion

The administration of intra-arterial chemotherapy is an infrequent occurrence but it has been used to achieve significant reductions in tumour size and improved survival. A decrease in systemic circulating levels of drugs and a lessening of side-effects to patients has been shown, although this is variable.

Do not hesitate to contact a radiologist if a problem is suspected as he/she is the expert in catheter placement and management of complications.

References and further reading

Bedford, R. F. (1978) Percutaneous radial artery cannulation. *Surgical News*, no. 4.
Consertino, F. (1987) Chapter 23. *Principles and Practice of Intravenous Therapy*, (eds A. Plumer & F. Consertino), 4th edn, pp. 477–504. Little, Brown & Co, Boston, USA.
Dorr, R. T. & Fritz, W. L. (1980) *Cancer Chemotherapy Handbook*. Kimpton, London.
Gilbertson, A. A. (1984) *Intravenous Technique and Therapy*. Heinemann, London.
Reymann, P. E. (1993) *Chemotherapy: Principles of Administration in Cancer Nursing. Principles and Practice*, (eds S. L. Groenwald, M. Goodman, M. H. Frogge & C. H. Yarbro), 3rd edn, Chapter 15. Jones & Bartlett Publishers, Boston.
von Roemeling, R. *et al.* (1986) Chemotherapy via implanted infusion pump. New perspectives for delivery of long-term continuous treatment. *Oncology Nursing Forum*, 13, 17–24.
Taylor, I. (1985) Hepatic arterial infusion of anti-cancer drugs. *Cancer Topics*, 5(5), 50–1.
Weinstein, S. M. (1993) *Plumer's Principles and Practice of Intravenous Therapy*, 5th edn. J. B. Lippincott, Philadelphia.

NURSING CARE PLAN

Problem	Action	Rationale
Haemorrhage.	Observe the dressing at regular intervals. Monitor pulse and blood pressure at least 4-hourly.	To prevent blood loss or detect haemorrhage at the earliest possible moment.
	Instruct the patient on the amount of movement permitted and to report any feeling of faintness, or oozing noted on dressing.	
	After removal of the catheter, vital signs and the dressing should be observed every 15 minutes for 2 hours. Whether the patient should remain on bedrest for 24 hours is dependent on the site that the patient has been catheterized.	
	If bleeding occurs, pressure should be applied immediately and a member of the medical staff contacted.	
Displacement of the catheter.	Do not disturb the dressing placed in the X-ray department.	To prevent displacement or detect it as early as possible, so reducing the likelihood of extravasation of drugs (see Guidelines: Management of extravasation, above).
	Instruct the patient on amount of movement permitted.	
	Check position daily, if requested by the doctor.	
Arterial occlusion.	Check vessel patency daily, if instructed to do so by medical staff. This may be done using a Doppler flowmeter or by manual location of distal pulses.	To prevent this occurring and ensure continued delivery of therapy to the patient.
	Report any abnormality to the doctor or radiologist.	
Infection.	Strict asepsis must be maintained for all procedures and manipulations of the arterial line.	To prevent both localized infection and septicaemia.
	Temperature must be taken every four hours and any pyrexia investigated.	To observe for pyrexia as it may indicate a developing infection.
Exsanguination/air embolism.	Luer-lock connections must be used throughout the pathway. These should be checked at regular intervals, and continuous flow maintained. Care must be	To prevent a major blood loss progressing to shock. To prevent an air embolus, although this is less likely.

Problem	Action	Rationale
	taken when changing equipment to prevent blood loss occurring or air entering the line, e.g. shut off tap, firm clamping, if necessary.	
	Care must be taken when injecting medications, as above.	
	The seriousness of an air embolus depends on the siting of the arterial line and whether it is a direct route to the carotid artery and so to the brain.	
Thrombosis/emboli.	The literature indicates that thrombosis occurs in over 40% of arteries catheterized for over 48 hours. However, this is dependent on the vessel used. Most used for chemotherapy delivery pose no problem and will remain patent for the treatment period. However, a resulting thrombus may embolize causing vascular insufficiency, distal or central embolism.	To detect this problem at the earliest possible moment, so preventing reduced blood flow to the limb or organ.
	When occlusion occurs due to thrombus formation or spasm, blood flow is usually maintained by collaterals until the vessel recovers.	
	Presence of a pulse and the colour of the area should be checked daily or a Doppler flowmeter may be used.	
	Any abnormality should be reported to the medical staff and radiologist.	
	The catheter should be removed by the doctor using firm, steady traction, in an attempt to prevent dislodging any thrombus present.	
	The condition of the patient and the limb/area should be observed carefully at the time that vital signs are measured.	
Damage to the artery, arteriovenous fistula, aneurysm formation.	The incidence of these is low and the likelihood of them occurring can be minimized by gentle handling of the catheter	To reduce the incidence of these complications, however rare, and to ensure that the medical staff are notified immediately.

Nursing care plan (cont'd)

Problem	Action	Rationale
	and immobilization of the limb/area as soon as appropriate.	
Extravasation of drugs/failure of drug to reach target area.	Both of these are very rare but can lead to significant morbidity. The incidence can be reduced by careful placement of the catheter and verification by X-ray or installation of dye.	As above.
	If there is any doubt concerning the placement of the catheter the doctor and radiologist should be notified, as extravasation of the drug may lead to ulceration and necrosis.	
Chemical hepatitis/bilary sclerosis.	The occurrence of these will be evident from elevated liver enzymes. Therefore, monitoring of liver function tests is important. Any elevation is usually transient.	To be aware that this may occur and of the significance.

CHAPTER 14

Discharge Planning

Definition

Discharge planning is the plan evolved before a patient is transferred from one environment to another (Jupp & Simms, 1986). It is a complex process which cannot be examined in isolation from what has occurred before or separated from the consequences that follow (Armitage, 1990).

The process can begin either in pre-admission clinics for pre-booked admissions, or on admission. It comprises an individualized assessment encompassing physical, psychological, social and economic needs, thereby promoting continuity and coordination of health care throughout admission and discharge. It involves not only patients, but also families, friends, the hospital, the multidisciplinary team and the community health care teams.

REFERENCE MATERIAL

Healthy individuals have sufficient self-care abilities to be able to meet their fundamental self-care needs. Individuals who experience illness or injury are subject to additional needs. They may be able to meet those needs with nursing assistance or may require a nurse to meet their needs for them until they are capable of resuming that self-care. In certain circumstances their needs may fluctuate due to their disease process and so self-care may not be a realistic goal. Discharge planning is therefore a vital procedure to assist these individuals who are in need of help to maintain their self-care or to help them with their care needs when they leave one care environment for another.

Despite well documented concern about the quality of procedures for the discharge of patients from hospital, shortcomings persist (Altschul, 1984; Jones, 1984; Armitage, 1985; Saddington, 1985; Jackson, 1990; Marks, 1994). Primary care teams often receive little or no notice that patients are being discharged, and patients and their carers may receive little or no information (Hurley & Chapman, 1991; Young et al., 1991; Marks, 1994).

The chronic nature of some cancers, coupled with episodes of acute life-threatening illness, due to complex treatments and the disease's natural process, can profoundly affect patients' and families' quality of life (Giacquinta, 1977; Sque, 1985). Ineffective discharge planning has been shown to have detrimental effects on patients' and families' psychological and physical well-being (Edstrom & Miller, 1981; Wingate & Lackey, 1989) and the days following discharge are recognized as a period of great vulnerability and anxiety (Waters, 1987). Planning care, providing adequate information and involving patients and families keep disruption and distress to a minimum (Oberst & Scott, 1988).

Inadequate communication networks and a lack of interpersonal cooperation between hospital and community have been identified as contributing to problems with discharge (Skeet, 1970; Armitage, 1990; Williams & Fitton, 1991; Curran et al., 1992; Meara et al., 1992; Closs & Tierney, 1993). With the discharge process spanning organizational and professional boundaries, what is required is effective communication (Bowling & Betts, 1984a,b; Ncill & Williams, 1992) and more multidisciplinary and joint approaches to planning. Invitations to community nurses (Guerrero, 1990) and local authority home care managers to participate in the discharge process facilitate closer links between care environments and promote continuity of care for patients (McMahon, 1988) and also ensure that services commence on discharge and that there are no delays in service contact (Victor & Vetter, 1988; Harding & Modell, 1989; Leigh-Smith et al., 1991; Closs & Tierney, 1993).

The role of hospital nurses in assessing and planning for discharge is vital. Kerston & Hackeniz (1991) commented that hospital nurses see their activities as ending formally at the hospital door, and do not necessarily appreciate the consequences of a hastily or badly prepared discharge. Continuous assessment of patients' needs and early liaison with the multidisciplinary team and the primary health care team are essential if appropriate care and a safe environment are to be provided in the community.

The NHS and Community Care Act 1990 has had major implications for professionals working in health and social care as well as for patients and their carers. It emphasizes the need for continuity of health and social care and promotes choice for consumers. It stresses that patients should not leave hospital until a community care package has been formulated and agreed to meet their needs. The Act also states that resources cannot be committed without prior agreement of the agencies involved. This has implications for health and social carers as it is often in the financial interests of the local authorities for patients to remain in hospital until their social care needs are reduced and it is in the hospital's interests to discharge patients early (Marks, 1994). Local agreements and contracts are therefore recommended to prevent a clash of interests between those agencies involved.

Audit and the discharge process

The Government white paper *Working for Patients* (Department of Health, 1989) defines audit as

'the systematic critical analysis of the quality of care including the procedures used for diagnosis and treatment, the use of resources and the resulting outcome and quality of life for the patient'.

Audit is therefore concerned with current practice and is central to any measures taken to improve quality of care for patients (Kinn *et al.*, 1994). However an integral part of audit is standard setting and this must be done as the initial part of the audit process. (An example of a patient's charter standard on the Discharge Procedure can be found in Appendix 1.)

The 1989 Department of Health circular (*HC(89)5*) states that it is the responsibility of health authorities in collaboration with social service departments to monitor the way in which discharges from hospitals are being undertaken and, if problems occur, to establish the reasons and to ensure that any necessary changes are made to address the local needs (Kinn *et al.*, 1994), for example, monitoring discharge failures (this information is required for most purchasers). Closs & Tierney (1993) indicate that negative outcome measures, such as readmission, morbidity and mortality rates, are not always appropriate evaluations of discharge planning, but suggest that patient/carer/professional satisfaction surveys appear to be the most useful form of obtaining audit information.

Aims of discharge planning

(1) To prepare the patient, partner and family physically and psychologically for transfer home or to an agreed environment.

(2) To facilitate a smooth transfer, by ensuring that all necessary health care facilities are prepared to receive the patient.

(3) To promote the highest possible level of independence for the patient, partner and family by encouraging self care activities.

(4) To provide continuity of care between the hospital and the agreed environment by facilitating effective communication.

Principles of good discharge planning

When planning discharges from one care environment to another certain principles should be followed. These include:

(1) Discharge procedures should be of a consistently high standard for all patients.

(2) Patients' needs should always be a priority when discharge is being planned.

(3) Patients should be discharged to a safe and adequate environment.

(4) Continuity of care between environments should be paramount.

(5) Discharge planning should commence on the initial contact with patients.

(6) Information about discharge arrangements should be disseminated between professionals and patients/carers.

(7) Patients' beliefs and culture should be considered when planning discharges.

Patients with particular care needs

All plans for patients' discharge should be of a high standard. However, particular attention should be given to:

(1) People who live alone.

(2) People who are frail and/or elderly.

(3) People whose carers may find difficulty coping.

(4) People with limited prognosis.

(5) People with serious illnesses, who may be returning to hospital for further treatments.

(6) People with continuing disability.

(7) People with learning difficulties.

(8) People with psychiatric disorders.

(9) People who have dependants.

(10) People with limited financial resources.

(11) Homeless people or those living in poor housing.

(12) People whose first language is not English.

Conclusion

From the patient's perspective, discharge remains one of the most important events of the hospital stay. The way in which the patient is transferred into the community directly influences the ability of the patient's family and friends to cope at home. It is essential, therefore, that discharge planning is considered as an integral part of the nursing and multidisciplinary process. Assessment, planning, implementation and evaluation of care from the initial contact with the patient in hospital, up to and including discharge, are essential if care is to be individualized and continuity of care achieved.

References and further reading

Altschul, A. (1984) Safe journey home. *Nursing Times*, 80(41), 18–19.

Armitage, S. (1985) Hospital to home – discharge referrals, who is responsible? *Nursing Times*, 81(8), 26–8.

Armitage, S. (1990) *Liaison and Continuity of Nursing Care. Executive Summary*. The Welsh Office, Cardiff.

Barrett, A. (1994) Collaborative care planning. *Journal of Community Nursing*, May, 9–10.

Booth, J. & Davis, C. (1991) Happy to be home? A discharge planning package for elderly people. *Professional Nurse*, March, 330–32.

Bowling, A. & Betts, G. (1984a) From hospital to home 1: communication on discharge. *Nursing Times*, 8 August, 31–3.

Bowling, A. & Betts, G. (1984b) From hospital to home 2: communication on discharge. *Nursing Times*, 15 August, 44–6.

Carlisle, D. (1993) From hospital to community. *Nursing Times*, 89(7), 37–9.

Cole, A. (1992) Confidence trick. *Social Work Today*, February, 25(5).

Closs, S. J. & Tierney, A. J. (1993) The complexities of using a structure, process and outcome framework: the case of an evaluation of discharge planning for elderly patients. *Journal of Advanced Nursing*, 18, 1279–87.

Corkery, E. (1989) Discharge planning and home care. What every staff nurse should know. *Orthopaedic Nursing*, 8(6), 18–26.

Curran, P. *et al.* (1992) Communication of discharge information for elderly patients in hospital. *Ulster Medical Journal*, 61(1), 56–8.

Department of Health (1989a) *Health Circular HC (89) 5. Discharge of Patients from Hospital*. HMSO, London.

Department of Health (1989b) *Working for Patients*. HMSO, London.

Department of Health (1990a) *NHS and Community Care Act*. HMSO, London.

Department of Health (1990b) *Community Care in the Next Decade and Beyond; Policy Guidance*. HMSO, London.

Department of Health (1994) *The Hospital Discharge Workbook. A Manual on Hospital Discharge Practice*. The Health Publication Unit, Heywood.

Downey, R. (1994) Community chaos. *Nursing Times*, 90(14), 21.

Edstrom, S. & Miller, M. (1981) Preparing the family to care for the cancer patient at home – a home care course. *Cancer Nursing*, 5(2), 49–52.

Edwards, O. (1991) Discharge home. *Journal of District Nursing*, August, 4–7.

Giacquinta, B. (1977) Helping families to face the crisis of cancer. *American Journal of Nursing*, 77(10), 1585–8.

Guerrero, D. (1990) Working towards a partnership. *Community Outlook*, September, 14–18.

Handcock, M. & Knight, D. (1992) Improving discharge planning standards. *Nursing Standard*, 6(21), 29–31.

Harding, J. & Modell, M. (1989) Elderly peoples' experiences of discharge from hospital. *Journal of the Royal College of General Practitioners*, 39, 17–20.

Henwood, M. (1994) Hospital discharge. *Health Service Journal*, March, 22–4.

Henwood, M. & Wistow, G. (1994) *Hospital Discharge and Community Care – Early Days*. NHS Management Executive, Nuffield Institute for Health and Community Care Division. HMSO, London.

Hurley, D. & Chapman, J. (1991) Coming or going. Discharge of elderly patients from Northwick Park Hospital. Quality improvement project. Northwick Park Hospital, London. In: *Seamless or Patchwork Quilt? Discharging Patients from Acute Hospital Care*, (L. Marks, *Research Report 17*, 1994). The King's Fund Institute, The King's Fund Centre, London.

Ingleton, C. & Faulknor, A. (1995) Quality assurance in palliative care: some of the problems. *European Journal of Cancer Care*, 4, 38–44.

Jackson, M. F. (1990) Use of community support services by elderly patients discharged from general medical and geriatric medical wards. *Journal of Advanced Nursing*, 15, 167–75.

Jones, I. H. (1984) Cause for complaint 2: lack of communication. *Nursing Times*, 80(32), 51–2.

Jupp, M. & Simms, S. (1986) Going home. *Nursing Times*, 82(33), 40–42.

Kersten, D. & Hackeniz, E. (1991) How to bridge the gap between hospital and home. *Journal of Advanced Nursing*, 16, 4–14.

King, C. & Macmillan, M. (1994) Documentation and discharge planning for elderly patients. *Nursing Times*, 90(20), 31–4.

Kinn, S. *et al.* (1994) *The Nursing Audit Handbook*. The University of Glasgow.

Leigh-Smith, J. *et al.* (1991) Discharged well? Bath CHC Research Project. In: *Seamless or Patchwork Quilt? Discharging Patients from Acute Hospital Care*, (L. Marks, *Research Report 17*, 1994). The King's Fund Institute, The King's Fund Centre, London.

McMahon, R. (1988) Home truths. *Geriatric Nursing and Home Care*, 8(9), 16–17.

Mamon, J. *et al.* (1992) Impact of hospital discharge planning on meeting the patients' needs after returning home. *Health Service Research*, 27(2), 155–75.

Marks, L. (1994) *Seamless or Patchwork Quilt? Discharging Patients from Acute Hospital Care. Research Report 17*. The Kings Fund Institute, The Kings Fund Centre, London.

Meara, J. R. *et al.* (1992) Home from hospital: a survey of hospital discharge arrangements in Northamptonshire. *Journal of Public Health Medicine*, 14(2), 145–50.

National Council for Hospice and Specialist Palliative Care Services (1993) *Care in the Community for People who are Terminally Ill. Guidelines for Health Authorities and Social Services Department*. National Council for Hospice and Specialist Palliative Care Services, London.

Naylor, M. D. (1990a) Comprehensive discharge planning for the elderly. *Research in Nursing and Health*, 13, 327–48.

Naylor, M. D. (1990b) Comprehensive discharge planning for the hospitalised elderly – a pilot study. *Nursing Research*, 39(3), 156–61.

Neill, J. & Williams, J. (1992) Leaving hospital – elderly people and their discharge to community care. Research Unit, National Institute for Social Work, London. In: *Seamless or Patchwork Quilt? Discharging Patients from Acute Hospital Care*, (L. Marks, *Research Report 17*, 1994). The King's Fund Institute, The King's Fund Centre, London.

Oberst, M. T. & Scott, D. W. (1988) Post discharge distress in surgically treated cancer patients and their spouses. *Research in Nursing and Health*, 11, 223–33.

Pearson, A. & Vaughan, B. (1989) *Nursing Models for Practice*. Heinemann, Oxford.

Royal College of Nursing (1992) *Good Practice in Early Discharge*. Royal College of Nursing, London.

Saddington, N. (1985) A communication breakdown. *Nursing Times*, 81(8), 31.

Skeet, M. (1970) *Home from Hospital. The Results of a Survey conducted among Recently Discharged Hospital Patients*. Dan Mason Nursing Research Sub-Committee of the National Florence Nightingale Memorial Committee of Great Britain and Northern Ireland. Macmillan Press, London.

Skeet, M. (1985) *Home from Hospital Providing Continuing Care for Elderly People*. In: *Seamless or Patchwork Quilt? Discharging Patients from Acute Hospital Care*, (L. Marks, *Research Report 17*, 1994). The King's Fund Institute, The King's Fund Centre, London.

Sque, M. (1985) What's in a name? *Nursing Mirror*, 160, 28–30.

Tierney, A. J. (1983) *Discharge of Patients from Hospital*. Nursing Research Unit, University of Edinburgh.

Tierney, A. J. (1993) An evaluation of hospital discharge. *Nursing Times*, 89(47), 11–12.

Tierney, A. J. *et al.* (1994) Discharge of patients from hospital – current practice and perceptions of hospital and community staff in Scotland. *Health Bulletin*, 52(6), 498–510.

United Kingdom Central Council for Nursing, Midwifery and Health Visiting. *Annexe One to Registrar's Letter (18/1995) Discharge of Patients from Hospital*. UKCC, London.

Victor, C. & Vetter, N. J. (1988) Preparing the elderly for discharge from hospital – a neglected aspect of neglected care. *Age and Ageing*, 17, 155–63.

Victor, C. & Vetter, N. J. (1989) Measuring outcomes after discharge from hospital for the elderly – a conceptual and emperical investigation. *Archives of Gerontology and Geriatrics*, 8, 87–94.

Waters, K. R. (1987) Discharge planning – an exploratory study of the process of discharge planning on geriatric wards. *Journal of Advanced Nursing*, 12, 71–83.

Williams, E. I. & Fitton, F. (1991) Use of nursing and social services by elderly patients discharged from hospital. *British Journal of General Practice*, 41, 72–5.

Wingate, A. L. & Lackey, N. R. (1989) A description of the needs of non-institutionalised cancer patients and their primary care givers. *Cancer Nursing*, 12(4), 216–25.

Young, E. *et al.* (1991) Older people at the interface. A study of the provision of services for older people within Parkside Health Authority. Occasional paper number 10. The Helen Hamlyn Research Unit, Department of General Practice, St Mary's Hospital Medical School, London. In: *Seamless or Patchwork Quilt? Discharging Patients from Acute Hospital Care*, (L. Marks, *Research Report 17*, 1994). The King's Fund Institute, The King's Fund Centre, London.

GUIDELINES: DISCHARGE PLANNING

PROCEDURE

Action	Rationale
1 The admitting nurse is responsible for ensuring that an initial assessment is completed when the patient is admitted and is documented in the multidisciplinary care plan. An expected date of discharge should be established.	To enable the physical, psychological and social care needs of the patient and carers to be identified at an early stage and planning for discharge to commence. To determine whether the patient will require community health service support and/or local authority service support on discharge.
2 Referrals should be made by the ward based nurse as appropriate to other members of the multidisciplinary team, e.g. physiotherapist, occupational therapist, as soon as possible after admission.	To give time for assessments to be completed and community services to be arranged in order to prevent discharge delays.

Patients identified as requiring local authority service support are referred to the Social Services department. Some NHS Trusts are using a 'trigger' form as an aid to assessment, an example of which can be found in Appendix 2.

To ensure early referral to the Social Services department for assessment.

3 A discharge planning 'area of care' should be commenced in the care plan: all members of the multidisciplinary team should document in the care plan their assessment, plans and action taken.

To facilitate multidisciplinary planning, coordination and communication.

4 Where there is a designated community liaison nurse/advisor, she/he can act as a resource offering support and education to the ward team in the preparation of discharge plans, especially for those patients requiring a complex package of care. An example of referral criteria is given in Appendix 3.

To facilitate effective discharge planning.

5 Ensure that the home address and telephone number of the patient are documented accurately in the care plan. Establish where the patient will be going on discharge and document the discharge address if different from the permanent address.

Personal information may not have been updated on previous nursing or medical records. It is crucial that this information is accurate when making referrals to community services.

6 Ensure that the patient is registered with a permanent general practitioner (GP) and with a GP on a temporary basis if going to a different address on discharge. Check the names, addresses and telephone numbers with the patient and document accurately.

Community nursing services may not wish to accept the patient without medical support. Accurate information is required to establish which district nurse will have responsibility for patient care. It is important for the patient that medical care can be provided at home.

7 Establish whether any statutory community health or Social Services have been involved before the patient's admission. Document names and telephone numbers. Include the health visitor when the patient has children under the age of 5 years.

To enable contact for exchange of information. Valuable information can be obtained from community services to assist in assessing potential needs on discharge.

Ensure that all services visiting the patient at home are informed of the patient's admission.

To prevent anxiety and wasted time for community services in trying to locate the client.

8 Check whether the patient has dependants, e.g. elderly relatives, children or a disabled or unwell partner. If so, establish who is looking after them and whether they are receiving any services.

Arrangements may need to be made for alternative care or an increase in services.

9 Establish who are the main care givers and sources of support for the patient and the degree of contact and care they are able to provide, e.g. partner, relatives, friends. Document appropriate names, addresses and telephone numbers and their relationship to the patient.

To assess the support that the patient and carers may require at home so that appropriate services can be mobilized.

10 Establish who else is involved in giving care/ support and the type of help given, e.g. local support group, voluntary agency, church.

To establish social network in order to coordinate care between voluntary and statutory agencies.

Guidelines: Discharge planning (cont'd)

Action

Rationale

11 Ascertain the type of accommodation the patient is living in, e.g. residential or nursing home, sheltered housing, private or local authority house, flat or bungalow.

To identify early potential housing problems which may entail social work intervention.

Document the names and telephone numbers of sheltered housing wardens or officers in charge of homes.

To enable contact to be made to establish that an appropriate degree of care and support can continue to be provided.

12 Assess the patient's ability to carry out activities of daily living at home prior to admission, e.g. was he/she able to climb stairs? Consider whether he/she is likely to experience difficulties as a result of treatment and current symptoms.

To establish at an early stage whether an occupational therapy assessment is required.

13 Refer to other hospital personnel as soon as potential need is recognized, e.g. occupational therapist, physiotherapist, dietitian. Referral as soon as possible after admission is essential – do not wait until treatment is completed and discharge is imminent.

To ensure multidisciplinary planning and coordination. Considerable time may be needed to arrange community services.

14 Formulate a discharge plan in conjunction with patient and carers and all involved hospital and community personnel and set discharge date.

To collate information and coordinate planning.

For complex discharges a discharge planning meeting should be held. Document planned action resulting from meeting.

15 The ward based nurse is responsible for arranging and coordinating community nursing services (including Macmillan and hospice home care) in consultation with the community liaison nurse if applicable.

To facilitate continuity of care between hospital and community.

16 Refer to the community nursing services with a minimum of 48 hours notice. If a complex package of care is being organized more notice will be required. Invite community nurses to visit the ward where appropriate.

Community nurses may wish to assess the patient's nursing care needs and ensure preparation of the home prior to discharge. They need time to liaise with other agencies to coordinate care and to obtain any equipment required.

17 Ascertain whether district nurses are able to carry out necessary clinical procedures in accordance with their health authority policy, e.g. care of skin-tunnelled catheters.

District nurses may not have been trained in certain procedures or may be unfamiliar with particular equipment.

Consider alternative arrangement if necessary. Give written information and instructions.

18 Complete the community care referral form. Allow time to complete it fully and accurately.

The district nurse requires full knowledge of the patient's history and nursing requirements. The

Action	Rationale
The form should be completed and signed by the same person. Provide a copy for the Macmillan/hospice home care team.	form may be inaccurate if insufficient time is allowed to complete it.
19 Ensure any essential medical/nursing aids or equipment have been obtained before discharge, e.g. oxygen, commode.	Some equipment may not be available or may take a long time to obtain. The patient may be at risk at home or suffer unnecessary discomfort and distress.
20 Patients requiring community nursing, physiotherapy, occupational therapy, stoma care, speech therapy and/or dietetic support on discharge will be referred by the appropriate hospital based health care professional to their equivalent in the community.	To ensure continuity of specialist care.
The ward based nurse should liaise with the appropriate disciplines regarding the arrangements that have been made for follow up in the community and the supply of appropriate equipment.	
21 Medical staff are responsible for assessing the patient's medical fitness for discharge and for liaising with other members of the multidisciplinary team regarding arrangements for meeting the patient's care needs in the community.	To ensure that both health and social care needs are taken into consideration when formulating discharge plans.
22 Ensure that medical staff have contacted the general practitioner by telephone when medical back-up will be required at home.	Lack of information makes it difficult for the GP to provide the medical care needed.
23 Notify the sheltered housing warden or officer in charge of the nursing/residential home of discharge date.	To ensure preparation of accommodation.
24 Ensure that patient and, with his/her agreement, carers, have full information regarding the patient's medical condition and care required.	To prepare carers and to enable patient and carers to support each other.
25 Teach the patient and carers any necessary skills, allowing sufficient time to practise before discharge.	To enable the patient to be as independent as possible and promote an understanding of self-care techniques.
26 Inform the patient and carers of potential side effects of treatment and management.	To alleviate anxiety and to promote patient comfort and knowledge.
27 Ensure that patient and carers have information on local support groups or national specialist organizations as appropriate.	Some patients benefit from the kind of support offered by these organizations.
28 Reinforce any special instructions with written information or by giving an approved education booklet.	To promote an understanding of disease and treatment.
29 Information on community services arranged, including names and telephone numbers and	To confirm arrangements made. To enable the patient to contact the appropriate services.

Guidelines: Discharge planning (cont'd)

Action	Rationale
expected date of first visit, should be given to the patient and carers prior to discharge. This information should also be documented in the patient's care plan.	
The social worker informs the patient and carers of local authority arrangements upon discharge, provides them with a summary of their care plan and gives contact names, including the care manager or equivalent in the patient's local social services department.	To confirm with patient and carers arrangements made upon discharge.
30 Ensure that arrangements have been made to provide patient with food at home on discharge and that there will be adequate heating.	To supply immediate needs.
31 Ensure that the patient has door key and can gain entrance to their residence. Wherever possible, ensure that someone is at home to receive the patient.	The patient may have left their key with a neighbour. It is helpful for someone to be available to welcome patient and attend to any immediate needs.
32 Book transport if required within 48 hours' notice, using relevant form. Specify if patient needs a stretcher or chair. Ensure that transport is also booked for return clinic appointment if necessary.	The patient may not have private transport facilities and may be too weak to use public transport.
Cancel transport if discharge date or outpatients department appointment is altered.	To prevent a waste of resources.
33 Patients should be given a supply of medication and, where necessary, a supply of wound management dressings or medical equipment.	To ensure the safe and continuous administration of medication and use of equipment at home. Time is needed to obtain items in the community.
If patients are being transferred to other institutions, e.g. hospice or nursing home, a supply of medication and equipment may be required.	
There may be restrictions on the amount supplied to patients depending on local policy.	
Ensure that the patient and carers are given verbal and written information on the dosage, route, frequency and side-effects of any medication, on the use of any equipment given and how to obtain further supplies.	
Patients should have been assessed during their hospital stay for their ability to self-medicate. If they are unable to do this, alternative arrangements will need to be made, i.e. the district nurse can set up a pill dispenser and arrange with carers for the administration of medication.	

34	Book outpatients clinic appointment and give the patient an appointment card.	To ensure the patient is followed up and to minimize any difficulty in attending.

If the patient had a previous appointment booked before admission, ensure this appointment is cancelled.

If patient requires appointments at different clinics, ensure they are spaced realistically, e.g. not on consecutive days when patient may have a long way to travel.

35	Discharge plans should not be altered without consultation with all the hospital personnel who have been involved in the planning, e.g. occupational therapist, social worker, community liaison nurse.	If there is no consultation this causes considerable confusion and stress for the patient, family and friends, and all involved services. It may result in the patient being unsupported at home.

36	If discharge is cancelled or postponed or if patient dies, ensure that all relevant community services are informed.	To avoid distress to relatives. To avoid wasted visits and promote good community relations.

37	*Weekend discharge*: patients who require a high level of health services and social services support should not be discharged home on a Friday or Saturday or a public holiday. This applies particularly to patients who were previously unknown to community services.	All community services will be operating at a reduced level and emergency medical back-up may be difficult to obtain.

Note: assessment and planning for weekend leave are as important as for final discharge.

GUIDELINES: PATIENTS TAKING THEIR OWN DISCHARGE

Action

Rationale

1	The hospital social work department, community liaison team or appropriate hospital based professional should be made aware of any patients wishing to take their own discharge against the advice of their doctor, nurse or therapist.	So that appropriate professionals in the community can be alerted.

2	Patients taking their own discharge against advice who have already been identified as being in need of community health services will be seen by the relevant hospital based professional and given information about the services available on discharge following consultation with their equivalent in the community. If it is not possible to make satisfactory arrangements at short notice following discharge, the patient will be advised of the various services that may be obtained privately, an example being the services of an agency nurse. The patient's GP (or on-call equivalent) will be contacted by a member of the medical staff.	To ensure that patients have information to enable them to access services in the community.

GUIDELINES: DELAYS IN DISCHARGE ARRANGEMENTS

Action	Rationale
1 The ward based nurse will inform other members of the multidisciplinary team of any delay in the arrangements for the discharge of a patient.	To discuss and agree a strategy for action to overcome the problem and to set a further discharge date.
2 Detailed documentation pertaining to the reasons for the failure to effect discharge must be maintained.	To ensure that accurate records are maintained for auditing purposes.
3 If delays occur involving external agencies the agreed local procedure should be followed, an example of which is shown in Appendix 4.	To ensure that appropriate action is taken to avoid further delay.
4 Delays in effecting discharge for patients should be monitored monthly on each clinical unit by ward staff and returned to the quality assurance team at the end of each month. This information is now required by most purchasing authorities on a quarterly basis, an example of a discharge delay monitoring form is shown in Appendix 5.	To provide information on the reasons for the failure to discharge patients home and for auditing purposes. To enable improvements in practice.

APPENDIX 1: THE ROYAL MARSDEN NHS TRUST CHARTER STANDARD 10

Ensure that appropriate arrangements have been made in association with voluntary, community or local authority services to provide continuing care following discharge from hospital.

IMPLEMENTATION

- Hospital Policy regarding the discharge of patients to be identified – arising from DoH Circular HC(89)5.
- Patients will be discharged only when agreed by all members of the multidisciplinary team and when satisfactory community arrangements have been made.
- Provide unambiguous comprehensible information to patients and carers about discharge and courses of action.
- Patient and carer(s) to receive relevant education and support to manage any specialist equipment, techniques, etc. required for home care.
- Patients to be provided with any appropriate equipment as required for home care.

- GPs and, if appropriate, community and social services to be informed of the patients' needs on discharge.
- GPs to be notified within 24 hours when a death has occurred.
- The relevance of information in discharge summaries to be reviewed with GPs and referring medical staff.
- Develop a standard time in which discharge letters must be sent following patients' discharge.

MONITORING

Medical Audit, Nursing and Rehabilitative Therapists Audit

- Ensure protocols are established and adhered to.
- Test GPs' satisfaction with the procedures and whether protocols are adhered to.
- Check pattern of dissatisfaction and whether improvements are made.

In-patient Survey

- Test patients' understanding of the procedures and satisfaction with the working of all aspects of the arrangements.

APPENDIX 2: TRIGGERS FOR INITIAL ASSESSMENT

The aim of this form is to ensure that hospital and social services staff organize a safe and timely discharge. The issues raised under 'medical condition' warrant an immediate referral to the social services department. Issues raised under 'social network' and 'environment' require careful consideration for referral at the point of admission and/or the multidisciplinary team meetings as they crucially influence the patients' and their families' ability to cope in the future.

Name of patient . . . .   Hospital No. . . . .
Ward . . . .   Referred by . . . .
Expected date of discharge . . . .

Medical condition

(1) A significant change in ability to look after self due to the effects of treatment or the debilitating symptoms of progressive disease, warranting daily home care. ☐

(2) End stage illness where a complex package of palliative medical and nursing care as well as community care is to be provided either in the patient's own home or within a combination of home and respite hospice care. ☐

(3) When complexity of nursing needs suggests nursing home as a placement option. ☐

Social network

(4) High dependency on a carer for all or most aspects of physical care. ☐

(5) Carer shows signs of stress, or questions own ability to continue caring. ☐

(6) Patient is a primary carer with dependant partner, parent or child. ☐

Environment

(7) Basic amenities unsuitable, e.g. poor housing, inadequate access between rooms, including WC; inadequate heating, electricity, water supply. ☐

(8) High risk home environment. ☐

(9) Homelessness or threat of homelessness. ☐

Please tick the appropriate boxes and contact the hospital social services department immediately if an 'initial assessment' is indicated. Alternatively, if no risk factors have been identified upon admission, tick here: ☐

APPENDIX 3: CRITERIA FOR REFERRAL OF PATIENTS TO COMMUNITY LIAISON NURSES

The aim of this form is to ensure that nursing staff are aware that the community liaison team acts as a resource when considering a patient's needs on discharge.

Below are listed (in order of priority) the categories of patient that the community liaison team needs to be aware of.

(Community nurse = district nurse/health visitor/ Macmillan nurse/specialist nurse/community psychiatric nurse.)

(1) Patients considered to be at risk

- Patients readmitted because of inability to cope at home.
- Patients who are unable to receive adequate community nursing services because of lack of provision or expertise.
- Patients or their carers who decline appropriate referral or on-going service from community nurses.
- Patients who require constant reassessment and on-going liaison with community nurses because of problems with supervision in the community, e.g. difficulties with treatment compliance, inability to self-care, non-attendance for follow-up appointments.
- Patients with psychological/psychiatric problems who require follow-up care in the community.
- Patients who take their own discharge and require nursing care in the community.

(2) Patients in need of emotional support/information

- Patients and carers who require emotional support.
- Patients and carers who are requesting information or expressing concern about the provision of community nursing care.

(3) Patients in need of physical support and nursing care

- Patients who require a high level of community nursing input (i.e. more than two visits in any 24-hour period).
- Patients who require pain and symptom control advice.
- Patients receiving IV chemotherapy at home.
- Patients with skin-tunnelled catheters who require support from community nurses.

- Patients receiving enteral/parenteral feeding who require support from community nurses.
- Patients who require monitoring by community nurses for side-effects of drugs or therapy.
- Patients with advanced disease on research protocols who are not already under the care of community nursing services.

- Patients who require respite or day care (e.g. hospice services).
- Patients who require nursing/medical equipment where there are difficulties in provision.

Note: Patients who fulfil the criteria on the social services 'trigger' form should also be brought to the attention of the community liaison team.

APPENDIX 4: DEALING WITH DELAYS IN DISCHARGE ARRANGEMENTS INVOLVING EXTERNAL AGENCIES

PROCEDURE
(Planned discharge date = Day 0.)

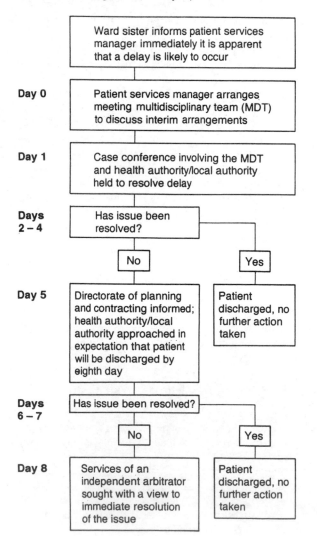

APPENDIX 5: DISCHARGE DELAY MONITORING FORM

Patient whose date for discharge was agreed by all members of the multidisciplinary team but whose discharge from The Royal Marsden NHS Trust was delayed by *one night or more.*

Name of patient . . . .
Hospital No. . . . .
Ward . . . .
Expected date of discharge . . . .
Actual date of discharge . . . .

Reason for delay . . . .
Signature . . . .

CHAPTER 15

Drug Administration

REFERENCE MATERIAL

The United Kingdom Central Council for Nursing, Midwifery and Health Visiting (UKCC) states that the administration of drugs is not a 'mechanistic task to be performed in strict compliance with the written prescription of a medical practitioner'. It is a process which requires thought and the application of professional judgement, the safety and well being of the patient being of paramount importance (UKCC, 1992a).

Whilst administering medicines the nurse must meet the requirements set out in the document *Standards for the Administration of Medicines* (UKCC, 1992a). This document provides guidance regarding the professional responsibility of the nurse involved in the administration of drugs.

Legislation

The manufacture, supply and use of medicines (and the interactive wound dressings) are controlled by two statutes, the 1968 Medicines Act and the 1971 Misuse of Drugs Act.

The Medicines Act 1968

This defines 'medicinal products' as substances sold or supplied for administration to humans (or animals) for medicinal purposes. Part 3 of the Act, and regulations and orders made under it, control the manufacture and sale or supply of medicines and for this purpose broadly classifies them into three groups:

(1) Prescription-only medicines (POM).
(2) Pharmacy medicines (P).
(3) General sales list medicines (GSL).

Different requirements apply to the sale, supply and labelling of medicines in each group. In NHS hospitals, adherence to the Act usually means that the purchasing and supply of medicines is supervised by a pharmacist, and that supply or administration to a patient is only on a doctor's prescription.

Sections 9, 10, and 11 of the Act exempt doctors, dentists, pharmacists and nurses, respectively, from many restrictions otherwise imposed by the act on the general public, and thus allow them to supply and use drugs in the practice of their respective professions.

The Misuse of Drugs Act 1971

This designates and defines as controlled drugs a number of 'dangerous or otherwise harmful' substances. These substances are all also by definition prescription-only medicines under the Medicines Act, 1968.

The controls imposed by the Misuse of Drugs Act are therefore additional to those under the Medicines Act.

The purpose of the 1971 Act is to prevent abuse of controlled drugs, most of which are potentially addictive or habit forming, by prohibiting their manufacture, sale or supply except in accordance with regulations made under the Act. Other regulations govern safe storage, destruction and supply to known addicts.

The level of control to be exercised is related to the potential for abuse or misuse of the substances concerned. Under the current (1985) regulations, controlled drugs are classified into five schedules, each representing a different level of control. The requirements of the Act as they apply to nurses working in a hospital with a pharmacy department are described in Table 15.1. Schedule 2 is the most relevant to everyday nursing practice.

Summary

Hospital wards and departments are authorized to hold a stock of controlled drugs. These are obtained by the use of a special duplicate order form signed by the nurse in charge who is then responsible for them. They should be stored in a locked cupboard used exclusively for this purpose. They may be administered only to a patient in that ward or department when prescribed by a doctor. Appropriate records of their use must be maintained. Completed registers and copies of orders should be kept for two years. Unwanted drugs should normally be destroyed in the pharmacy but may, under some circum-

Table 15.1 Summary of the legal requirements for the handling of controlled drugs as they apply to nurses in hospitals with a pharmacy.

	Schedule 1	*Schedule 2*	*Schedule 3*	*Schedule 4*	*Schedule 5*
Drugs in schedule	Cannabis + derivatives but excluding nabilone, LSD (lysergic acid diethylamide)	Most opioids in common use including: alfentanyl amphetamines cocaine diamorphine methadone morphine papaveretum fentanyl phenoperidine pethidine codeine dihydrocodeine pentazocine	Minor stimulants. Barbiturates (but excluding: hexobarbitone thiopentone methohexitone). Diethylpropion. Buprenorphine. Temazepam[7] injections only	Benzodiazepines	Some preparations containing very low strengths of: cocaine codeine morphine pholcodine and some other opioids
Ordering	Possession and supply permitted only by special licence from the Secretary of State issued (to a doctor only) for scientific or research purposes	A requisition must be signed in duplicate by the nurse in charge. The requisition must be endorsed to indicate that the drugs have been supplied. Copies should be kept for two years	As Schedule 2	No requirement[1]	No requirement[1]
Storage[5]	As Schedule 2	Must be kept in a suitable locked cupboard to which access is restricted	Buprenorphine and diethylpropion: as Schedule 2. All other drugs: no requirement	No requirement[1]	No requirement[1]
Record keeping	As Schedule 2	Controlled drugs[3] register must be used	No requirement	No requirement[1]	No requirement[1]
Prescriptions	As Schedule 2	See below for detail of requirements[4]	As Schedule 2 except for phenobarbitone[2]	No requirement[1]	No requirement[1]
Administration to patients	As Schedule 2. Under special licence only	A doctor or dentist or anyone acting on their instructions may administer these drugs to anyone for whom they have been prescribed	As Schedule 2	No requirement[1]	No requirement[1]

[1] 'No requirement' indicates that the Misuse of Drugs Act imposes no legal requirements additional to those imposed by the Medicines Act 1968.

[2] All references to phenobarbitone should be taken to include all preparations of phenobarbitone and phenobarbitone sodium. Because of its use as an anti-epileptic, phenobarbitone is exempt from the handwriting requirements only of the full prescription requirements (see 4 below).

[3] *Record keeping.*

There is no legal requirement for the nurse in charge or acting in charge of a ward or department to keep a record of Schedule 1 or 2 controlled drugs obtained or supplied. However the Aitken Report (1958) recommended that this should be done and in practice a controlled drug register is invariably kept according to the following guidelines:

(a) Each page should be clearly headed to indicate the drug and preparation to which it refers. Records for different classes of drug should be kept on separate pages.

Table 15.1 *Continued*

(b) Entries should be made as soon as possible after the relevant transaction has occurred and always within 24 hours.

(c) No cancellations or obliteration of an entry should be made. Corrections should be made by means of a note in the margin or at the foot of the page and this should be signed, dated and cross-referenced to the relevant entry.

(d) All entries should be indelible.

(e) The register should be used for controlled drugs only and for no other purposes.

(f) A completed register should be kept for two years from the date of the last entry.

[4] *Prescription requirements.*

(a) The prescription *must* state:

    (i)   The name and address of the patient.

    (ii) The drug, the dose, the form of preparation (e.g. tablet).

    (iii) The total quantity of drug, or the total number of dosage units to be supplied. This quantity must be stated in *words* and *figures*.

        All of the above must be written indelibly in the prescriber's own handwriting and he/she must sign the prescription.

    (iv) The date of the prescription.

    (v) If the prescription is to be dispensed in instalments, the number of instalments and the intervals between them.

    It is illegal to write or dispense a prescription which does not comply with these requirements.

(b) The full handwriting requirements and statement of quantity to be supplied do not apply to prescriptions for hospital inpatients if the controlled drugs concerned are administered from ward or department stocks. They do, however, apply to prescription for drugs 'to take home' or for outpatients.

[5] *Storage and safe custody.*

(a) All controlled drugs should be stored in a suitably secure (usually metal) cupboard which is kept locked and to which access is restricted. This cupboard (which may be within a second outer cupboard) should be used only for the storage of controlled drugs.

(b) The Aitken Report (1958) recommends that all controlled drug record entries be checked by two nurses. In conjunction with the pharmacy a procedure should be developed to ensure regular checking of records and reconciliation of receipts and issues.

(c) A programme for regular stock checking should be established and adhered to.

[6] *Destruction.*

Unwanted or unused controlled drugs in Schedule 2 should normally be returned to the pharmacy.

[7] Temazepam preparations are exempt from record keeping and prescription requirements, but are subject to storage requirements.

stances be disposed of on the ward under the supervision of a pharmacist. An appropriate entry should then be made in the ward register.

Types of medicinal preparations of drugs

Preparations for oral administration

Tablets

These come in a great variety of shapes, sizes, colours and types. The formulation may be very simple and result for instance in a plain, white, uncoated tablet, or complex and designed with specific therapeutic aims. Sugar coatings are used to improve appearances and palatability. In cases where the drug is a gastric irritant or is broken down by gastric acid, an enteric coating may be used. This is designed to allow the tablet to remain intact in the stomach and to pass unchanged into the small bowel where the coating dissolves and hence the drug is released and absorbed. Tablets may be formulated specifically to achieve control of the rate of release of drug from the tablet as it passes through the alimentary tract. Terms such as 'sustained-release', 'controlled-release' and 'modified-release' are used by manufacturers to describe these preparations. Tablets may also be formulated specifically to dissolve readily ('soluble' or 'effervescent'), to be chewed or to be held under the tongue ('sublingual'). Unscored or coated tablets should not be crushed or broken, nor should most 'slow-release' or 'sustained action' tablets, since this can alter the rate of release of drug from the tablet.

Capsules

These consist of a gelatin shell in which is contained the drug powder or granules. They offer a useful method of formulating drugs which are difficult to make into a tablet or are particularly unpalatable. Slow-release capsule formulations also exist. Capsules should not normally be broken or opened.

Lozenges and pastilles

These are designed to be sucked for local treatment of the mouth and throat.

Linctuses, elixirs, syrups

These are usually sweet, syrup-like solutions used to treat coughs or where, in children for instance, a tablet or capsule may be inappropriate.

Mixtures

These are flavoured solutions or suspensions of drugs. It is particularly important the suspensions are thoroughly mixed by shaking before each dose is measured. This ensures that the measured volume always contains the correct amount of drug.

Rectal and vaginal preparations

Enemas

These are solutions which are instilled into the rectum as laxatives or to obtain other localized therapeutic effects, or for diagnostic purposes.

Suppositories

These are solid wax pellets for rectal administration. They may either melt at body temperature or dissolve or disperse in the mucous secretions of the rectum. They may be used to obtain local effect (e.g. as laxatives) or for systemic therapy. Many drugs, such as the opioids for example, are well absorbed when administered this way. Suppositories sometimes offer a useful alternative to injections for very sick patients unable to take drugs orally.

Pessaries

These are solid pellets for vaginal administration and are usually designed to have a local therapeutic action.

Topical preparations

Creams

These are semi-solid emulsions containing a high proportion of water. When applied they are quickly absorbed into the skin leaving little or no greasy residue. They may be used as a 'base' in which a variety of drugs may be applied for local therapy.

Ointments

These are similar to cream but contain a higher proportion of oil. They are absorbed more slowly into the skin and leave a greasy residue. They have similar uses to creams, and are particularly suitable for dry, scaly lesions.

Injections

Injections are sterile solutions, emulsions or suspensions. They are prepared by dissolving, emulsifying or suspending the active ingredient and any added substances in water for injections, in a suitable non-aqueous liquid or in a mixture of these vehicles (*European Pharmacopoeia*, 1990).

Single-dose preparations

The volume of the injection in a single-dose container is sufficient to permit the withdrawal and administration of the nominal dose using a normal technique.

Multi-dose preparations

Multi-dose aqueous injections contain a suitable antimicrobial preservative at an appropriate concentration except when the preparation itself has adequate antimicrobial properties. When it is necessary to present a preparation for parenteral use in a multidose container, the precautions to be taken for its administration and more particularly for its storage between successive withdrawals are given.

Parenteral infusions

Parenteral infusions are sterile, aqueous solutions or emulsions with water as the continuous phase; they are free from pyrogens and are usually made isotonic with blood. They are principally intended for administration in large volume. Parenteral infusions do not contain any added antimicrobial preservative (*European Pharmacopoeia*, 1990).

Inhalations

The term 'inhalation' once referred solely to the inhalation of volatile constituents of such preparations as compound tincture of benzoin. In modern therapeutics two techniques – nebulization and aerosolization – permit the inhalation of a range of drugs with the aim of a localized therapeutic effect.

Nebulization involves the passage of air (or sometimes oxygen) through a solution of the drug concerned to create a fine spray. Some antibiotics and bronchodilators may be given in this way.

Aerosolization involves the use of a solution of drug in an inert diluent. Passing a metred volume of this solution through a valve under pressure allows the delivery to the patient of a measured dose of drug in a very fine spray of controlled particle size. Bronchodilators and steroids are administered commonly in this way. Although a very small total dose of drug is administered, the concentration achieved at the site of action is high. Rapid and effective control of symptoms is achieved but without the side-effects commonly associated with an equivalent systemic (oral or parenteral) dose of the drug(s).

There are now available on the market aerosol and non-aerosol inhaler devices. Each device has its own advantages and disadvantages dependent on the particular situation.

Storage

Certain general principles apply to the storage of medicinal preparations (Department of Health, 1988).

Principle	Rationale
1 *Security*: locked cupboards. When not in use drug trolleys should not only be kept locked but should also be secured to a wall and thus immobilized.	To prevent unauthorized access and deter abuse and/or misuse.
2 *Separate storage*: for medicines and non-medicines.	To prevent confusion and hence danger to patients.
Separate storage: for preparations for oral use and those for topical use.	To prevent errors and therefore danger to the patient.
3 *Stability*: no medicinal preparation should be stored where it may be subject to substantial variations in temperature, e.g. not in direct sunlight or over a radiator.	To maintain efficacy of the medicines.
Stability: some preparations require storage under well-defined conditions, e.g. 'below 10°C' or 'store in a refrigerator'.	To maintain efficacy of the medicines.
4 *Labelling*: the wording of labels is chosen carefully to convey clearly all essential information. Printed labels should always be used.	To ensure that the user has all the necessary information.
5 *Containers*: the type of container used may have been chosen for specific reasons.	The design and material of which the container is made may significantly influence the stability of the contents.
Medicinal preparations should never be transferred (in bulk) from one container to another except in the pharmacy.	As above. Inadequate labelling of repackaged medicines is dangerous.
6 *Stock control*: a system of stock rotation must be operated (e.g. 'first in, first out') to ensure that there is no accumulation of 'old' stocks. Regular stock checks should be carried out, if possible by pharmacy staff.	All medicinal preparations, even when stored correctly retain activity only for a limited period of time.

The label on the pack should in most cases give guidance about storage conditions for individual preparations. The term 'a cool place' is normally interpreted as meaning between 1° and 15°C for which a refrigerator (between 2° and 8°C) will normally suffice. 'Room temperature' allows a range of approximately 15° to 25°C.

If you are in any doubt about the storage requirements for any preparation you should check with a pharmacist, but the following points are noteworthy:

(1) Aerosol containers should not be stored in direct sunlight or over radiators – there is a risk of explosion if they are heated.

(2) Creams may deteriorate rapidly if subjected to extremes of temperature.

(3) Eye drops and ointments may become contaminated with micro-organisms during use and thus pose a danger to the recipient. Therefore in hospitals, eye preparations should be discarded seven days after they are first opened. For use at home this limit is extended to 28 days.

(4) Mixtures may have a relatively short shelf-life. Most antibiotic mixtures require refrigerated storage and even then have a shelf-life of only 7–14 days. Always check the label for details.

(5) Tablets and capsules are relatively stable but are

susceptible to moisture unless correctly packed. They should be stored only in the containers in which they were supplied by the pharmacy.

(6) Vaccines and similar preparations usually require refrigerated storage and may deteriorate rapidly if exposed to heat.

Administration

The effective and safe administration of drugs to patients demands a partnership between the various health professionals concerned, i.e. doctors, pharmacists and nurses. The nurse is responsible for the correct administration of prescribed drugs to patients in his/her care. To achieve this the nurse must have a sound knowledge of the use, action, usual dose and side-effects of the drugs being administered. Various studies have shown that this is not always the case.

Institutional policies and procedures also assist the nurse to administer drugs safely and a sound knowledge of local procedures is essential, since most errors in hospital are the result of procedural error (Malseed, 1990). The importance of reporting errors to the appropriate authority can never be underestimated as recent research suggests that many undeclared medication errors are made by nurses. One survey demonstrated that of every ten medication errors that occurred only one was reported (Kuhn, 1989).

It must be recognized, however, that errors in drug administration can have traumatic consequences for the individual nurse involved and that disciplinary procedures invoke fear in most nurses (Arndt, 1994). The UKCC has stated that there should be a distinction made between errors which result from a serious pressure of work as opposed to those which are a result of reckless practice (UKCC, 1992b).

Prescriptions should be written legibly in ink or otherwise as to be indellible. Also, nurses should record in the appropriate documents that the prescribed medication has been administered.

Single nurse administration of medicines

Certain nurses may administer drugs by themselves provided it is the policy of the health authority by whom they are employed. Some authorities have policies which require that nurses have received specific training, both in theory and practice, and are in possession of a certificate stating their proficiency in the technique.

It is felt that this will result in greater care being given since that one nurse will be aware that she/he is solely responsible and accountable.

Those nurses who wish or need to have their administration supervised will retain the right to do so until such time as all parties agree that the requested level of proficiency has been achieved.

Self-administration of medicines

Hospital patients approaching discharge, who will continue on a prescribed regime of medicines at home, benefit significantly from the opportunity to adjust to the responsibility of self-administration whilst still having access to professional support (UKCC, 1992a).

Teaching patients to take their own medication correctly forms part of their programme of rehabilitation, which should begin with the first multidisciplinary assessment on their arrival in hospital (Crome *et al.*, 1980). However, repeated studies have shown high levels of non-compliance resulting in inadequate control of symptoms, hoarding of drugs and errors of over- or underdosage and incorrect dosing times. Non-compliance can result in slower recovery from illness, reduced health potential, and poorer quality of life (Williams, 1991).

Ultimately it is often patients themselves who are responsible for administering prescribed medicines at home. Health professionals can no longer assume that people are passive recipients of care (Kennedy, 1981). Bird (1990) suggests that

'for the majority of hospital patients, self-administration of drugs would appear to be a more appropriate method than the conventional system. Self-administration is not merely the process of patients taking their own drugs, it can also help clients retain or regain control over their health.'

Patients taught to self-administer their drugs in hospital are encouraged to regain independence and to participate in their own care. Problems which would otherwise only arise after discharge may be identified earlier and addressed before discharge. Although, by definition, self-administration of medicines shifts the balance of responsibility for this part of care firmly towards the patient, it in no way diminishes the fundamental professional duty of care. It is therefore essential that local policies, procedures and records are adequate to ensure that this duty is, and can be shown to be, discharged.

Observation of the patient receiving medication is important. No drug produces a single effect. The combined effect of two or more drugs taken together may be different from the effects when taken separately. The effectiveness of any drug should be noted and any signs of resistance or dependence reported. Side-effects may vary from slight symptoms to severe reaction and any signs must be brought to the attention of the appropriate personnel.

Injections

Injections can be described as the act of giving medication by use of a syringe and needle.

Newton & Newton (1979) identify eight routes for the use of parenteral injection:

(1) Intra-arterial.   (5) Intralesional.
(2) Intra-articular.   (6) Intramuscular.
(3) Intracardiac.   (7) Intravenous.
(4) Intradermal.   (8) Subcutaneous.

In addition, intrathecal routes are employed when the prescribed drug is unable to cross the blood–brain barrier. These authors also include a useful table of the tissues, sites and types of needle used, the amount of medication usually injected and the medications commonly administered via these routes.

Sites of injection

Site selection is predetermined for intra-arterial, intra-articular, intracardiac, intralesional and intrathecal injections. The choice of the remaining sites will normally depend on the desired therapeutic effect and the patient's safety and comfort.

Intra-arterial

This special technique allows the delivery of a high concentration of drug to the tissues supplied by a particular artery. This route can be used for the administration of chemotherapy, vasodilators and diagnostic purposes. Injection of drugs into an artery is a rare and hazardous procedure. The introduction of the cannula or catheter must be performed with care as the vessel may go into spasm, causing pain and occlusion. This could result in necrosis of an organ or part of a limb. Injection of irritant chemicals increases the risk of spasm and its sequentiae. In patients with some forms of cancer, however, arterial catheterization is occasionally performed when it is desirable to deliver a high concentration of a drug to a tumour mass. The most common procedures are catheterization of the hepatic artery and isolated limb perfusion.

Intra-articular

This may be used in the treatment of acute local inflammatory conditions. Corticosteriods are absorbed locally reducing toxicity but using this route can be painful for the patient.

Intrathecal

This may be used when the drug concerned does not penetrate the blood–brain barrier. The intrathecal route can be used for the administration of local anaesthetics, antibiotics, X-ray or contrast media and cytotoxic therapy which necessitates administration into the cerebral spinal fluid (CSF) (Malseed, 1990).

Intravenous

The administration of intravenous medications is an area in which the role of the nurse is being increasingly extended. For further information see Chapter 23, Intravenous Management.

Intradermal

Chosen sites are the ventral forearms and the scapulae. Observation of an inflammatory reaction is a priority, so the best sites are those that are highly pigmented, thinly keratinized and hairless. This site is used mainly for diagnostic tests, e.g. Mantoux. The injection sites most commonly used are the medial forearm area. The injections are best performed using a 26 g needle with a volume of 0.5 ml or less (Malseed, 1990).

Subcutaneous

This is given beneath the epidermis into the fat and connective tissue underlying the dermis. Chosen sites are the lateral aspects of the upper arms and thighs, the abdomen in the umbilical region, the back and lower loins. Absorption from these sites through the capillary network is slower than that of the intramuscular route. Rotation of these sites decreases the likelihood of irritation and ensures improved absorption. Subcutaneous injections given in the upper arm tend to be less painful since there are fewer large blood vessels and less pain sensations in these areas. A 25 g needle should be used, the maximum volume tolerable using this route is 2 ml, and drugs must be highly soluble to prevent irritation (Kuhn, 1989).

Intramuscular

Many drugs may be administered by this route provided they are not irritant to soft tissues and are sufficiently soluble. Absorption is usually rapid and can produce blood levels comparable to those achieved by intravenous bolus injection. Intramuscular injections should, where possible, be avoided in thrombocytopaenic patients.

Intramuscular injections are given at five sites (see Fig. 15.1 for some examples):

(1) *Mid-deltoid*: used for the injection of such drugs as narcotics, sedatives, absorbed tetanus toxoid, vaccines, epinephrine in oil and vitamin B_{12}. It has the advantage of being easily accessible whether the patient is standing, sitting or lying down. It is also a better site than the gluteal muscles for small-volume (less than 2 ml), rapid onset injections because the deltoid has the greatest blood flow of any muscle routinely used for intramuscular injections. However, as the area is small, it limits the number and size of the injections that can be given at this site.

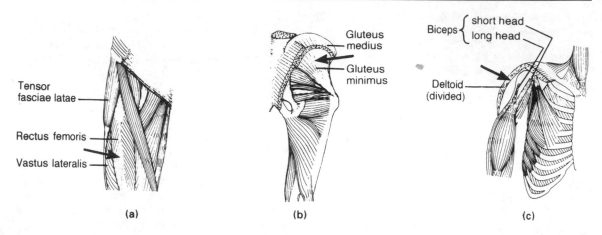

Figure 15.1 Sites for intramuscular injections. (a) Rectus femoris. (b) Gluteus medius and gluteus minimus. (c) Mid-deltoid.

Volumes of up to 5 ml can be given via this route using 20–23 g needles.

(2) *Gluteus medius*: used for deep intramuscular and Z-track injections. The gluteus muscle has the lowest drug absorption rate. The muscle mass is also likely to have atrophied in elderly, non-ambulant and emaciated patients. This site carries with it the danger of the needle hitting the sciatic nerve and the superior gluteal arteries. The Z-track method involves pulling the underlying skin to one side of the injection site, inserting the needle at a right angle to the skin, injecting and withdrawing the needle quickly while releasing the pulled back skin at the same time. This manoeuvre seals off the puncture tract. This method is used for medications which may cause subcutaneous irritation should they leak and preparations such as iron which may discolour the skin (Malseed, 1990).

(3) *Gluteus minimus*: used for antibiotics, anti-emetics, deep intramuscular and Z-track injections in oil, narcotics and sedatives. It is best used when large-volume intramuscular injections are required and for injections in the elderly, non-ambulant and emaciated patient as the site is away from major nerves and vascular structures.

(4) *Rectus femoris*: used for anti-emetics, narcotics, sedatives, injections in oil, deep intramuscular and Z-track injections. It is the preferred site for infants and for self-administration of injections.

(5) *Vastus lateralis*: used for deep intramuscular and Z-track injections. This site is free from major nerves and blood vessels. It is a large muscle and can accommodate repeated injections. This is the site used for small children since the muscle mass will be greater in this area, and needle length should be smaller than that used for adults.

Skin preparation

McConnell (1982) quotes the two most common solutions for preparing the skin for injection as ethyl alcohol and the iodophors, such as povidone-iodine. If using the iodophors, the nurse must check beforehand that the patient is not allergic to iodine. An iodophor must not be used to prepare the skin for an intradermal injection as the solution discolours the skin and this makes it difficult to assess any expected reaction.

When cleaning the skin, the use of friction together with a circular motion is recommended. The nurse should begin at the centre of the chosen site and progress outwards. The antiseptic must be allowed to dry thoroughly before injection, otherwise the antiseptic may be forced into the tissue with the injection.

The practice at the Royal Marsden NHS Trust is to continue to clean the skin prior to injection because patients are immunocompromised and the risk of contamination from the patient's skin flora is increased.

Research, however, has questioned the value of skin preparation before injection. Dann (1969) has shown that there is no experimental evidence that skin bacteria are introduced into the deeper tissues by injection, thereby causing infection. Antiseptics in current use cannot act in the time allowed in practice (five seconds on average) and cannot possibly cause complete sterility. Over a period 6 years, during which time more than 5000 injections were given to unselected patients via all the injection routes, without using any form of skin preparation, no single case of local and/or systemic infection was reported. Only before injections where strict asepsis is needed, as in intrathecal or intra-articular injections, is skin preparation required. Koivistov & Felig (1978) carried out a survey into the need for skin preparation before giving an insulin injection and found that skin preparation did reduce skin bacterial count but was not necessary to prevent infection at the injection site.

Needle bevel

Three categories of needle bevel are available:

(1) *Regular*: for all intramuscular and subcutaneous injections.
(2) *Intradermal*: for diagnostic injections and other injections into the epidermis.
(3) *Short*: rarely used.

Needle size

Lenz (1983) states that when choosing the correct needle length for intramuscular injections it is important to assess the muscle mass of the injection site, the amount of subcutaneous fat and the weight of the patient. Without such an assessment, most injections intended for gluteal muscle are deposited in gluteal fat. The following are suggested by the author as ways of determining the most suitable size of needle to use:

Deltoid and vastus lateralis muscles

The muscle to be used should be grasped between the thumb and forefinger to determine the depth of the muscle mass or the amount of subcutaneous fat at the injection site. One half of the distance between the thumb and forefinger will be the appropriate length of the needle required to penetrate into that muscle.

Gluteal muscles

The layer of fat and skin above the muscle should be gently lifted with the thumb and forefinger for the same reasons as before. Use the patient's weight to calculate the needle length required. Lenz (1983) recommends the following guide:

31.5–40 kg	2.5 cm needle
40.5–90 kg	5–7.5 cm needle
90+ kg	10–15 cm needle

Injections and pain

McConnell (1982) and Newton & Newton (1979) set out, in point form, techniques which may reduce the discomfort experienced by the patient. Kruszewski *et al.* (1979) focus on ways in which positioning can help to minimize pain. Field (1981) attempts to answer the question of what it is like to give an injection, and goes on to explore the meaning and use of language relating to injections, the feelings involved in preparing and administering injections, and the meaning of the patient's response to the nurse.

References and further reading

Adamson, L. (1978) Control of medicines in the UK. *Nursing Times*, 74, 973–5.

Arndt, M. (1994) Research and practice: how drug mistakes affect self-esteem. *Nursing Times*, 90(15), 27–31.

Bayliss, P. F. C. (1980) *Law on Poisons, Medicines and Related Substances*, 3rd edn. Ravenswood Publications, London.

Bird, C. (1990) A prescription for self-care. *Nursing Times*, 86(43), 52–5.

Brock, A. M. (1979) Self-administration of drugs in the elderly. *Nursing Forum*, 18(4), 340–57.

Central Health Services Council (1958) *Report of Joint Sub-Committee on the Control of Dangerous Drugs and Poisons in Hospitals* (Chairman J. K. Aitken). HMSO, London.

Crome, P. *et al.* (1980) Drug compliance of elderly hospital in-patients. *The Practitioner*, 224, 728.

Dale, J. R. & Appelbe, G. E. (1983) *Pharmacy, Law and Ethics*, 3rd edn. The Pharmaceutical Press, London.

Dann, T. C. (1969) Routine skin preparation before injection: an unnecessary procedure. *Lancet*, 2, 96–7.

David, J. A. (1983) *Drug Round Companion*, Chapters 3, 7 and 8. Blackwell Science, Oxford.

Department of Health (1988) *Guidelines for the Safe and Secure Handling of Medicines* (The Duthie Report). HMSO, London.

Dorr, T. & Von Hoff, D. (1993) *Cancer Chemotherapy Handbook*, 2nd edn. Appleton & Lange, Hemel Hempstead.

Downie, G. *et al.* (1987) *Drug Management for Nurses*. Churchill Livingstone, Edinburgh.

Drugs and Therapeutics Bulletin (1977) Storage and shelf life of drugs: when is it important? *Drugs and Therapeutics Bulletin*, 15(21), 81–3.

European Pharmacopoeia (1990) 2nd edn, Monograph 520. Maisonneuve sa.

Falconer, M. (1971) Self administered medication. *Hospital Administration in Canada*, 13(5), 28–30.

Field, P. A. (1981) A phenomenological look at giving an injection. *Journal of Advanced Nursing*, 6(4), 291–6.

Fink, J. L. (1983) Preventing lawsuits. *Nursing Life*, 3(2), 27–9.

Francis, G. (1980) Nurses' medication errors: a new perspective. *Supervisor Nurse*, 11(8), 11–13.

Hopkins, S. J. (1987) *Drugs and Pharmacology for Nurses*, 9th edn. Churchill Livingstone, Edinburgh.

Kennedy, B. (1981) Self-medication. *Cancer Nursing*, 77, 336–7.

Koivistov, V. A. & Felig, P. (1978) Is skin preparation necessary before insulin injection? *Lancet*, 1, 1072–3.

Kuhn, M. M. (1989) *Pharmacotherapeutics. A Nursing Process Approach*, 2nd edn. F. A. Davis, Philadelphia.

Kruszewski, A. Z. *et al.* (1979) Effect of positioning on discomfort from intramuscular injections in the dorsogluteal site. *Nursing Research*, 28(2), 103–5.

Lenz, C. L. (1983) Make your needle selection right to the point. *Nursing (US)*, 13(2), 50–1.

Loebl, S. *et al.* (1980) *The Nurse's Drug Handbook*, 2nd edn. John Wiley, Chichester, pp. 10–22.

Lydiate, P. W. H. (1977) *The Law Relating to the Misuse of Drugs*. Butterworth, London.

McConnell, E. A. (1982) The subtle art of really good injections. *Research Nurse*, 45(2), 25–34.

Malseed, R. T. (1990) *Pharmacology. Drug Therapy and Nursing Considerations*, 3rd edn. J. B. Lippincott, Philadelphia.

Markowitz, J. S. *et al.* (1981) Nurses, physicians, and pharmacists: their knowledge of hazards of medication. *Nursing Research*, 30(6), 366–70.

Newton, D. W. & Newton, M. (1979) Route, site and technique: three key decisions in giving parenteral injections. *Nursing (US)*, 9(7), 18–25.

Nurses Action Group (1981) Health and safety 3. Beware the drug. *Nursing Mirror*, 152, 22–5.

Pearson, R. M. & Nestor, P. (1977) Drug interactions. *Nursing Mirror*, 145, Supplement XI.

Powys Health Authority (1984) *All Wales Working Party of Review of the Administration of Drugs by Nurses*. Powys Health Authority, Bronllys.

Roberts, R. (1978) Self medication trial for the elderly. *Nursing Times*, 74(23), 976–7.

Thomas, S. (1979) Practical nursing – medicines: care and administration. *Nursing Mirror*, 148, 28–30.

United Kingdom Central Council for Nursing, Midwifery and Health Visiting (1992a) *Standards for the Administration of Medicines*. UKCC, London.

United Kingdom Central Council for Nursing, Midwifery and Health Visiting (1992b) *The Scope of Professional Practice*. UKCC, London.

Wade, A. (1980) *Pharmaceutical Handbook*, 19th edn. The Pharmaceutical Press, London.

Wandless, I. & Davie, J. W. (1977) Can drug compliance in the elderly be improved? *British Medical Journal*, 1, 359–61.

Whincup, M. H. (1982) *Legal Rights and Duties in Medical and Nursing Service*, 3rd edn. Ravenswood Publications, London.

Wieck, L. *et al.* (1986) *Illustrated Manual of Nursing Techniques*, 3rd edn. J. B. Lippincott, Philadelphia.

Williams, A. (1984) Medicine management. *Nursing Mirror*, 159(12), Supplement 1, i–viii.

Williams, B. (1991) Medication education. *Nursing Times*, 87(29), 50–52.

GUIDELINES: ORAL DRUG ADMINISTRATION

PROCEDURE

Action	Rationale
1 Wash hands with bactericidal soap and water or bactericidal alcohol hand rub.	To prevent cross-infection.
2 Before administering any prescribed drug, check that it is due and has not been given already. Check that the information contained in the prescription chart is complete, correct and legible.	To protect the patient from harm.
3 Before administering any prescribed drug, consult the patient's prescription sheet and ascertain the following: (a) Drug. (b) Dose. (c) Date and time of administration. (d) Route and method of administration. (e) Diluent as appropriate. (f) Validity of prescription. (g) Signature of doctor. (h) The prescription is legible.	To ensure that the patient is given the correct drug in the prescribed dose using the appropriate diluent and by the correct route. To protect the patient from harm. To comply with UKCC standards for administration of medicines.
4 Select the required medication and check the expiry date.	Treatment with medication that is outside the expiry date is dangerous. Drugs deteriorate with storage. The expiry date indicates when a particular drug is no longer pharmacologically efficacious.
5 Empty the required dose into a medicine container. Avoid touching the preparation.	To prevent cross-infection. To prevent harm to the nurse.

| 6 | Take the medication and the prescription chart to the patient. Check the patient's identity and the dose to be given. | To prevent error. |

| 7 | Evaluate the patient's knowledge of the medication being offered. If this knowledge appears to be faulty or incorrect, offer an explanation of the use, action, dose and potential side-effects of the drug or drugs involved. | A patient has a right to information about treatment. |

| 8 | Administer the drug as prescribed. | |

| 9 | Offer a glass of water, if allowed, to facilitate swallowing the medication. | |

| 10 | Record the dose given in the prescription chart and in any other place made necessary by legal requirement or hospital policy. | To meet legal requirements and hospital policy. |

| 11 | Administer irritant drugs with meals or snacks. | To minimise their effect on the gastric mucosa. |

| 12 | Administer drugs that interact with foods, or drugs destroyed in significant proportions by digestive enzymes, between meals or on an empty stomach. | To prevent interference with the absorption of the drug. |

| 13 | Do not break a tablet unless it is scored. Break scored tablets with a file. | Breaking may cause incorrect dosage, gastrointestinal irritation or destruction of a drug in an incompatible pH. |

| 14 | Do not interfere with time-release capsules and enteric coated tablets. Ask patients to swallow these whole and not to chew them. | The absorption rate of the drug will be altered. |

| 15 | Sublingual tablets must be placed under the tongue and buccal tablets between gum and cheek. | To allow for correct absorption. |

| 16 | When administering liquids to babies and young children, or when an accurately measured dose in multiples of 1 ml is needed for an adult, an oral syringe should be used in preference to a medicine spoon or measure. | A syringe is much more accurate than a measure or a 5 ml spoon. Use of a syringe makes administration of the correct dose much easier in an uncooperative child. Special syringes are available for this purpose: (a) They are washable and re-usable; the graduations do not readily rub off. (b) They have a non-luer fitting to which it is impossible to attach a needle in error. |

| 17 | In babies and children especially, correct use of the syringe is very important. The tip should be gently pushed into and towards the side of the mouth. The contents are then *slowly* discharged towards the inside of the cheek, pausing if necessary to allow the liquid to be swallowed. In difficult children it may help to place the end of the barrel between the teeth! | To prevent injury to the mouth and eliminate the danger of choking the patient.

To get the dose in and to prevent the patient spitting it out. |

Guidelines: Oral drug administration (cont'd)

Controlled drugs

Action	Rationale

1 Consult the patient's prescription sheet, and ascertain the following:
   (a) Drug.
   (b) Dose.
   (c) Date and time of administration.
   (d) Route and method of administration.
   (e) Diluent as appropriate.
   (f) Validity of prescription.
   (g) Signature of doctor.

To ensure that the patient is given the correct drug in the prescribed dose using the appropriate diluent and by the correct route.

2 Select the correct drug from the controlled drug cupboard.

3 Check the stock against the last entry in the ward record book. (At The Royal Marsden NHS Trust, a second person is required to check the stock level.)

To comply with hospital policy (Department of Health, 1988).

4 Check the appropriate dose against the prescription sheet.

5 Return the remaining stock to the cupboard and lock the cupboard.

6 Enter the date and the patient's name in the ward record book.

7 Take the prepared dose to the patient, whose identity is checked.

To prevent error and confirm patient's identity.

8 Administer the drug after checking the prescription chart again. Once the drug has been administered, the prescription chart is signed by the nurse responsible for administering the medication.

9 Complete any documentation required.

GUIDELINES: ADMINISTRATION OF INJECTIONS

EQUIPMENT

1 Clean tray or receiver in which to place drug and equipment.
2 21g needle(s) to ease reconstitution and drawing up.
3 21, 23 or 25g needle, size dependent on route of administration.
4 Syringe(s) of appropriate size for amount of drug to be given.
5 Swabs saturated with isopropyl alcohol 70%.
6 Sterile topical swab, if drug is presented in ampoule form.
7 Drug(s) to be administered.

8 Patient's prescription chart, to check dose, route, etc.
9 Recording sheet or book as required by law or hospital policy.
10 Any protective clothing required by hospital policy for specified drugs, such as antibiotics or cytotoxic drugs.

PROCEDURE

Action	Rationale
1 Collect and check all equipment..	To prevent delays and enable full concentration on the procedure.
2 Check that the packaging of all equipment is intact.	To ensure sterility. If the seal is damaged, discard.
3 Wash hands with bactericidal soap and water or bactericidal alcohol hand rub.	To prevent contamination of medication and equipment.
4 Prepare needle(s), syringe(s), etc. on a tray or receiver.	
5 Inspect all equipment.	To check that none is damaged; if so, discard.
6 Consult the patient's prescription sheet, and ascertain the following: (a) Drug. (b) Dose. (c) Date and time of administration. (d) Route and method of administration. (e) Diluent as appropriate. (f) Validity of prescription. (g) Signature of doctor.	To ensure that the patient is given the correct drug in the prescribed dose using the appropriate diluent and by the correct route.
7 Check all details with another nurse if required by hospital policy.	To minimize any risk of error.
8 Select the drug in the appropriate size or dosage and check the expiry date.	To reduce wastage. To prevent an ineffective or toxic compound being administered to the patient.
9 Proceed with the preparation of the drug, using protective clothing if advisable.	
10 Evaluate the patient's knowledge of the medication being offered. If this knowledge appears to be faulty or incorrect, offer an explanation of the use, action, dose and potential side-effects of the drug or drugs involved.	A patient has a right to information about treatment.
11 Administer the drug as prescribed.	

Single-dose ampoule: solution

Action	Rationale
1 Inspect the solution for cloudiness or particulate matter. If this is present, discard	To prevent the patient from receiving an unstable or contaminated drug.

Guidelines: Administration of injections (cont'd)

Action	Rationale
and follow hospital guidelines on what action to take, e.g. return drug to pharmacy.	
2 Tap the neck of the ampoule gently.	To ensure that all the solution is in the bottom of the ampoule.
3 Cover the neck of the ampoule with a sterile topical swab and snap it open. If there is any difficulty a file may be required.	To aid asepsis. To prevent aerosol formation or contact with the drug which could lead to a sensitivity reaction. To prevent injury to the nurse.
4 Inspect the solution for glass fragments; if present, discard.	To prevent injection of foreign matter into the patient.
5 Withdraw the required amount of solution, tilting the ampoule if necessary.	To avoid drawing in any air.
6 Replace the guard on the needle and tap the syringe to dislodge any air bubbles. Expel air.	To prevent aerosol formation, etc. To ensure that the correct amount of drug is in the syringe.
7 Alternatives to expelling the air with the needle guard in place include the following: (a) Covering the needle tip with sterile topical swab. (b) Using the ampoule or vial to receive any air and/or drug.	
8 Change the needle.	To reduce the risk of infection. To avoid tracking medications through superficial tissues. To ensure that the correct size of needle is used for the injection.

Single-dose ampoule: powder

Action	Rationale
1 Tap the neck of the ampoule gently.	To ensure that any powder lodged here falls to the bottom of the ampoule.
2 Cover the neck of the ampoule with a sterile topical swab and snap it open. If there is any difficulty a file may be required.	To aid asepsis. To prevent contact with the drug which could cause a sensitivity reaction. To prevent injury to the nurse.
3 Add the correct diluent carefully down the wall of the ampoule.	To ensure that the powder is thoroughly wet before agitation and is not released into the atmosphere.
4 Agitate the ampoule and inspect the contents.	To dissolve the drug. To detect any glass fragments or any other particulate matter. If present, continue agitation or discard as appropriate.
5 When the solution is clear withdraw the prescribed amount, tilting the ampoule if necessary.	To avoid drawing in air.
6 Replace the guard on the needle and tap the syringe to dislodge any air bubbles. Expel air.	To prevent aerosol formation, etc. To ensure that the correct amount of drug is in the syringe.

Note: Replacing the guard should NOT be confused with resheathing used needles.

| 7 | Change the needle. | To reduce the risk of infection. To avoid tracking medications though superficial tissues. To ensure that the correct size of needle is used for the injection. |

Multi-dose vial: solution

Action   **Rationale**

| 1 | Inspect the solution for cloudiness or particulate matter. If this is present, discard. Follow hospital guidelines on what action to take, e.g. return drug to pharmacy. | To prevent patient from receiving an unstable or contaminated drug. |

| 2 | Clean the rubber cap with an appropriate antiseptic and let it dry. | To prevent bacterial contamination of the drug. |

| 3 | Insert a 19g needle into the cap to vent the bottle (Fig. 15.2a). | To prevent pressure differentials which can cause separation of needle syringe. |

| 4 | Withdraw the prescribed amount of solution, and inspect for pieces of rubber which may have 'cored out' of the cap (Fig. 15.2b). | To prevent the injection of foreign matter into the patient. |

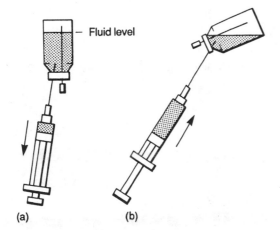

(a) (b)

Figure 15.2 (a) To remove reconstituted solution, insert syringe needle and then invert vial. Ensure that tip of second needle is above fluid, and withdraw solution. (b) Remove air from syringe without spraying into the atmosphere by injecting air back into vial.

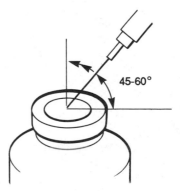

Figure 15.3 Method to minimize coring.

Note: Coring can be minimized by inserting the needle into the cap, bevel up, at an angle of 45° to 60°. Before complete insertion of the needle tip, lift the needle to 90° and proceed (Fig. 15.3).

| 5 | Replace the guard on the needle and tap the syringe to dislodge any air bubbles. Expel air. | To prevent aerosol formation. To ensure that the correct amount of drug is in the syringe. |

Guidelines: Administration of injections (cont'd)

Action

| 6 | Change the needle. |

Rationale

To reduce the risk of infection. To avoid possible trauma to the patient if the needle has barbed. To avoid tracking medications through superficial tissues. To ensure that the correct size of needle is used for the injection.

Multi-dose vial: powder

Action

| 1 | Clean the rubber cap with the chosen antiseptic and let it dry. |

| 2 | Insert a 21 g needle into the cap to vent the bottle (Fig. 15.4a). |

| 3 | Add the correct diluent carefully down the wall of the vial. |

| 4 | Remove the needle and the syringe. |

| 5 | Place a sterile topical swab over the venting needle (Fig. 15.4b). |

| 6 | Proceed to the patient. |

Rationale

To prevent bacterial contamination of the drug.

To prevent pressure differentials, which can cause separation of needle and syringe.

To ensure that the powder is thoroughly wet before it is shaken and is not released into the atmosphere.

To prevent contamination of the drug or the atmosphere.

Note: The nurse may encounter other presentations of drugs for injection, e.g. vials with a transfer needle, and should follow the manufacturer's instructions in these instances.

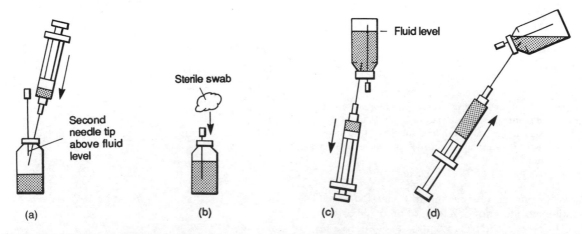

Figure 15.4 Suggested method of vial reconstitution to avoid environmental exposure. (a) When reconstituting vial, insert a second needle to allow air to escape when adding diluent for injection. (b) When shaking the vial to dissolve the powder, push in second needle up to Luer connection and cover with a sterile swab. (c) To remove reconstituted solution, insert syringe needle and then invert vial. Ensuring that tip of second needle is above fluid, withdraw the solution. (d) Remove air from syringe without spraying into the atmosphere by injecting air back into vial.

Subcutaneous injections

Action	Rationale

1 Explain and discuss the procedure with the patient.

To ensure that the patient understands the procedure and gives his/her valid consent.

2 Consult the patient's prescription sheet, and ascertain the following:
(a) Drug.
(b) Dose.
(c) Date and time of administration.
(d) Route and method of administration.
(e) Diluent as appropriate.
(f) Validity of prescription.
(g) Signature of doctor.

To ensure that the patient is given the correct drug in the prescribed dose using the appropriate diluent and by the correct route.

3 Assist the patient into the required position.

4 Expose the chosen site.

5 Choose the correct needle size.

To minimize the risk of missing the subcutaneous tissue and any ensuing pain.

6 Clean the chosen site with a swab saturated with isopropyl alcohol 70%.

To reduce the number of pathogens introduced into the skin by the needle at the time of insertion. (For further information on this action see 'Skin preparation', above.)

7 Grasp the skin firmly.

To elevate the subcutaneous tissue.

8 Insert the needle into the skin at angle of 45° and release the grasped skin.

Injecting medication into compressed tissue irritates nerve fibres and causes the patient discomfort (Malseed, 1990).

9 Pull back the plunger. If no blood is aspirated, depress the plunger and inject the drug slowly. If blood appears, withdraw the needle completely, replace it and begin again. Explain to the patient what has occurred.

To confirm that the needle is in the correct position. To prevent pain and ensure even distribution of the drug.

10 Withdraw the needle rapidly. Apply pressure to any bleeding point.

To prevent haematoma formation.

11 Record in the appropriate documents that the injection has been given.

12 Ensure that all sharps and non-sharp waste are disposed of safely and in accordance with locally approved procedures. For example, sharps into sharps bin and syringes into yellow clinical waste bag.

To ensure safe disposal and to avoid laceration or other injury to staff.

Intramuscular injections

Action	Rationale

1 Explain and discuss the procedure with the patient.

To ensure that the patient understands the procedure and gives his/her valid consent.

Guidelines: Administration of injections (cont'd)

Action	Rationale
2 Consult the patient's prescription sheet, and ascertain the following: (a) Drug. (b) Dose. (c) Date and time of administration. (d) Route and method of administration. (e) Diluent as appropriate. (f) Validity of prescription. (g) Signature of doctor.	To ensure that the patient is given the correct drug in the prescribed dose using the appropriate diluent and by the correct route.
3 Assist the patient into the required position.	
4 Expose the chosen site.	
5 Clean the chosen site with a swab saturated with isopropyl alcohol 70%.	To reduce the number of pathogens introduced into the skin by the needle at the time of insertion. (For further information on this action see 'Skin preparation', above.)
6 Stretch the skin around the chosen site.	To facilitate the insertion of the needle and to displace the subcutaneous tissue.
7 Holding the needle at an angle of 90°, quickly plunge it into the skin. Leave a third of the shaft of the needle exposed.	To ensure that the needle penetrates the muscle. To facilitate removal of the needle should it break.
8 Pull back the plunger. If no blood is aspirated, depress the plunger and inject the drug slowly. If blood appears, withdraw the needle completely, replace it and begin again. Explain to the patient what has occurred.	To confirm that the needle is in the correct position. To prevent pain and ensure even distribution of the drug.
9 Withdraw the needle rapidly. Apply pressure to any bleeding point.	To prevent haematoma formation.
10 Record in the appropriate documents that the injection has been given.	
11 Ensure that all sharps and non-sharp waste are disposed of safely and in accordance with locally approved procedures, e.g. put sharps into sharps bin and syringes into yellow clinical waste bag.	To ensure safe disposal and to avoid laceration or other injury to staff.

GUIDELINES: ADMINISTRATION OF RECTAL AND VAGINAL PREPARATIONS

EQUIPMENT

1 Disposable gloves.
2 Topical swabs.

3 Lubricating jelly.
4 Prescription chart.

PROCEDURE

Rectal preparations

For further information about the administration of rectal medication see the relevant sections in Chapter 8, Bowel Care.

Vaginal pessaries

Action	Rationale
1 Explain and discuss the procedure with the patient.	To ensure that the patient understands the procedure and gives his/her valid consent.
2 Consult the patient's prescription sheet, and ascertain the following: (a) Drug. (b) Dose. (c) Date and time of administration. (d) Route and method of administration. (e) Diluent as appropriate. (f) Validity of prescription. (g) Signature of doctor.	To ensure that the patient is given the correct drug in the prescribed dose using the appropriate diluent and by the correct route.
3 Select the appropriate pessary and check it with the prescription chart.	To ensure that the correct medication is given to the correct patient at the appropriate time.
4 Assist the patient into the appropriate position, either left lateral with buttocks to the edge of the bed or supine with the knees drawn up and legs parted.	To facilitate the correct insertion of the pessary.
5 Wash hands with bactericidal soap and water or bactericidal alcohol hand rub, and put on gloves.	To prevent cross-infection.
6 Apply lubricating jelly to a topical swab and from the swab on to the pessary.	To facilitate insertion of the pessary and ensure the patient's comfort.
7 Insert the pessary along the posterior vaginal wall and into the top of the vagina. Note: This procedure is best performed late in the evening when the patient is unlikely to get out of bed.	To ensure that the pessary is retained and that the medication can reach its maximum efficiency.
8 Wipe away any excess lubricating jelly from the patient's vulval and/or perineal area with a topical swab.	To promote patient comfort.
9 Make the patient comfortable and apply a clean sanitary pad.	To absorb any excess discharge.
10 Record in the appropriate documents that the pessary has been given.	

GUIDELINES: TOPICAL APPLICATIONS OF DRUGS

EQUIPMENT

1 Flat wooden spatulae.
2 Sterile topical swabs.
3 Applicators.

PROCEDURE

Action	Rationale
1 Explain and discuss the procedure with the patient.	To ensure that the patient understands the procedure and gives his/her valid consent.
2 Check the patient's prescription chart. (See note 2 on page 243.)	To ensure that the patient is given the correct drug.
3 Use aseptic technique if the skin is broken.	To prevent local or systemic infection.
4 Remove semi-solid or stiff preparations from their containers with a flat wooden spatula. Use a different spatula each time if more of the preparation is required.	To prevent cross-infection.
5 If the medication is to be rubbed into the skin, the preparation should be placed on a sterile topical swab. The wearing of gloves may be necessary.	To prevent cross-infection. To protect the nurse.
6 If the preparation causes staining, advise the patient of this.	To ensure that adequate precautions are taken beforehand and to prevent unwanted stains.

GUIDELINES: ADMINISTRATION OF DRUGS IN OTHER FORMS

PROCEDURE

Inhalations

Action	Rationale
1 Explain and discuss the procedure with the patient.	To ensure that the patient understands the procedure and gives his/her valid consent.
2 Seat the patient in an upright position if possible.	To permit full expansion of the diaphragm.
3 Consult the patient's prescription sheet, and ascertain the following: (a) Drug. (b) Dose. (c) Date and time of administration. (d) Route and method of administration.	To ensure that the patient is given the correct drug in the prescribed dose using the appropriate diluent and by the correct route.

(e) Diluent as appropriate.
(f) Validity of prescription.
(g) Signature of doctor.

4	Administer only one drug at a time unless specifically instructed to the contrary.	Several drugs used together may cause undesirable reactions or they may inactivate each other.
5	Measure any liquid medication with a syringe.	To ensure the correct dose.
6	Clean any equipment used after use.	To prevent infection.
7	Correct use of inhalers is essential (see manufacturer's information leaflet) and will be achieved only if this is carefully explained and demonstrated to the patient. If further advice is required, contact the hospital pharmacist.	Incorrect use may result in most of the dose remaining in the mouth and/or being expelled almost immediately. This renders treatment ineffective.

Gargles

Action   Rationale

1	Throat irrigations should not be warmer than body temperature.	Any liquid warmer may cause discomfort or damage tissue.

Nasal drops

Action   Rationale

1	Explain and discuss the procedure with the patient.	To ensure that the patient understands the procedure and gives his/her valid consent.
2	Consult the patient's prescription sheet, and ascertain the following: (a) Drug. (b) Dose. (c) Date and time of administration. (d) Route and method of administration. (e) Diluent as appropriate. (f) Validity of prescription. (g) Signature of doctor.	To ensure that the patient is given the correct drug in the prescribed dose using the appropriate diluent and by the correct route.
3	Have paper tissues available.	To wipe away secretions and/or medication.
4	Clean the patient's nasal passages, with tissues or damp cotton bud.	To ensure maximum penetration for the medication.
5	Hyperextend the patient's neck.	To obtain the best position for insertion of the medication.
6	Avoid touching the external nares with the dropper.	To prevent the patient from sneezing.
7	Request the patient to maintain his/her position for one or two minutes.	To ensure full absorption of the medication.
8	Each patient should have his/her own medication and dropper.	To prevent cross-infection.

Guidelines: Administration of drugs in other forms (cont'd)

Eye medications

For information on eye care see Chapter 20.

Ear drops

Action	Rationale
1 Explain and discuss the procedure with the patient.	To ensure that the patient understands the procedure and gives his/her valid consent.
2 Consult the patient's prescription sheet, and ascertain the following: (a) Drug. (b) Dose. (c) Date and time of administration. (d) Route and method of administration. (e) Diluent as appropriate. (f) Validity of prescription. (g) Signature of doctor.	To ensure that the patient is given the correct drug in the prescribed dose using the appropriate diluent and by the correct route.
3 Ask the patient to lie on his/her side with the ear to be treated uppermost.	To ensure the best position for insertion of the drops.
4 Warm the drops to body temperature if allowed.	To prevent trauma to the patient.
5 Pull the cartilagenous part of the pinna backwards and upwards.	To prepare the auditory meatus for instillation of the drops.
6 Allow the drop(s) to fall in direction of the external canal.	To ensure that the medication reaches the target.
7 Request the patient to remain in this position for 1 or 2 minutes.	To allow the medication to reach the eardrum and be absorbed.

Note: Further guidance on proficiency can be found in the *Scope of Professional Practice* (UKCC, 1992b).

GUIDELINES: SELF–ADMINISTRATION OF DRUGS

PROCEDURE

Action	Rationale
1 Take a drug history from the patient on admission.	To ensure an accurate record of: all medicines being taken (prescribed or otherwise); allergies or hypersensitivities; understanding of current medicines; possible problems with self-administration.
2 Review proposed (inpatient) prescription and compare with details given by patient and medicines in their possession.	If frequent changes of drug or dose are expected, immediate self-administration may be undesirable and/or impractical.

Appropriate medicines already in the patient's possession may be used, subject to local policy and agreement with the pharmacist.

3 Consider whether there are any constraints on self-administration, and if so, how they might be overcome. Discuss this with appropriate members of the multidisciplinary team.

To promote successful and safe self-administration and ensure that medicines are dispensed and labelled appropriately for the patient's needs.

Constraints such as physical or visual handicap must be addressed. Changes in performance status may result from the underlying condition or its treatment, and must be allowed for.

If a compliance aid such as a 'Dosette' box is to be used, responsibility for filling and labelling the aid, especially whilst used on the ward, must be agreed and documented in local policies.

4 Discuss self-administration with the patient and prepare a jointly agreed plan for: teaching; secure storage of drugs; monitoring and recording progress.

To promote the informed commitment and involvement of patients in their own care. To ensure that treatment is received as intended.

Teach any special skills required, e.g. correct use of aerosol inhalers.

5 Check that drugs are taken as intended, and that the necessary records are kept.

To discharge the nurse's overall responsibility for patient care and well-being. To maintain a record of responsibilities undertaken.

Particular care with record keeping is needed in the period of gradual transition from nurse administration to self-administration. Any problems encountered must be addressed.

The detail and format of the record may vary according to: the patient's needs and performance status; the complexity of treatment; and local circumstances and policy.

6 Monitor changes in the patient's prescription.

To ensure that: changes are put into effect promptly; drugs are properly relabelled or redispensed; any discontinued drugs are retrieved from the patient

7 Check when drug supplies are expected to run out and make arrangements for re-supply. Order TTOs (drugs 'to take out') as far in advance as possible.

To ensure that drugs are represcribed and dispensed in time to allow uninterrupted treatment and to facilitate planned discharge.

8 Evaluate the effectiveness of the self-administration teaching programme and record any difficulties encountered and interventions made.

To identify further learning and teaching needs and modify care plan accordingly.

CHAPTER 16

Ear Syringing

Definition

Ear syringing is the irrigation of the external auditory canal of the ear with water at body temperature using an ear syringe or electronic pulsed water unit. It is usually carried out by practice nurses to remove ear wax (cerumen), but it is also performed to remove exudate or pus and, in some circumstances, foreign bodies. Irrigation of the ear should be prescribed by a medical practitioner and only undertaken by an appropriately qualified practitioner.

REFERENCE MATERIAL

Anatomy of the ear

The ear can be divided into three parts: the external ear, the middle ear and the inner ear. Syringing is directed only at the external ear. The pinna (or auricle), the external auditory meatus and the tympanic membrane (ear drum) make up the external ear (Fig. 16.1).

The *pinna* is the prominent, visible part of the external ear which sits over the temporal bone of the skull. It consists of cartilage covered by perichondrium and skin. The *external auditory meatus* is an S-shaped canal which leads down from the pinna to the tympanic membrane. It is covered with epithelium continuous with the tympanic membrane. The inner two-thirds of the canal are formed by bone, while the outer third consists of fibrocartilage which is an inward extension of the pinna (Marshall & Attia, 1983). The surface of this part of the canal is dotted with hairs and sebaceous glands. Cerumen is produced in this area by modified sweat glands or apocrine glands (known as ceruminous glands). The *tympanic membrane* (or ear drum) forms the inner end of the external auditory canal. It is normally a smooth, pearly-grey, moderately translucent membrane, which may be opaque in scarred areas (Becker *et al.*, 1994). As part of the normal ageing process, the ear drum becomes whiter and duller (Webber-Jones, 1992). Some structures of the middle ear are faintly visible through the normal tympanic membrane.

Foreign bodies

Foreign bodies are sometimes inserted into the external canal and may become lodged. Alternatively, insects or debris may be blown into the ear (Beare & Myers, 1994). If the foreign body is composed of vegetable matter, irrigation and the use of liquids (e.g. mineral oil) are contraindicated because vegetable matter (e.g. peas, beans) is absorbent and swells up on contact with the liquid. Once swollen, the foreign body becomes more firmly lodged and therefore more difficult to remove.

Insects may be removed by instilling mineral oil, vegetable oil or diluted alcohol into the ear. The insect is usually killed and floats to the entrance of the auditory canal where it can be retrieved with ear forceps. Vegetable matter should be removed from the ear by a medical practitioner using a curette or suction (Beare & Myers, 1994). Attempting this procedure without the necessary skills may result in the foreign body being forced into the bony portion of the canal, the skin in the canal being perforated, or the eardrum being perforated (Brunner & Suddarth, 1989). Occasionally (for example if the patient is very young) general anaesthesia is required to remove foreign bodies.

Foreign bodies should only be removed by specialised medical staff.

Impaction of cerumen

Cerumen is continuously produced by ceruminous glands. It lubricates the external ear and exerts a bacteriostatic effect. Cerumen protects the ear by trapping debris. It is gradually moved towards the entrance of the auditory canal by the action of muscles used in chewing and talking. Hooper (1991) points out that 'people seem to be unaware that wax is necessary to protect the external auditory meatus and view its presence as a sign of poor personal hygiene'. Using cotton-tipped swabs ('cotton buds') in an attempt to remove ear wax frequently pushes wax further into the canal and causes it to become impacted (Webber-Jones, 1992).

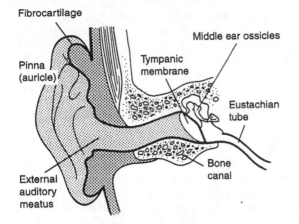

Figure 16.1 External auditory canal. The external one-third is formed of fibrocartilage; the inner two-thirds are bony.

If cerumen production is excessive, or if an obstruction prevents it moving towards the entrance to the auditory canal, the canal may become blocked with wax which hardens over time. People with large amounts of hair in their ears, or who work in dusty or dirty atmospheres, are more likely to experience excessive build-up of ear wax (Beare & Myers, 1994).

Routine cleaning of the ear

In normal circumstances ear hygiene can be maintained by washing the pinna and external auditory meatus with soap and water and a face cloth. Patients should be advised not to insert anything into the ear further than the part that can be seen from the outside (Beare & Myers, 1994). Cotton buds, match sticks and hairpins can damage the wall of the canal, cause wax to become impacted, increase the likelihood of otitis externa or perforate the tympanic membrane.

Examining the outer ear

The external auditory meatus and tympanic membrane must be examined with an otoscope by a qualified practitioner before the decision to irrigate the ear can be made. An otoscope consists of a changeable ear speculum, and a powerful, low-voltage, built-in light source giving magnification of between 1.5 and 2 times (Becker *et al.*, 1994).

It is also important to allow patients to describe their symptoms in detail. If pressure or movement of the pinna is painful, the patient may have an infection of the outer ear (otitis externa). Otitis externa is also associated with redness, scaling, itching, swelling, watery discharge and crusting of the external ear (Long *et al.*, 1993). Pain and hearing loss together may indicate an infection of the middle ear (otitis media) (Blakely & Swanson, 1989).

Otitis media is also associated with headache, loss of appetite and nausea and vomiting (Brunner & Suddarth, 1992). If an infection of the outer or middle ear is suspected, advice from a specialized medical practitioner should be sought. Blockage of the ear with impacted cerumen may cause a feeling of pressure or fullness, muffled hearing, whistling, squeaking and crackling noises and discomfort (rarely pain).

Otoscopic examination using an appropriately sized speculum is carried out by first pulling the pinna upwards and backwards, which stretches the cartilaginous part of the external meatus (Fig. 16.2). The otoscope is held in the dominant hand whilst the pinna is gently pulled up and back by the non-dominant hand. The external auditory canal can be inspected as the speculum is carefully inserted into the ear. The walls of the canal are very sensitive and fragile. Rough contact with the end of the speculum is painful, and should be avoided. Holding the otoscope so that the ulnar surface of the hand is stabilized on the patient's temple (when the otoscope is reversed) or the patient's jaw or occiput (when the otoscope is upright) prevents scratching of the auditory canal with the speculum if the patient moves (Webber-Jones, 1992).

In infants and young children the pinna is pulled down and back. The cartilaginous part of the external auditory meatus is proportionately smaller, and only a

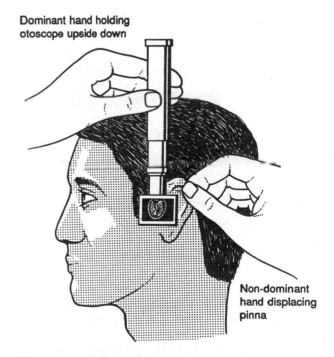

Dominant hand holding otoscope upside down

Non-dominant hand displacing pinna

Figure 16.2 Technique for otoscopic examination.

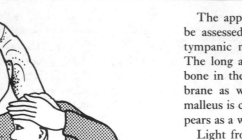

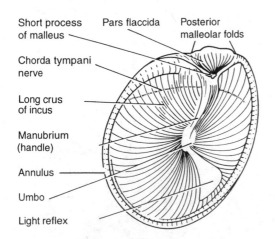

Figure 16.3 Holding a small child for examination of the ear.

Short process of malleus
Pars flaccida
Posterior malleolar folds
Chorda tympani nerve
Long crus of incus
Manubrium (handle)
Annulus
Umbo
Light reflex

Figure 16.4 Right tympanic membrane.

small, narrow speculum can be used. Otoscopic examination is therefore difficult. It is important that young patients have their head held gently and firmly by a skilled practitioner or trusted carer (Fig. 16.3) to avoid sudden movements and possible painful grazing of the ear with the otoscope (Becker *et al.*, 1994).

The appearance of the tympanic membrane should be assessed (Fig. 16.4). In normal circumstances the tympanic membrane is intact (without perforations). The long and short processes of the malleus (a small bone in the middle ear) are visible through the membrane as white markings, and the umbo, where the malleus is connected with the tympanic membrane, appears as a white spot.

Light from the otoscope is reflected off the normal tympanic membrane from a triangle formed by the annulus and the umbo (the 'light reflex'). If the light is reflected in an uneven way, the light reflex is said to be diffuse, and is abnormal.

Changes in the colour of the tympanic membrane, which is normally shiny, translucent and pearly grey, and the shape, which is normally slightly concave, may indicate an infection of the middle ear. Otitis media may make the tympanic membrane red; serous otitis may cause it to be dull or retracted. A bulging tympanic membrane indicates the presence of exudate in the middle ear.

Normally, the surface of the tympanic membrane is smooth and unmarked. Scarring is caused by previous infections and/or perforations. If perforations are present, or if a patient has a history of perforations, instillations and irrigations should not be used (Beare & Myers, 1994). Perforations hidden behind a plug of wax should be excluded by a careful history (Becker *et al.*, 1994). The presence of grommets also contraindicates irrigation. Impacted ear wax can be removed with a blunt curette ('cerumen spoon') but this procedure should only be carried out by a specialist.

Any abnormality identified in the external ear should be brought to the attention of appropriate medical staff, and advice on further action sought.

Irrigation of the external auditory canal

Irrigation is carried out with tap water at body temperature (37°C) using an ear syringe. Water that is too cold or too hot is uncomfortable, may damage tissues and can cause nausea, vomiting and dizziness by triggering the vestibular reflex. Approximately 300 ml are used in total, although no more than 50–70 ml are instilled at one time (Ignatavicius *et al.*, 1995).

Electronic pulsed water units (e.g. the *Propulse* syringe) are available. These incorporate variable pressure settings, and are operated either by foot or hand controls. Detailed guidelines for the *Propulse* syringe have been published by the Primary Ear Care Agency, Rotherham Health Authorities.

A cerumenolytic product or baby oil, mineral oil or olive oil may be prescribed to soften ear wax that is too thick or dry to be removed immediately. Softening agents often take 3 or 4 days to take effect (Beare & Myers, 1994). Ignatavicius *et al.* (1995) point out that

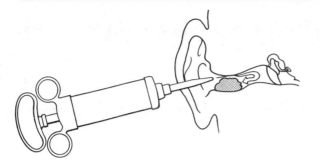

Figure 16.5 Irrigation of the ear with an ear syringe. A low-pressure stream of water is directed at the roof of the canal.

removal of wax is a slow process, and may not be completed in one session.

Patients should be seated where there is a good source of light. Having assembled and prepared the equipment (see *Guidelines*, below) the tap water is warmed to body temperature. It is important to ensure that the ear syringe nozzle is firmly secured. An otoscopic examination of the external meatus is carried out to check the position of the ear wax and to confirm that the tympanic membrane is intact and there are no signs of external ear or middle ear infection. A waterproof covering is placed around the patient's neck and shoulder, and a receiver or Noots tank placed or held (by an assistant or the patient) under the ear. A Noots tank is a conical metal container shaped on one side of the rim to fit under the ear, and on the other to allow the syringe to be angled upwards.

The syringe is filled with 50–70 ml water. With the patient's head in an upright position, the ear is gently pulled upwards and backwards (downwards and backwards in children) and the tip of the syringe placed at an angle so that a low-pressure stream of water is directed at the roof of the auditory canal (Fig. 16.5). The tip of the syringe should not occlude the meatus. In this way, the stream of water will flow along the roof behind the cerumen plug and back along the canal, washing out the obstruction. The returning fluid should be examined for traces of the cerumen plug. Irrigation should be repeated with a further 50–70 ml of water. The ear should be examined again with the otoscope to ascertain the position of the wax plug and the condition of the external meatus. Irrigation may cause the tympanic membrane to appear pink. If the patient becomes nauseous or dizzy at any point during the procedure irrigation should be discontinued. If the cerumen has not been removed, irrigate with a further 50–70 ml. If it cannot be dislodged, medical advice about a suitable softening agent should be sought. A suitably qualified physician or nurse may, alternatively, remove the wax with a blunt curette.

Following the irrigation procedure, the canal should be examined to assess the effect of the irrigation and then dried. The head should be tilted to allow water and remaining debris to drain out. A cotton swab should be placed beneath, but not over the meatus to absorb the fluid (Jameson *et al.*, 1992; Webber-Jones, 1992; Beare & Myers, 1994; Ignatavicius *et al.*, 1995).

Follow-up and prevention

Lewis-Cullinan & Janken (1990) suggest that impacted cerumen is a common condition in the hospitalized elderly. Of a random sample of 226 patients, 35% were found to have either bilateral or unilateral cerumen impaction. Improved hearing was demonstrated in 75% of ears after cerumen had been removed. On the basis of this study the researchers suggest that the hearing health of the elderly can be promoted by routine otoscopic examinations by nurses in acute care of the elderly settings, followed by ear canal irrigation when impacted cerumen is found.

A patient with recurring build-up and plugging of excess cerumen may be taught to use a prescribed non-irritant softener regularly. They may also require planned irrigations from a health care professional (Beare & Myers, 1994).

References and further reading

Beare, P. G. & Myers, J. L. (eds) (1994) *Principles and Practice of Adult Health Nursing.* Mosby, St Louis.

Becker, W. *et al.* (1994) *Ear, Nose, and Throat Diseases: A Pocket Reference.* Thieme Medical Publications, New York.

Birrell, J. F. (1986) *Paediatric Otolaryngology.* Wright, Bristol.

Blakely, B. W. & Swanson, R. W. (1989) *Otolaryngology for the House Officer.* Williams & Wilkins, Baltimore.

Browning, G. G. (1994) *Updated ENT.* Butterworth-Heinemann, Oxford.

Brunner, L. S. & Suddarth, D. S. (1989) *The Lippincott Manual of Medical-Surgical Nursing.* Harper & Row, London.

Brunner, L. S. & Suddarth, D. S. (1992) *The Textbook of Adult Nursing.* Chapman & Hall, London.

Hampson, G. D. (1994) *Bolden & Takle's Practice Nurse Handbook*, 3rd edn. Blackwell Scientific, Oxford.

Hooper, M. (1991) Aural hygiene and the use of cotton swabs. *Nursing Times*, 6(12), 38–9.

Ignatavicius, D. D. *et al.* (eds) (1995) *Medical-Surgical Nursing: A Nursing Process Approach.* W. B. Saunders, Philadelphia.

Jameson, E. M. *et al.* (1992) *Guidelines for Clinical Nursing Practices: Related to a Nursing Model.* Churchill Livingstone, Edinburgh.

Lewis-Cullinan, C. & Janken, J. K. (1990) Effect of cerumen removal on the hearing ability of geriatric patients. *Journal of Advanced Nursing*, 15, 594–600.

Long, B. C. *et al.* (eds) (1993) *Medical-Surgical Nursing: A Nursing Process Approach.* Mosby, St Louis.

Marshall, K. G. & Attia, E. L. (1983) *Disorders of the Ear: Diagnosis and Management.* John Wright/PSG, Boston.

Webber-Jones, J. (1992) Doomed to deafness? *American Journal of Nursing*, November, 37–9.

GUIDELINES: IRRIGATING THE EXTERNAL AUDITORY CANAL

Irrigation of the external auditory canal to remove impacted cerumen is normally carried out by nursing staff, particularly practice nurses. Only suitably qualified nurses should perform this procedure.

EQUIPMENT

1 Lamp.
2 Tray.
3 Otoscope and range of specula.
4 200–300 ml tap water in suitable container.
5 Lotion thermometer.
6 Waterproof covering.
7 Ear syringe/pulsed water unit.
8 Receiver/Noots tank.
9 Cotton swabs.
10 Yellow clinical waste bag.

PROCEDURE

Action	Rationale
1 Explain and discuss the procedure with the patient.	To ensure that the patient understands the procedure and gives his/her valid consent.
2 Position the patient's chair and direct the lamp.	To allow the nurse to move freely and to illuminate the ear clearly.
3 Examine the ear with the otoscope.	To confirm position of the cerumen and that there are no contraindications to irrigation (e.g. perforations in ear drum; infection; vegetable matter foreign body; grommets).
4 Ask the patient to sit with head in upright position.	To facilitate drainage of irrigation fluid.
5 Arrange waterproof covering over patient's neck and shoulder.	To protect clothing from irrigation fluid and debris.
6 Ask assistant or patient to hold the receiver or Noots tank below the ear, close to the head.	To catch irrigation fluid and debris.
7 Check temperature of water with lotion thermometer.	Irrigation fluid should be at body temperature to avoid triggering vestibular reflex.
8 Draw up water into the ear syringe and holding the nozzle upwards, expel any air. Or, run water through tubing of the pulsed water unit.	To ensure an even flow of water without air bubbles. To expel any air or cold water remaining in the tubing.
9 Make sure the syringe nozzle or tip of the pulsed water unit is firmly secured.	The auditory canal may be damaged or the ear drum perforated if the nozzle or tip flies off under pressure from the water.
10 Pull ear gently upwards and backwards (adults); downwards and backwards (children).	To stretch and straighten external auditory canal; to hold the ear steady to prevent injury.

11	Place tip of ear syringe at entrance to meatus but do not occlude it; direct low-pressure stream of water (50–70 ml) towards the top and back of the canal.	Water should flow behind the cerumen plug and back along the canal to wash it out; too forceful a stream of water may force the plug back along the canal or rupture the tympanic membrane.
12	If the patient experiences dizziness or nausea, discontinue the irrigation.	To prevent further triggering of the vestibular reflex.
13	Observe solution in receiver/Noots tank for traces of dislodged ear wax.	To evaluate effect of irrigation.
14	Examine external auditory meatus with otoscope.	To determine position and size of cerumen plug and monitor condition of ear.
15	Irrigate ear with 50–70 ml water once or twice more if necessary.	To remove remaining ear wax.
16	Ask patient to tilt head to allow water to drain, and place cotton swab below meatus.	To dry ear without irritating or damaging canal.
17	Carry out final examination of ear with otoscope.	To confirm removal of cerumen, and monitor condition of external meatus and tympanic membrane.
18	If any abnormality is observed, refer patient to medical practitioner.	Medical advice is required if cerumen plug has not been removed, or further treatment is necessary.
19	Remove waterproof covering and ensure patient is comfortable.	
20	Wash the aural speculum and syringe nozzle in hot soapy water, and dry.	To maintain hygiene.
21	To disinfect equipment, wash in hot soapy water, dry and then immerse in 70% ethanol. Dry equipment after immersion.	To reduce the risk of cross-infection. 70% ethanol does not penetrate organic matter.
22	If equipment can be autoclaved, it may be sterilized by this method.	Autoclaving is the most effective sterilization method.
23	Wipe over the syringe plunger with instrument lubricating oil.	To ensure free movement when the plunger is depressed.

CHAPTER 17

Entonox Administration

Definition

Entonox is a gaseous mixture of 50% oxygen and 50% nitrous oxide which acts as an analgesic agent when inhaled. The mixture remains stable at temperatures of above −6°C.

The Entonox cylinder is coloured blue and has a white band on the shoulder. The apparatus needed for administration consists of the cylinder, the Bodok seal, inhalation tubing and the handpiece. Either a mask or a mouthpiece may be used.

Indications

The use of Entonox is indicated before and during a number of painful procedures because it has several advantages:

(1) It has a rapid onset of analgesic effect.
(2) It has a very short half-life thus wears off within 2–5 minutes.
(3) The gas has no depressive effects on respiratory or cardiovascular functions. It should be considered for the following procedures:
   (a) Changing or removing packs, drains and dressings.
   (b) Removal of sutures from sensitive areas, e.g. the vulva.
   (c) Re-dressing burns, wounds or pressure ulcers.
   (d) Invasive procedures such as catheterization and sigmoidoscopy.
   (e) Childbirth.
   (f) Removal of radioactive intracavity gynaecological applicators.
   (g) Altering the position of a patient who has pain on movement, e.g. during the process of symptom control.
   (h) Manual evacuation of the bowel in severe constipation.
   (i) Traumatic injuries.
   (j) Applying orthopaedic traction; from our experience this is particularly relevant in cases of pathological fractures.
   (k) Physiotherapy procedures, particularly postoperatively. In addition, the use of Entonox is found to have been particularly useful for some of the above indications in the palliative care setting.

Contraindications

Its use is contraindicated in the following cases and situations:

(1) Maxilofacial injuries – as the patient may not be able to hold the mask tightly to the face or use the mouthpiece adequately. There is a risk of causing further damage to facial wounds and there may also be a significant risk of blood inhalation.
(2) Head injuries with impairment of consciousness.
(3) Heavily sedated patients – as they would firstly be unable to breathe in the Entonox on demand and to potentiate sedation further may be hazardous.
(4) Intoxicated patients – as drowsiness and aspiration would be a hazard in the event of vomiting.
(5) Pneumothorax – as it will increase the problem. Nitrous oxide diffuses into gas-filled cavities with a resulting build-up of pressure.
(6) Decompression illness or a recent dive (the 'bends') – as nitrous oxide escapes into the blood stream and increases the size of the nitrogen bubbles in the tissues.
(7) Laryngectomy patients – as they will be unable to use the apparatus.
(8) Temperatures of below −6°C as separation of the gases occurs.

Caution

The very young and very old may require additional care in the administration of Entonox due to possible mask fitting difficulties or inability to understand instructions for use. Entonox should be used with caution in patients with bowel obstruction or abdominal distension due to diffusion effects (Toulson, 1990). Consideration should be given to the patient's ability to use the Entonox, for example very dyspnoeic patients or those with reduced lung capacity may not be able to tolerate deep inhalation of the gas.

REFERENCE MATERIAL

Despite increasing awareness of pain control by health professionals and the availability of a wide variety of analgesic agents, the area of pain control for patients undergoing painful procedures is often inadequate. There are many reasons for this including inadequate assessment, prior to a procedure, underestimation of a patient's pain and difficulty of judging at the outset how painful a procedure will prove to be. Hollinworth (1995) describes poor assessment and management of pain control at wound dressing changes and discusses the difficulties clinicians may have in assessing pain, which during a dressing change may be brief but intense (Entonox is recommended in this situation). This is often true for many other procedures, and Entonox provides an effective analgesia which can be self-administered to provide immediate pain relief.

Nurses, midwives and physiotherapists may be able to administer Entonox (according to local policy) without a written prescription from a doctor. Entonox also provides patients with some control over their pain during painful procedures with minimal side-effects.

To wait for a doctor to prescribe analgesia or to wait for a prescribed analgesic to take effect is sometimes difficult or unacceptable. In these situations an analgesic which could be prescribed and administered by other qualified health care professionals, which would take immediate effect, which would be equally rapidly excreted from the body and which would have few side-effects is the ideal (Diggory, 1979). Entonox fulfils these criteria but is underutilized. Hollinworth (1995) advocates wider availability of Entonox and staff training through workshops to improve its use and heighten awareness of health professionals to its potential (see Table 17.1 for a comparison between opiates and Entonox).

Principle of administration

Entonox is designed for self-administration by the patient. The apparatus works as a demand unit, i.e. gas can be obtained only by the patient inhaling from the mouthpiece or mask and producing a negative pressure (Fig. 17.1). The gas flow stops when the patient removes the mouthpiece or mask from their face. Therefore, the patient must hold the mask firmly over the face or mouthpiece to the lips to produce an airtight fit and breathe in before the gas will flow. Expired gases escape by the expiratory valve on the handpiece. It is essential to adhere to this method of self-administration as it is impossible for patients to overdose themselves because if they become drowsy they will relax their grip on the handset

Table 17.1 Comparison of opiates and Entonox.

Opiates	Entonox
(1) Usually have to be given by injection – an added discomfort for the patient. There is also the risk of local or systemic infection.	Inhaled, i.e. a painless procedure.
(2) May take up to 1 hour to become effective.	Rapid onset, i.e. $1\frac{1}{2}$–2 minutes.
(3) Effects that last for approximately 1 hour or more.	Effects wear off rapidly, i.e. in approximately 2–5 minutes.
(4) Need to be prescribed by a doctor.	May be prescribed by an appropriately qualified trained nurse or physiotherapist according to local policy.
(5) Side-effects include respiratory and cardiovascular depression, emesis, drowsiness and thus an inability to cooperate.	Side-effects are few and self-limiting as the gas is self-administered. Recovery from side-effects such as drowsiness and amnesia is rapid.
	The main complications following the use of nitrous oxide are those due to varying degrees of hypoxia. Prolonged administration has been followed by megaloblastic anaemia and peripheral neuropathy (Reynolds, 1993).
(6) Tend to decrease peripheral circulation in patients suffering from shock due to their effect on the cardiovascular system.	The extra oxygen in Entonox increases peripheral circulation oxygenation in patients suffering from shock.

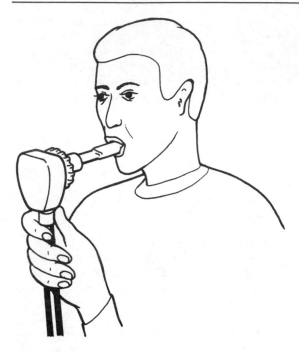

Figure 17.1 A patient administering Entonox through a mouthpiece. (Courtesy of B.O.C. Medical Gases.)

and the gas flow will cease when no negative pressure is applied.

Entonox has an oxygen content two-and-a-half times that of air and is, therefore, a good way of giving extra oxygen as well as providing analgesia.

References and further reading

Diggory, G. (1979) Entonox and its role in nursing care. *Nursing*, April, 28–31.

Hollinworth, H. (1995) Nurses' assessment and management of pain at wound dressing changes. *Journal of Wound Care*, 4(2), 77–83.

Msi, J. (1981) The use of Entonox for the relief of pain experienced by cancer patients. In: *Cancer Nursing Update*, (ed. R. Tiffany). Baillière Tindall, London.

Pritchard & Mallett (1992) *The Royal Marsden Hospital Manual of Clinical Nursing Procedures*, 3rd edn. Blackwell Science, Oxford.

Reynolds, J. E. F. (ed. Martindale) (1993) *The Extra Pharmacopoeia*, 13th edn. The Pharmaceutical Press, London.

Toulson, S. (1990) More than a lot of hot air. *Nursing*, 4(2), 23–6.

GUIDELINES: ENTONOX ADMINISTRATION

EQUIPMENT

1 Entonox cylinder and head.
2 Face mask and/or mouthpiece.

PROCEDURE

Action	Rationale
1 Check to see if there is gas in Entonox cylinder by turning the tap in an anticlockwise direction.	
2 Examine the gauge to determine how much gas is in the cylinder.	To ensure an adequate supply of gas throughout the procedure.
3 Ensure that the patient is in as comfortable a position as possible.	
4 Demonstrate how to use the apparatus by holding the mask tightly to your face. Explain to the patient that when they breathe in and out regularly and deeply a hissing sound will be heard, indicating that the gas in being inhaled.	To ensure that the patient understands what to do and what to expect before any painful procedure commences.
5 Allow the patient to practise using the apparatus.	To enable the patient to adopt the correct technique and observe the analgesic effect of the gas before the procedure commences.

| 6 | Encourage the patient to breathe gas in and out for at least 2 minutes before commencing any painful procedure. | To allow sufficient time for an adequate circulatory level of nitrous oxide to provide analgesia. (When the patient inhales, gas enters first the lungs then the pulmonary and systemic circulations. It takes 1–2 minutes to build up reasonable concentrations of nitrous oxide in the brain.) |

| 7 | During the procedure encourage the patient to breathe in and out regularly and deeply. | To maintain adequate circulatory levels, thus providing adequate analgesia. |

| 8 | At the end of the procedure observe the patient until the effects of the gas have worn off. | Some patients may feel a transient drowsiness or giddiness and should be discouraged from getting out of bed until these effects have worn off. It is rare for the patient to experience transient amnesia (Pritchard & Mallett, 1992). |

| 9 | Evaluate the effectiveness of Entonox with the patient throughout and following procedures by verbal questioning and encouraging the patient to self-assess the analgesic effect. | To establish whether the Entonox has been a useful analgesia for the procedure. This should then be documented to assist any subsequent procedures, e.g. dressing changes. |

| 10 | Turn off Entonox supply from the cylinder by turning the tap in a clockwise direction. The gauge should read 'Empty'. | To avoid potential seepage of gas from the apparatus. |

| 11 | Depress the diaphragm under the valve. | To remove residual gas from tubing. |

| 12 | Wash the face mask, expiratory valve and handpiece in hot soapy water. | To reduce the risk of cross-infection. |

Note: if the patient is known or suspected to be infected, e.g. hepatitis B or MRSA, then the equipment must be sent to the Sterile Services Department for disinfection.

NURSING CARE PLAN

Problem	Cause	Suggested action
Patient not experiencing adequate analgesic effect.	Entonox cylinder empty. Apparatus not properly connected.	Check before procedure commences.
	Patient not inhaling deeply enough.	Encourage the patient to breathe in until a hissing noise can be heard from the cylinder. Reassess suitability of patient for Entonox use. May not be strong enough or have reduced lung capacity to inhale deeply.
	Patient inhaling pure oxygen, i.e. cylinder has been stored below −6°C and nitrous oxide has liquified and settled at the	Initially safe, but later the patient may inhale pure nitrous oxide and be asphyxiated. Discontinue the procedure. Ensure adequate

Nursing care plan (cont'd)

Problem	Cause	Suggested action
	bottom of the cylinder. (All cylinders should be stored horizontally at a temperature of 10°C or above for 24 hours before use.)	warming of the cylinder and inversion of the cylinder to remix the gases adequately.
	Not enough time has been allowed for nitrous oxide to exert its analgesic effect.	Allow at least two minutes of Entonox use before commencing the procedure.
Patient experiences generalized muscle rigidity.	Hyperventilation during inhalation.	Discontinue Entonox and allow the patient to recover. Explain the procedure again, stressing deep and regular inspiration. Try a mouthpiece instead of a mask.
Patient unable to tolerate a mask.	Smell of rubber, feeling of claustrophobia.	Try a mouthpiece.
Patient feels nauseated, drowsy or giddy.	Effect of nitrous oxide accumulation.	Discontinue Entonox administration – the effect will then rapidly disappear.
Patient afraid to use Entonox.	Associates gases with previous hospital procedures, e.g. anaesthesia before surgery.	Reassure patient and reiterate instructions for use and short-term effects.

CHAPTER 18
Epidural Analgesia

Definition

This is the administration of analgesics and anti-inflammatory drugs into the epidural space. Analgesic drugs may be divided into two categories:

(1) Local anaesthetics, which provide a conduction block for sensory stimuli.
(2) Opiates which act within the central nervous system by attaching to specific opiate receptors in the substantia gelatinosa and the thalamus (Marieb, 1992).

Both groups of drugs provide excellent analgesia and each has its own specific side-effects:

(1) Local anaesthetics. The main side-effects are related to sympathetic and motor neuronal blockade. Sympathetic blockade may result in hypotension, due to vascular dilatation, requiring treatment with volume expanders and/or vasoconstrictors such as ephedrine. Motor blockade will result in temporary paralysis of muscle groups supplied by the affected segments.
(2) Opiates. The main side-effect is that of respiratory depression, which may require treatment with intravenous naloxone and respiratory therapy. A further minor, though significant, side-effect can be pruritis, requiring treatment with antihistamine and calamine (McNair, 1990).

A side-effect common to both classes of analgesics is urinary retention which may require catheterization.

Indications

(1) Provision of analgesia during labour.
(2) As an alternative to general anaesthesia, e.g. in severe respiratory disease or for patients with malignant hyperthermia.
(3) As a supplement to general anaesthesia.
(4) Provision of post-operative analgesia.
(5) Provision of analgesia resulting from trauma, e.g.

fractured ribs, which may result in respiratory failure due to pain on breathing.
(6) Management of chronic intractable pain, e.g. from bone metastases.
(7) To relieve muscle spasm and pain resulting from lumbar cord pressure due to disc protrusion or local oedema and inflammation.

Contraindications

These may be absolute or relative

Absolute:

(1) Patients with coagulation defects, which may result in epidural haematoma formation and spinal cord compression, e.g. iatrogenic (anticoagulated patient) or congenital (haemophiliacs).
(2) Local sepsis at the site of proposed epidural injection; the result might be meningitis or epidural abscess formation.
(3) Proven allergy to the intended drug.
(4) Unstable spinal fracture.
(5) Patient refusal to consent to the procedure.

Relative:

(1) Unstable cardiovascular system.
(2) Spinal deformity.
(3) Raised intracranial pressure (a risk of coning if a dural tap occurs).
(4) Certain neurological conditions (Morgan, 1989).

REFERENCE MATERIAL

Anatomy of the epidural space

The epidural space lies between the spinal dura and ligamentum flavum. Its average diameter is 0.5 cm and it is widest in the midline posteriorly in the lumbar region. The contents of the epidural space include a rich venous plexus, spinal arterioles, lymphatics and extradural fat.

259

Spinal nerves traverse the epidural space laterally. There are 31 pairs of spinal nerves of varying size. The two main groups of nerve fibres are:

(1) Myelinated – myelin is a thin, fatty sheath which insulates the fibres, preventing impulses being transmitted to adjacent fibres. Myelin also protects fibres and speeds of impulses.
(2) Unmyelinated – delicate fibres, more susceptible to hypoxia and toxins than myelinated fibres.

The spinal nerves are composed of a posterior and anterior root, which join to form a spinal nerve:

(1) Posterior root – transmits ascending sensory impulses from the periphery to the spinal cord.
(2) Anterior root – transmits descending motor impulses from the spinal cord to the periphery by means of its corresponding spinal nerve.

Principal insertion technique

(1) The patient is positioned either in the left or right lateral position, with the knees curled into the abdomen and the chin into the chest (the 'fetal' position), or seated on the edge of the trolley with the feet on a stool and bent forward onto a pillow placed across the knees.
(2) Full asepsis is observed, i.e. the operator is scrubbed, gowned and gloved.
(3) The skin is prepared with an alcoholic solution (chlorhexidine or betadine).
(4) The site of injection is isolated with a fenestrated towel.
(5) Local anaesthetic is injected at the site of epidural injection.
(6) The skin is punctured at the site with an appropriate needle, and the 16 gauge Tuohy needle is inserted as far as the ligamentum flavum. This is identified by applying pressure on the plunger of a glass syringe filled with air or saline, which meets with resistance while the needle tip lies within the ligamentum flavum. Needle and syringe are then advanced with a constant pressure being applied to the syringe plunger, which will suddenly plunge 'home' when the tip of the Tuohy needle enters the epidural space, i.e. loss of resistance technique.
(7) The epidural catheter is then passed by means of the Tuohy needle into the epidural space, the needle is withdrawn and the catheter length adjusted so that there are approximately 4 or 5 cm left in the space (Fig. 18.1).
(8) The catheter is aspirated to exclude accidental insertion into an epidural vein.
(9) The catheter is taped into position.

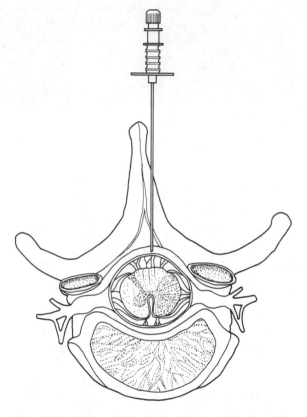

Figure 18.1 Diagram showing positioning of Tuohy needle. (Courtesy of Crul, B. & Delhaas, E. (1991) Technical complications during long-term subarachnoid or epidural administration of morphine in terminally ill cancer patients. *Regional Anaesthesia*, 16, 209–13.)

Common solutions used

(1) Local anaesthetics – either plain or with adrenaline 1 : 200 000:
    (a) Lignocaine 0.5–2%: rapid onset, short duration (one to two hours).
    (b) Bupivacaine: slower onset of action, but longer duration (two to eight hours).
(2) Opiates: diamorphine, morphine and fentanyl are the most commonly used opiates.

Spread of local anaesthetic solutions
Spread of local anaesthetic solutions is influenced by the following:

(1) Volume injected.
(2) Age of patient (any degenerative disease may interrupt local anaesthetic spread).
(3) Force of injection.
(4) Level of catheter.
(5) Drug concentration.

Mode of injection

(1) Bolus injections.
(2) Continuous infusions.
(3) Combined infusion/bolus method, i.e. background infusion with boluses as required if analgesia inadequate.

Methods of administration

(1) Bolus administered by nurse or doctor, when required.
(2) Patient-controlled administration using a microprocessor-controlled infusion device.

Complications of epidural analgesia

(1) Paraplegia is a rare occurrence. It may be caused by cord infarction.
(2) Intraocular haemorrhage has been reported after rapid injection of 30 ml of fluid. This is thought to raise cerebrospinal fluid pressure with resultant intraocular bleeding.
(3) Backache has been produced occasionally from local irritation caused by the needle or catheter.
(4) Extradural abscess may take up to 16 days to develop. Extradural abscess or haematoma should be drained on diagnosis otherwise paraplegia may result (Pritchard & David, 1988).

Epidural analgesia in chronic pain

Epidural analgesia may be chosen for patients with intractable pain. As the catheter will need to remain *in situ* sometimes for several months, long-term fixation needs to be addressed. Different centres have various ways of addressing this need, but the commonest ways are:

(1) Skin tunnelling.
(2) Fixation externally with a 'glue' based fixation device.

Once inserted and stabilized, patients can receive their epidural analgesia in the community provided there are adequate resources and a support network. These patients should be advised to check the puncture sites daily for any redness, inflammation or swelling and to contact their GP if they develop the signs of a raised temperature. Any sign of infection should be taken seriously because of the danger of ascending infection and meningitis (Crul & Delhaas, 1991).

References and further reading

Adam, S. (1985) Epidural anaesthesia. *Nursing Mirror*, 160(10), 38–41.

Atkinson, R. S. *et al.* (1982) *A Synopsis of Anaesthesia*, 9th edn. John Wright, Bristol.

Bibbings, J. (1984) Epidural analgesia. *Nursing Times*, 80(35), 53–5.

de Boek, R. *et al.* (1990) *Patient-Controlled Analgesia*, The Royal Marsden Hospital (Patient Information Series) (unpublished), London.

Brown, E. (1990) Narcotics via the epidural route (Part 1). *Nursing Standard*, 4(38), 24–39; Part II, *Nursing Standard*, 4(39), 37–9.

Crul, B. & Delhaas, E. (1991) Technical complications during long-term subarachnoid or epidural administration of morphine in terminally ill cancer patients. *Regional Anesthesia*, 16, 209–13.

Marieb, E. N. (1992) *Human Anatomy and Physiology*. Benjamin/Cummings Publishing Co., Wokingham.

McNair, N. D. (1990) Epidural narcotics for post-operative pain – nursing implications. *Journal of Neuroscience Nursing*, 22(5), 275–9.

Morgan, M. (1989) The rational use of intrathecal and extradural opioids. *British Journal of Anaesthetists*, 63, 165–8.

Owen, H. *et al.* (1988) The development and clinical use of patient-controlled analgesia. *Anaesthetic Intensive Care*, 16, 437–47.

Pritchard, A. P. & David, J. (1988) *The Royal Marsden Hospital Manual of Clinical Nursing Procedures*, 2nd edn. Harper & Row, London.

Sheargold, L. (1986) Epidural and spinal anaesthetics. *Nursing Times*, 82(27), 44–5.

The Royal College of Surgeons of England & The College of Anaesthetists (1990) *Report of the Working Party on Pain After Surgery*, pp. 15–17.

Ward, M. E. (1978) Epidural analgesia. *Nursing*, May, No 2, 78–81.

Yarde, A. (1989) Epidural analgesia. *Professional Nurse*, September, Vol. 4, Part 12, 608–13.

GUIDELINES: EPIDURAL ANALGESIA

Note: patients undergoing epidural analgesia should always have venous access or an intravenous infusion *in situ* before the procedure.

EQUIPMENT

1 Chlorhexidine in 70% isopropyl alcohol.
2 Local anaesthetic.

Guidelines: Epidural analgesia (cont'd)

3 Selection of needles and syringes.
4 Sterile dressing pack.
5 Face mask.
6 Tuohy needle or assorted gauge lumbar puncture needles.
7 Epidural catheter.
8 Bacterial filter.
9 Waterproof dressing and plastic adhesive dressing to tape catheter securely.

PROCEDURE

Action	Rationale
1 Explain and discuss the procedure with the patient.	To ensure that the patient understands the procedure and gives his/her valid consent.

2 Assist the patient into the required position:
(a) Lying:
  Position pillow under patient's head.
  Firm surface.
  On side with knee drawn up to the abdomen and clasped by the hands.
  Support the patient in this position.
(b) Sitting:
  Patient sits on firm surface with arms resting on a table, and with the head resting on the arms.
	To ensure maximum widening of the intervertebral spaces, providing easier access to the epidural space.
	
	To prevent sudden movement.
	
	Allows proper identification of the spinal processes and therefore invertebral spaces.

3 Support, encourage and observe the patient throughout the procedure.	As procedure takes place behind the patient, reassurance is very important.
4 Assist the doctor as required. The doctor will proceed as follows: (a) Clean the skin with alcohol-based solution (e.g. chorhexidine in 70% isopropyl alcohol) or povidone–iodine solution. (b) Identify the area to be punctured and inject the skin and subcutaneous layers with local anaesthetic. (c) Introduce Tuohy or spinal needles usually between third and fourth lumbar vertebrae. (d) Ensure epidural space has been entered. (e) Inject test dose of drug (may be performed). (f) Thread epidural catheter through barrel of Tuohy needle. (g) Attach the bacterial filter. (h) Apply dressing and tape to the catheter insertion site. (i) Inject solution into epidural space via catheter.	To maintain asepsis. To prevent anaesthesia being given directly into spinal cord or intravenously by means of the dural veins. To ensure the position of the needle. To facilitate intermittent topping-up of anaesthesia and to allow greater control. To prevent injection of contaminants into epidural space. To prevent the catheter being dislodged. To provide anaesthesia.

5	Position the patient according to the doctor's instructions, tilting if appropriate.	To ensure spread of solution to provide optimum effect.
6	Take vital signs observations: blood pressure and respirations every 5 minutes for 30 minutes, and then 15 minutes for next 90 minutes. Take pulse every 15 minutes for 2 hours, or more frequently if the patient's condition dictates.	To monitor for signs of hypotension and respiratory depression.
7	Make the patient comfortable. Usually the patient is nursed flat for the first 3–6 hours, then slowly elevated into a sitting position. Bedclothes should not constrict the feet.	To prevent the development of footdrop.

GUIDELINES: TOPPING UP EPIDURAL ANALGESIA

Usually performed by the doctor. Local anaesthetic agents *or* opioids may be given by nursing staff as part of an extended role, according to local policy. This should follow an agreed period of education and supervised practice.

EQUIPMENT

1 Antiseptic cleaning agent.
2 Syringes and needles.
3 Drug as prescribed.
4 Water or 0.9% sodium chloride for injection as necessary.
5 Patient's prescription chart.
6 Sterile hub/bung.

PROCEDURE

Action		Rationale
1	Wash hands with bactericidal soap and water or bactericidal alcohol hand rub.	To reduce risk of cross-infection.
2	Check the drug to be administered and diluents, according to policy.	To ensure the correct drug, amount and concentration is administered to the correct patient.
3	Draw up the drug.	
4	Clean the access portal of the bacterial filter.	To prevent the introduction of contaminants and micro-organisms into the epidural space.
5	Inject drug as prescribed.	
6	Make the patient comfortable.	
7	Monitor vital signs, blood pressure and respirations every 5 minutes for 30 minutes, then every 15 minutes for 90 minutes. Take pulse	To monitor signs of hypotension and respiratory depression.

Guidelines: Topping up epidural analgesia (cont'd)

Action	Rationale
every 15 minutes for 2 hours or more frequently if the patient's condition dictates.	
8 Dispose of the equipment appropriately.	
9 Maintain pain control assessment.	To ensure optimum pain control.

GUIDELINES: REMOVAL OF AN EPIDURAL CATHETER

EQUIPMENT

1 Dressing pack.
2 Skin cleansing agent, i.e. 0.9% sodium chloride.
3 Spray dressing (moisture vapour permeable), i.e. Opsite.
4 Occlusive dressing.

PROCEDURE

Action	Rationale
1 Wash hands with bactericidal soap and water or bactericidal alcohol hand rub.	To minimize cross-infection.
2 Open dressing pack.	
3 Remove tape and dressing from catheter insertion site.	
4 Gently, in one swift movement, remove catheter. Check that it is removed intact by observing marks along the catheter.	To ensure the catheter is removed intact with the minimum of discomfort to the patient.
5 Apply spray dressing (moisture vapour permeable), e.g. Opsite with povidone–iodine.	As prophylaxis against infection along the catheter tract.
6 Apply an occlusive dressing and leave *in situ* for 24 hours.	To prevent inadvertent access of micro-organisms along the tract.

The epidural tip may be sent for culture and sensitivity if infection is suspected, or according to local policy.

NURSING CARE PLAN

Problem	Cause	Suggested action
Rapid fall in blood pressure.	Sympathetic blockade producing hypotension.	Turn off infusion pump if in progress.

		If systolic blood pressure falls below 70–80 mmHg:
		    Summon duty anaesthetist or doctor.
		    Tilt the patient's head down unless contraindicated.
		    Give oxygen 4 litres per minute via a mask.
		To prevent hypoxia caused by reduction in cardiac output:
		
		(1) Increase intravenous infusion (unless contraindicated, i.e. congestive cardiac failure).
		(2) Prepare 15–30 mg ephedrine for intravenous injection which may be requested urgently by medical staff. Ephedine increases heart rate and therefore cardiac output.

Respiratory depression.	Opiate analgesia.	Call for medical assistance. Turn off infusion pump or patient-controlled analgesia (PCA) pump if in progress. Prepare naloxone 0.4 mg intravenously. If prescribed, give dose according to criteria, i.e. respiratory rate <8 per minute. Dosage counteracts respiratory depression and might also reverse the analgesic effect. If no improvement, administer second dose. A further 0.4 mg naloxone intravenously can be given 5–10 minutes after first. Prepare emergency equipment to support respiration. The patient's respiratory rate, pattern and depth should be observed at all times. Maintain continuous monitoring of tissue oxygen saturation, e.g. with pulse oximeter. Access to blood gas machines should be available. Observe pupil constriction.
Total spinal anaesthesia.		Prepare emergency equipment to support respiration. Call for medical assistance. Turn patient into the supine position.

Nursing care plan (cont'd)

Problem	Cause	Suggested action
		Ventilate the lungs. Elevate the legs. Prepare emergency drugs. Open intravenous infusion. Prepare equipment for intubation.
Total central neurological blockade: (1) Marked hypotension. (2) Apnoea. (3) Dilated pupils. (4) Loss of consciousness.		Call for medical assistance and begin emergency procedures.
Toxicity due to injected drug: (1) Disorientation. (2) Twitching. (3) Convulsions. (4) Apnoea.		Call for medical assistance and institute emergency procedures.
Nausea or vomiting.	Side-effect of opiates. Due to stimulation of the vomiting centre in the brain stem and stimulation of the chemoreceptor zone in the fourth ventricle of the brain.	Administer antiemetics as prescribed. Inform an anaesthetist.
Headache.	May be caused by accidental dural puncture.	Administer systemic analgesia. Lie patient flat. Oral and intravenous fluids may be increased to encourage cerebrospinal fluid formation.
Pruritis, especially of the face and/or neck.	Histamine release following administration of opiates.	Inform anaesthetist. Administer antihistamine as prescribed. Keep patient cool. Use calamine lotion.
Urinary retention.	Due to parasympathetic block at the sacral level of the spinal cord.	Inform anaesthetist. Catheterize as required. The majority of patients on an intensive therapy unit or high dependency unit are catheterized.
Infection.		Check temperature 4-hourly. Check catheter entry site for inflammation or exudate. Remove epidural cannula if appropriate.

Assess pain regularly using a visual analogue scale or pain chart if appropriate. Observe the patient's movements and facial expressions. Discuss insufficient or ineffective analgesia with the anaesthetist.

PATIENT-CONTROLLED ANALGESIA AND INFUSIONS

Patient-controlled analgesia (PCA) is a technique developed over the last 20 years which allows patients to administer their own analgesia. The PCA syringe pump can deliver an opioid analgesic, e.g. diamorphine, in three different ways:

(1) By pressing a button, the patient can deliver a programmed *bolus dose* as required. A *lockout period* is set so that the syringe pump will not respond to further pressing of the button for the set amount of time. This allows time for each dose to work before patients can give themselves another bolus. This mechanism prevents the occurrence of overdosage.
(2) A continuous *background infusion* can be delivered by the pump just as by any continuous syringe driver.
(3) A combination of *background infusion* and *bolus dose* can be used.

For patient safety, all patients receiving epidural analgesia should be nursed on a high dependency unit by skilled staff with appropriate equipment.

Continuous monitoring and observation is essential.

Facilities for resuscitation should be readily available for all of these patients. The patient should be the *only* person who operates the patient-controlled analgesia pump. Inappropriate pressing of the button by nursing staff or doctors may lead to oversedation and respiratory arrest.

Patient-controlled analgesia may not be suitable for all patients and it is important that every patient is assessed carefully by the nursing and medical staff.

The use of pain charts is advocated in most units. Patients can be assessed 30 minutes after commencing therapy, then at designated times according to local policy.

Continuous in-service training of staff is essential in order to detect rare cases of equipment malfunction and to minimize error.

Continuous infusions

An increasing number of units are using a combination of one or more drugs as a continuous infusion. Drugs used vary according to the clinical situation. A variety of opiates may be used, e.g. diamorphine, fentanyl.

In most cases, a 30 cc or 60 cc syringe containing the selected drug is run at a rate prescribed by the anaesthetic team. The rate can be increased or decreased as necessary.

The syringe pump should be monitored and marked hourly to ensure that the correct dose is given and that the pump is working accurately.

The most important, and potentially fatal, complication of spinal opiates is respiratory depression, which may be considerably delayed many hours after these infusions commence.

All patients must be observed constantly and their respiratory rate, depth and pattern recorded. The use of pulse oximeters to continually display oxygen saturation is now employed in most units. Blood gases may need to be taken and oxygen therapy administered if appropriate (McNair, 1990).

CHAPTER 19

External Compression and Support in the Management of Chronic Oedema

Definition

'Support may be defined as the retention and control of tissue without the application of compression . . . Compression implies the deliberate application of pressure' (Thomas, 1991a). The application of both support and compression results in pressure; the differences between the two techniques are, firstly, that the resulting pressure arises from different mechanisms and, secondly, that the relationship between resting pressures and active pressures is different (Thomas, 1991b).

In the case of support, pressure arises from the body tissues pushing outwards against the stocking or bandage. The pressure from compression results from the forces in the stocking or bandage exerting pressure on the tissues beneath. Thus it is the type of material from which stockings or bandages are made that determines whether support or compression is being applied. Short-stretch or extensible bandages and the more rigid types of hosiery will result in support, as the tissues push out against the firm rigid casing provided by the stocking/bandage. Elastic hosiery or bandages will result in compression, as the elastic properties of the material pull in against the tissues (Thomas, 1991b).

Under support the resting pressure is relatively low and the active pressure relatively high, resulting in a massaging effect on the tissues beneath. Under compression the difference between the resting and active pressure is less pronounced and the massaging effect diminished (Thomas, 1991b).

Indications

External graduated pressure is the mainstay of the conservative management of moderate to severe oedema. It is important for several reasons:

(1) It ensures that fluid in the limb travels towards the root of the limb.
(2) It limits the formation of fluid in the tissues.
(3) It contains the tissues of the swollen limb and helps to maintain a normal shape to the limb.

(4) It helps to maximize the effect of the muscle pump (Leduc et al., 1990; Olszewski & Engeset, 1990).

Compression is primarily indicated in the maintenance phase of treatment, when the oedema has been reduced and the drained tissues must be contained to prevent fluid re-accumulating. It may also be used in cases of mild oedema (i.e. the swollen limb volume is more than 20% greater than the contralateral normal limb) as long as the oedema is soft and pitting.

Support is indicated in the reduction of moderate to severe oedema (i.e. the swollen limb volume is greater than 20%), and is always the technique of choice if fibrosis of the subcutaneous tissues is present, when the massaging effect of the low resting and high active pressures appears most effective.

Contraindications for compression

(1) Arterial disease in the arm or leg.
(2) Acute stages of deep vein thrombosis in the leg.

REFERENCE MATERIAL

Chronic oedema (of which lymphoedema is just one form) is defined as 'tissue swelling due to a failure of lymph drainage' (Mortimer, 1990). Lymph drainage commonly fails in cancer patients as a result of damage to lymph nodes from surgery and/or radiotherapy, or from the obstructive effects of local tumour. A study carried out at the Royal Marsden NHS Trust (Kissen et al., 1986) found an incidence of lymphoedema of 25% in 200 patients following treatment for breast cancer. The incidence rose to 38% in patients who had received both surgery and radiotherapy to the axilla.

The incidence of leg oedema following treatment for abdominal and pelvic tumours is not known, nor is the incidence in patients with soft tissue sarcoma or melanoma. However, lymphoedema is not uncommon in these patients.

Lymphoedema can affect any part of the body including the head, but it most commonly affects the limbs

(Mortimer, 1990). The high protein concentration of lymphoedema causes skin and tissue changes in the oedematous limb, leading to the characteristic deepened skin folds, distorted limb shape and hyperkeratosis associated with longstanding lymphoedema. There is an increased risk of infection in the affected limb (fungal infections, cellulitis) and recurrent acute inflammatory episodes are common (Mortimer, 1990).

Chronic venous disease of the lower limbs, commonly seen in the elderly, can result in oedema usually affecting the lower legs. This oedema often has a lymphatic component (Prasad *et al.*, 1990). The increased load on the lymphatic system from the outpouring of fluid from incompetent veins leads to lymphatic failure. Dependency or gravitational oedema is another problem commonly seen in the immobile, elderly patient. It arises from a lack of propulsion to venous blood flow and lymph flow (Levick, 1991).

There is no cure for lymphoedema but it is possible to reduce the size of the swollen limb and, in the patient free of active cancer, to control the swelling in the long term (Badger & Twycross, 1988). For patients with recurrent or advanced cancer, treatment can be modified with the aim of palliating the symptoms associated with oedema (Badger, 1987).

MAINTENANCE PHASE OF TREATMENT

Types of compression and support

Compression and support can be applied in many ways. In the management of chronic oedema compression is usually applied in the form of elastic compression hosiery during the maintenance phase of treatment. Prescribing and fitting compression hosiery is a skilled job and it should only be attempted by health care professionals who have the necessary experience and training.

Elastic hosiery is available in a wide range of off-the-shelf sizes and designs. Ready-made stockings come in three compression classes:

(1) Class 1: 20–30 mm Hg at the ankle.
(2) Class 2: 30–40 mm Hg at the ankle.
(3) Class 3: 40–50 mm Hg at the ankle.

Lymphoedema usually calls for the use of class 3 stockings, while classes 1 and 2 are more appropriate for mixed lympho-venous oedema or dependency oedema where the swelling is usually soft and pitting in nature. Class 1 and 2 stockings are available on general prescription, while class 3 hosiery has to be obtained through a hospital appliance department. Elastic sleeves, like class 3 stockings, are not available on general prescriptions and must also be obtained through the hospital appliance department. These, too, come in a range of sizes and designs but are limited to one compression class (between 30 and 40 mm Hg). Anti-embolism stockings are designed to improve blood flow in the lower limbs and are inappropriate for the treatment of oedema, but shaped, elasticated surgical tubular stockinette may be used in situations where class 1 hose is called for. Hosiery is used to maintain improvement in limb size following bandaging. Ideally, it should be applied before the patient gets out of bed in the morning or, if this is not feasible, as soon after rising as possible. At night, when the limb is in a horizontal position, there is no need for the patient to wear hosiery and the stocking or sleeve is removed. An elastic sleeve or stocking should always feel comfortable and supportive. It should not cause pain or trauma and, while it should be firm-fitting, it should not constrict the limb. Hosiery may also be used as the initial treatment for mild, uncomplicated oedema, or to provide support in the palliative treatment of oedema.

Support is provided in the reduction phase of the treatment of chronic oedema using a specialized technique of bandaging known as multi-layer bandaging. The reduction phase of treatment consists of a multi-faceted approach, including a range of different treatments of which multi-layer bandaging is just one example. This phase of treatment is best left in the hands of specialists in the field. Multi-layer bandaging should only be carried out by practitioners with the necessary experience since, if applied incorrectly, damage may result to the skin and/or superficial lymphatics.

Assessment

A full and careful assessment will highlight the patient's main problems and any co-existing complications. This information is then used to set realistic treatment goals and to determine the initial treatment approach. Assessment should establish:

(1) The cause and type of oedema (lymphoedema, venous oedema).
(2) The degree and extent of the swelling.
(3) The duration of the swelling.
(4) Any distortion in limb shape.
(5) The condition of the skin.
(6) The degree of mobility in the limb.
(7) Any obstruction to blood flow.
(8) Symptoms and causes of pain.
(9) Neurological impairment.

In order to monitor the effectiveness of support or compression in the management of chronic oedema, a reliable method of assessing response to treatment is the measurement of limb volume.

References and further reading

Badger, C. M. A. (1987) Lymphoedema: Management of patients with advanced cancer. *Professional Nurse*, 2(4), 200–2.

Badger, C. M. A. & Regnard, C. F. B. (1989) Oedema in advanced disease: a flow diagram. *Palliative Medicine*, 3, 213–15.

Badger, C. M. A. & Twycross, R. G. (1988) *The Management of Lymphoedema – Guidelines*. Sobell Study Centre, Oxford.

Foldi, M. (1983) Lymphology today. *Angiology*, February, 84–90.

Foldi, E. *et al.* (1985) Conservative treatment of lymphoedema of the limbs. *Angiology*, 36, 171–80.

Kissen, M. W. *et al.* (1986) Risk of lymphoedema following the treatment of breast cancer. *British Journal of Surgery*, 73, 580–4.

Leduc, O. *et al.* (1990) Bandages: scintigraphic demonstration of its efficacy on colloidal protein reabsorbtion during muscle activity. In: *Progress in Lymphology – XII: Excerpta Medica*, (eds M. Nishi, S. Uchino & S. Yabuki), pp. 421–3. Elsevier, Tokyo.

Levick, J. R. (1991) *An Introduction to Cardiovascular Physiology*, Chapter 9, Section 9.9. Butterworths, London.

Mortimer, P. S. (1990) Investigation and management of lymphoedema. *Vascular Medicine Review*, 1, 1–20.

Olszewski, W. L. & Engeset, A. (1990) Peripheral lymph dynamics. *Progress in Lymphology – XII, Excerpta Medica*, (eds M. Nishi, S. Uchino & S. Yabuki), pp. 213–14. Elsevier, Tokyo.

Prasad, A. *et al.* (1990) Leg ulcers and oedema: a study exploring the prevalence, aetiology and possible significance of oedema in venous ulcers. *Phlebology*, 5, 181–7.

Stillwell, G. K. (1973) The law of Laplace: some clinical applications. *Mayo Clinic Proceedings*, December, 48, 863–9.

Stillwell, G. K. (1977) Management of arm oedema. In: *Breast Cancer Management: Early and Late*, (ed. B. A. Stoll). Royal Free Hospital, London.

Thomas, S. (1991a) Bandages and bandaging: the science behind the art. *CARE Science and Practice*, 8(2), 56–60.

Thomas, S. (1991b) Bandages and bandaging. *Nursing Standard*, Special Supplement 8, 4(39), 4–6.

MEASUREMENT OF LIMB VOLUME CALCULATED FROM SURFACE MEASUREMENTS

Definition

The measurement of limb volume is calculated from a series of circumference measurements taken along the length of a limb, using the formula for the volume of a cylinder.

Indications

To monitor the size of oedematous limbs, thereby determining the effectiveness of interventions designed to reduce the size of limbs.

REFERENCE MATERIAL

A variety of methods exists, including:

- Volume measured by water displacement (Kettle *et al.*, 1958; Engler & Sweat, 1962);
- Volume measured electronically (Fischbach *et al.*, 1986; Blume *et al.*, 1992); and
- Volume calculated from surface measurements (Lennihan & Mackereth, 1973; Kuhnke, 1978; Stranden, 1981).

Each method could be said to have its own advantages and disadvantages. Volume calculated from surface measurements is described here since it is a method that is uncomplicated, requires no expensive equipment and, providing care is taken with the procedure for measurement, is a method that is accurate and reproducible (Badger, unpublished observations).

A number of formulae can be used to calculate volume from circumferences, the method described here uses the formula for volume of a cylinder (Fig. 19.1). This formula assumes that one cylinder has a height of 4 cm. It is important to note that measurement of body weight taken alongside limb measurements will allow a more accurate interpretation of any changes seen in limb size over time. Volume measurements are preferred to single measurements of the girth of the limb since measurement of the total volume of the limb provides a great deal more information than measurement of a single point (Stillwell, 1977).

The formula for calculating the volume of a cylinder is $\dfrac{circumference^2}{\pi}$. The formula must be applied to each circumference measurement ($circ_1$, $circ_2$, ... $circ_n$) in order to calculate the volume of each segment; the volumes are totalled to give the total limb volume.

$$\text{So} \left(\frac{circ_1 \times circ_1}{3.1415} \right) + \left(\frac{circ_2 \times circ_2}{3.1415} \right) + \left(\frac{circ_3 \times circ_3}{3.1415} \right)$$
$$+ \ldots \text{etc.}$$

Use of a programmable calculator will speed up the process of calculation.

Figure 19.1 Procedure for calculating volume from circumferences.

At the start of treatment volume measurements can be used to determine:

(1) The total excess volume of the swollen limb compared to the patient's contralateral normal limb.
(2) The distribution of the swelling along the limb.

Once treatment has begun measurement can be used to determine:

(1) Changes in the size of the swollen limb over time.
(2) The distribution of any loss or gain in the size of the limb.

Treatment can be adapted to take account of any of the above changes.

In order to ensure reproducibility and accuracy when measuring, particularly if more than one person is involved in carrying out measurements, adherence to a set protocol is essential. The following points should be borne in mind when establishing a protocol.

The position of the limb will affect the measurements taken from it: the degree to which muscles are flexed or relaxed will affect the shape and size of the limb at any particular point. Once a standard position has been decided upon, the same position must be adopted by the patient for all subsequent measurements. The positions suggested here are comfortable for both subject and measurer and are easily reproduced.

The limb should be marked afresh when measuring on consecutive days. The previous day's marks cannot be relied upon, since they will have shifted if the limb has increased or decreased in size.

No tension should be exerted on the tape measure by the measurer since no two people will use the same amount of tension. A tape measure fitted with weights or a pre-tensioned tape measure are two simple ways of overcoming the problem of varying tension.

A standard format for recording measurements should be decided upon. Information should be presented in such a way as to be easily read, with the key points of interest, such as the percentage bigger than normal, loss or gain in volume, etc., clearly identified. Make sure that everyone involved in measuring uses the record charts in the same way. The starting point for measurements, at the wrist or ankle, should always be

recorded accurately since even a small error here will throw out all other measurements along the limb.

The patient's normal limb (in cases of unilateral swelling) would not be expected to change significantly in volume except when there has been significant weight loss or gain, vigorous exercise immediately prior to measurement or a significant change in the ambient temperature; it therefore acts as the patient's own control.

References

Blume, J. *et al.* (1992) Quantification of oedema using the Volometer technique: therapeutic application of Daflon 500 mg in chronic venous insufficiency. *Phlebology*, Supplement 2, 37–40.

Engler, H. S. & Sweat, R. D. (1962) Volumetric arm measurements: technique and results. *American Surgery*, 28, 465–8.

Fischbach, J. U. *et al.* (1986) Messungen von Armödemen durch optoelektronische Volumetrie. In: *Phlebologie und Proktologie, Ergebnisse aus Klinik und Praxis*, (ed. H. Fischer). Schattauer Verlag, Stuttgart.

Kettle, J. H. *et al.* (1958) Measurement of upper limb volumes: a clinical method. *Australian and New Zealand Journal of Surgery*, 27, 263–70.

Kuhnke, E. (1978) Statistischer Wirksamkeitsnachweis der Manuellen Lymphdrainage nach Vodder-Asdonk. In: *Lympho-Kinetics – Proceedings of the International Colloquium, Brussels*, (eds A. Leduc & P. Lievens). Birkhauser Verlag, Stuttgart.

Lennihan, R. & Mackereth, M. (1973) Calculating volume changes in a swollen extremity from surface measurements. *American Journal of Surgery*, 126, 649–52.

Stillwell, G. K. (1977) Management of arm oedema. In: *Breast Cancer Management: Early and Late*, (ed. B. A. Stoll). Royal Free Hospital, London.

Stranden, E. (1981) A comparison between surface measurements and water displacement volumetry for the quantification of leg oedema. *Journal of Oslo City Hospital*, 31, 153–5.

GUIDELINES: THE APPLICATION OF ELASTIC HOSIERY AND ELASTICATED SURGICAL TUBULAR STOCKINETTE

The application of hosiery is made easier by applying any necessary moisturizing creams at night-time, rather than in the morning just before putting on a sleeve or stocking. A very light layer of talcum powder applied to hot, sticky skin will also ease application. If this is the first time a patient has worn compression hosiery, explain that the feeling of pressure may seem strange for the first few hours but that it should not cause pain.

PROCEDURE FOR APPLYING HOSIERY TO THE LEG

Action	Rationale
1 Explain and discuss the procedure with the patient.	To ensure that the patient understands the procedure and gives his/her valid consent.

Guidelines: The application of elastic hosiery and elasticated surgical tubular stockinette (cont'd)

Action	Rationale
2 If possible, position the patient seated upright on a bed or couch and raise the height to a comfortable level.	To ensure the comfort of both the patient and nurse.
3 Turn the stocking inside-out to the heel.	This makes it easier to ease the stocking up.
4 Pull the foot of the stocking over the patient's foot.	
5 Turn the top of the stocking back over the foot and up the leg.	
6 Ask the patient to keep the leg straight and if possible to push against the nurse.	
7 Starting at the foot, gradually ease the stocking over the heel and up the leg a bit at a time.	
Do not pull from the top. Remember that since it is the material of the stocking that provides the pressure, it must be distributed evenly to ensure an even distribution of pressure.	This will cause the stocking top to become overstretched and will lead to an uneven distribution of the stocking material.
8 Once the stocking is in place, check that there are no creases or wrinkles, particularly around the joints.	Wrinkles cause chafing of the skin and constricting bands of pressure.
9 Check that the patient finds the stocking comfortable and ask that any feelings of pain, tingling or numbness be reported.	Pain, tingling or numbness indicate that the stocking has been either inappropriately applied or fitted.
10 To remove the stocking, simply peel off the limb from the top downwards. Do not roll it down.	Rolling the stocking can result in tight bands of material forming, which are difficult to move.

PROCEDURE FOR APPLYING HOSIERY TO THE ARM

Action	Rationale
1 Explain and discuss the procedure with the patient.	To ensure that the patient understands the procedure and gives his/her valid consent.
2 The patient may be seated or standing.	
3 Turn the sleeve inside-out to the wrist. Pull over the patient's hand.	
Note: If the handpiece is separate from the sleeve, always put the handpiece on before the sleeve.	To avoid increasing swelling in the hand.
4 Turn the top of the sleeve back over the hand and up the arm.	
5 Ask the patient to grip something stable, such as a towel rail or the back of a chair.	This steadies the arm and gives the patient something to pull against.

| 6 | Working from the hand or wrist, gradually ease the sleeve up the arm. | This will cause the top to become overstretched and will result in an uneven distribution of pressure. |

Do not pull up from the top. Remember that since it is the material that provides the pressure, it must be evenly distributed to ensure an even distribution of pressure.

| 7 | Once the sleeve is in place, check that there are no creases or wrinkles, particularly around the joints. | Wrinkles and creases cause chafing of the skin and constricting bands of pressure. |

| 8 | Check that the patient finds the sleeve comfortable and ask that any signs of pain, tingling or numbness be reported. | |

| 9 | To remove the sleeve simply peel off the limb from the top. Do not roll it down. | Rolling the sleeve down can lead to tight bands of material forming which are difficult to move. |

GUIDELINES: CALCULATION OF LIMB VOLUME

EQUIPMENT

1 Ruler, preferably 30 cm or longer.
2 Tape measure; avoid those made from fabric which tends to stretch.
3 Felt tip pen for marking the limb.
4 Record chart and pen.

PROCEDURE FOR MEASURING LOWER LIMBS

Action

1 Place the patient in a sitting position with the legs outstretched horizontally, preferably on a firm couch with adjustable height.

2 Standing on the outside of the leg, ask the patient to flex the foot to a right angle. Measure the distance from the base of the heel to the ankle, along the inside of the leg; mark the ankle, allowing at least 2 cm of leg to lie below the mark, and record the distance on the chart.

3 Ask the patient to relax the foot. From the starting point mark the inside of the leg at 4 cm intervals along the length of the leg up to the groin; use the ruler for this.

4 Place the tape measure around the limb and measure the circumference at each marked point, recording each measurement on the chart. Make sure that the tape lies smoothly around the relaxed limb and that it does not lie at an angle. Decide at the outset whether the tape is to be placed above, below or on the mark and keep to the same position every time.

Rationale

The lower limbs are relaxed and supported and the adjustable height means that the measurer can work without straining the back.

This establishes a reproducible fixed starting point for all subsequent measurements.
Note: The marks represent a point midway through each cylinder segment, they do not represent the base of the cylinder, therefore at least half the segment (i.e. 2 cm) must lie below the mark

Reducing the limb to 4 cm segments improves the accuracy of measurement since these segments resemble a cylinder more closely than does the whole limb. The formula used here assumes that the measurements are 4 cm apart.

Ensuring that there are no gaps between the limb and the tape and ensuring that the procedure is the same each time reduces error.

Guidelines: Calculation of limb volume (cont'd)

Action	Rationale
5 Repeat the process on the other leg, whether or not it is swollen.	If only one limb is affected the normal limb acts as the patient's own control.
6 If desired, a circumference measurement may be taken of the foot but this is *not* included in the calculation of volume.	The foot cannot be considered to be a cylinder and it is therefore inappropriate to include it in the calculation of volume.

PROCEDURE FOR MEASURING UPPER LIMBS

Action	Rationale
1 Sit the patient in a chair with the arms extended in front and resting on the back of a chair. The arms should be as close to an angle of 90° to the body as possible.	The arms are supported and accessible at a standard height. Changing the angle of the arms to the body will result in changes in the measurements.
2 Measure the distance from the tip of the middle finger to the wrist. Mark the wrist, allowing at least 2cm from where the hand joins the arm, and note down the distance.	This establishes a reproducible fixed starting point for all subsequent measurements. *Note:* The marks represent a point midway through each cylinder segment, they do not represent the base of the cylinder, therefore at least half the segment (i.e. 2cm) must lie below the mark.
3 From the starting point mark along the length of the arm at 4cm intervals up to the axilla; use the ruler for this.	Reducing the limb to 4cm segments improves the accuracy of measurement since these segments resemble a cylinder more closely than does the whole limb.
4 Place the tape measure around the limb and measure the circumference at each marked point, recording each measurement on the chart. Make sure that the tape lies smoothly around the relaxed limb and that it does not lie at an angle. Decide at the outset whether the tape is to be placed above, below or on the mark and keep to the same position every time.	Ensuring that there are no gaps between the limb and the tape and ensuring that the procedure is the same each time reduces error.
5 Repeat the process on the other arm whether or not it is swollen.	If only one limb is affected the normal limb acts as the patient's own control.
6 If desired, a circumference measurement may be taken of the hand but this is *not* included in the calculation of volume.	The hand cannot be considered to be a cylinder and it is therefore inappropriate to include it in the calculation.

REDUCTION PHASE OF TREATMENT

A number of treatments are used in combination during the management of chronic oedema. Their choice and usefulness is determined by the therapist following a careful physical, psychological and psychosocial assessment of the patient which should include how the patient feels about the swelling and the influence that it may have upon his or her role in life. Information acquired during this assessment enables treatment of the swelling to be planned realistically around the needs of the patient (Woods, 1995).

Indications

Elements of treatment used in the management of chronic oedema:

(1) External graduated pressure: to improve or maintain the size, shape and condition of the swollen limb.
(2) Manual lymph drainage/simple self-massage: to stimulate lymphatic vessels and move excess fluid away from the root of the swollen limb and the adjacent quadrant of the trunk.
(3) Skin care: to preserve skin integrity and prevent infection.
(4) Limb movement and positioning: to enhance lymph drainage using the force of gravity and gentle muscle movement.
(5) Exercises: to promote joint mobility and lymph drainage using the pumping action of the muscles (Hodkinson, 1992).

A combination of these elements of treatment should be used if results are to be achieved. The choice will depend upon the degree and extent of the swelling in addition to the patient's ability and motivation.

Treatment can be approached in two phases: the reduction or intensive phase of treatment and the maintenance phase (Badger, 1992). The difference between the phases is primarily focused upon the choice of external graduated pressure applied to the swollen limb. In the reduction phase of treatment, external support is provided with short-stretch extensible bandages whilst in the maintenance phase of treatment, elastic hosiery is used to provide compression. Not all patients will follow both phases of treatment and many may only need to follow the maintenance phase.

The intensive or reduction phase should always be carried out by a skilled therapist with the necessary experience to apply bandages to the swollen limb, ensuring that pressure is graduated towards the root of the limb and applied evenly. Damage to the skin and tissues can occur if bandages are incorrectly or inappropriately applied (Thomas, 1990).

Indications for the reduction or intensive phase of treatment:

(1) Large limbs: containment hosiery used on large swollen limbs may be ineffective due to the difficulties of applying sufficient tension to compress the limb (Stillwell, 1973).
(2) Misshapen limbs: containment hosiery will promote the development of deep skin folds when the limb is awkwardly shaped. Foam or soft padding under bandages will smooth out the folds and restore normal shape to the limb.
(3) Severe lymphoedema: large limbs with long-standing oedema require high pressures to break down tissue fibrosis. Bandages provide a low resting and high active pressure which enables hardened tissues to soften.
(4) Lymphorrhoea: the leakage of lymph fluid from the skin responds readily to external pressure provided by bandages.
(5) Damaged or fragile skin: containment hosiery can cause damage to fragile skin. Bandages should be used until the skin condition improves (Mortimer et al., 1993).

Palliative care

Bandaging can be versatile and extremely useful in the palliative care setting when volume reduction may be unrealistic or not indicated. Support and comfort can be provided to a limb using a low level of pressure with a modified technique of bandaging designed around the patient's needs. The bandages can be left in place for 2–3 days and should not prevent the patient from maintaining full movement in their bandaged limb (Mortimer et al., 1993).

Principles to be followed in multi-layer bandaging

Low-stretch bandages should always be used. These provide a low resting pressure to the swollen limb when the muscle is inactive and a high working pressure during activity when the muscle is pumping against the resistance created by the bandage (Staudinger, 1993). The bandages should provide an even pressure around the circumference of the limb (Thomas, 1990). In awkwardly shaped limbs this can be achieved with the use of soft foam or padding to smoothe out skin folds and promote a suitable profile. The pressure from the bandages should be graduated towards the root of the limb with the greatest pressure over the hand or foot, gradually reducing as the limb is bandaged upwards. This is achieved by controlling the amount of bandage tension and overlap used. Moderate tension only should be maintained on the bandages. The bandages should never be stretched to their maximum length.

The bandages should be left in place day and night and removed once every 24 hours. This enables skin hygiene to be attended to and the condition of the skin to be checked. Re-application of the bandages then ensures that effective compression is maintained on the changing limb shape (Staudinger, 1993).

The bandages should be comfortable for the patient and removed at any time if they cause any pain, numbness or discoloration (blueness) in the fingers or toes. This may indicate a variety of causes including too great a compression on the limb. A satisfactory outcome of treatment should be achieved within 2–3 weeks. The patient may then begin the maintenance phase of treatment where containment hosiery is fitted.

Evaluation of the bandaging procedure

Evaluation of each stage of the bandaging procedure is essential to ensure that the bandage and padding have been used appropriately and correctly.

The process of evaluation must be thorough and exhaustive and should include:

(1) Continuous attention to the colour of the digits. Too much pressure will result in compromised circulation.
(2) Continuous attention to the sensations experienced in the bandaged limb. The bandages should not cause pain, numbness or tingling.
(3) The shape of the limb. A cylindrical contour should be achieved with the use of soft foam and padding.
(4) The overlap of the bandages. This should be even and consistent with no gaps in the bandages.
(5) The pressure achieved. This should feel even to the patient and there should be no creases in the bandages. Layers should be used appropriately.

Patient evaluation

The patient should feel comfortable and able to move their limb. Information should be given concerning when and how to remove the bandages if necessary.

References

Badger, C. (1992) *Lymphoedema: Assessment and Management.* Educational Leaflet No 13, Wound Care Society, Northampton.

Caseley-Smith, J. & Caseley-Smith, J. R. (1994) *Modern Treatment for Lymphoedema.* The Henry Thomas Laboratory, University of Adelaide, Adelaide.

Hodkinson, M. (1992) Lymphoedema: applying physiology to treatment. *European Journal of Cancer Care*, 1(2), 19–23.

Mortimer, P. *et al.* (1993) Lymphoedema. In: *Textbook of Palliative Medicine*, (eds D. Doyle, G. Hanks & N. McDonald). Oxford Medical Publications, Oxford.

Staudinger, P. (1993) Compression bandaging for lymphoedema. *National Lymphoedema Network Newsletter USA*, 5(3), 5–6.

Stemmer, R. *et al.* (1980) Compression Treatment of the Lower Extremities particularly with Compression Stockings. *The Dermatologist*, 31, 355–65.

Stillwell, G. K. (1973) The law of Laplace: some clinical applications. *Mayo Clinic Proceedings*, 48, 863–9.

Thomas, S. (1990) Bandages and bandaging. *Nursing Standard*, 4(39).

Woods, M. (1995) Sociological factors and psychosocial implications of lymphoedema. *International Journal of Palliative Nursing*, 1(1), 17–20.

GUIDELINES: STANDARD MULTI-LAYER COMPRESSION BANDAGING

This procedure should not be attempted by anyone who has not had specialist education in this area. The swollen limb should be clean and well moisturized with a bland cream (e.g. E45) before being bandaged. Pressure must be applied in a graduated profile, i.e. highest over the hand or foot, and gradually reducing as the limb is bandaged upwards, to ensure that fluid is encouraged to drain towards the root of the limb. The degree of pressure is influenced by:

1 The circumference of the limb – pressure will be highest over a small circumference and lowest over a large circumference (Laplace's law (Stillwell, 1973)).
2 The amount of tension placed on the bandage.
3 The amount of bandage overlap.
4 The number of bandage layers (Thomas, 1990).

Thus, on a normally shaped limb, maintaining the same amount of bandage tension and the same amount of bandage overlap all the way up the limb will result in a natural graduation of pressure due to the gradual increase in the size of the limb from ankle to groin, or wrist to axilla. In cases where swelling has distorted the shape of the limb, additional padding is used to create a suitable profile on which to bandage, and adjustments may be needed in bandage tension and bandage overlap. Very large limbs may also require extra layers of bandage to be used in order to ensure that sufficient pressure is applied (Badger & Twycross, 1988).

EQUIPMENT FOR BANDAGING AN ARM

1 Stockinette.
2 Light retention bandages, 6 cm and 10 cm to bandage digits and to hold foam padding in place.

3 Padding, 6 cm roll.
4 Foam.
5 Low-stretch compression bandages, 6 cm and 8 cm.
6 Tape.
7 Scissors.

PROCEDURE

Action	Rationale

1 Explain and discuss the procedure with the patient.

To ensure that the patient understands the procedure and gives his/her valid consent.

2 If possible, the patient should be seated in a chair. The nurse should be positioned in front of the patient.

To ensure the comfort of both the patient and nurse.

3 Cut a length of stockinette long enough to fit the patient's arm. Cut a small hole for the thumb and slip over the patient's arm.

To protect the skin from chafing.

4 The fingers must be bandaged (Fig. 19.2). Using a narrow light retention bandage anchor the bandage loosely at the wrist and bring across the back of the hand to the thumb. Bandage around the thumb from the tip downwards (start at the level of the nail bed). Do not pull the bandage tight but go gently and firmly. Take the bandage under the wrist and back over the back of the hand to the index finger (Fig. 19.3). Again, bandage from the nail bed down to the webs of the finger. Repeat the same procedure for all fingers. Finish by tucking in the end of the bandage (Fig. 19.4).

To reduce or prevent swelling.

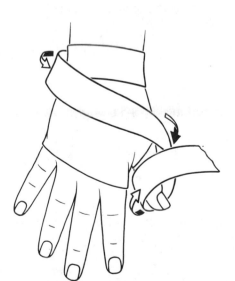

Figure 19.2 Bandaging swollen fingers.

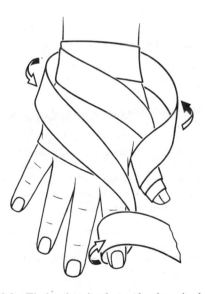

Figure 19.3 The bandage is taken under the wrist, back over the hand, to the index finger.

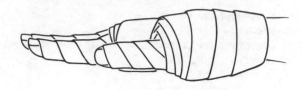

Figure 19.5   The palm and back of the hand are padded out.

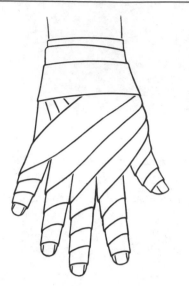

Figure 19.4   The finished bandage.

Guidelines: Standard multi-layer compression bandaging (cont'd)

Action	Rationale
5 Check the colour and temperature of the tips of the fingers.	To ensure that the blood supply is not compromised.
6 Check that the patient can move the fingers and make a fist.	To check that the bandage is not too tight.
7 Using the roll of padding, cover the hand in a figure of eight, padding out the palm and back of the hand (Fig. 19.5).	Padding out the hand ensures even pressure distribution and protects the bony areas of the hand.
8 Cut foam to fit the length of the arm from the wrist to axilla. Ensure that the width is sufficient to encircle the arm with a small overlap.	To protect the elbow joint and provide a smooth, even profile on which to bandage.
9 Wrap the foam around the arm, securing with a light retention bandage. Finish by tucking in the end of the bandage (Fig. 19.6).	
10 Take a 6 cm compression bandage and start by anchoring it loosely at the wrist. Bandage the hand firmly in a figure of eight until all of the hand is covered (Fig. 19.7). Continue the rest of the bandage up the forearm in a spiral, covering half of the bandage with each turn. Keep the bandage as smooth as possible.	To avoid constriction at the wrist.
11 Take an 8 or 10 cm bandage and, starting at the wrist, bandage in a spiral, still covering half of the bandage with each turn, up to the top of the arm (Fig. 19.8).	Two layers are used on the forearm to ensure that pressure is highest distally.
12 Secure the end of the bandage with tape.	

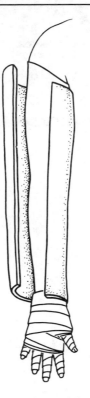

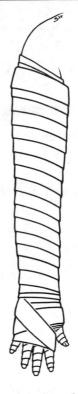

Figure 19.6 Foam is wrapped around the arm, secured with a light retention bandage.

Figure 19.8 Starting at the wrist, an 8 cm or 10 cm bandage is used to cover to the top of the arm, in a spiral fashion.

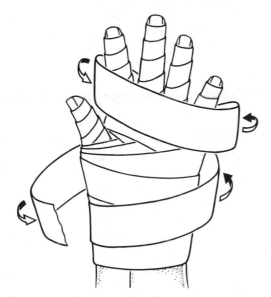

Figure 19.7 The hand is bandaged firmly in a figure of eight using a 6 cm compression bandage.

Guidelines: Standard multi-layer compression bandaging (cont'd)

Action	Rationale
13 Once again, check the colour and sensations of the finger tips and check that the patient can move all joints.	To check that the blood flow is not compromised.
14 Remind the patient to use the limb as normally as possible and to report any feelings of discomfort, tingling or numbness.	To ensure good lymph flow.

EQUIPMENT FOR BANDAGING A LEG

1 Stockinette.
2 Light retention bandages, 6 cm and 10 cm or 12 cm.
3 Padding, 10 cm and 20 cm.
4 Foam.
5 Low-stretch compression bandages, 8 cm, 10 cm and 12 cm.
6 Tape.
7 Scissors.

PROCEDURE FOR BANDAGING A LEG AND THE TOES

Action	Rationale
1 Explain and discuss the procedure with the patient.	To ensure that the patient understands the procedure and gives his/her valid consent.
2 If possible, the patient should be seated upright on a bed or treatment couch. Raise the bed or couch to a comfortable height.	To ensure the comfort of both the patient and nurse.
3 Cut a length of stockinette long enough to fit the patient's leg. Slip over the leg.	To protect the skin from chafing.
4 If the toes are swollen or have a tendency to swell they must be bandaged. The little toe can be omitted.	To reduce or prevent swelling. To prevent friction to and around the little toe.
Using a narrow light retention bandage anchor the bandage around the foot and bring across the top of the foot to the big toe (Fig. 19.9). Bandage around the toe from the tip downwards (start at the level of the nail bed). Do not pull the bandage tight but gently and firmly. Take the bandage under the foot and back over the top of the foot to the next toe (Fig. 19.10). Repeat the same procedure for each toe that needs to be bandaged. Finish by tucking in the end of the bandage (Fig. 19.11).	
5 Cut the foam into pads to fit over the dorsum of the foot, around the ankle (Fig. 19.12) and behind the knee (Fig. 19.13).	To protect bony prominences and joint flexures.
6 Secure the pads firmly in place with light retention bandages.	

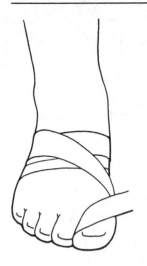

Figure 19.9

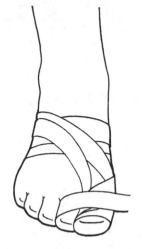

Figure 19.10

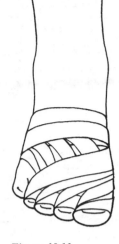

Figure 19.11

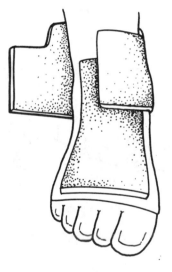

Figure 19.12 Foam is used to cover the dorsum of the foot and around the ankle.

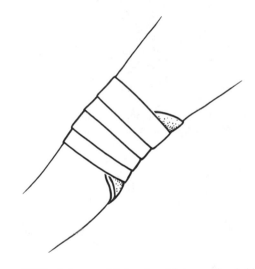

Figure 19.13 A foam pad is bandaged into position behind the knee.

7 Using a 10 cm roll of padding, apply firmly in a spiral up the leg, starting around the foot. Use the 20 cm padding over the thigh (Fig. 19.14).

To protect the skin and create a smooth profile on which to bandage.

8 Take an 8 cm compression bandage and start by anchoring it loosely at the ankle. Bandage the foot, starting as close as possible to the toes (Fig. 19.15). Use a spiral over the instep, covering half of the bandage with each turn, and use a figure of eight over the heel and ankle.
Bandage firmly and do not leave any gaps.

To avoid constriction at the ankle.

Fluid will accumulate in any unbandaged areas.

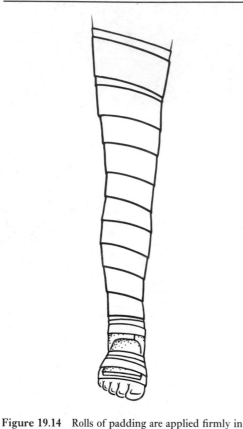

Figure 19.14 Rolls of padding are applied firmly in a spiral up the leg, starting around the foot.

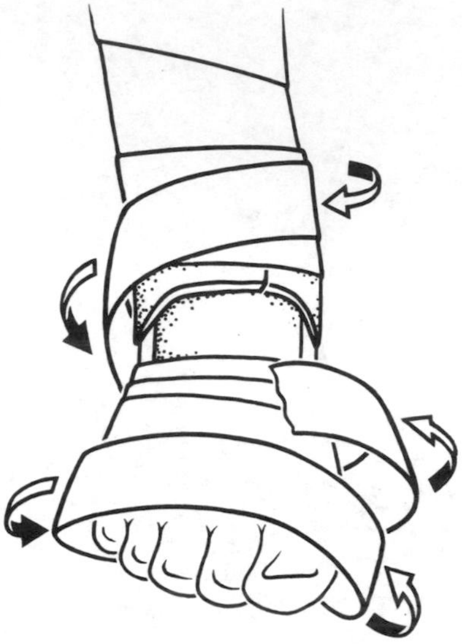

Figure 19.15 Bandaging the foot using an 8 cm compression bandage and starting close to the toes.

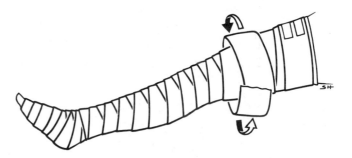

Figure 19.16 Applying a second layer of bandage, from ankle to thigh.

Guidelines: Standard multi-layer compression bandaging (cont'd)

Action	Rationale
9 Using a 10 cm bandage, continue from where the first bandage finished, using a spiral up the leg and covering half of the bandage with each turn. Remember to bandage firmly. Use the widest bandage over the thigh. Secure the end of the last bandage with tape.	
10 Apply a second layer of bandage, from ankle to thigh, using a figure of eight. Secure the end with tape (Fig. 19.16).	
11 Check the colour and temperature of the patient's toes. It may be difficult for the	To check that the blood flow is not compromised.

patient to flex the knee at first but this should get easier as the bandages loosen slightly.

12 Remind the patient to use the limb as normally as possible and to report any feelings of discomfort, tingling or numbness.

To ensure good lymph flow.

CHAPTER 20

Eye Care

Indications

Eye care may be necessary under the following circumstances:

(1) To relieve pain and discomfort.
(2) To prevent infection.
(3) To prevent any further injury to the eye.
(4) Early detection of disease.
(5) Early detection of drug induced toxicities (Cloutier, 1992).

REFERENCE MATERIAL

Patients should be encouraged after instruction to carry out for themselves many of the procedures involved in eye care. However, the nurse is often involved in caring for the post-operative, very ill or unconscious patient. Infection can easily be transmitted, by careless technique, from one eye to another. In some cases this can lead to loss of sight.

Anatomy and physiology

The eyeball is protected from injury by the bony cavity of the orbit, the conjunctiva, the lacrimal apparatus, the eyebrows and the eyelashes.

The eyeball itself has three layers (Fig. 20.1):

(1) The outermost, composed of the cornea and sclera.
(2) The middle, composed of the choroid, ciliary body and iris (uveal tract).
(3) The innermost, composed of the retina, macula lutea (yellow spot) and fovea centralis.

The function of the outer coat is protective. The middle layer is vascular and pigmented, while the innermost layer contains the light-sensitive nerve endings concerned with vision, i.e. the rods and cones.

The blood vessels of the retina are seen readily with an ophthalmoscope. Abnormal changes in these vessels can be indicative of both generalized diseases, such as diabetes and hypertension, and diseases of the eye itself (Tortora & Anagnostakos, 1992).

The optic nerve (cranial II) has two tracts which cross over at the optic chiasma. Each tract supplies the opposite side of the body. These tracts enter the eyeball to the side of the macula lutea. This area is known as the optic disc and is an area of no vision (blind spot) (Fig. 20.2).

An additional blind spot or scotoma may be indicative of a brain tumour. In 90% of pituitary tumours there is a defect in the field of vision (Tortora & Anagnostakos, 1992).

The inside of the eye is divided by the lens into two chambers: the aqueous chamber anterior to the lens (containing clear, watery fluid called aqueous humour); and the vitreous chamber posterior to the lens, filled with a jelly-like substance, the vitreous humour, or vitreous body. The aqueous chamber is divided into anterior and posterior chambers, located in front of, and behind the iris, respectively (Marieb, 1989) (Fig. 20.3).

The aqueous humour is secreted into the posterior chamber by choroid plexuses of the ciliary processes of the ciliary bodies behind the iris. This fluid then permeates the posterior chamber and passes between the iris and the lens, through the pupil, into the anterior chamber. From the anterior chamber the aqueous humour, which is produced continually, is drained off into the scleral venous sinus (canal of Schlemm) and then into the blood. The intraocular pressure is produced mainly by the aqueous humour, which together with the vitreous humour helps to counteract the pull of the extrinsic eye muscles and maintain the shape of the eyeball. Glaucoma is a disease which can cause degeneration of the retina and blindness due to the excessive intraocular pressure. The aqueous humour also acts as the principal link between the cardiovascular system, the lens and the cornea (Marieb, 1989).

The tears are produced in the lacrimal gland (Fig. 20.4). Their function is to wash over the eyeball, removing any foreign substances and providing antisepsis by the action of the enzyme lysozyme. Lysozymes can rupture the cell walls of some bacteria and cause their lysis

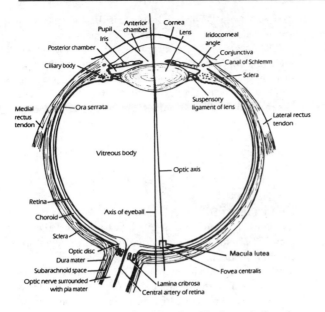

Figure 20.1 Horizontal section through the eyeball at the level of the optic nerve. The optic axis and the axis of the eyeball are included.

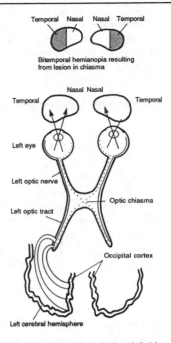

Figure 20.2 Visual pathways and visual fields.

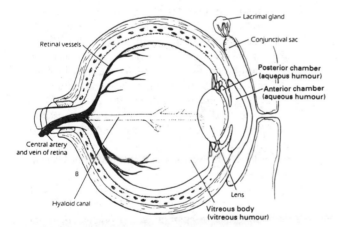

Figure 20.3 The anterior cavity in front of the lens is incompletely divided into the anterior chamber (anterior to the iris) and the posterior chamber (behind the iris), which are continuous through the pupil. Aqueous humour, which fills the cavity, is formed by the ciliary processes and reabsorbed into the venous blood by the canal of Schlemm.

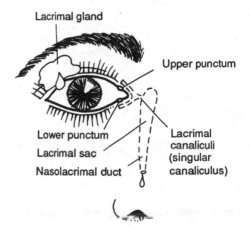

Figure 20.4 Lacrimal apparatus.

or death (e.g. Gram-negative bacteria). The tears drain through the lacrimal puncti into the nasolacrimal duct. In health, the surface of the eye should always be slightly moist. The cornea has no blood vessels and is dependant on tears and aqueous humour for its nourishment (Marieb, 1989).

General principles of eye care
Aseptic technique is necessary only in certain circumstances, for example, when the eye is damaged or following ophthalmic surgery.

Position of the patient

Where possible, the patient should be lying down with the head tilted backwards and the chin pointing upwards. This enables ease of access to the eyes and is a good position for patient comfort and ease of compliance.

Position of the light source

A good light source before commencing eye procedures is necessary in order to be able to assess carefully the state of the eyes and to avoid damaging their delicate structures during the procedure. The positions of the patient and the nurse in relation to the light source are vital in order for the procedure to be carried out safely and efficiently. The light should be above and behind the nurse or to the side. Light should never be allowed to shine directly into the patient's eyes as this will be painful for the patient.

Instillation of drops

Most types of drops are instilled into the outer rim of the lower fornix (part of the conjunctiva overlying the cornea) as the conjunctiva is less sensitive than the cornea, and the outer rim avoids loss of the drops into the nasolacrimal passage. Exceptions to this are as follows:

(1) *Drugs used to lubricate the cornea*: these should be directed into the lower fornix. Oil-based drops produce less corneal reaction than aqueous ones as they do not feel as cold to the cornea when administered.
(2) *Anaesthetic drops*: the first drop should be instilled into the conjunctiva for absorption and then directly onto the cornea one drop at a time until the patient is no longer able to feel the drops.
(3) *Drops used to treat the nasal passages*: these should be instilled at the punctal end of the eye.

The number of drops used depends on the type of solution used and its purpose. Usually, one drop only is ordered and will be sufficient if it is instilled in the correct manner. The exceptions to the 'one drop' rule are:

(1) Oil-based solutions: these are used for lubricating the eyeball, one drop being instilled and repeated as required.
(2) Anaesthetic drops: it is usual to instil two or three drops at a time at intervals, until the drop cannot be felt on the eye.

The dropper should be held as close to the eye as possible without touching either the lids or the cornea. This will avoid corneal damage and the risk of infection. If the drop falls from too great a height it is difficult to control and will also be uncomfortable for the patient.

There are a variety of droppers and bottles available, including pipettes, pipettes incorporated into the eye-drop bottle, plastic bottles and single-dose packs. Pipettes are easy to use but need drying and sterilizing between doses. Plastic bottles can be squeezed and so avoid the need for a pipette and are cheaper than glass bottles with a dropper. Ideally, single-dose containers should be used if they do not prove to be too expensive for routine use.

Eye irrigation

The most common use of eye irrigation is for the removal of caustic substances from the eye, e.g. domestic cleaning agents or (in the hospital setting) medications, particularly cytotoxic material. This should be done as soon as possible to minimize damage. The procedure is also used as a pre-operative preparation or to remove infected material. The lotion most commonly used is 0.9% sodium chloride. In an emergency tap water may be used (McConnell, 1991).

Care of the insensitive eye

Any interference with the sensory nerve supply to the eye, such as unconsciousness, will cause the eye reflex to become insensitive. The blink reflex is often lost, the eye's surface becomes dry and the cornea may be damaged. Corneal ulcers, infection, scarring and loss of vision may be the end result. When the patient has lost these protective reflex measures, the nurse must institute measures to replace them. The surface of the eye should be kept clean and moist by gentle swabbing of the eye with sterile saline and the instillation of artificial tears where necessary.

If there is no blink reflex the eyelids should be kept closed by the use of hypoallergenic tape or by the application of hydrogel preparations, e.g. Geliperm. If the eyes become infected the relevant medication should be applied.

With each of these measures care must be taken not to spread infection between the eyes. Any alteration to the appearance of the eye must be reported to the doctor.

Eye medications

Drugs may be given either systemically or topically to exert an effect on the eye. However, if given systemically the prescribing doctor needs to take account of the physiological barrier and the blood-aqueous barrier which exists within the eye and which is selective in allowing drugs to pass into the intraocular fluids. Perme-

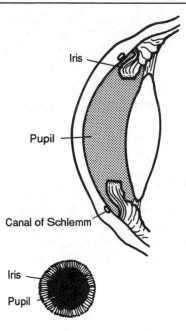

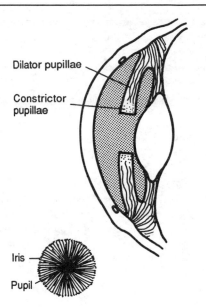

Figure 20.6   Effect of miotics.

Figure 20.5   Effect of mydriatics.

ability of this barrier may be altered in inflammatory conditions and following paracentesis.

Drugs applied locally meet some resistance at the tear film. The cornea allows the passage of water but not of drugs. This resistance may alter where there are corneal epithelial changes. Wetting agents may be employed to alter corneal permeability.

Many drugs will produce similar effects on a diseased or a healthy eye. Drugs for use in the eye are usually classified according to their action.

Mydriatics and cycloplegics

These drugs produce their effects by paralysing the ciliary muscle, by stimulating the dilator muscle of the pupil or by a combination of both (Fig. 20.5). They are used mainly for diagnostic purposes and most have an anticholinergic action. The most commonly used preparations are cyclopentolate 1% and tropicamide 1%.

Miotics

These drugs produce their effects by constricting the pupil and contracting the ciliary muscle (Fig. 20.6). Miotics help in the drainage of aqueous humour and are used primarily in the treatment of glaucoma.

Local anaesthetics

These render the eye and the inner surfaces of the lids insensitive. They are used before minor surgery,

removal of foreign bodies and tonometry. Cocaine is less used now as some patients develop an idiosyncrasy to it and may suddenly collapse after its use. Its effects do not wear off for at least half an hour after administration.

Anti-inflammatories

These may be steroids, antihistamines or pyrazole derivatives, such as oxyphenabutazone 10%. The most commonly used preparations are dexamethasone, prednisolone and betamethasone.

Corticosteroid eye drops should be used with caution as they can cause a serious rise in intraocular pressure in a small percentage of people (especially if they have a history of glaucoma).

Antibiotics

Antibiotics can be used in the active treatment of infection and as prophylactics both pre- and post-operatively, following removal of a foreign body or following an injury. Antibiotic preparations in common use are framycetin 0.5%, neomycin 0.5% and chloramphenicol 0.5%.

Artificial tears

Where tear deficiency exists due to disease processes, treatment with radiation or reduction of the blink reflex, artificial lubricants such as methyl cellulose or hypromellose may be used.

Toxic effects of common systemic drugs on the eye

As the eye may be the first place to show signs of systemic disease, so some systemic drugs may now show their toxic effects in the eye. These effects range from pruritis, irritation, redness, excess tear formation with overflow (epiphora), photophobia and blepharoconjunctivitis, to disturbance of vision (Cloutier, 1992). Particular effects of specific drugs are listed below:

(1) *Methotrexate and related antimetabolites*: these drugs can affect the Meibomian glands, causing blepharoconjunctivitis, and produce photophobia, epiphora, periorbital oedema and conjunctival hyperaemia.

(2) *5-Fluorouracil (5-FU)*: 5-FU can cause canalicular fibrosis and oculomotor disturbances (probably secondary to a local neurotoxicity affecting the brainstem).

(3) *Antihistamines*: these drugs decrease tear production and may lead to 'dry eye', especially in patients with Sjogren's syndrome or ocular pemphigus, in patients who wear contact lenses and in the elderly.

(4) *Tamoxifen*: this drug can cause subepithelial whirl-like, corneal deposits and retinal lesions.

(5) *Indomethacin*: this can cause corneal deposits and retinal pigmentary toxicity.

(6) *Oral contraceptives*: these can stimulate corneal steeping and intolerance to contact lenses.

(7) *Atropine, scopalamine and belladonna-like substances*: such drugs cause mydriasis and cycloplegia.

(8) *Corticosteroids*: prolonged use of corticosteroids produces posterior subcapsular cataracts.

(9) *Chloramphenicol*: chloramphenicol treatment can lead to optic neuritis.

(10) *Ethambutol*: this drug can cause damage to the optic nerve.

(11) *Rifampicin*: stains soft contact lenses.

(12) *Digoxin*: in overdose results in blurred vision and yellow/green vision.

(13) *Oxygen*: in neonates, high concentrations for a long period can cause retrolental fibroplasia.

Tumours of the orbit and eye

Orbital tumours are rare, but in children rhabdomyosarcoma is the most common primary tumour and in adults the commonest type seen is lymphoma (Char, 1993). Rarer tumours are meningiomas, soft tissue sarcoma, nerve and nerve sheath tumours, including optic nerve gliomas (Souhami & Tobias, 1987; Char, 1993). Primary and secondary tumours occur in the orbit, but it is a less common site of metastases than the eye (Henderson, 1980). Presentation of metastases to the orbit is indicative of a latent carcinoma elsewhere, and varies from a rapidly developing mass often incorporating adjacent tissue infiltration and bone destruction to slow scaring of soft tissue (Tijl *et al.*, 1992). Metastatic deposits are likely to be from carcinoma of the thyroid, bronchus, breast, prostate, kidney or skin (Souhami & Tobias, 1987; Tijl *et al.*, 1992).

The orbit

To appreciate spread of disease and clinical features of orbital and eye malignancies it is important to know the relationship of the orbit to other vital structures. The anterior cranial fossa lies superiorly, the nasal cavity and ethmoid labyrinth medially, the maxillary antrum inferiorly, and the infratemporal and middle cranial fossae laterally (Lund, 1987).

The average volume of the orbital cavity is 26 ml, and because the orbit is a fixed bony cavity an increase of orbital volume of 4 ml produces 6 mm of proptosis (Gorman, 1978).

Signs and symptoms

Most orbital tumours push the eye away from its normal visual axis in a sagittal or vertical plane. Displacement of the eye is a common diagnostic feature of an orbital tumour, and in almost all cases the direction of displacement is opposite to the position of the growing tumour (Moeloek, 1993). Proptasis is the main clinical feature. Lack of room for growth due to the bony cavity causes the eye to proptose, often to a large degree, which is both disfiguring and distressing for the patient (Lund, 1987; Souhami & Tobias, 1987; Tijl *et al.*, 1992; Char, 1993; Moeloek, 1993).

Panopthalmitis (inflammation of tissues of the eyeball) can cause perforation of the globe, and unilateral blindness is common with advanced tumours (Souhami & Tobias, 1987). Opthalmoplegia (paralysis of some or all of the muscles of the eye) could occur if there is interference with the external ocular muscles or due to third nerve palsy (Souhami & Tobias, 1987). Chemosis (swelling of the conjunctival tissue around the cornea) and infection are common and could lead to a misdiagnosis of cellulitis (Souhami & Tobias, 1987).

Visual changes occur with tumours that involve the optic nerve, or its sheath, or that externally press against its surface. Diplopia, tearing, a visible tumour mass, ptosis (dropping of the upper eyelid due to loss of control by the III cranial nerve), epiphora (persistent overflow of tears) and pain are other clinical features (Lund, 1987; Souhami & Tobias, 1987; Tijl *et al.*, 1992; Char, 1993; Moeloek, 1993).

Tumours of the eyelid and conjunctiva

Basal cell and squamous cell carcinomas (SCC) are fairly common tumours of the eyelid, the lower lid and inner canthus being the commonest areas affected. Tumours frequently occur in the elderly (Henk, 1976).

Melanoma and squamous cell carcinoma are occasionally found in the conjunctiva. Early diagnosis is essential as small lesions may be effectively treated by radiotherapy, conserving the eye and preserving vision. However, in most cases local surgical excision is advised, with post-operative radiation. It is essential that a specialist opinion is sought to differentiate a true melanoma from precancerous ocular melanosis (a diffuse flat pigmented lesion), which can be clinically diagnosed with confidence, and observed without biopsy, because any malignant change could take years to develop. The overall prognosis of conjunctival melanoma is good, with a 5 year survival of about 75%. Patients presenting with bulky lesions have a high risk of early fatal dissemination. Those patients with SCC have an improved prognosis if early diagnosis and correct treatment of surgery and/or radiotherapy is given (Souhami & Tobias, 1987).

Tumours of the globe

Retinoblastoma (hereditary malignant tumour of the retina) and uveal (choroidal) melanoma are the two main tumours. The choroid is a vascular membrane, containing large branched pigment cells, which lies between the retina and sclera of the eye. The commonest intra-ocular tumour of adults is malignant melanoma of the uveal tract, 6 per 1 000 000 annually. Blood-borne metastases are common, but may not present clinically for some years; 15% occur in the ciliary body and iris, they present earlier because they are more visible; 85% of the total are choroidal melanomas. Initially they may cause no symptoms unless the tumour is at the macula. Retinal detachment could be a feature. Diagnosis is mostly confirmed upon inspection. Primary choroidal melanomas must be distinguished from any secondary deposits as the choroid is a common site of metastases of cutaneous melanoma (Souhami & Tobias, 1987).

Investigations

Comprehensive clinical examination by a specialist consultant is imperative. Techniques available include:

- Plain X-ray
- Hypocyloidal tomography
- Computerized tomography
- Magnetic resonance imaging
- Orbital venography
- Carotid angiography
- Ultrasound.

The last three techniques have become less popular with the advent of computerized tomography and magnetic resonance imaging (Lund, 1987). Where possible, biopsy should be obtained to provide a histological confirmation. Surgical biopsy may be difficult, risking tumour spillage, haemorrhage and blindness. If the tumour is encapsulated, it may be best to excise it entirely (Souhami & Tobias, 1987).

Treatment

Treatment of orbital metastases depends on the type of primary tumour, the general opthamological status and the condition of the patient.

Patients with metastatic breast cancer to the orbit are given radiotherapy in the first instance, or chemotherapy with or without hormone therapy (Tijl et al., 1992). Prostate cancer is radiosensitive so metastases would also be treated with radiotherapy. Thyroid metastases can be treated with radiotherapy, or iodine if receptive (Tijl et al., 1992). These palliative measures are appropriate if the patient is well enough to tolerate treatment, and can help to preserve vision, reduce pain and consequently improve the quality of life.

Recently a more conservative approach has been adopted, particularly in the elderly. For example, small melanomas may be observed, and surgery performed only when the tumour enlarges (Souhami & Tobias, 1987). Treatment is then by photocoagulation, cryotherapy, local irradiation with high dose radiation or surgery (Souhami & Tobias, 1987).

Preservation of orbital contents must be founded on a clear, unemotional decision that will not jeopardize prognosis, and if preserved, the eye will have aesthetic and functional capabilities (Lund, 1987). This applies to radiotherapy, where blindness can occur, as well as surgery.

Enucleation may be necessary for large tumours, macular optic nerve involvement, retinal detachment and secondary glaucoma (Souhami & Tobias, 1987). Orbital exenteration is also of importance if it prevents pain and marked proptosis and, in combination with total maxillectomy, allows control of any residual tumour by laser or cryosurgery (Lund, 1987).

Summary

Like most disfigurements of the head and neck, orbital tumours are also difficult to camouflage. Commonly patients will wear tinted glasses, or wear an eye pad/ protector so that it looks more like protection than camouflage. Eye patches are occasionally worn, but most patients feel that this is indicative of eye loss.

Patients with orbital disease need skilled emotional support. These patients not only live with disfigurement and dysfunction, but also the threat to their survival from the disease process. Specialist hospital centres will have knowledge of comprehensive community support networks, and ensure that the patient is also referred to a specialist prosthetic department.

Nursing intervention will fundamentally be observation, and early detection, of any orbital irregularities and clinical care of any symptoms, as described in the chapter. This mostly involves ensuring that the patient is free from pain, keeping the eye clean and comfortable, administering topical medication as prescribed and covering the eye if necessary for either patient comfort, camouflage or protection should a paralysis or other dysfunction be present.

References and further reading

Bryant, W. M. (1981) Common toxic effects of systemic drugs on the eye. *Occupational Health Nursing*, 29, 15–17.

Char, D. H. (1993) Management of orbital tumours. *Mayo Clinical Practice*, 68, 1081–96.

Chilman, A. M. & Thomas, M. (1987) *Understanding Nursing Care*, 3rd edn. Churchill Livingstone, Edinburgh.

Cloutier, A. O. (1992) Occular side effects of chemotherapy: nursing management. *Oncology Nursing Forum*, 8(19), 1251–9.

Darling, V. H. & Thorpe, M. R. (1981) *Ophthalmic Nursing*, 2nd edn. Baillière Tindall, London.

Gorman, C. A. (1978) The presentation and management of endocrine opthalmopathy. *Clinics in Endocrinology and Metabolism*, 7, 67–96.

Henderson, J. W. (1980) Metastatic carcinoma. In: *Orbital Tumours*, (ed. J. W. Henderson), 2nd edn, pp. 451–71. Decker, New York.

Henk, J. M. (1976) Neoplasms of the head and neck. In: *Radiotherapy in Modern Clinical Practice*, (ed. H. F. Hope-Stone), pp. 108–42. Crosby Lockwood Staples, London.

Lund, V. J. (1987) The orbit. In: *Otolarygology*, (ed. A. G. Kerr), 5th edn. Butterworth, London.

Marieb, E. N. (1987) *Human Anatomy and Physiology Laboratory Manual.* Benjamin Cummings, California.

Marieb, E. N. (1989) *Human Anatomy and Physiology.* Benjamin Cummings, California.

Moeloek, N. F. (1993) Updates in orbital tumours. *Eye Science*, 9(1), 40–44.

McConnell, E. A. (1991) How to irrigate the eye. *Nursing 91*, March, 28.

Phillips, M. (1982) Ophthalmic preparations. *Nursing Mirror*, 155, 69–71.

Rooke, E. C. E. *et al.* (1980) *Ophthalmic Nursing – Its Practice and Management.* Churchill Livingstone, Edinburgh.

Smith, J. & Nachazel, D. P. (1980) *Ophthalmologic Nursing*, Little, Brown, Boston.

Souhami, R. & Tobias, J. (1987) *Cancer and its Management*, pp. 175–8. Blackwell Scientific Publications, Oxford.

Tijl, J. *et al.* (1992) Metastatic tumours to the orbit – management and prognosis. *Graefe's Archive for Clinical and Experimental Opthalmology (Amsterdam)*, 230, 527–30.

Tortora, G. J. & Anagnostakos, N. P. (1992) *Principles of Anatomy & Physiology*, 7th edn. Harper & Row, London, pp. 373–85.

GUIDELINES: EYE SWABBING

EQUIPMENT

1 Sterile dressing pack.
2 Sterile water.

PROCEDURE

Action	Rationale
1 Explain and discuss the procedure with the patient.	To ensure that the patient understands the procedure and gives his/her valid consent.
2 Assist the patient into the correct position: (a) Head well supported and tilted back. (b) Preferably the patient should be in bed or lying on a couch.	The patient needs to be discouraged from flinching or making unexpected movements and so should be in the most comfortable position possible at the start of the procedure.
3 Ensure an adequate light source, taking care not to dazzle the patient.	To enable maximum observation of the eyes without causing the patient harm or discomfort.
4 Wash hands thoroughly using bactericidal soap and water or bactericidal alcohol hand rub, then dry hands.	Use a non-touch technique where the patient has a damaged eye or has just had an operation on the eye. Infection can lead to loss of an eye.

5	Always treat the uninfected or uninflamed eye first.	To avoid cross-infection.
6	Always bathe lids with the eyes closed first.	To avoid damage to the cornea.
7	Using a slightly moistened low-linting swab, ask the patient to look up and swab the lower lid from the nasal corner outwards.	If the swab is too wet the solution will run down the patient's cheek. This increases the risk of cross-infection and causes the patient discomfort. Swabbing from the nasal corner outwards avoids the risk of swabbing discharge into the lacrymal punctum, or even across the bridge of the nose into other eye.
8	Ensure that the edge of the swab is not above the lid margin.	To avoid touching the sensitive cornea.
9	Using a new swab each time, repeat the procedure until all the discharge has been removed.	To reduce risk of infection.
10	Swab the upper lid by slightly everting the lid margin and asking the patient to look down. Swab from the nasal corner outwards and use a new swab each time until all discharge has been removed.	To effectively remove any foreign material from eye. To reduce the risk of infection.
11	Once both eyelids have been cleansed and dried, make the patient comfortable.	
12	Remove and dispose of equipment.	
13	Wash hands.	To reduce the risk of cross-infection.
14	Record the procedure in the appropriate documents.	To monitor trends and fluctuations.

Note: For information about obtaining an eye swab for pathological investigations, see the appropriate section in Chapter 38, Specimen Collection.

GUIDELINES: INSTILLATION OF EYE DROPS

EQUIPMENT

1 Sterile dressing pack.
2 Sterile water.
3 Appropriate eye drops. (Any preparation must be checked against the doctor's prescription.)
4 Low-linting swab.

PROCEDURE

Action

Rationale

1	Explain and discuss the procedure with the patient.	To ensure that the patient understands the procedure and gives his/her valid consent.

Guidelines: Instillation of eye drops (cont'd)

Action	Rationale
2 If there is any discharge, proceed as for eye swabbing.	To remove any infected material and thus ensure adequate absorption of the drops.
3 Check the following: (a) Prescription against bottle label. (b) For which eye the drops are prescribed. (c) Expiry date on bottle.	To ensure that appropriate drops are instilled. To avoid cross-infection and instillation of the drug into the wrong eye. To ensure that medication has not expired.
4 Assist the patient into the correct position, i.e. head well supported and tilted back.	To ensure that drops are instilled beneath the lower lid into the fornix and to avoid excess solution running down the patient's cheek.
5 Wash hands thoroughly using bactericidal soap and water or bactericidal alcohol hand rub, and dry them.	Asepsis is essential, particularly when the patient has a damaged eye or has just had an operation on the eye. Infection can lead to loss of an eye.
6 Place a wet low-linting swab on the lower lid against the lid margin.	To absorb any excess solution which may be irritating to the surrounding skin.
7 Ask the patient to look up immediately before instilling the drop.	This opens the eye and allows the drop to be instilled into the outer side of the lower fornix. If done too soon the patient may blink as the drop is instilled.
8 Ask the patient to close the eye. Keep the wet low-linting swab on the lower lid.	To ensure absorption of the fluid and to avoid excess running down the cheek.
9 Make the patient comfortable.	
10 Remove and dispose of equipment.	
11 Wash hands with bactericidal soap and water.	To avoid cross-infection.
12 Record the procedure in the appropriate documents.	To monitor trends and fluctuations.

GUIDELINES: INSTILLATION OF EYE OINTMENT

EQUIPMENT

1 Sterile dressing pack.
2 Sterile water.
3 Appropriate eye ointment. (Any preparation must be checked against the doctor's prescription.)

PROCEDURE

Action	Rationale
1 Explain and discuss the procedure with the patient.	To ensure that the patient understands the procedure and gives his/her valid consent.

2	If there is any discharge, and to remove any previous application of ointment, proceed as for eye swabbing.	To remove any infected material and previous ointment to allow for absorption of ointment.
3	Check the following: (a) Prescription against tube of ointment. (b) For which eye the ointment is prescribed. (c) Expiry date on tube.	To ensure that appropriate ointment applied. To avoid cross-infection and administration of an inappropriate treatment. To ensure that medication has not expired.
4	Wash hands thoroughly using bactericidal soap and water or bactericidal alcohol hand rub.	To avoid infection.
5	Place a wet low-linting swab on the lower lid against the lid margin.	To absorb excess ointment which may be irritating to the surrounding skin.
6	Slightly evert the lower lid by pulling on the low-linting swab. Ask the patient to look up immediately before applying the cream.	To allow the application to be made inside the lower lid into the lower fornix.
7	Apply the ointment by gently squeezing the tube and, with the nozzle 2.5 cm above the lower lid, drawing a line along the inner edge of the lower lid from the nasal corner outward.	To avoid possible contamination and trauma.
8	Ask the patient to close the eye and remove excess ointment with a new wet low-linting swab.	To avoid excess ointment irritating the surrounding skin.
9	Warn the patient that, when the eye is opened, vision will be a little blurred for a few minutes.	To prepare patient and to avoid anxiety.
10	Make the patient comfortable.	
11	Remove and dispose of equipment.	
12	Wash hands with bactericidal soap and water.	To avoid infection.
13	Record the procedure in the appropriate documents.	To monitor trends and fluctuations.

GUIDELINES: EYE IRRIGATION

EQUIPMENT

1 Sterile dressing pack.
2 Irrigation fluid (usually sterile 0.9% sodium chloride but, in an emergency, tap water may be used).
3 Receiver.
4 Towel.
5 Plastic cape.
6 Irrigating flask.
7 Hot water in a bowl to warm irrigating fluid to tepid temperature.
8 Anaesthetic drops.

Guidelines: Eye irrigation (cont'd)

PROCEDURE

Action	Rationale
1 Explain and discuss the procedure with the patient.	To ensure that the patient understands the procedure and gives his/her valid consent.
2 Instil anaesthetic drops if required.	To avoid any discomfort.
3 Prepare the irrigation fluid to the appropriate temperature.	Tepid fluid will be more comfortable for the patient. The solution should be poured across the inner aspect of the nurse's wrist to test the temperature.
4 Assist the patient into the appropriate position: (a) Head comfortably supported with chin almost horizontal. (b) Head inclined to the side of the eye to be treated.	To avoid the solution running either over the cheek into the eye or out of the eye and down the side of the nose.
5 Wash hands using bactericidal soap and water or bactericidal alcohol hand rub, and dry.	To reduce risk of infection.
6 Remove any discharge from the eye by swabbing.	To prevent washing the discharge down the lacrimal duct or across the cheek.
7 Ask the patient to hold the receiver against the cheek below the eye being tested.	To collect irrigation fluid as it runs away from the eye.
8 Position the towel and plastic cape.	To protect the patient's clothing.
9 Hold the patient's eyelids apart, using your first and second fingers, against the orbital ridge.	The patient will be unable to hold the eye open once irrigation commences.
10 Do not press on the eyeball.	To avoid causing the patient discomfort or pain.
11 Warn the patient that the flow of solution is going to start and pour a little onto the cheek first.	To allow time for adjustment of feeling of water flow.
12 Direct the flow of the fluid from the nasal corner outwards.	To wash away from the lacrimal punctum and prevent contaminating other eye.
13 Ask the patient to look up, down and to either side while irrigating.	To ensure that the whole area is washed.
14 Evert lids while irrigating.	To ensure complete removal of any foreign body.
15 Keep the flow of irrigation fluid constant.	To ensure swift removal of any foreign body.
16 When the eye has been thoroughly irrigated, ask the patient to close the eyes and use a new swab to dry the lids.	For patient comfort.

17	Take the receiver from the patient and dry the cheek.	If the receiver is removed first, solution may run down the patient's neck.
18	Make the patient comfortable.	
19	Remove and dispose of equipment.	
20	Wash hands with bactericidal soap and water.	To avoid infection.
21	Record the procedure in the appropriate documents.	To monitor trends and fluctuations.

CHAPTER 21

Gastric Decontamination

Definition

Gastric decontamination is the removal of poisonous substances from the stomach by induced emesis or gastric lavage, or by activated charcoal which will absorb various toxins or drugs, thus preventing gastrointestinal absorption. This is undertaken to prevent further absorption of ingested toxins or drugs in the case of overdose.

There has been much debate and a great deal of controversy about the roles each of these methods (induced emesis, gastric lavage and activated charcoal) has in the management of ingested poisons. They have been the subject of research; however, as yet no clear conclusions have been reached (Davis, 1991; Olson, 1994).

Gastric lavage

Gastric lavage is the irrigation or washing out of the stomach with repeated flushings of an appropriate fluid, usually water. It is most commonly used to remove ingested poisons or other harmful substances that may have been swallowed either deliberately or accidentally, thus preventing further absorption. It may also be used to empty the stomach before surgery or investigations such as endoscopy (Eaves, 1988) or to test for gastrointestinal haemorrhage (Robinson & Stott, 1980).

Indications

Gastric lavage may be used under the following circumstances:

(1) If the patient is seen within 4 hours of ingesting poisons or harmful substances. It is of doubtful value if performed more than 4 hours after ingestion of most poisons.
(2) If the patient is unconscious and the time of ingestion is not known.
(3) In all cases of salicylate poisoning up to 24 hours post-ingestion (Paynter, 1993).
(4) If the patient has swallowed any substance that slows gastric emptying such as trycylic antidepressants

which may be recovered up to 8 hours post-ingestion (Paynter, 1993).
(5) To administer activated charcoal to patients unwilling or unable to swallow them (Olson, 1994).
(6) For gastrointestinal haemorrhage (Evans, 1981).
(7) Before surgery in patients with pyloric obstruction.

Induced emesis may be used under the following circumstances:

(1) If the patient is alert and the development of drowsiness and lethargy is unlikely.
(2) If the patient is seen within one hour of ingesting most poisons – after this time emesis is not very effective, less than half the gastric content is removed (Olson, 1994).

Activated charcoal is used to absorb many different drugs, chemicals and gases (Davis, 1991).

REFERENCE MATERIAL

The decontamination debate

The reliability of gastric lavage is debatable, advice on its use is conflicting, and its value is questionable (Burstom, 1970; Matthew, 1971; Stoddart, 1975; Goth & Vesell, 1984). Blake *et al.* (1978) attempted to identify those factors that influenced the decision to perform gastric lavage in 236 cases of deliberate self-poisoning seen over a period of 6 months in one hospital. Of patients seen within 4 hours of ingesting the poison, 87% had a lavage performed irrespective of the number of tablets and the nature of the drug taken. Overall, 77% had a gastric lavage. Most of the late lavages were carried out for salicylate ingestion. The authors concluded that given the changing pattern of drugs used for attempted self-poisoning, at least 50% of patients were subjected to gastric lavage unnecessarily.

Gastric lavage is most effective if carried out within an hour to an hour and a half post-ingestion of poisons (Paynter, 1993). Patients need to be carefully assessed before this procedure is carried out; the amount and type of poisons ingested need to be taken into account. However lavage may not be indicated if the risk of toxicity is small (Hall, 1987), if only a small to moderate amount of substance is ingested (Olson, 1994) or if the patient presents too late (Hall, 1987).

This procedure has been found to be unreliable in removing undissolved pills or pill fragments, especially sustained release or enteric coated preparations (Olson, 1994). Post-mortem examinations have revealed concentrations of drugs trapped within mucosal folds in the stomachs of patients who had undergone apparently thorough lavage procedures (Davis, 1991). Lavage fluid has been found to push poisons through the pylorus and into the small intestine where there is increased absorption and consequently increased toxicity (Davis, 1991; Olson, 1994).

There are a number of complications associated with gastric lavage (Paynter, 1993; Olson, 1994). These include:

- Oesophageal perforation;
- Stomach perforation;
- Inadvertent tracheal intubation;
- Aspiration of gastric content;
- Aspiration pneumonitis;
- Laryngospasm;
- Cardiac arrhythmias.

In view of these complications gastric lavage should not be undertaken lightly. Patients who are comatosed or who have a depressed or absent gag reflex must be intubated with a cuffed oral endotracheal tube to protect the airway before lavage is undertaken (Paynter, 1993).

Gastric lavage is generally carried out by medical staff assisted by nurses. Registered general nurses in specialized units, mainly accident and emergency departments, may carry out the procedure without medical involvement after initial assessment.

Ipecacuanha is the most convenient way of inducing emesis. It is a centrally acting drug, its site of action being the chemotrigger zone in the medulla oblongata. It also has an irritant effect on the lining of the stomach. It can take up to 20 minutes to produce an effect: if this fact is not appreciated, repeated doses may be given before the first dose has had time to work. This may result in protracted vomiting. However, if after 20 minutes no emesis has occurred, a further dose can be given. It is recommended by the manufacturing company that a glass of water is taken following a dose of ipecacuanha.

Ipecacuanha should not be given if: corrosive or petroleum distillate agents have been taken, or medications which could cause a rapid onset of symptoms (especially fitting), or agents that depress the central nervous system.

Induced emesis should be used only when the patient is alert and when the development of lethargy and coma is unlikely. Unless the patient is awake, the cough reflex may be depressed and this may result in the patient inhaling the vomitus. When a drug with strong anti-emetic properties has been ingested, e.g. chlorpromazine, induced emesis will have little or no effect, and gastric lavage may become the method of choice.

If syrup of ipecacuanha is unavailable and a hospital is more than a 15 minute drive away, a soapy solution may be used as an alternative. A solution of two tablespoons of standard washing up liquid or lotion soap in a glass of water will induce emesis (Olson, 1994). Powdered laundry or dish-washing detergents or their concentrated liquid preparations *should not be used* as they are corrosive. In addition, manual digital stimulation, which is relatively ineffective and may result in trauma, copper sulphate, salt water and mustard water which have toxic effects (Lawson, 1986) should not be used to induce emesis.

Syrup of ipecacuanha may cause protracted vomiting in some patients which if very forceful may lead to haemorrhagic gastritis or a Mallory–Weiss tear (Olson, 1994). Nausea and fatigue are also side-effects of this treatment (Davis, 1991).

Activated charcoal is a tasteless, odourless, finely divided back powder which is made from a distillation of wood pulp (Davis, 1991; Olson, 1994). It has a very large surface area and is highly effective in absorbing a wide variety of drugs, chemicals and gases (Davis, 1991). There are a few substances that are poorly absorbed by charcoal – these include iron, lithium, methanol and potassium (Olson, 1994). Activated charcoal therefore prevents gastrointestinal absorption of various drugs and toxins. It is thought that it may also absorb drugs back from the bloodstream into the gastrointestinal tract. The effectiveness of this treatment decreases with time, the longer the period of time that has elapsed post-ingestion of substance, the less effective the charcoal is (Davis, 1991).

The usual recommended initial dose of activated charcoal is 50–100 g for adults and 15–20 g for children or 1 g/1 kg (Davis, 1991). One or two additional doses may be given at hourly intervals, particularly if a large amount of poisons were ingested. The side-effects are few and include distention of the stomach, vomiting, constipation and black faeces. Activated charcoal is not very palatable, it may be administered via a lavage tube, a nasogastric tube or by mouth as a slurry in water. Its grittiness, colour and lack of flavour are cited as reasons why individuals find it unpalatable. Manufacturers are trying to produce a solution that is more acceptable to patients (Davis, 1991), although some patients find this method more favourable than more traditional approaches.

Activated charcoal may be given prior to a gastric lavage so that it may begin absorbing toxins straight away, and a second dose administered after the lavage procedure to 'mop up' any drug that has not been recovered (Burton *et al.*, 1984). Burton *et al.* (1984) also suggest that it is administered post-gastric lavage so that a large dose of charcoal can be given. Kulig *et al.* (1985) and Tenenbein *et al.* (1987) recommend that activated charcoal be given as the sole treatment.

It is not possible, with the research evidence available, to state which of these three methods is the most effective. Each individual case of ingested poisoning should be assessed carefully. Attention should be paid to the patient's general condition, the time of ingestion and the type and amount of poison ingested before a treatment strategy is decided.

Further information

For more specific information on the ingestion of poisons, and whenever there is any doubt about the management of such patients, the Poisons Information Centres should be contacted:

Poisons Information Services:

(1) Belfast (01232 240503).
(2) Birmingham (0121 554 3801).
(3) Cardiff (01222 709901).
(4) Dublin (003531 8379964).
(5) Edinburgh (0131 229 2477; 0131-228 2441) – Viewdata, a service whereby information on drugs can be assessed via a computer. It is free to NHS hospitals, which have to provide their own computer systems.
(6) Leeds (0113 2430715 *or* 0113 2923547).
(7) London (0171 635 9191).
(8) Newcastle (0191 232 5131).

References and further reading

Arena, J. (1974) *Poisoning: Toxicology, Symptoms, Treatment*, 3rd edn. Charles C. Thomas, Springfield, Ill.

Beckett, A. & Rowland, M. (1965) Urinary excretion kinetics of amphetamine in man. *Journal of Pharmacy and Pharmacology*, 17, 628.

Blake, D. R. *et al.* (1978) Is there excessive use of gastric lavage in the treatment of self-poisoning? *Lancet*, 2, 1362–4.

Budassi, S. A. & Barber, J. M. (1985) *Emergency, Nursing: Principles and Practice*. C. V. Mosby, St Louis.

Burstom, G. R. (1970) *Self-poisoning*. Lloyd-Luke, London.

Burton, B. T. *et al.* (1984) Comparisons of activated charcoal and gastric lavage in the prevention of asprin absorption. *Journal of Emergency Medicine*, 1(5), 411–16.

Chazan, J. & Cohen, J. (1969) Clinical spectrum of glutethimide intoxication. *Journal of the American Medical Association*, 208, 837.

Cosgriff, J. H. (1978) *An Atlas of Diagnostic and Therapeutic Procedures for Emergency Personnel*. J. B. Lippincott, Philadelphia.

Cosgriff, J. H. *et al.* (1984) *The Practice of Emergency Nursing*, 2nd edn. J. B. Lippincott, Philadelphia.

Danel, V. *et al.* (1988) Activated charcoal, emesis and gastric lavage in aspirin overdose (study). *British Medical Journal*, 296, 1507.

Davis, J. E. (1991) A consideration not to be overlooked. Activated charcoal in acute drug overdoses. *Professional Nurse*, 6(12), 710–14.

Eaves, D. (1988) Making sense of gastric lavage. *Nursing Times and Nursing Mirror*, 84(20), 52–3.

Evans, R. (1981) *Emergency Medicine*. Butterworth, London.

Goth, A. & Vesell (1984) *Medical Pharmacology: Principles and Concepts*, 11th edn. C. V. Mosby, St Louis.

Hall, A. H. (1987) *Current Therapy in Emergency Medicine*. Philadelphia Press, Philadelphia, PA.

Hall, A. H. & Krenzelok, E. (1991) Gastrointestinal decontamination. *Emergency Medicine Reports*, 12, 19, 21, 3.

Kulig, K. *et al.* (1985) Management of acutely poisoned patients without gastric emptying. *Annals of Emergency Medicine*, 14(6), 562–7.

Lawson, A. (1986) Acute poisoning: common errors of management. *Care of the Critically Ill*, 2(2), 71–80.

Matthew, H. (1971) Acute poisoning: some myths and misconceptions. *British Medical Journal*, 1, 521.

Olson, K. R. (1994) *Poisoning and drug overdose*, 2nd edn. Appleton & Lange, Newalk.

Paynter, M. (1993) Gastric lavage in accident and emergency. *Nursing Standard*, 20(7), 32–3.

Robinson, R. & Stott, R. (1980) *Medical Emergencies, Diagnosis and Management*, 3rd edn. Heinemann Medical Books, London.

Stoddart, J. C. (1975) *Intensive Therapy*. Blackwell Scientific Publications, Oxford.

Tenenbein, M. *et al.* (1987) Efficacy of ipecac-induced emesis, orogastric lavage and activated charcoal for acute drug overdose. *Annals of Emergency Medicine*, 16(8), 838–41.

GUIDELINES: GASTRIC LAVAGE

EQUIPMENT

1 Clean gastric tube with connector.
2 Connecting tubing.

 3 Lubricating jelly.
 4 Tape.
 5 Syringe (50 ml) .
 6 Receiver.
 7 Litmus paper.
 8 Mouth gag.
 9 Funnel.
10 Jug.
11 Tepid water or prescribed irrigation fluid.
12 Plastic sheet.
13 Disposable paper sheets.
14 Disposable plastic aprons.
15 Disposable plastic gloves.
16 Bucket.
17 Suction equipment.
18 Emergency resuscitation equipment.

PROCEDURE

Action	Rationale
1 Explain and discuss the procedure with the patient whenever possible.	To ensure that the patient understands the procedure and gives his/her valid consent. (The efficacy of explanations is questionable, however, on the basis that an adult who has ingested a toxic substance deliberately is unlikely to want to cooperate with agents whose aim is to prevent suicidal gestures. Tact must be employed in these circumstances.)
2 Unconscious patients must be intubated.	To maintain a clear airway.
3 Place the patient on a firm surface, lying in the left lateral position, with the head down (Fig. 21.1). (A standard emergency department trolley should be available ideally.)	To maintain a clear airway.

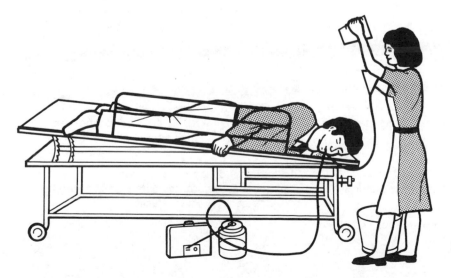

Figure 21.1   Gastric lavage.

Guidelines: Gastric lavage (cont'd)

Action

Rationale

4 Remove any prostheses from the buccal cavity. Remove debris and/or vomitus from the buccal cavity with suction.

To maintain a clear airway.

5 Have emergency resuscitation equipment available.

Strong vagal stimulation can induce cardiac dysrhythmias and cardiopulmonary arrest.

6 Place a disposable sheet under the patient's head and a plastic sheet over the floor.

To protect nurse and patient should vomiting occur.

7 Lubricate the tube with lubricating jelly.

To facilitate passage of the tube.

8 If the patient is able to cooperate ask him/her to sit up and swallow sips of water.

Swallowing will cause the epiglottis to close and prevent accidental passage of the tube into trachea.

9 Secure the tube with tape once inserted.

To prevent dislodgement of the tube.

10 Either aspirate the tube before lavage begins and test the aspirate with litmus paper, or listen with a stethoscope over the stomach as air is introduced into the tube via a syringe.

To ensure that the tube is in the stomach.

11 Retain a specimen of aspirate in a labelled specimen bottle.

For analysis.

12 Instil, via a funnel, water or the prescribed irrigation fluid, in volumes of 100–500 ml.

Approximately 500 ml of fluid are necessary to flatten out the rugae of the stomach so that the fluid may reach all parts of the mucous membrane.

13 Any fluid instilled must be tepid.

To prevent a sudden lowering of body temperature and possible shock.

14 Hold the funnel below the level of the patient. Once the required amount of fluid has been poured into the funnel, raise it gradually until the fluid empties into the stomach. Do not allow the contents of the funnel to empty.

To control the rate at which the fluid is instilled. A siphoning action is needed to return the contents of the stomach.

15 Lower the funnel and observe all the contents as they return from the stomach. Empty the contents into a bucket. If blood returns, stop the procedure and inform the medical staff. Otherwise lavage until the returning fluid is clear.

16 Once lavage is completed, pinch the tube off and remove the tube quickly. Have suction at hand.

Gagging and possible vomiting may occur when the tube is removed. As the tube reaches the pharynx, any fluid left may escape and infiltrate into the lungs.

17 Check buccal cavity for signs of trauma. Provide oral hygiene facilities as required.

To maintain a clean, moist mouth. To prevent the accumulation of oral secretions. To prevent the development of mouth infections.

18 Explain to patient that procedure is completed and ensure patient comfort.

CHAPTER 22

Intrapleural Drainage

Definition

Intrapleural drainage is an underwater-seal system of drainage that prevents the entry of air into the pleural space, thus avoiding pneumothorax.

Indications

(1) To remove matter from the pleural space or thoracic cavity:
   (a) Solids, e.g. fibrin or clotted blood.
   (b) Liquids, e.g. serous fluids, blood, pus, malignant effusion, chyle or gastric juice.
   (c) Gas, e.g. air from the lungs, trachea or oesophagus.
(2) To allow the lung to re-expand following surgery (Oh, 1995).

REFERENCE MATERIAL

Anatomy and physiology

The pleura is a thin sheet of tissue covering the undersurface of the ribs, diaphragm and the structures of the mediastinum. It continues over the surface of both lungs, thus forming a space known as the pleural space. The layer in contact with the surface of the lungs is known as the visceral pleura; that in contact with the thoracic wall, the parietal pleura. These two membranes are continuous with each other but are separated by a thin serous fluid that allows the pleurae to slide smoothly over each other during respiration. In health the pleural space is a potential space only. This space has a negative pressure normally. The elastic tissues of the lungs and the chest wall continually pull in opposite directions, the lungs tending to recoil inwards and the chest wall outwards. As these opposing forces attempt to pull the visceral and parietal pleurae apart, they create a negative pressure in the pleural space. Pressures in the pleural space are approximately 8 mm water during inspiration and 2 mm water on expiration. A negative pressure of 54 mm water can be measured during forced inspiration; during expiration, e.g. coughing, a positive pressure of approximately 68 mm water develops (Marieb, 1994).

Any opening of the thoracic cavity results in a loss of negative pressure and the lungs collapse. Collections of fluids or materials can also cause the lung to collapse as these substances are incompressible and restrict expansion of the lungs and inhibit cardiopulmonary function.

When a tube is inserted to remove air it is normally inserted fairly high in the intrapleural space, usually through the second anterior intercostal space, as air will rise. If a tube is inserted to remove liquid or debris, it is usually inserted fairly low through the sixth or seventh intercostal space to achieve satisfactory drainage (Hinds, 1987). If more than one tube is inserted, e.g. following intrathoracic surgery, to remove air and fluid or debris the higher tube, known as the apical drain, is used to remove air, and the lower tube, known as the basal drain, is used to remove liquid and debris.

Types of chest drain

Any system must be capable of removing whatever collects in the pleural space more rapidly than it accumulates (Fig. 22.1). The choice of chest drain to be used is dictated by ease of insertion, patency over time, and patient comfort. A blunt insertion technique is now favoured.

The choice of drainage and collection systems employed will depend on the clinical application and total volume of drainage. The most frequently used systems are those utilizing a single drain, or those where extra pressure is applied with the aid of a pump.

Single-bottle water-seal system

In this system the end of the drainage tube from the patient's chest is covered by a layer of water that permits drainage and prevents lung collapse by stopping

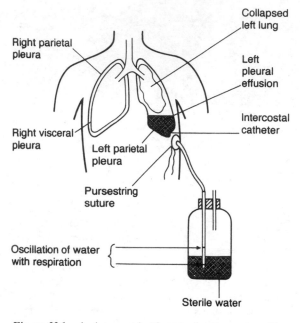

Figure 22.1   An intercostal catheter and underwater seal bottle are used to drain a left pleural effusion.

atmospheric air entering the pleural space. If the tube is not deep enough under the water level, there is a danger of it emerging above the water line if the bottle is moved. If the tube is too deep, a higher intrapleural pressure is required to expel air. Drainage depends on gravity, the mechanics of respiration and, if necessary, suction by the addition of a controlled vacuum. The tube from the patient should extend approximately 2.5 cm below the level of the water in the container (Fig. 22.2).

Two-bottle water-seal system

This system consists of the same water seal chamber with the addition of a manometer bottle. Effective drainage depends on gravity and the amount of suction added as controlled by the manometer bottle.

Use of pump or suction apparatus

If there is no response to the above method of drainage, external suction apparatus can be applied. The addition of a low-suction pump ensures continuous suction, thus improving drainage with the minimum of risk to the patient. Suction at approximately 15–20 cm water pressure can be used via a pump such as the Roberts' pump.

References and further reading

Brunner, L. S. & Suddarth, D. S. (1986) *The Lippincott Manual of Nursing Practice*, 4th edn. J. B. Lippincott, Philadelphia.

Cohen, S. & Stack, M. (1980) Programmed instruction: how to work with chest tubes. *American Journal of Nursing*, 80, 685–712.

Erickson, R. (1981) Chest tubes: they're really not that complicated. *Nursing* (US), 11(5), 34–43.

Erickson, R. (1981) Solving chest tube problems. *Nursing* (US), 11(6), 62–8.

Gordon, D. B. & Lorenz, B. L. (1991) A simple way to treat simple pneumothorax . . . Heimlich chest drain valve. *RN*, 54(12), 50–52.

Hinds, C. J. (1987) *A Concise Textbook of Intensive Care*, pp. 164–5, 235. Baillière Tindall, London.

Marieb, E. N. (1994) *Human Anatomy and Physiology*. Benjamin Cummings, California.

Mumford, S. P. (1986) Draining the pleural cavity. *Professional Nurse*, 1(9), 240–2.

Oh, T. E. (1995) *Intensive Care Manual*. Butterworths, Sydney, Australia.

One-bottle system

Two-bottle system

Figure 22.2   One- and two-bottle chest drainage systems.

GUIDELINES: MANAGEMENT OF UNDERWATER-SEAL DRAINAGE

EQUIPMENT

1 Sterile chest drainage bottle.
2 Sterile disposable tubing.

3 Drainage bottle holder, if available.
4 Suction pump, if required.
5 Two pairs of large artery forceps (tips covered with rubber).

PROCEDURE

Action	Rationale
1 Attach the intrapleural drain to the drainage tube. *Note*: This should lead to the long tube whose end is situated below water level.	Water-seal drainage provides for the escape of air, fluid and debris into a drainage bottle. The water acts as a seal and keeps the air from being drawn back into the pleural space.
2 Ensure that drainage tubing is 2.5cm below the water level (Fig. 22.3).	To prevent re-entry of air leading to a collapsed lung.
3 The other, shorter tube, is: (a) Left open to the atmosphere. (b) Attached to a controlled suction apparatus.	To allow air to be expelled. Although drainage of liquids and/or debris relies on gravity and the mechanics of respiration, additional controlled suction may be necessary to accelerate the process.
4 Establish the original level of fluid by: (a) Marking with a piece of tape. (b) Filling to a preset amount. *Note*: All bottles used should, preferably, be calibrated.	This provides a baseline for measurement of fluid drainage. To ensure any change in drainage is observed and monitored.
5 When recording fluid drainage: (a) Note the date and time. (b) Mark hourly or daily increments, or more frequently if there is excessive drainage, by taping the level on the drainage bottles. *Note*: When using tape specify whether the upper, mid or lower border of the tape is the level to be measured at (Fig. 22.4).	This marking will show the amount of fluid loss and how fast fluid is collecting in the drainage bottle. If the fluid is blood, it serves as a basis for retransfusion or reoperation, if following surgery. Inaccuracies of 100–200ml can occur if the incorrect border is used.
6 Secure tubing to the bed clothes by the use of tape and safety pins.	This will prevent kinking, looping or pressure on the tubing which may cause reflux of fluid into the pleural space or impede drainage, causing blocking of the intrapleural drain by debris.
7 Ensure that artery clamps are in close proximity to patient, i.e. taped to the wall,	In the event of accidental disconnection of the drainage tubing from the intrapleural drain, the

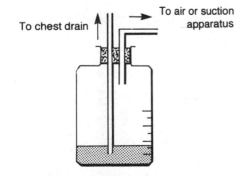

Figure 22.3   Underwater–seal drainage.

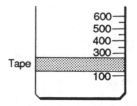

Figure 22.4   Specify whether the upper, mid- or lower level of the tape is to be measured.

Guidelines: Management of underwater-seal drainage (cont'd)

Action

clamped to the bed clothes or on the bedside locker.

Rationale

artery clamps should be applied immediately to the intrapleural drain to prevent entry of air (on inspiration) into the pleural space – leading to pneumothorax. When moving the patient, the drainage tubing is more likely to become disconnected, therefore the artery clamps should be readily available. There may be medical advice to apply the clamps, at set intervals, to delay drainage; e.g. following instillation of drugs or radioactive substances it is normal to clamp the tubing for 24 hours.

8   Ensure that the patient is sitting in a comfortable position which allows optimum drainage. Encourage the patient to change position frequently. This may be enhanced by adequate pain control, using drugs which do not depress respiration, as patient's respiration may already be compromised.

Correct poisitioning aids drainage by gravity and by ensuring that the patient breathes freely, to promote gaseous exchange. Changing position also promotes better drainage as well as avoiding discomfort and pressure sores.

9   Ask the physiotherapist to help encourage the patient with mobility, chest and arm exercises.

To promote drainage and avoid the complications of pressure ulcers and stiffness of the arm on the side of drain insertion.

10   Ensure patency of tubing by 'milking' tubing towards the drainage bottle, if necessary. Take care not to disconnect tubing while executing this manoeuvre.
Note: This is only necessary if draining fluid.

'Milking' the tubing prevents it from becoming clogged with clots or fibrin. Constant attention to maintaining the patency of the tube will facilitate prompt expansion of the lung and minimize complications.

11   Ensure that there is fluctuation (swinging) of the fluid level in the drainage tube leading from the patient (which terminates below the water level).

Fluctuation of the water level in the tube shows that there is effective communication between the pleural cavity and the drainage bottle, provides a valuable indication of the patency of the drainage system, and is a gauge of intrapleural pressure.

12   Ensure that the drainage bottle remains at floor level, except when the patient is being helped to move. The drainage bottle should never be raised above the level of the intrapleural drain, unless it is clamped.

To prevent backflow of fluid and debris into the pleural space.

13   Caution visitors and ancillary staff against handling any part of the system or displacing the drainage bottle.

To prevent backflow and to guard against accidental disconnection of the tubing which would allow air entry.

GUIDELINES: CHANGING DRAINAGE TUBING AND BOTTLES

EQUIPMENT

1 Sterile drainage bottle.
2 Sterile water.

3 Two pairs of artery clamps (tips covered with rubber).
4 Chlorhexidine in 70% spirit.
5 Sterile tubing.

PROCEDURE

Action	Rationale
1 Explain and discuss the procedure with the patient.	To ensure that the patient understands the procedure and gives his/her valid consent.
2 Wash hands with bactericidal soap and water or bactericidal alcohol hand rub.	To minimize the risk of infection.
3 Prepare drainage bottle by putting in a set amount (enough to cover the end of the long arm of the drainage tubing) of sterile water and taking note of that level. Mark this level with tape. If tubing is to be changed, attach clean tubing to the prepared drainage bottle.	To provide an underwater seal. Enough water should be in the bottle to ensure maintenance of the seal (usually 500 ml). Too much water creates pressure and reduces the capacity of the bottle for drainage. It is essential to note the amount of water added to the bottle for accurate measurement of drainage.
4 Take the equipment to the bedside.	
5 Clamp the intrapleural drain using both artery clamps, before changing the bottle or tubing.	To avoid tension pneumothorax occurring when the water seal is broken.
6 Clean hands with a suitable solution, e.g. bactericidal alcohol hand rub.	To minimize the risk of infection.
7 Remove the bung with the drainage tubing from the underwater-seal bottle and replace it in the clean bottle. Ensure that there is an airtight connection between the bung and bottle. If tubing is being changed, the bung will already be in place in the sterile bottle.	To prevent air entry and reduce the risk of infection.
8 Take the clamps off the intrapleural drainage tube.	To re-establish drainage.
9 Ensure that there is fluctuation (swinging) of the fluid level in the drainage tube leading from the patient (which terminates below the water level).	To establish that there is communication between pleural cavity and the drainage bottle.
10 Make the patient comfortable.	
11 Remove equipment.	
12 Record in appropriate documentation the amount of drainage, deducting the amount of water originally in the bottle.	For accurate measurement and recording of the amount of drainage.
13 Empty and clean the bottle and return it to the central sterile supplies department.	To reduce risk of cross-infection between patients.

Note: if an underwater-seal drain is established to drain air from the pleural space, there is probably no need to change either connection tubing or bottle. However, if fluid and debris are drained the bottle may

Guidelines: Changing drainage tubing and bottles (cont'd)

need changing frequently (at least daily), depending on the amount drained. The tubing need be changed only if there is a copious amount of debris and there is a danger of it becoming blocked. Changing the tubing or the bottle breaks the closed system and provides a potential portal of entry for bacteria.

GUIDELINES: REMOVAL OF AN INTRAPLEURAL DRAIN

EQUIPMENT

1 Sterile dressing pack.
2 0.9% sodium chloride.
3 Surgical gloves.
4 Stitch cutter.
5 Collodion lotion.
6 Adhesive tape, waterproof and hypoallergenic.
7 Plaster remover.

PROCEDURE

This procedure is usually carried out by a member of the nursing or medical staff who has been instructed and supervised in the removal of intrapleural drains.

Action		Rationale
Doctor/First nurse	*Assisting nurse*	
1 Explain and discuss the procedure with the patient and allow the patient to practise the procedure beforehand.	Wash hands with bactericidal soap and water or bactericidal alcohol hand rub.	To ensure that the patient understands the procedure and gives his/her valid consent. Speed and accuracy are essential in this procedure so all equipment must be at hand.
2 Establish patient is not allergic to tape or collodion.		To avoid allergic reactions.
3 Wash hands with bactericidal soap and water or bactericidal alcohol hand rub.		To reduce the risk of infection.
4 Prepare equipment using strict aseptic technique.	Assist in preparation of equipment without causing contamination.	
5 Remove the old dressing.		
6 Cut the knot from the pursestring suture.		Allows mobility of the suture.
7 Cut the suture holding the drain in place.	Hold the drain in place.	To prevent the drain falling out.

| 8 | Tie the purse-string suture lightly to skin level. | | To enable rapid tightening of the suture when the drain is removed. |

| 9 | Instruct the patient to breathe in to the maximum and to hold the breath. This manoeuvre should have been practised beforehand. | | To minimize the risk of tension pneumothorax occurring as the drain is removed. Prior preparation of the patient ensures full co-operation. |

| | | Steadily pull out the drain. | If the drain is pulled out too quickly, tension pneumothorax may occur through further rupture of the pleura. |

| 10 | As the drain leaves the skin, tighten the pursestring suture and tie a firm double-knot. Speed is essential. Cut the end to 1.25 cm. | | The purse-string suture must be tightened immediately the drain leaves the chest to prevent air from re-entering the pleural cavity and creating a tension pneumothorax. |

| 11 | Place gauze with collodion over the suture. | Strap the gauze firmly in place. | To provide a tight seal. |

| 12 | Tell the patient that he/she may exhale and relax. | | |

| | | Remove any debris from the site of the wound and ensure that the patient is comfortable. | |

| | | Clear equipment away. | |

| | | Wash hands with bactericidal soap and water. | To reduce risk of cross-infection. |

| | | Measure fluid drained. | |

| | | Empty and clean the drainage bottles and send them to the central sterile supplies department. | |

| | | Record the amount of drainage in appropriate documents. | To provide an accurate record. |

NURSING CARE PLAN

Problem	Cause	Suggested action
Lack of drainage.	Kinking, looping or pressure on the tubing may cause reflux of fluid into the intrapleural space or may impede drainage, causing blocking of the intrapleural drain.	Check the system and straighten tubing as required. Secure the tubing to prevent a recurrence of the problem.

Nursing care plan (cont'd)

Problem	Cause	Suggested action
No fluctuation of fluid in tubing from the underwater seal.	Re-expansion of the lung.	Ask medical staff if the drain may be removed following chest X-ray. The purpose of the drain has been fulfilled. Keeping the drain in any longer than necessary may lead to hazards from infection or air re-entry.
	Tubing is obstructed by blood clots or fibrin.	'Milk' the tubing towards the drainage bottle to try to dislodge the obstruction and re-establish patency.
	Tubing is looped or kinked.	Straighten tubing as required. Secure the tubing to prevent a recurrence.
	Failure of the suction apparatus.	Disconnect the suction apparatus and ensure drain is patent.
Constant bubbling of fluid in the drainage bottle.	An air leak in the system.	Clamp the intrapleural drain, momentarily, close to the chest wall and establish whether there is a leak in the rest of the system. Clamping the tubing shows whether the leak is below the level of the clamp. However, if the clamp is left on for too long, and the leak is at thoracic level, i.e. air is entering the pleura, this will increase the patient's pneumothorax. Inform medical staff as leaking and trapping of air in the pleural space can result in tension pneumothorax.
Patient shows signs of rapid, shallow breathing, cyanosis, pressure in the chest, subcutaneous emphysema or haemorrhage.	Tension pneumothorax; mediastinal shift; postoperative haemorrhage; severe incisional pain; pulmonary embolus or cardiac tamponade.	Observe, record and report any of these signs to a doctor immediately.
Incisional pain.		Provide adequate analgesia, as prescribed, to minimize the patient's discomfort and to enable deep-breathing exercises to be performed. Mobilization to ensure adequate drainage and to avoid complications.
Accidental disconnection of the drainage tubing from the intrapleural drain.		Apply an artery clamp to the drain immediately in order to avoid air entering the pleural

	space. Re-establish the connection as soon as possible in order to re-establish drainage. If necessary, use a clean, sterile drainage tube; tubing may have been contaminated when it became disconnected. Report to the doctor, who may wish to X-ray. Record the incident in the relevant records. The patient may have been upset by the incident and will need reassurance.
Patient needs to be moved to another area, e.g. X-ray department.	Place the drainage bottle below the level of the intrapleural drain, as close to the floor as possible, in order to prevent reflux of fluid into the pleural space. Clamp drain if this has been discussed and agreed with medical colleagues. Ensure clamps are readily available in case of accidental disconnection *en route*.
Intrapleural drain falls out.	Pull the purse-string suture immediately to close the wound. Cover the wound with an occlusive sterile dressing. Inform a doctor. The objective is to minimize the amount of air entering the pleural space. The drain will probably need reinserting. Reassure the patient with appropriate explanations.

CHAPTER 23

Intravenous Management

The aim of intravenous management is the safe, effective delivery of treatment without discomfort or tissue damage to the patient, and without compromising venous access, especially if long-term therapy is proposed.

DRUG ADMINISTRATION

REFERENCE MATERIAL

The involvement of nursing staff in the administration of intravenous drugs was formally recognized in the mid-1970s following the publication of the Breckenridge Report (Department of Health and Social Security, 1976). A working party had been established in 1974 under the chairmanship of Professor Breckenridge as a result of the increasing use of the intravenous route for drug administration. There was concern that hazards such as microbial contamination and drug incompatibilities were not fully appreciated and that the staff participating were not adequately trained in the procedures used.

The terms of reference of the working party were as follows:

(1) To identify and investigate the problems associated with this form of intravenous therapy.
(2) To consider the responsibilities of the various parties involved.
(3) To consider modification of nurse training to ensure safe practice.
(4) To produce guidelines for the three main professions, i.e. doctor, pharmacists and nurses.
(5) To assess the value of various aids, e.g. charts for reference.

The working party received evidence from a number of sources and considered pharmaceutical data. In 1976 the findings were published by the Department of Health and Social Security. The report proposed a rational approach to intravenous drug administration, established

guidelines for documentation and outlined the responsibilities of health authorities and health professionals. The responsibility of medical staff was to ensure that the drug was administered by the most effective and safest route and that the instructions to facilitate this were clearly written.

An intravenous additive service provided by pharmacists was favoured. In situations where this was not practical, pharmacists were to act as an information source for other personnel. It was accepted that nursing staff could undertake the addition and administration of intravenous drugs. The nurse, however, should be qualified (i.e. should be a registered general nurse or an enrolled nurse) and have undergone a period of training and assessment in both the theoretical knowledge and practical procedures involved in such drug administration. Guidance on the scope of professional practice, published by the United Kingdom Central Council (UKCC, 1992), states that 'the nurse must endeavour always to achieve, maintain and develop knowledge, skill and competence to respond to the needs and interests of the patient or client'.

In all intravenous therapy the nurse's responsibility continues to include the following:

(1) Checking the infusion fluid and container for any obvious faults or contamination.
(2) Ensuring the administration of the prescribed drug or fluid to the correct patient.
(3) Observing whether the intravenous line remains patent.
(4) Inspecting the site of insertion and reporting abnormalities.
(5) Controlling the rate of flow as prescribed.
(6) Monitoring the condition of the patient and reporting any changes.
(7) Maintaining appropriate records.

Permitted methods of intravenous drug administration by nurses were identified:

(1) Continuously, or intermittently, by addition to an intravenous infusion in a bottle, bag or burette. This method may include the use of a variety of equipment, e.g. a small-volume syringe pump or a Y administration set.

(2) Intermittently by injection into the latex rubber section of an intravenous administration set.

(3) Intermittently by injection into a cannula or winged infusion device. The device's patency may be maintained by:
  (a) Injecting heparinized 0.9% sodium chloride.
  (b) Injecting 0.9% sodium chloride.
  (c) Placing a stylet in the cannula.

(4) Intermittently by injection via a three-way tap or stopcock. This method is not advised, however, due to the increased risk of contamination associated with these devices. Streamlined adaptors are now available and are preferred (Cheeseborough & Finch, 1984; Brismar et al., 1984).

Additional guidelines

Guidelines were also issued in 1976 about general intravenous management related to the area of nursing involvement. These included the following:

(1) The infusion container should not hang for more than 24 hours. This was reduced to 8 hours in the case of blood or blood products.

(2) The administration set must be changed every 24 hours (Department of Health and Social Security, 1973). However, recent research indicates that changing sets every 48 or 72 hours is not associated with an increase in infection and could result in considerable savings for hospitals (Band & Maki, 1979; Josephson et al., 1985; Maki & Ringer, 1987). It is desirable to record the time and date that the set is due to be changed.

(3) The site of the infusion should be inspected at least daily for complications such as infiltration or inflammation.

(4) The sterile dressing covering the insertion site must be changed daily, at the time of inspection or whenever it is touched, e.g. at the time of administration of an intravenous injection.

Further recommendations in the light of recent research have shown that it is desirable that a closed system of infusion is maintained wherever possible, with as few connections or stopcocks as is necessary for its purpose (Speechley, 1986). This reduces the risk of extrinsic bacterial contamination, especially if three-way taps or their equivalent are excluded. The dead space in this equipment has been identified as a reservoir for microorganisms which may be released into the circulation (Weinbaum, 1987).

In the largest European study to date, Nystrom et al. (1983) provided evidence of the increased risk of infection to patients with an intravenous device. As the majority of sepsis is device related (Maki, 1991) and both infective and non-infective complications have been shown to increase substantially after the device has been in place for 72 hours (Maki, 1977; Goodison et al., 1988), routine resiting of peripheral cannulae every 48–72 hours is advised.

In order for the insertion site to be readily available for inspection, it may be necessary for the nurse to assume responsibility for taping the cannula in place as well as dressing the insertion site. Non-sterile tape should not cover the site, the equivalent of an open wound, and a method must be devised so that the site remains visible and the cannula is stable. The procedure shown in Fig. 23.1 is recommended: the site is visible during drug administration, and the tape does not cover the insertion site. Previous research has shown that dry sterile gauze and transparent dressings are associated with similar rates of skin colonization (Maki & Ringer, 1987; Hoffman et al., 1992). Recent developments in the moisture permeability rate of transparent dressings appear to show a reduction in skin colonization and the ability for the dressing to remain in place for 5–7 days (Maki, 1991; Keenleyside, 1993).

The purpose of all recommendations is to reduce the complications associated with intravenous therapy. Competent, informed management of and adherence to basic principles will ensure this.

Removal of the intravenous device or cannula should be an aseptic procedure. The cannula must be taken out gently in order to prevent damage to the vein and pressure should be applied immediately. This pressure should be firm and not involve any rubbing movement. A haematoma will occur if the needle is carelessly removed, causing discomfort and a focus for infection. Pressure should be applied until bleeding has stopped, then a light sterile dressing applied (Weinstein, 1993).

ADMINISTRATION OF DRUGS

Drugs are used for three basic purposes:

(1) Diagnostic purposes, e.g. assessment of liver function or diagnosis of myasthenia gravis.

(2) Prophylaxis, e.g. heparin to prevent thrombosis or antibiotics to prevent infection.

(3) Therapeutic purposes, e.g. replacement of fluids or vitamins, supportive purposes (to enable other treatments, such as anaesthesia), palliation of pain and cure (as in the case of antibiotics).

Drugs administered intravenously also fall within the above-mentioned categories.

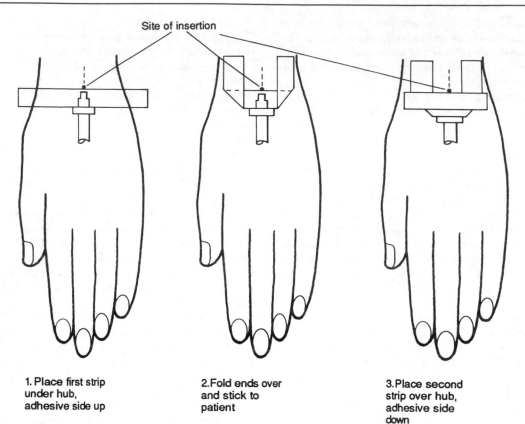

1. Place first strip under hub, adhesive side up

2. Fold ends over and stick to patient

3. Place second strip over hub, adhesive side down

Figure 23.1   Site of insertion.

Advantages of using the intravenous route

(1) An immediate, therapeutic effect is achieved due to rapid delivery of the drug to its target site, which allows a more precise dose calculation and therefore more reliable treatment.

(2) Pain and irritation caused by some substances when given intramuscularly or subcutaneously are avoided.

(3) The vascular route affords a route of administration for the patient who cannot tolerate fluids or drugs by the gastrointestinal route.

(4) Some drugs cannot be absorbed by any other route; the large molecular size of some drugs prevents absorption by the gastrointestinal route, while other drugs, unstable in the presence of gastric juices, are destroyed.

(5) The intravenous route offers a better control over the rate of administration of drugs; prolonged action can be provided by administering a dilute infusion intermittently or over a prolonged period of time (Weinstein, 1993).

Disadvantages of using the intravenous route

(1) There is an inability to recall the drug and reverse the action of it. This may lead to increased toxicity or a sensitivity reaction.

(2) Insufficient control of administration may lead to speed shock. This is characterized by a flushed face, headache, congestion, tightness in the chest, etc.

(3) Additional complications may occur, such as the following:
   (a) Microbial contamination (extrinsic or intrinsic).
   (b) Vascular irritation, e.g. chemical phlebitis.
   (c) Drug incompatibilities and interactions if multiple additives are prescribed.

Principles to be applied throughout preparation and administration

Asepsis
Aseptic technique must be adhered to throughout all intravenous procedures to prevent extrinsic bacterial

contamination. The nurse must employ good hand washing and drying techniques using a bactericidal soap or a bactericidal alcohol hand rub as an alternative. Injection sites or bungs should be cleaned using an alcohol-based antiseptic, allowing time for it to dry (Maki, 1991). A non-touch technique should be employed when changing infusion bags or bottles and these procedures should be completed as quickly as possible (Sager & Bomar, 1980; BNF, 1995). If asepsis is not maintained, local infection, septic phlebitis or septicaemia may result (Nystrom *et al.*, 1983; Maki, 1992). Any indication of infection, e.g. redness at the insertion site of the device or pyrexia, requires removal of the cannula and further investigation (Maki, 1981; Goodison, 1990b).

Inspection of fluids, drugs, equipment and their packaging must be undertaken to detect any points where contamination may have occurred during manufacture and/or transport. This intrinsic contamination may be detected as cloudiness, discoloration or the presence of particles (Sager & Bomar, 1980; BNF, 1995).

Sterility will ensure that the patient does not receive an injection or infusion of microbes.

Safety

All details of the prescription and all calculations must be checked carefully in accordance with hospital policy in order to ensure safe preparation and administration of the drug(s). The volume required can be calculated using the following calculation:

$$\frac{\text{strength required}}{\text{stock strength}} \times \text{volume of stock solution}$$
$$= \text{volume required}$$

(Gatford, 1990). The nurse must also check the compatibility of the drug with the diluent or infusion fluid. The nurse should be aware of the types of incompatibilities, and the factors which could influence them. These include pH, concentration, time, temperature, light and the brand of the drug. If insufficient information is available, a reference book (e.g. *The British National Formulary*) or the product data sheet must be consulted. If the nurse is unsure about any aspect of the preparation and/or administration of a drug, she should not proceed and should consult with a senior member of staff (UKCC, 1992). Constant monitoring of both the mixture and the patient is important. The preferred method and rate of intravenous administration must be determined.

Drugs should never be added to the following: blood; blood products i.e. plasma or platelet concentrate; mannitol solutions; sodium bicarbonate solution, etc. Only specially prepared additives should be used with fat emulsions or amino acid preparations.

Accurate labelling of additives and records of administration are essential.

Any protective clothing which is advised should be worn.

Comfort

Both the physical and psychological comfort of the patient must be considered. By maintaining high standards throughout, the patient's physical comfort should be assured. Comprehensive explanation of the practical aspects of the procedure together with balanced information about the effects of treatment will contribute to reducing anxiety (Wilson-Barnett & Carrigy, 1978; Wilson-Barnett & Batehup, 1992) and will need to be tailored to each patient's individual needs.

Methods of administering intravenous drugs

There are three methods of administering intravenous drugs: continuous infusion, intermittent infusion and intermittent injection.

Continuous infusion

Continuous infusion may be defined as the intravenous delivery of a medication or fluid at a constant rate over a prescribed time period, ranging from a number of hours to days (Reville & Almadrones, 1989).

A continuous infusion may be used when:

(1) The drugs to be administered must be highly diluted.
(2) A maintenance of steady blood levels of the drug is required.

Pre-prepared infusion fluids with additives such as those containing potassium chloride should be used whenever possible. This reduces the risk of extrinsic contamination, which can occur during the mixing of drugs (Weinstein, 1993). Only one addition should be made to each bottle or bag of fluid after the compatibility has been ascertained. More additions can increase the risk of incompatibility occurring, e.g. precipitation (Weinstein, 1993). The additive and fluid must be mixed well to prevent a layering effect which can occur with some drugs. The danger is that a bolus injection of the drug may be delivered. To safeguard this, any additions should be made to the infusion fluid before the fluid is hung on the infusion stand. The infusion container should be labelled clearly after the addition has been made. Constant monitoring of the infusion fluid mixture (Weinstein, 1993) for cloudiness or presence of particles should occur, as well as checking the patient condition and IV site for patency, extravasation or infiltration.

Intermittent infusion

Intermittent infusion is the administration of a small-volume infusion, i.e. 50–250 ml, over a period of between 20 minutes and 2 hours. This may be given as a specific dose at one time or at repeated intervals during 24 hours.

An intermittent infusion may be used when:

(1) A peak plasma level is required therapeutically.
(2) The pharmacology of the drug dictates this specific dilution.
(3) The drug will not remain stable for the time required to administer a more dilute volume.
(4) The patient is on a restricted intake of fluids.

Delivery of the drug by intermittent infusion may utilize a system such as a Y set, if the simultaneous infusion is of a compatible fluid, or a burette set with a chamber capacity of 100 or 150 ml. A small-volume infusion may also be connected to a cannula to keep the vein open, if no fluids are required between doses.

All the points considered when preparing for a continuous infusion should be taken into account here, e.g. pre-prepared fluids, single additions, adequate mixing, labelling and monitoring.

Direct intermittent injection

Direct intermittent injection is a procedure for the introduction of a small volume of drug(s) into the cannula or the injection site of the administration set using a needle and syringe. Most must be administered slowly anywhere from a few minutes up to 30 minutes depending on the drug (Weinstein, 1993).

A direct injection may be used when:

(1) A maximum concentration of the drug is required to vital organs. This is a 'bolus' injection which is given rapidly over seconds, as in an emergency.
(2) The drug cannot be diluted due to pharmacological or therapeutic reasons or does not require dilution. This is given as a controlled 'push' injection over a few minutes.
(3) A peak blood level is required and cannot be achieved by small-volume infusion.

Rapid administration could result in toxic levels and an anaphylactic-type reaction. Manufacturers' recommendations of rates of administration (i.e. millilitres or milligrams per minute) should be adhered to. In the absence of such recommendations, administration should proceed slowly.

Delivery of the drug by direct injection may be via the cannula through a resealable latex bung, extension set or via the injection site of an administration set. Whatever method is chosen, the same procedure prior to injecting the drug should be followed. This includes the following:

(1) Removal of any bandage or dressing present to inspect the insertion of the cannula.
(2) Confirmation of the patency of the vein and its ability to accept an extra flow of fluid or irritant chemical.

Administration into the injection site of a fast-running drip may be advised if the infusion in progress is compatible. Alternatively, a stop–start procedure may be employed if there is doubt about venous integrity. This allows the nurse to constantly check the patency of the vein and detect early signs of extravasation. If the infusion fluid is incompatible with the drug, the line may be switched off and a syringe of 0.9% sodium chloride used as a flush.

In some centres a 'heparin' lock may be utilized. This means maintaining the patency of the cannula using a weak solution of heparin. A plug with a resealable injection cap is inserted into the end of the intravenous device. Sufficient heparin to fill the 'dead space' and of a concentration to prevent fibrin formation is injected. The cannula can then be left for a number of hours before reheparinization is required. The time is dependent on the strength of heparin used. After every use, reheparinization is required.

The advantage of using a heparin lock are as follows:

(1) It reduces the risk of circulatory overload.
(2) It reduces the risk of vascular irritation.
(3) It decreases the risk of bacterial contamination as it eliminates a continuous intravenous pathway.
(4) It increases patient comfort and mobility.
(5) It may reduce the cost of intravenous equipment.

One of the disadvantages is the necessity for constant vigilance and regular flushing (Weinstein, 1993).

Research has shown that flushing with 0.9% sodium chloride can also adequately maintain the patency of the cannula (Epperson, 1984; Dunn & Lenihan, 1987; Hamilton et al., 1988; Barrett & Lester, 1990; Goode et al., 1991). Using 0.9% sodium chloride avoids side-effects such as local tissue damage, drug incompatibilities and iatrogenic haemorrhage, which can occur with heparin (Goode et al., 1991). Using 0.9% sodium chloride as a flushing solution could reduce the cost of maintaining peripheral devices and prevent potentially harmful side-effects. However, it has been suggested that one of the most important aspects of maintaining patency is the method of flushing. The intravenous device should be flushed briskly using the positive pressure technique. This is accomplished by clamping the catheter or extension set while flushing before the syringe completely empties. Alternatively, pressure can be maintained on the plunger of the syringe while withdrawing the syringe from the injection cap – thus preventing reflux of blood into the tip of the device (Baranowski, 1993).

If a number of drugs are being administered, 0.9% sodium chloride must be used to flush in between each drug to prevent interactions. 0.9% sodium chloride should also be used at the end of the administration to ensure that all of the drug has been delivered.

The insertion site of the device should be observed throughout the administration for signs of redness or swelling. Patients must be consulted constantly about any pain or discomfort they may be experiencing. These signs and symptoms will enable the nurse to detect extravasation of the drug and act appropriately to reduce the likelihood of tissue damage.

Summary

The nurse is responsible for administering intravenous drugs safely by the methods listed. In order to do this he/she requires a thorough knowledge of the principles and their application, and a responsible attitude which ensures that intravenous medications are not given without full knowledge of immediate and late effects, toxicities and nursing implications. The nurse must also be able to justify any actions taken and be prepared to be accountable for the action taken (UKCC, 1992).

References and further reading

Band, J. & Maki, D. (1979) Safety of changing intravenous delivery systems at longer than 24-hour intervals. *Annals of Internal Medicine*, 90, 173–8.

Baranowski, L. (1993) Central venous access devices, current technologies, uses and management strategies. *Journal of Intravenous Nursing*, 16(3), 167–94.

Barrett, P. & Lester, R. (1990) Heparin versus saline flushing solutions in a small community hospital. *Hospital Pharmacy*, 25, 115–18.

Brismar, B. *et al.* (1984) Bacterial contamination of intravenous cannula injection ports and stopcocks. *Clinical Nutrition*, 3, 23–6.

British Medical Association/Pharmaceutical Society of Great Britain (1988) *British National Formulary*. BMA, London.

British National Formulary (BNF) (1995) *British Medical Association and Royal Pharmaceutical Society of Great Britain*, No 30, September, Appendix 6, 584–94.

Cheeseborough, J. S. & Finch, R. (1984) Side ports – an infection hazard? *British Journal of Parenteral Therapy*, July, 155–7.

Clarkson, D. (1995) The future of infusion. *Hospital Equipment and Supplies*, June, 17.

Cyganski, J. *et al.* (1987) The case for the heparin flush. *American Journal of Nursing*, 87, 796–7.

Department of Health and Social Security (1973) *Medicines Commission Report on Prevention of Microbial Contamination of Medicinal Products*. HMSO, London.

Department of Health and Social Security (1976) *Health Services Development, Addition of Drugs to Intravenous Fluids, HC(76)9 (Breckenridge Report)*. HMSO, London.

Dunn, D. & Lenihan, S. (1987) The case for the saline flush. *American Journal of Nursing*, 87(6), 798–9.

Epperson, E. L. (1984) Efficacy of 0.9% sodium chloride injection with and without heparin for maintaining indwelling intermittent injection sites. *Clinical Pharmacy*, 3, 626–9.

Gatford, J. D. (1990) *Nursing Calculations*, 3rd edn. Churchill Livingstone, Edinburgh.

Goode, C. J. *et al.* (1991) A meta analysis of effects of heparin flush and saline flush – quality and cost implications. *Nursing Research*, 40(6), 324–30.

Goodison, S. M. (1990a) The risks of IV therapy. *Professional Nurse*, February, 235.

Goodison, S. M. (1990b) Keeping the flora out. *Professional Nurse*, August, 572.

Goodison, S. M. (1990c) Good practice insures minimum risk factors. *Professional Nurse*, December, 175.

Goodison, S. *et al.* (1988) A survey of intravenous catheters and other inserts. *Proceedings of Second International Conference on Infection Control*, 13–80.

Hamilton, R. A. *et al.* (1988) Heparin sodium vesus 0.9% sodium chloride injection for maintaining patency of indwelling intermittent infusion devices. *Clinical Pharmacy*, 7, 439–43.

Haynes, S. (1989) Infusion phlebitis and extravasation. *The Professional Nurse*, December, 160–61.

Hecker, J. (1988) Improved technique in IV therapy. *Nursing Times*, 84(34), 28–33.

Hoffman, K. K. *et al.* (1992) Transparent polyurethane film as an intravenous catheter dressing – a meta analysis of the infection risks. *Journal of American Medical Association*, 267(15), 2072–6.

Hook, M. (1990) Heparin vs 0.9% sodium chloride. Letters to the Editor, *Journal of Intravenous Nursing*, 13(3), 150–1.

Hudek, K. (1986) Compliance in intravenous therapy. *Journal of Canadian Intravenous Nursing Association*, 2(3), 7–8.

Josephson, A. *et al.* (1985) The relationship between intravenous fluid contamination and the frequency of tubing replacement. *Infection Control*, 9, 367–70.

Keenleyside, D. (1993) Avoiding an unnecessary outcome. *Professional Nurse*, February, 288–91.

Maki, D. (1977) A semi-quantative culture method for identifying intravenous catheter-related infections. *New England Journal of Medicine*, 296, 1305–6.

Maki, D. G. (1991) *Proceedings of International Congress and Symposium*, Royal Society of Medicine (Series 179).

Maki, D. G. (1992) Infections due to infusion therapy. In: *Hospital Infections*, (eds J. V. Bennett & P. S. Bradman), 3rd edn, Chapter 40. Little, Brown & Co, Boston.

Maki, D. G. & Ringer, M. (1987) Evaluation of dressing regimens for prevention of infection with peripheral intravenous catheters. *Journal of the American Medical Association*, 256(17), 2396–2403.

Maki, D. *et al.* (1987) Prospective study replacing administration sets for intravenous therapy, at 48 to 72 hour intervals. *Journal of the American Medical Association*, 258(13), 1777–81.

Nystrom, B. *et al.* (1983) Bacteraemia in surgical patients with intravenous devices: a European multicentre incidence study. *Journal of Hospital Infection*, 4, 338–49.

Oldman, P. (1991) A sticky situation? *Professional Nurse*, 6(5), 265–9.

Ostrow, L. S. (1981) Air embolism and central venous lines. *American Journal of Nursing*, 81(11), 2036–9.

Parish, P. (1982) Benefits to risks of IV therapies. *British Journal of Intravenous Therapy*, 3(6), 10–19.

Peters, J. *et al.* (1984) Peripheral venous cannulation: reducing the risks. *British Journal of Parenteral Therapy*, 5(2), 56–68.

Plumer, A. L. (1987) *Principles and Practice of Intravenous Therapy*, 4th edn. Little Brown & Co, Boston, USA.

Reville, B. & Almadrones, L. (1989) Continuous infusion chemotherapy in the ambulatory setting: the nurse's role in patient selection and education. *Oncology Nursing Forum*, 16, 529–35.

Sager, D. & Bomar, S. (1980) *Intravenous Medications*. J. B. Lippincott, Philadelphia.

Sager, D. & Bomar, S. (1983) *Quick Reference to Intravenous Drugs*. J. B. Lippincott, Philadelphia.

Smith, R. (1985a) Extravasation of intravenous fluids. *British Journal of Parenteral Therapy*, 6(2), 30–5.

Smith, R. (1985b) Prevention and treatment of extravasation. *British Journal of Parenteral Therapy*, 6(5), 114–19.

Smolders, C. (1988) Infusion phlebitis. *Canadian Intravenous Nurses Association*, 4(2), 20–22.

Speechley, V. (1984) The nurse's role in intravenous management. *Nursing Times*, 2 May, 31–2.

Speechley, V. (1986) Intravenous therapy: peripheral/central lines. *Nursing*, 3(3), 95–100.

Speechley, V. & Toovey, J. (1987) Factsheets: problems in IV therapy 1, 2, 3. *Professional Nurse*, 2(8), 240–2; 2(12), 413; 3(3), 90–1.

United Kingdom Central Council for Nursing, Midwifery and Health Visiting (1992) *Scope of Professional Practice*. UKCC, London.

Weinbaum, D. L. (1987) Nosocomial bacterias. In *Infection Control in Intensive Care*, (ed. B. F. Faser), pp. 39–58. Churchill Livingstone, New York.

Weinstein, S. M. (ed.) (1993) *Plumer's Principles and Practices of Intravenous Therapy*, 5th edn. J. B. Lippincott, Philadelphia.

Wilson-Barnett, J. & Carrigy, A. (1978) Factors influencing patients' emotional reactions to hospitalization. *Journal of Advanced Nursing*, 3, 221–9.

Wilson-Barnett, J. & Batehup, L. (1992) *Patients' problems: A Research Base for Nursing Care*, Chapter 3. Scutari Press, London.

Wright, A. *et al.* (1985) Use of transdermal glyceryl trinitrate to reduce failure of intravenous infusion due to phlebitis and extravasation. *Lancet*, 11, 1148–50.

GUIDELINES: ADMINISTRATION OF DRUGS BY CONTINUOUS INFUSION

This procedure may be carried out by the infusion of drugs from a bag, bottle or burette.

EQUIPMENT

1 Clinically clean receiver or tray containing the prepared drug to be administered.
2 Patient's prescription chart.
3 Recording sheet or book as required by law or hospital policy.
4 Protective clothing as required by hospital policy for specific drugs.
5 Container of appropriate intravenous infusion fluid.
6 Swab saturated with isopropyl alcohol 70%.
7 Drug additive label.

PROCEDURE

Action	Rationale
1 Explain and discuss the procedure with the patient.	To ensure that the patient understands the procedure and gives his/her valid consent.
2 Inspect the infusion.	To check it is running satisfactorily and if the patient is experiencing any discomfort at the site of insertion.
3 Wash hands with bactericidal soap and water or bactericidal alcohol hand rub, and assemble the necessary equipment.	

4 Prepare the drug for injection described in the procedure (see Chapter 15, Drug Administration).

5 Check the name, strength and volume of intravenous fluid against the prescription chart.

To ensure that the correct type and quantity of fluid are administered.

6 Check the expiry date of the fluid.

To prevent an ineffective or toxic compound being administered to the patient.

7 Check that the packaging is intact.

To maintain asepsis.

8 Inspect the container and contents in a good light for cracks, punctures, air bubbles, discolouration, haziness and crystalline or particulate matter

To maintain asepsis. To prevent any toxic or foreign matter being infused into the patient.

9 Check the identity and amount of drug to be added. Consider:
   (a) Compatibility of fluid and additive.
   (b) Stability of mixture over the prescription time.
   (c) Any special directions for dilution, e.g. pH, optimum concentration, etc.
   (d) Sensitivity to external factors such as light.
   (e) Any anticipated allergic reaction.
If any doubts exist about the listed points, consult the pharmacist or appropriate reference works.

To minimize any risk of error. To ensure safe and effective administration of the drug. To enable anticipation of toxicities and the nursing implications of these.

10 Any additions must be made immediately before use.

To prevent any possible microbial growth or degradation.

11 Wash hands thoroughly using bactericidal soap and water or bactericidal alcohol hand rub.

To maintain asepsis.

12 Expose the injection site on the container by removing any seal present.

13 Clean the site with the swab and allow it to dry.

To maintain asepsis.

14 Inject the drug using a new sterile needle into the bag, bottle or burette. A 23 or 25 g needle should be used.

To enable resealing of the latex or rubber injection site.

15 If the addition is made into a burette at the bedside:
   (a) Avoid contamination of the needle and inlet port.
   (b) Check that the correct quantity of fluid is in the chamber.
   (c) Switch the infusion off briefly.

To maintain asepsis and prevent incompatibility, etc.

To ensure the correct dilution.

To ensure a bolus injection is not given.

16 Invert the container a number of times, especially if adding to a flexible infusion bag.

To ensure adequate mixing of the drug.

17 Check again for haziness, discolouration, etc. This can occur even if the mixture is

To detect any incompatibility or degradation.

Guidelines: Administration of drugs by continuous infusion (cont'd)

Action	Rationale
theoretically compatible, thus making vigilance essential.	
18 Complete the drug additive label and fix it on the bag, bottle or burette.	To identify which drug has been added, when and by whom.
19 Place the container in a clinically clean receptacle. Wash hands and proceed to the patient.	To maintain asepsis.
20 Check the identity of the patient with the prescription chart and infusion bag.	To minimize the risk of error and ensure the correct infusion is administered to the correct patient.
21 Check again that the infusion is running well and that the contents of the previous container have been delivered.	To confirm that the vein and/or cannula remain patent. To ensure that the preceding prescription has been administered
22 Switch off the infusion and hang the new container quickly using a non-touch technique.	To achieve a safe and aseptic change-over.
23 Restart the infusion and adjust the rate of flow as prescribed.	To ensure that the infusion will be delivered at the correct rate over the correct period of time.
24 If the addition is made into a burette, the infusion can be restarted immediately following mixing and recording and the infusion rate adjusted accordingly.	
25 Ask the patient if any abnormal sensations, etc. are experienced.	To ascertain whether there are any problems and refer to medical staff where appropriate.
26 Discard waste, making sure that it is placed in the correct containers, e.g. 'sharps' into a designated receptacle.	To ensure safe disposal and avoid injury to staff. To prevent re-use of equipment.
27 Complete the patient's recording chart and other hospital and/or legally required documents.	To maintain accurate records. To provide a point of reference in the event of any queries. To prevent any duplication of treatment.

GUIDELINES: ADMINISTRATION OF DRUGS BY INTERMITTENT INFUSION

This procedure is carried out via a heparinized cannula or when patency is maintained by a stylet.

EQUIPMENT

Equipment for this procedure is as described for the previous procedure (i.e. items 1–7), together with the following:
  8 Intravenous administration set.
  9 Intravenous infusion stand.
10 Clean dressing trolley.
11 Clinically clean receiver or tray.

12 Sterile needles and syringes.
13 0.9% sodium chloride, 20 ml for injection.
14 Heparin, in accordance with hospital policy, plus, sterile bung or sterile stylet.
15 Alcohol-based lotion for cleaning injection site, e.g. chlorhexidine in 70% alcohol.
16 Alcohol-based hand wash solution.
17 Sterile dressing pack.
18 Hypoallergenic tape.

PROCEDURE

Action	Rationale
1 Explain and discuss the procedure with the patient.	To ensure that the patient understands the procedure and gives his/her valid consent.
2 Prepare the intravenous infusion and additive as described for the previous procedure (i.e. items 2–11) .	
3 Prime the intravenous administration set with infusion fluid mixture and hang it on the infusion stand.	
4 Draw up 10 ml of 0.9% sodium chloride for injection in two separate syringes, using an aseptic technique.	
5 Draw up flushing solution, as required by hospital policy.	
6 Place the syringes in a clinically clean receiver or tray on the bottom shelf of the dressing trolley.	
7 Collect the other equipment and place it on the bottom shelf of the dressing trolley.	
8 Place a sterile dressing pack on the top of the trolley.	
9 Check that all necessary equipment is present.	To prevent delays and interruption of the procedure.
10 Wash hands thoroughly using bactericidal soap and water or bactericidal alcohol hand rub before leaving the clinical room.	To maintain asepsis
11 Proceed to the patient. Check patient's identity with prescription chart and prepared drugs.	To minimize the risk of error and ensure the correct drug is given to the correct patient.
12 Open the sterile dressing pack.	To maintain asepsis.
13 Add lotion for cleaning the skin to the gallipot in order to wet the low-linting swabs.	
14 Wash hands with bactericidal soap and water or with a bactericidal alcohol hand rub.	To maintain asepsis.
15 Remove the patient's bandage and dressing.	To observe the insertion site.

Guidelines: Administration of drugs by intermittent infusion (cont'd)

Action	Rationale
16 Inspect the insertion site of the cannula.	To detect any signs of inflammation, infiltration, etc. If present, take appropriate action.
17 Wash hands as above (see item 14).	To maintain asepsis.
18 Put on gloves, if appropriate.	To protect against contamination with hazardous substances, e.g. cytotoxic drugs.
19 Place a sterile towel under the patient's arm.	To create a sterile area on which to work.
20 Remove the injection bung or stylet from the cannula while applying digital pressure at the point in the vein where the cannula tip rests. This may be achieved more easily using a sterile low-linting swab.	To prevent blood spillage.
21 Inject gently 10 ml of 0.9% sodium chloride for injection.	To confirm the patency of the cannula.
22 Check that no resistance is met, no pain or discomfort is felt by the patient, no swelling is evident, no leakage occurs around the cannula and there is a good back-flow of blood on aspiration.	To ensure the cannula is patent.
23 Connect to the infusion.	To commence treatment.
24 Open the control valve.	To check free flow.
25 Check the insertion site and ask the patient if he/she is comfortable.	To confirm that the vein can accommodate the extra fluid flow and that the patient experiences no pain, etc
26 Adjust the flow rate as prescribed.	To ensure that the correct speed of administration is established.
27 Tape the administration set in a way that places no strain on the cannula, which could in turn damage the vein.	To reduce the risk of mechanical phlebitis or infiltration
28 Cover the cannula with a sterile topical swab and tape it in place.	To maintain asepsis.
29 Remove gloves, if used.	
30 If the infusion is to be completed within 40 minutes, bandaging is unnecessary and the patient may be instructed to keep the arm resting on the sterile towel.	
31 If the infusion is to be in progress for longer than 40 minutes a bandage should be applied.	To reduce the risk of dislodging the cannula.
32 The equipment must be cleared away and reassembled at the end of the infusion.	To ensure that the equipment used is sterile prior to use.

33	Return at frequent intervals.	To check the flow rate, the patient's comfort and for signs of infiltration.

34 When the infusion is complete, wash hands using bactericidal soap and water or bactericidal alcohol hand rub, and recheck that all the equipment required is present.

To maintain asepsis and ensure that the procedure runs smoothly.

35 Stop the infusion when all the fluid has been delivered

To ensure that all of the prescribed mixture has been delivered

36 Wash hands with bactericidal soap and water or bactericidal alcohol hand rub.

To maintain asepsis.

37 Put on gloves, if appropriate.

To protect against contamination with hazardous substances.

38 Disconnect the infusion set and flush the cannula with 10 ml of 0.9% sodium chloride for injection. (A 'minibag' may be used to flush the drug through the tubing but the cost implications of this as well as the risk to patients on restricted intake should be considered before this is adopted routinely.)

To flush any remaining irritating solution away from the cannula.

39 Attach a new sterile injection cap.

40 Flushing must follow.

To maintain the patency of the cannula.

41 Clean the injection site of the bung with a swab saturated with chlorhexidine in 70% alcohol.

To maintain asepsis.

42 Administer flushing solution (using a 23 or 25 g needle) using the positive pressure technique.

To maintain the patency of the cannula and enable reseal of the latex injection site.

43 Cover the insertion site and cannula with a new sterile low-linting swab. Tape it in place.

To minimize the risk of contamination of the insertion site.

44 Apply a bandage.

To reduce the risk of dislodging the cannula.

45 Ensure that the patient is comfortable.

46 Discard waste, placing it in the correct containers, e.g. 'sharps' into a designated container.

To ensure safe disposal and avoid injury to staff. To prevent re-use of equipment.

47 Remove gloves, if used.

GUIDELINES: ADMINISTRATION OF DRUGS BY DIRECT INJECTION, BOLUS OR PUSH

This procedure may be carried out via any one of the following:

Guidelines: Administration of drugs by direct injection, bolus or push (cont'd)

1 The injection site of an intravenous administration set.
2 An adaptor or injection cap into a cannula or winged infusion device (patency may be maintained by stylet or by flushing).
3 An extension set, multiple adaptor or stopcock (one-, two- or three-way).

EQUIPMENT

1 Clinically clean receiver or tray containing the prepared drug(s) to be administered.
2 Patient's prescription chart.
3 Recording sheet or book as required by law or hospital policy.
4 Protective clothing as required by hospital policy or specific drugs.
5 Clean dressing trolley.
6 Clinically clean receiver or tray.
7 Sterile needles and syringes.
8 0.9% sodium chloride, 20 ml for injection.
9 Flushing solution, in accordance with hospital policy, or a sterile intravenous stylet.
10 Alcohol-based solution for cleaning injection site, e.g. chlorhexidine in 70% alcohol.
11 Sterile dressing pack.
12 Hypoallergenic tape.
13 Sharps container.

PROCEDURE

Action	Rationale
1 Explain and discuss the procedure with the patient.	To ensure that the patient understands the procedure and gives his/her valid consent.
2 Check any infusion in progress.	To see if it is running satisfactorily, and that the patient is not experiencing any discomfort at the site of insertion.
3 Wash hands with bactericidal soap and water or bactericidal alcohol hand rub, and assemble necessary equipment.	To minimize the risk of infection.
4 Prepare the drug for injection as per procedure described earlier.	
5 Prepare a 20-ml syringe of 0.9% sodium chloride for injection, as described, using aseptic technique	To use for flushing between each drug.
6 Draw up flushing solution, as required by hospital policy.	
7 Place syringes in a clinically clean receptacle on the bottom shelf of the dressing trolley, along with the receptacle containing any drug(s) to be administered.	
8 Collect the other equipment and place it on the bottom of the trolley.	
9 Place a sterile dressing pack on top of the trolley.	

10	Check that all necessary equipment is present.	To prevent delays and interruption of the procedure.
11	Wash hands thoroughly (see item 3, above).	To minimize the risk of infection.
12	Proceed to the patient and check identity with prescription chart and prepared drug.	To minimize the risk of error and ensure the correct patient.
13	Open the sterile dressing pack. Add lotion to wet the low-linting swab.	
14	Wash hands with bactericidal soap and water or with bactericidal alcohol hand rub.	To reduce the risk of infection.
15	Remove the bandage and dressing.	To observe the insertion site.
16	Inspect the insertion site of the cannula.	To detect any signs of inflammation, infiltration, etc. If present, take appropriate action.
17	Observe the infusion, if in progress.	To confirm that it is infusing as desired.
18	Check if the infusion fluid and the drugs are compatible. If not change the fluid to 0.9% sodium chloride.	To prevent drug interaction. Some manufacturers may recommend that the drug is given into the injection site of a rapidly running infusion.
19	Wash hands or clean them with an alcohol hand rub.	To minimize the risk of infection.
20	Place a sterile towel under the patient's arm.	To create a sterile field.
21	Clean the injection site with a swab saturated with chlorhexidine in 70% alcohol and allow to dry.	To reduce the number of pathogens introduced by the needle at the time of the insertion.
22	Switch off the infusion or close the fluid path of a tap or stopcock	To prevent excessive pressure within the vein. To prevent contact with an incompatible infusion fluid. To allow the nurse to concentrate on the site of insertion and injection.
23	Use a sterile 23 or 25g needle if the injection is made through a resealable latex site and gently inject 0.9% sodium chloride. This may not be necessary if the patient has a 0.9% sodium chloride infusion in progress.	To enable resealing of the site at the end of the injection. To confirm patency of the vein. To prevent contact with an incompatible infusion solution.
24	Change syringes and inject the drug smoothly in the direction of flow at the specified rate.	To prevent excessive pressure within the vein. To prevent speed shock.
	Ensure used needles and syringes are disposed of immediately into appropriate sharps container (or are returned to tray). Do not leave uncapped sharps on pack.	To reduce the risk of needlestick injury and to prevent contamination of pack.
25	Observe the insertion site of the cannula throughout.	To detect any complications at an early stage, e.g. extravasation or local allergic reaction.
26	Blood return and/or 'flashback' must be checked frequently throughout the injection.	To confirm that the device is correctly placed and that the vein remains patent.

Guidelines: Administration of drugs by direct injection, bolus or push (cont'd)

Action	Rationale
27 Consult the patient during the injection about any discomfort, etc.	To detect any complications at an early stage, and ensure patient comfort.
28 If more than one drug is to be administered, flush with 0.9% sodium chloride between administrations by restarting the infusion or changing syringes.	To prevent drug interactions.
29 At the end of the injection, flush with 0.9% sodium chloride by restarting the infusion or changing syringes.	To flush any remaining irritant solution away from the cannula site.
30 Open the control clamp of the giving set fully. Inject the drug at a speed sufficient to slow but not stop the infusion	To prevent a back-flow of drug up the tubing.
31 Observe the insertion site of the cannula carefully.	To detect any complications at an early stage. Extra pressure within the vein caused by both fluid flow and injection of the drug may cause rupture.
32 After the final flush of 0.9% sodium chloride adjust the infusion rate as prescribed or open the fluid path of the tap/stopcock or use flushing solution or an intravenous stylet.	To continue delivery of therapy. To maintain the patency of the cannula.
33 Cover the insertion site with new sterile topical dressing and tape it in place.	To minimize the risk of contamination of the insertion site.
34 Apply a bandage.	To reduce the risk of dislodging the cannula.
35 Make sure that the patient is comfortable.	
36 Record the administration on appropriate sheets .	To maintain accurate records, provide a point of reference in the event of any queries and prevent any duplication of treatment.
37 Once injection has been administered, place all used syringes with needle unsheathed directly into 'sharps' container. Do not disconnect needle from syringe prior to disposal. Other waste should be placed into the appropriate plastic bags.	To avoid needlestick injury.

NURSING CARE PLAN

The problems associated with injection and infusion of intravenous fluids and drugs fall into two categories:

1 Local venous complications associated with the cannula insertion site.
2 Systemic problems which affect the whole patient, exerting effects on vital organs and their functions.

The nurse must observe regularly the insertion site, the infusion and the patient to detect any complications at the earliest possible moment and to prevent progression to more serious conditions. Early detection is aided by paying attention to the patient's comments of discomfort or pain. The patient's symptoms and physical signs both constitute reasons for a resiting of the cannula or discontinuation of the infusion. Signs and symptoms are used as problem headings.

Problem	Possible causes	Preventive nursing measures	Suggested action
Infusion slows or stops.	Change in position of the following:		
	(a) Patient.	Check the height of the fluid container if the patient is active, as all infusions run by gravity.	Adjust the height accordingly.
	(b) Limb.	Tape, bandage or splint the limb if infusion is sited at a point of flexion. Instruct the patient on the amount of movement permitted. Continued movement could result in mechanical phlebitis.	Move the arm or hand until infusion starts again. Retape, bandage or splint the limb again carefully in the desired position.
	(c) Administration set.	Check for kinks and/or compression if the patient is active or restless.	Correct accordingly.
	(d) Cannula.	Tape the cannula firmly to prevent movement. It may come into contact with the vein wall or a valve. Infusions sited in small veins are prone to this problem.	Remove the bandage and dressing and manoeuvre the cannula gently until the infusion starts again. Retape carefully.
	Technical problems:		
	(a) No air inlet in the rigid container.	Ensure that the container is vented.	Vent if necessary, using venting needle.
	(b) Empty container.	Check fluid levels regularly.	Replace the fluid container before it runs dry.
	(c) Venous spasm due to chemical irritation or coldness.	Dilute drugs as recommended. Remove solutions from the refrigerator a short time before use.	Apply a warm compress to soothe and dilate the vein, increase blood flow and dilute the infusion mixture.
	(d) Injury to the vein.	Detect any injury early as it is likely to progress and cause more serious conditions (see below).	Stop the infusion and request a resiting of the cannula.
	(e) Occlusion of the cannula due to fibrin formation.	Maintain a continuous, regular fluid flow or ensure that patency is maintained by flushing or by placement of a stylet. Instruct the patient to keep limb at waist level or below if ambulant.	Remove extension set/ injection cap and attempt to flush the cannula gently using a 1 ml syringe of 0.9% sodium chloride. If resistance is met, stop and request a re-siting of the cannula.

Nursing care plan (cont'd)

Problem	Possible causes	Preventive nursing measures	Suggested action
	(f) The cannula has become displaced either completely or partially, i.e. it has 'tissued'.	Tape the cannula and the giving set so that no stress is placed on them. Instruct the patient on the amount of movement permitted.	Confirm that infiltration has/has not occurred by: (i) inspecting the site for leakage, swelling, etc.; (ii) testing the temperature of the skin – it will be cooler if infiltration has occurred; (iii) comparing the size of the limb with the opposite limb; (iv) applying a tourniquet above the cannula site or lowering the infusion below the height of the limb. If the vein is patent, blood will flow back into the giving set. Once infiltration has been confirmed, stop the infusion and request a resiting of the cannula. If the infusion is allowed to progress, discomfort and tissue damage will result. Apply cold or warm compresses to provide symptomatic relief. Reassure the patient by explaining what is happening.
Erythema or inflammation around the insertion site.	Phlebitis due to:		
	(a) Sepsis.	Adhere to aseptic techniques when performing all intravenous procedures (Maki, 1991)	Stop the infusion and request a resiting of the cannula. Follow hospital policy about sending equipment for bacterial analysis. Clean the area and apply a sterile dressing. Check regularly.
	(b) Chemical irritation.	Dilute drugs according to instructions. Check compatibilities carefully	Stop the infusion and request a resiting of the cannula. If the infusion is

	to reduce the risk of particulate formation. Be aware of the factors involved, e.g. pH (Wright *et al.*, 1985; Smolders, 1988; Haynes, 1989). Apply a glycerol trinitrate (GTN) patch to aid vasodilation (Wright *et al.*, 1985; Hecker, 1988).	allowed to progress, tissue damage and severe pain will result. Apply cold or warm compresses to provide symptomatic relief. Encourage movement of the limb. Reassure the patient by explaining what is happening.
(c) Mechanical irritation.	Tape, bandage or splint the limb if the infusion is sited at a point of flexion. Use an extension set to minimize direct handling if cannula sited in awkward position. Instruct the patient on the amount of movement permitted (Hecker, 1988; Goodison, 1990a).	Stop the infusion and request a resiting of the cannula. Although inflammation of this type progresses more slowly, it will cause discomfort. Provide symptomatic relief as above. Encourage movement and reassure the patient by explaining what is happening. Failure to detect and act when phlebitis is at an early stage, for whatever reason, will result in painful and incapacitating thrombophlebitis. Dislodgement of a thrombus could cause a pulmonary embolus (Weinstein, 1993).
Infection with or without discharge.	Adhere to aseptic techniques when performing all intravenous procedures. Observe all recommendations for equipment changes, etc.	Stop the infusion and request a resiting of the cannula. Follow hospital policy about sending equipment for bacterial analysis. Clean the area and apply a sterile dresing. Check regularly. Observe the patient for signs of systemic infection.
Cellulitis due to: (a) Sepsis. (b) Non-specific sterile inflammation.	As above.	As above. Due to the nature of the connective tissue any infection or inflammation spreads

Nursing care plan (cont'd)

Problem	Possible causes	Preventive nursing measures	Suggested action
			quickly, especially if the limb is oedematous.
	Local allergic reaction.	Ask if the patient has any allergies before administration of any drugs or fluids, including sensitivities to topical solutions. Check whether the particular medication is commonly associated with local or venous flushing.	Observe the patient for systemic reaction. Treat the local area symptomatically. Reassure the patient. Inform medical staff.
Local oedema.	During infusion: (a) Infiltration. (b) Phlebitis. (Haynes, 1989)	Tape the cannula and giving set so that no stress is placed on the cannula. Use an extension set. Instruct the patient on the amount of movement permitted. Check regularly for swelling, e.g. tightness of bandages or a wedding ring.	Stop the infusion and request a resiting of the cannula before proceeding. Apply cold or warm compresses to provide symptomatic relief. Reassure the patient by explaining what is happening.
	During injection: (a) Extravasation of medication. (Haynes, 1989)	Observe the patient carefully throughout drug administration.	Stop the injection immediately extravasation is suspected. Act in accordance with hospital policy. Some drugs may cause inflammation and supportive, symptomatic relief will be required. Others may have the potential to cause necrosis of tissue and further action may be necessary.
Oedema of the limb.	Infiltration.	Tape the cannula and giving set so that no stress is placed on the cannula, which in turn can lead to damage of the vein. Use an extension set. Instruct the patient on the amount of movement permitted. Check regularly for swelling, as above.	Stop the infusion and request a resiting of the cannula. Provide symptomatic relief and support. Reassure the patient.

	Circulatory overload.	Administer infusion fluids at the prescribed rate and do not make sudden alterations of flow. Be aware of the patient's renal and cardiac status. Monitor intake and output routinely (Speechley & Toovey, 1987).	Slow the infusion. Monitor vital signs for increase in blood pressure and respirations. Place the patient in an upright position and keep him/her warm to promote peripheral circulation and relieve stress on the central veins. Reassure the patient. Notify a doctor immediately.
Pain at the insertion site.	All of the previous listed conditions may be accompanied by soreness or pain.	As previously listed.	Provide local symptomatic relief, e.g. warm pack, as required. Administer systemic analgesia, as prescribed, if necessary.
Pyrexia, rigors, tachycardia.	Septicaemia.	Adhere to aseptic techniques when performing all intravenous procedures. Inspect all equipment, infusion fluids, etc., before use. Observe recommendations for additives, equipment changes and general management. Avoid the use of equipment that can increase the risk of contamination, e.g. stopcocks (Cheeseborough & Finch, 1984).	Notify a doctor immediately. Follow hospital policy about sending equipment for bacterial analysis.
Decrease in blood pressure, tachycardia, cyanosis, unconsciousness.	Embolism: (a) Air.	Check the containers and change before they run dry, especially bottles. Clear all air from tubing before commencing infusion. Check all connections regularly and make sure they are secure.	Turn the patient onto left side and lower the head of the bed to prevent air from entering the pulmonary artery. Notify a doctor immediately. Administer oxygen (Ostrow, 1981; Weinstein, 1993). Reassure the patient by explaining what is happening.
	(b) Particle.	Check all infusion fluids before and after any additions have been made. Check drug	As above, but also change the container and giving set. Replace with new equipment and

Nursing care plan (cont'd)

Problem	Possible causes	Preventive nursing measures	Suggested action
		compatibility and stability. Observe the solution throughout the infusion for precipitate formation (Speechley & Toovey, 1987).	0.9% sodium chloride infusion from a different batch. Follow hospital policy about sending contaminated fluid and equipment for bacterial analysis.
Itching, rash, shortness of breath.	Allergic reaction due to sensitivity to an intravenous fluid, additive or drug.	Ask the patient if he/she has any allergies *before* administration of any drugs or fluids. Check whether the particular medication is commonly associated with any allergic reactions and observe the patient more closely.	Stop drug infusion or injection and maintain the patency of the intravenous line using 0.9% sodium chloride Notify a doctor immediately. Reassure the patient. Ensure that hydrocortisone and adrenaline are available.
Flushed face, headache, congestion of the chest, possibly progressing to loss of consciousness.	Speed shock due to too rapid administration of drugs.	Administer drugs and infusion at the correct rate. Check the flow rate frequently. Use mechanical aids if the delivery rate is crucial.	As above.

FLOW CONTROL

Definition
The delivery of intravenous fluids and medications at an appropriate rate and in a constant, accurate manner, to achieve the desired therapeutic response and to prevent complications. The nurse has a responsibility to determine the correct rate in individual circumstances and to maintain that rate throughout the infusion.

Indications
The following should be considered when a decision on flow control is to be made.

Complications associated with over-infusion include:

(1) Fluid overload with accompanying electrolyte imbalance.
(2) Metabolic disturbances during parenteral nutrition, mainly related to serum glucose levels.

(3) Toxic concentrations of medications, which may result in a shock-like syndrome ('speed shock').
(4) Air embolism, due to containers running dry before expected.
(5) An increase in venous complications, e.g. chemical phlebitis, caused by reduced dilution of irritant substances (Weinstein, 1993).

Complications associated with under-infusion include:

(1) Dehydration.
(2) Metabolic disturbances, as above.
(3) A delayed response to medications, or below therapeutic dose.
(4) Occlusion of a cannula/catheter due to slow cessation of flow (Weinstein, 1993).

Delivery of fluids and medications should be constant over a period with no major adjustments to 'catch up' Small alterations are permissible.

Calculations of accurate rate of administration (continuous or intermittent)

The rate of administration of a continuous or intermittent infusion may be calculated from the following equation (Gatford, 1990):

$$\frac{\text{No of millilitres to be infused}}{\text{No of hours over which infusion is to be delivered}} \times \frac{\text{No of drops per millilitre}}{60 \text{ minutes}}$$

$$= \text{No of drops to be delivered per minute}$$

In this equation, 60 is a factor for the conversion of the number of hours to the number of minutes; the number of drops per millilitre is dependent on the administration set used and the viscosity of the infusion fluid. Increased viscosity causes the size of the drop to increase. For example, crystalloid fluid administered via a solution set is delivered at the rate of 20 drops/ml; the rate of packed red cells given via a blood set will be calculated at 15 drops/ml.

REFERENCE MATERIAL

Factors affecting infusion flow rates

Fluid and container

The type of fluid, viscosity and the temperature at which it is delivered affect the rate of flow (Sager & Bomar, 1980). The amount of fluid within the container exerts a pressure which falls as delivery continues. Therefore, adjustments in height may be required. The optimum height of the container above the patient is 0.9m and consequently changes in the patient's position may mean further adjustment (Auty, 1989).

Flow control clamps

The roller clamps used to control fluid flow may slip, loosen or distort the tubing causing a phenomenon known as 'cold flow'. Any marked tension or stretching of the tubing, due to movement by the patient, can render the clamp ineffective (Sager & Bomar, 1980; Luken & Middleton, 1990).

Cannula/catheter/intravenous line

The flow rate may be affected by any of the following:

(1) The condition and size of the vein.
(2) The gauge of the cannula/catheter.
(3) The position of the device within the vein.
(4) The site of the intravenous device, e.g. it may be positional.
(5) Kinking, pinching or compression of the cannula/catheter or tubing of the administration set may cause variation in the set rate.

(6) Occlusion of the cannula/catheter due to clot formation.
(7) Inclusion of other in-line devices e.g. filters may also affect the flow (Weinstein, 1993).

The drop calibration of the administration set limits flow rate and when slower delivery is required microdrip sets should be used.

The patient

Patients occasionally tamper with the control clamp or other parts of the delivery system, e.g. adjusting the height of the infusion container, thereby making flow unreliable.

Complications associated with flow control

To determine the flow rate intelligently, the nurse must have knowledge of the solutions and their effects and understand other factors which influence the speed of the infusion. Certain groups of patients may be more at risk and these include:

(1) Infants and young children.
(2) The elderly.
(3) Patients with compromised cardiovascular status.
(4) Patients with impairment or failure of organs, e.g. kidneys.
(5) Patients with major sepsis.
(6) Patients suffering from shock, whatever the cause.
(7) Postoperative or post-trauma patients.
(8) Stressed patients, whose endocrine homeostatic controls may be affected.
(9) Patients receiving multiple medications, whose clinical status may change rapidly (Weinstein, 1993).

Fluid/electrolyte imbalance

The most common disorder of fluid and electrolyte balance is circulatory overload, that is isotonic fluid expansion. It is caused by infusion of excessive quantities of isotonic fluids such as 0.9% sodium chloride. No flow of fluid from the extracellular to the intracellular compartment occurs and, therefore, the extracellular volume increases (Weinstein, 1993).

Due to electrolyte concentration, no extra water is available to enable the kidneys selectively to excrete and restore the balance. Early clinical manifestations of this condition are (Weinstein, 1993):

(1) Weight gain.
(2) An increase in fluid intake over output.
(3) A high bounding pulse pressure indicates a high cardiac output.
(4) Raised central venous pressure measurements.
(5) Peripheral hand vein emptying time longer than normal. (Peripheral veins will usually empty in 3–5

seconds when the hand is elevated and will fill in the same length of time when the hand is lowered to a dependent position) (Weinstein, 1993).

(6) Peripheral oedema.
(7) Hoarseness.

Progression will lead to dyspnoea and cyanosis, due to pulmonary oedema, and neck vein engorgement (Weinstein, 1993).

The nurse needs to recognize the condition early so that fluid can be withheld until excesses have been excreted. Careful monitoring should continue to prevent isotonic contraction occurring (Weinstein, 1993).

If a patient is receiving large quantities of electrolyte free water, such as glucose 5% in water, to replace losses from gastric suction, vomit, diarrhoea, diuresis or insensible loss, hypotonic expansion may develop. This involves both extracellular and intracellular compartments (Weinstein, 1993).

This condition is more frequently seen in the early postoperative period and in the elderly patient. Signs which differentiate hypotonic from isotonic expansion are:

(1) The pulse and blood pressure usually remain normal.
(2) Intracranial pressure is raised causing headache, nausea, vomiting, muscle twitching and confusion.
(3) Tibial oedema is present.

Fluids will be withheld and careful correction of electrolyte balance undertaken. In severe hyponatremia, it may be necessary to administer small quantities of hypertonic saline to increase the osmotic pressure and the flow of water from the cells to the extracellular compartment for excretion by the kidneys (Weinstein, 1993).

Metabolic disturbance

Metabolic disturbances are related to total parenteral nutrition and most commonly to glucose intolerance. This may result in either a hyper- or hypoglycaemic state. Signs of hypoglycaemia include weakness, headache, thirst and a cold clammy skin. Hyperglycaemia will lead rapidly to coma (Weinstein, 1993).

Disturbances in fat metabolism may occur if too rapid infusion takes place. These are most likely in patients with disordered liver function, major infections or other conditions which create physiological stress.

Accurate control of flow rates of all feeding solutions is essential and the *maximum* recommended adjustment of flow is four drops per minute every 15 minutes.

Administration of drugs

Rapid, uncontrolled administration of drugs will result in toxic concentrations reaching vital organs. Toxicity may be manifested by an exaggeration of the usual phar-macological actions of the drug or by signs and symptoms specific for that drug or class of drugs. The most extreme toxic response which can occur if a drug is given at a dose or rate exceeding that recommended, is the lethal response.

Signs of speed shock include:

(1) Flushed face.
(2) Headache.
(3) Congestion of the chest.
(4) Tachycardia, fall in blood pressure.
(5) Syncope.
(6) Shock.
(7) Cardiovascular collapse (Weinstein, 1993).

Administration must be slowed down or discontinued, and the medical staff notified (see Nursing care plan).

Paediatric intravenous therapy

Paediatrics is an area where extra care is required. The heart and circulatory system are smaller, therefore fluid and electrolyte imbalance and circulatory overload can occur more rapidly. Maintenance of flow is usually achieved by the use of special sets. Accurate intake requires precision in IV administration. It is paramount that the rate of IV fluids be delivered at a constant rate. Even the smallest error can cause serious problems especially in the compromised child (Sager & Bomar, 1980).

For example:

Intake
(1) An hourly record of the amount and type of fluid.
(2) A running total of the amount administered.
(3) Regular checks of the infusion device and the rate of flow.
(4) Recording the volume of diluent used in drug reconstitution.
(5) Checking the electrolyte content of drug presentations, especially sodium and potassium.
(6) Consideration of additional water needs due to a faster metabolic rate, and a greater loss in urine due to immature renal function.

Output
(1) Careful recording all output, including weighing nappies.
(2) Recording any other drainage, e.g. from a wound site.
(3) Adjustments to allow for insensible loss via a greater surface area.

Other observations include weight and general condition and behaviour, e.g. tachycardia, raised blood pressure and respirations, oedema, headache, abdominal cramps.

Dose calculations of medications should be checked carefully as micrograms are frequently used, and amounts often include a decimal point.

Principles of equipment selection and application

Choice of an infusion system

Many infusions are controlled adequately using the simple gravity drip. A measured volume ('burette') set may be used (for smaller amounts of fluid or greater accuracy). However, over recent years, mechanical infusion devices have been used more frequently to ensure the highest possible degree of accuracy. To meet increased demand manufacturers have developed a number of new products from the basic to the advanced. When choosing infusion equipment nurses must consider.

(a) The reasons for choosing the equipment;
(b) The benefits to be gained from a particular device; and,
(c) The problems that might occur, and anticipate them if possible.

(Leggett, 1990.)

It is also important to assess:

• Which device is most appropriate;
• How accurate the device is;
• Whether the device is user-friendly;
• Whether equipment should be standardised;
• The initial cost and running costs of the device.

Factors to consider when choosing an appropriate infusion system for a particular situation

• Risk to the patient of:
  over-infusion
  under-infusion
  uneven flow
  high delivery pressure
  inadvertent bolus
  extravascular infusion
• Delivery parameters:
  infusion rate and volume required
  accuracy required (long- and short-term)
  alarms required
  ability to infuse into site chosen (venous, arterial, subcutaneous)
  suitability for infusing given drug (viscosity, half-life)
• Environmental features:
  ease of operation
  frequency of observation and adjustment
  type of patient (neonate, child, very sick)
  mobility of patient

(Wittig & Semmler-Bertanzi, 1983; Medical Devices Agency, 1995.)

Types of device

• Simple gravity drip, including measured volume sets.
• Controllers: drip rate/volumetric.
• Infusion pumps: drip rate/volumetric.
• Syringe pumps.
• Ambulatory infusion pumps.

Simple gravity drip

Gravity flow depends on head pressure; roller clamps used to adjust and to maintain rates of flow on gravity infusions vary considerably in their efficiency and accuracy (Clarkson, 1995). The indications for use are:

• Delivery of fluids without additives.
• Administration of drugs or fluids where adverse effects are not anticipated if the infusion rate varies slightly.
• Where the patient's condition does not give cause for concern and no complication is predicted.

Advantages
• Lowest cost.
• Familiar to all staff.
• Simple to set up.
• Infusion of air is less likely.
• Minimizes risk of extravascular infusion.

Disadvantages
• Cannot be used for arterial infusions.
• Require frequent observation and adjustment.
• Variability of drop size.
• Infusion rates limited, especially with viscous fluids and small catheters.
• Risk of free flow (open roller clamps).
• User may need to convert between volume to be infused (VTBI) and drop rate.

Gravity controllers

A controller is a mechanical device that operates by gravity, there is no pumping action. It controls the flow of the infusion at the desired rate by constricting the infusion line (Auty, 1989; Luken & Middleton, 1990; Medical Devices Agency, 1995). There are two types:

(1) Drip rate controllers – the desired flow is set in drops per minute. They are suitable for the majority of lower risk infusions in which volumetric accuracy is of lesser importance.

Advantages
• Fairly inexpensive.
• Used with standard gravity solution sets.
• Simple to operate.

- Very quick alarms, no bolus.
- Infusion of air unlikely.
- Very low infusion pressure.
- Minimize risk of extravascular infusion.
- Flow status gives early warning of problems.
- Count drops very accurately.

Disadvantages
- Cannot be used for arterial infusions.
- Infusion rates limited, especially with viscous fluids and small catheters.
- Not accurate volumetrically unless calibrated with known solution sets and fluids.
- User may need to convert between VTBI and drop rate.

(2) Volumetric controllers – the desired flow is set in millilitres per hour. These devices can compensate for drop size and so volumetric accuracy is dependent upon the compensation being correct under all circumstances.

Advantages
- Calibrated in ml/h.
- Fairly easy to operate.
- Very quick alarms, no bolus.
- Very low infusion pressure.
- Infusion of air unlikely.
- Flow status gives early warning of impending problems.
- Minimizes risk of extravascular infusion.

Disadvantages
- More expensive to purchase than drip-rate controllers.
- Dedicated set usually required.
- Cannot be used for arterial infusions.
- Infusion rates limited, especially with viscous fluids and small catheters.
- Volumetric accuracy very much dependent on how the manufacturer has overcome the problems of conversion of drops to volumes.

Infusion pumps

Common to all pumps is the ability to overcome resistance to flow by increased delivery pressure. Pumps do not rely on gravity and can therefore be placed in almost any reasonable position relative to the infusion site. If a catheter becomes occluded or displaced, delivery pressures can rise to high values leading to the risk of extravascular infusion. However the default pressure is usually limited and some pumps include a facility for setting very low occlusion alarm pressures (Medical Devices Agency, 1995). The performance of these pumps is predictable, however these devices are associated with a number of risks. There are two types:

(1) Drip rate pumps – the flow rate is selected in drops per minute and a drop sensor attached to the drip chamber counts drops. As controls are few and simple, with poor response to alarms, the Medical Devices Agency (1995) does not recommend this type of pump for use in its present form.

Advantages
- None.

Disadvantages
- Very high occlusion alarm pressures.
- Potentially dangerous should extravascular infusion occur.
- Very long alarm delays and high bolus on release of occlusion.
- High delivery pressure can burst solution sets.
- Can pump dangerous amounts of air if no air detector fitted.
- Very few alarms.
- Not accurate on a volumetric basis.

(2) Volumetric pumps – these are the preferred pumps for medium and large flow rate and large volume infusions; the rate is selected in millilitres per hour. Most use a linear peristaltic pumping mechanism or a cassette. They have the capability of developing high delivery pressures but the pressure is limited to a preset value, above which the pump will alarm.

Advantages
- Calibrated in ml/h.
- Good volumetric accuracy.
- Wide flow rate range.
- Many features and facilities designed to ensure very safe operation.
- Comprehensive alarm systems.
- Air-in-line detection.
- Many have low occlusion alarm pressure settings.
- Some have delivery pressure sensing.
- Secondary infusion facility often available.
- Can be used for both venous and arterial infusions.
- Keep vein open (KVO) facility.
- Neonatal versions available.

Disadvantages
- More expensive than most other pumps.
- Dedicated sets required.
- Some can be complicated to set up.
- Incorrect set can be loaded and pump appears to work.

Syringe pumps

These are low volume, high accuracy devices designed to infuse at low flow rates and are calibrated in millilitres per hour, typically 0.1–99 ml/h. Many pumps will accept different sizes and brands of syringe. They are mains and/or battery powered and tend to cost less than volumetric pumps. Patient controlled analgesia (PCA) pumps are often syringe pumps, but the difference is that a PCA pump has the provision of a facility to enable patients to deliver a bolus dose themselves. Access by the patient to the pump settings can be prevented and a basal rate delivery of solution outside the control of the patient may be provided (Medical Devices Agency, 1995).

Advantages
- Usually calibrated in ml/h
- Smooth and precise delivery at low flow rates.
- Easy to operate.

Disadvantages
- Free flow possible on older models, without plunger clamps.
- There can be problems with mechanical backlash (slackness which causes start-up and alarm delays).
- Occlusion alarm pressure settings on earlier models are sometimes rather high, which would result in a poor occlusion response.
- Earlier models are prone to incorrect fitting of syringe.

Ambulatory pumps These pumps are small and light enough to be carried around by the patient without unduly interfering with most every day activities (Boutin & Hagar, 1992; Koeppen & Caspers, 1994). Due to their size the available battery capacity tends to be low. Most give an output in the form of a small bolus delivered every few minutes. There are two types:

(1) Syringe driver – these devices appear to be easily worn or carried (Nicolson, 1986; Hawkett & Nicolson, 1987). Most are battery powered, have few controls and the minimum of alarms. They can be used to give subcutaneous infusions, e.g. diamorphine or insulin, or for intravenous infusions, e.g. cytotoxic chemotherapy where small volumes are to be infused over days rather than hours. They usually accept syringes of between 2 and 10 ml and are able to achieve very low rates of delivery. They often require the rate to be set in millimetres per hour or per 24 hours. The volumetric accuracy can be variable.

Advantages
- Small, pocket sized, lightweight.
- Usually accept standard syringes.
- Fairly easy to use.

Disadvantages
- Few alarms on older models.
- User may need to convert between VTBI and drive rate.

- High occlusion alarm pressures leading to poor occlusion response.
- Usually a pulsatile output only.

(2) Ambulatory infusion pumps – these devices use removable reservoirs which contain the solution within the pump. Some may offer a large variety of programming options and alarms (Medical Devices Agency, 1995).

Advantages
- Small, pocket sized, lightweight.
- Usually calibrated in ml/h
- Reservoir may hold up to 250 ml.
- Good alarm systems (on newer models).

Disadvantages
- Few alarms on older models.
- Usually dedicated sets required.
- Usually a pulsatile output only.

Summary
Careful calculation and control of flow rates are essential as delivery of fluids and medications may be critical due to any of the factors mentioned above. There are many infusion control devices available to assist the nurse in this task, ranging from the simple to the complex. A knowledge of these systems and of their application is necessary to ensure appropriate choices are made (Manley, 1992). Although these devices provide a valuable aid to patient care they do not replace the need for good nursing assessment and intervention (Leggett, 1990).

References and further reading
Auty, B. (1989) Choice of instrumentation for controlled IV infusion. *Intensive Therapy & Clinical Monitoring*, 10(4), 117–22.
British Medical Association/Pharmaceutical Society of Great Britain (1987) *British National Formulary No. 14*. BMA, London.
British National Formulary (BNF) (1995) *British Medical Association and Royal Pharmaceutical Society of Great Britain* (1995), No. 30, September, Appendix 6, 584–94.
Boutin, J. & Hagar, E. (1992) Patients' preference regarding portable pumps. *Journal of Intravenous Nursing*, 15(4), 230–32.
Clarkson, D. (1995) The future of infusion. *Hospital Equipment and Supplies*, June, 17.
Department of Health and Social Security (1990) *Health Equipment Information Evaluation Issue No. 198*. HMSO, London.
Gatford, J. D. (1990) *Nursing Calculations*, 3rd edn. Churchill Livingstone, Edinburgh.
Hawkett, S. & Nicolson, R. (1987) Syringe drivers. *Journal of District Nursing*, February, 2–4.
Hudek, K. (1986) Compliance in intravenous therapy.

Journal of Canadian Intravenous Nurses Association, 2(3), 7–8.

Koeppen, M. A. & Caspers, S. M. (1994) Problems identified with home infusion pumps. *Journal of Intravenous Nursing*, 17(3), 151–6.

Leggett, A. (1990) Intravenous infusion pumps. *Nursing Standard*, 4 April, 4(28), 24–6.

Leggett, A. (1990) Looking at infusion devices. *Nursing Standard*, 18 April, 4(30), 29–31.

Luken, J. & Middleton, J. (1990) Intravenous infusion controllers. *Nursing Standard*, 11 April, 4(29), 30–2.

Manley, K. (1992) Flow control in intravenous therapy. *Surgical Nurse*, 12–15.

Medical Devices Agency (1995) Infusion systems. *Device Bulletin, MDA DB 9503*, May. Department of Health, London.

Miller, J. (1989) Intravenous therapy in fluid and electrolyte imbalance. *Professional Nurse*, February, p. 237.

Nicolson, H. (1986) The success of the syringe driver. *Nursing Times*, 9, 49–51.

Plumer, A. L. (1987) *Principles and Practice of Intravenous Therapy*, 4th edn. Little, Brown & Co, Boston.

Sager, D. & Bomar, S. (1980) *Intravenous Medications*. J. B. Lippincott, Philadelphia.

Sepion, B. (1990) Intravenous care for children. *Paediatric Nursing*, April, 14–16.

Weinstein, S. M. (ed.) (1993) *Principles and Practices of Intravenous Therapy*, 5th edn. J. B. Lippincott, Philadelphia.

Wittig, P. & Semmler-Bertanzi, D. J. (1983) Pumps and controllers: a nurse's assessment guide. *American Journal of Nursing*, 7, 1023–5.

PROBLEM SOLVING

Problem	Possible causes	Preventive nursing measures	Suggested action
Pump alarming (a) Air	Air bubbles in giving set.	Ensure all air is removed from all equipment prior to use.	Remove all air from giving set and restart infusion.
	Wrongly loaded set.	Ensure set is loaded correctly.	Check that set is loaded correctly and reload if necessary.
(b) Occlusion	Occlusion in device or giving set.	Ensure the device remains patent and flushed.	Check the device for patency and remove occlusion prior to restarting infusion.
	Kinking of tubing.	Ensure that tubing is taped to prevent kinking. Reposition tubing whenever set is removed from a pump to prevent crushing.	If tubing kinked, reposition and tape.
Pump malfunctioning (electrical/mechanical)	Not charging at mains. Low battery.	Ensure that the device is kept plugged in where appropriate.	Change device and remove pump from use until fully charged. Send to works department to check plug.
	Technical fault.	Ensure all pumps are serviced regularly.	Remove pump from use and contact clinical nurse specialist IV services/company.
	Device soiled inside mechanism.	Maintain equipment and keep clean and free from contamination.	Remove giving set and wipe pump, reload.

Unstable pump	Attached to old, poorly maintained stands.	Ensure that stands are maintained and kept clean. Replace old stands.	Remove device from stand. Remove stand and send to works department for repair.
	Attached to incorrect stands.	Ensure the correct stands are used.	Check the stand and change to appropriate stand.
	Equipment not balanced on stand.	Ensure that all equipment is balanced around the stand.	Remove devices and attach to two stands if necessary. Balance equipment.
Under/over infusion	Technical fault with equipment.	Ensure regular servicing of devices.	Remove device from use immediately and label to prevent further use. Report incident to medical staff and nursing staff and inform clinical nurse specialist IV Services of problem and serial number.
	Incorrect rate setting.	Ensure that the rate is calculated prior to commencing infusion. Check infusion rate hourly and at start of each shift to ensure correct rate is set.	Check patient's condition. Inform medical staff and senior member of nursing staff.

CHAPTER 24

Last Offices

'It is the fundamental right, of every human being, not to be afraid of death, or life: to die at peace, surrounded by wise, dear, and tender care, and to find ultimate happiness that can only come from understanding the measure of mind and of reality.'

(Rinpoche, 1992)

REFERENCE MATERIAL

The United Kingdom today is a multicultural, multiracial and multireligious society. This offers a great challenge to all areas of health care, but none more so than nursing. It is incumbent upon nurses to be aware of the different religious and cultural rituals which accompany the death of a patient. Nurses are also required to possess the information pertinent to the legal requirements for the care of the dead.

The subject of 'death with dignity' has received much prominence of late in the health care press (Hayes & van der Poel, 1990; Helman, 1990; Green & Green, 1992) and rightly so, for it is the execution of last offices with care and dignity that concludes the care which has been offered. From the viewpoint of many bereaved relatives, the way that a deceased loved one is treated forms an important part of their memory of a hospital's care.

It is essential than that the correct procedures are followed during last offices, and that every effort is made to accommodate the wishes of patients' relatives (Neuberger, 1978; Olivant, 1986; Hospital Chaplaincies Council, 1992; Speck, 1978). This is central to the concept of holistic care for the patient, and if we disregard such procedures for our patients, we also disregard both patients' and families' dignity (McGilloway & Myco, 1985; Wald, 1986; Speck, 1988; Spector, 1991).

The bibliography set out below is by no means exhaustive, but may be used by nurses to deepen their understanding of issues surrounding death, and broaden their knowledge of and respect for other cultures and faiths.

References and further reading

General

Bishop, P. & Danton, M. (1987) *The Encyclopaedia of World Religions.* Macmillan-Orbis, London.

Crowther, C. E. (1991) *AIDS – A Christian Handbook.* Epworth, London.

Department of Social Security (1990) *What to do after Death.* DSS, London.

Furman, E. (1974) *A Child's Parent Dies.* Yale University Press, New Haven.

Green, J. & Green, M. (1992) *Dealing with Death: Practices and Procedures.* Chapman & Hall, London.

Grolman, E. A. (ed.) (1985) *Explaining Death to Children.* Beacon Press, Boston.

Hayes, H. (OSF) & van der Poel, C. J. (CSSp) (eds) (1990) *Health Care Ministry: A Handbook for Chaplains.* Paullist Press, Mawah.

Helman, C. J. (1990) *Culture, Health and Illness,* 2nd edn. Wright, London.

Hospital Chaplaincies Council (1992) *Our Ministry and Other Faiths.* HCC, London.

Housely, J. (ed.) (1992) *Death Customs.* Wayland, Hove.

Karmi, G. (ed.) (1992) *The Ethnic Health Fact File.* NW/NE Thames Regional Health Authority, London.

Kübler-Ross, E. (1990) *Living with Dying and Death.* Souvenir, London.

McGilloway, O. & Myco, F. (eds) (1985) *Nursing and Spiritual Care.* Harper & Row, London.

Neuberger, J. (1978) *Caring for People of Different Faiths.* Austin Cornish, London.

Olivant, P. (1986) Coping with death: last offices . . . steps nurses should take to help bereaved relatives. *Nursing Times,* 82(12), 32–3.

Pricket, J. (ed.) (1980) *Death.* Lutterworth, Guildford.

Racial Equality Council (1992) *Religions and Cultures.* Lothian, Edinburgh.

Rankin, J. *et al.* (1993) *Ethics and Religions.* Longman, London.

Rinpoche, S. (1992) *Tibetan Book of the Living and Dying.* Rider, London.

Sambi, S. P. & Cole, W. O. (1990) Caring for Sikh patients. *Palliative Medicine,* 4, 229–33.

Sharma, D. L. (1990) Hindu attitudes towards suffering, dying and death. *Palliative Medicine,* 4, 235–8.

Shepherd, C. (1977) *Jewish Holy Days*. Loizeaux, Neptune.

Speck, P. (1978) *Loss and Grief in Medicine*. Ballière-Tindall, London.

Speck, P. (1988) *Being There: Pastoral Care in Time of Illness*. SPCK, London.

Spector, R. (1991) *Cultural Diversity in health and Illness*, 3rd edn. Appleton and Lange, Connecticut.

Storr, E. (1986) The cost of dying: practical details the relatives have to face. *Geriatric Medicine*, 16(16), 40–44.

Wald, F. S. (ed.) (1986) *In Quest of the Spiritual Component of Care for the Terminally Ill*. Yale University Press, New Haven.

Weymont, G. (1982) The Howie Report. *Nursing Times*, 78(35), *Journal of Infection Control Nursing*, Supplement 16.

Which? (1987) *What to do when Someone Dies*. Hodder, London.

Williams, A. (1982) *Procedures Following Deaths in Hospitals*. Institute of Health Services Administrators, London.

Zaehner, R. C. (ed.) (1979) *The Concise Encyclopaedia of Living Faiths*. Hutchinson, London.

Specific

Bahai

The Pattern of Bahai Life. Bahai Publishing Trust, London.

Buddhism

Humphreys, C. (1976) *Buddhism*. Penguin, London.

Humphreys, C. (1976) *Zen Buddhism*. Penguin, London.

Swindler, F. (1985) *Buddhism Made Plain*. Orbis, New York.

Williams, P. (1989) *Mahayana Buddhism*. Routledge, London.

Christianity

Cross, F. L. (ed.) (1988) *The Oxford Dictionary of the Christian Church*. Oxford University Press, Oxford.

Feiner, J. & Fisher, L. (1975) *The Common Catechism*. Search Press, London.

Searle, M. (1989) *Christening, the Making of Christians*. Kevin Mayhew, Leigh on Sea.

Hinduism

Johnson, R. & Killingley, D. (1988) *Approaches to Hinduism*. John Murray, London.

Mascaro, J. (trans.) (1980) *The Bhagavad Gita*. Penguin, London.

Mascaro, J. (trans.) (1982) *The Upanishads*. Penguin, London.

Sen, K. N. (1976) *Hinduism*. Penguin, London.

Jainism

Oldfield, K. (1989) *Jainism, the Path of Purity and Peace*. CEM, Derby.

Jehovah's Witnesses

Hoekma, A. A. (1979) *Jehovah's Witnesses*. Paternoster, Exeter.

Judaism

Borowitz, E. (1979) *Understanding Judaism*. Union of Hebrew Congregations, New York.

Epstein, I. (1980) *Judaism*. Penguin, London.

Jacobs, L. (1984) *The Book of Jewish Belief*. Behrman, New York.

Mormons

Hoekma, A. A. (1977) *Mormonism*. Paternoster, Exeter.

Muslim (Islam)

Dawood, N. J. (1990) *The Koran*. Penguin, London.

Nasr, S. (1986) *The Ideals and Realities of Islam*. George Allen, London.

Rastafarianism

Barrett, L. (1979) *Rastafarians*. Sangster, Kingston.

Morrish, I. (1987) *Obeah, Christ and Rastaman*. Clark, Cambridge.

Sikhism

Avora, R. (1986) *Sikhism*. Wayland, Hove.

Dhanja, B. (1987) *Sikhism*. Batsford, London.

Zoroastrianism

Hinnels, J. R. (1981) *Zoroastrians and the Parsees*. Ward Lock, London.

GUIDELINES: LAST OFFICES

EQUIPMENT

1 Bowl, soap, towel, two face cloths.
2 Razor (electric or disposable), comb, nail scissors.
3 Equipment for oral toilet including equipment for cleaning dentures.
4 Identification labels.
5 Documents required by law or hospital policy, e.g. notification of death cards.
6 Shroud or patient's personal clothing: night-dress, pyjamas, clothes previously requested by patient, or clothes which comply with family/cultural wishes.

Guidelines: Last offices (cont'd)

7 Body bag if required (i.e. in event of actual or potential leakage of bodily fluids and/or infectious disease).
8 Tape or Sellotape.
9 Dressing pack, tape and bandages if wounds present.
10 Valuables or property book.
11 Plastic bag for waste.

PROCEDURE

Action	Rationale
1 Inform medical staff. Confirmation of death must be given. This is usually done by medical staff. If an expected death occurs during the night, the senior nurse on duty sometimes confirms death if an agreed policy has been implemented.	A registered medical practitioner who has attended the deceased person during the last illness is required to give a medical certificate of the cause of death. The certificate requires the doctor to state the last date on which he/she saw the deceased alive and whether or not he/she has seen the body after death.
An unexpected death must be confirmed by the attending medical officer.	
Confirmation of death must be recorded in a patient's medical and nursing notes.	
2 Inform the appropriate senior nurse.	To maintain continuity of care, and to allow preparations for care of relatives/friends to continue.
Inform and offer support to relatives and/or next of kin.	To ensure relevant individuals are aware of patient's death. To provide sensitive care.
3 Lay the patient on his/her back. Close his/her eyelids. Remove all but one pillow. Support the jaw by placing a pillow or rolled-up towel on the chest underneath the jaw. Remove any mechanical aids such as syringe drivers, heel pads, etc. Straighten the limbs.	For the patient's dignity, as *rigor mortis* occurs 4–6 hours after death.
4 Drain the bladder by pressing on the lower abdomen. Pack orifices if fluid secretion continues or may be anticipated. Wear gloves and plastic apron.	Leaking orifices pose a health hazard to staff coming into contact with the body. If leakage has occurred, or is anticipated, a body bag must be used.
5 Remove dressings, drainage tubes etc., unless otherwise instructed. Open wounds or drainage sites may need to be sealed with an occlusive dressing (e.g. Tegaderm) and adhesive tape.	If a post-mortem is required, because, for example, the patient dies within 24 hours of surgery or the cause of death is unclear or suspicious.
6 Wash the patient, unless requested not to do so for religious/cultural reasons (please refer to section on individual faiths in this chapter).	For hygienic and aesthetic reasons.
It may be important to family and carers to assist with washing, to continue to provide the care given in the period before the death.	It is an expression of respect and affection, part of the process of adjusting to loss and expressing grief.

7	Remove all jewellery, in the presence of another nurse, unless requested to do otherwise.	To meet with legal requirements and relatives' wishes.
8	Dress patient in shroud, or specified clothing, unless requested to do otherwise.	For religious or cultural reasons and to meet family's or carers' wishes.
9	Label one wrist and one ankle with an identification label. Complete any documents such as notification of death cards. Copies of such cards are usually required (refer to hospital policy for details). Tape one securely to shroud.	To ensure correct and easy identification of the body in the mortuary.
10	Wrap the body in a mortuary sheet, ensuring that the face and feet are covered and that all limbs are held securely in position.	To avoid possible damage to the body during transfer and to prevent distress to colleagues, e.g. portering staff.
11	Secure the sheet with tape.	Pins must not be used as they are a health hazard to staff.
12	If body is to be placed in a body bag, first wrap in a disposable sheet.	Actual or potential leakage of fluid, whether infection is present or not, poses a health hazard to all those who come into contact with the deceased patient. The sheet will absorb excess fluid.
13	Tape the second notification of death card to the outside of the sheet (or body bag).	For ease of identification of the body in the mortuary.
14	Request the portering staff to remove the body.	Decomposition occurs rapidly particularly in hot weather and in overheated rooms, and may create a bacterial hazard for those handling the body. Autolysis and growth of bacteria are delayed if the body is cooled. Avoid causing unnecessary distress to other patients and relatives.

Screen off the appropriate area.

15	Check the patient's property with a second nurse. List the property in the valuables or property book. Lock the property in a safe place.	To ensure that all property can be accounted for.
16	Amend appropriate nursing documentation.	To record the time of death, names of those present, and names of those informed.
17	Transfer property, patient records etc. to the appropriate administrative department.	The administrative department cannot begin to process the formalities such as the death certificate or the collection of property by the next-of-kin until the required documents are in its possession.

NURSING CARE PLAN

Problem	Suggested action
Death occurring within 24 hours of an operation.	All tubes and/or drains must be left in position. Spigot any cannulae or catheters. Treat stomas as open wounds. Leave any endotracheal or tracheostomy tubes in place. Post-mortem

Nursing care plan (cont'd)

Problem	Suggested action
	examination will be required to establish the cause of death. Any tubes, drains, etc. may have been a major contributing factor to the death.
Unexpected death.	As above. Post-mortem examination of the body will be required to establish the cause of death.
Unknown cause of death.	As above.
Patient brought in dead.	As above, unless patient seen by a medical practitioner within 14 days before death. In this instance the attending medical officer may complete the death certificate if he/she is clear as to the cause of death.
Patient with leaking wounds/orifices with or without infection present.	Follow procedures outlined in section on hepatitis B (Chapter 5, Barrier Nursing).
Patient with hepatitis B or who is HIV positive.	For further information see the procedures in the sections on hepatitis B and AIDS (Chapter 5).
Patient who dies after receiving systemic radioactive iodine.	For further information, see the procedure on iodine-131 (Chapter 37, Sealed and Unsealed Radioactive Sources Therapy).
Patient who dies after insertion of gold grains or colloidal radioactive solution. Patient who dies after insertion of caesium needles or applicators or irridium wires or hair pins.	Inform the physics department as well as appropriate medical staff. Once a doctor has verified death, the sources are removed and placed in a lead container. A Geiger counter is used to check that all sources have been removed. This reduces the radiation risk when completing the last offices procedures. Record the time and date of removal of the sources.
Relatives not present at the time of the patient's death.	Inform the relatives as soon as possible of the death. Consider also that they may want to view the body before last offices are completed.
Relatives or next-of-kin not contactable by telephone or by the general practitioner.	If within UK, local police will go to next-of-kin's house. If abroad, the British Embassy will assist.
Relatives want to see the body after removal from the ward.	Inform the mortuary staff in order to allow time for them to prepare the body. The body will normally be placed in the hospital's chapel of rest. As required, religious artefacts should be removed from or placed in the non-denominational chapel of rest. The nurse should check that all is ready before accompanying the relatives into the chapel. The relatives may want to be alone with the deceased but the nurse should wait outside the chapel in order that support may be provided should the relatives become distressed. After the relatives have left, the nurse should contact the portering service who will return the body to the mortuary.

Relatives want the body to be placed in the hospital's chapel of rest.

The environment of the mortuary may cause great distress to the relatives. A sympathetic and understanding attitude to grief may help to alleviate some anxieties and if they wish to view the body (see above).

GUIDELINES: REQUIREMENTS FOR PEOPLE OF DIFFERENT RELIGIOUS FAITHS

The following are only guidelines: individual requirements may vary even among members of the same faith. Varying degrees of adherence and orthodoxy exist within all the world's major faiths. The given religion of a patient may occasionally be offered to indicate an association with particular cultural and national roots, rather than to indicate a significant degree of adherence to the tenets of a particular faith.

Bahai

1 Bahai relatives may wish to say prayers for the deceased person, but normal last offices performed by nursing staff are quite acceptable.
2 Bahai adherents may not be cremated or embalmed, nor may they be buried more than an hour's journey from the place of death.
3 Bahais have no objection to post-mortem examination and may leave their bodies to scientific research or donate organs if they wish.
4 Further information can be obtained from the nearest Assembly of the Bahais (see telephone directory). Alternatively, contact:

   National Spiritual Assembly of the Bahais of the United Kingdom
   27 Rutland Gate
   London SW7 1PD

Buddhism

1 There is no prescribed ritual for the handling of the corpse of a Buddhist person, so customary laying out is appropriate. However, a request may be made for a Buddhist monk or nun to be present.
2 There are a number of different schools of Buddhism. It is important to confirm which school the patient belongs to, as ritual requirements differ.
3 When the patient dies, inform the monk or nun if required (the patient's relatives often take this step). The body should not be moved for at least one hour if prayers are to be said.
4 The patient's body should be wrapped in an unmarked sheet.
5 For further information contact:

   The Buddhist Society
   58 Ecclestone Square
   London SW1
   Tel: 0171-834 5858

Christianity

1 There are many denominations and degrees of adherence within the Christian faith. In most cases customary last offices are acceptable.
2 Relatives may wish staff to call the hospital chaplain, or minister or priest from their own church to either perform last rites or say prayers.

Guidelines: Requirements for people of different religious faiths (cont'd)

3 Some Roman Catholic families may wish to place a rosary in the deceased patient's hands and/or a crucifix at the patient's head.
4 Some orthodox families may wish to place an ikon (holy picture) at either side of the patient's head.
5 For further information, consult the telephone directory for the local denominational minister or priest. Alternatively, contact:

Hospital Chaplaincies Council
Church House
Dean's Yard
Westminster
London SW1
Tel: 0171-222 9011

or
Apostolate of the Sick (Roman Catholic)
Tel: 0171-222 9011

or
Eastern (oriental) and orthodox Christians:

Fellowship of St Alban and St Sergius
52 Ladbroke Grove
London W10
Tel: 0171-727 7713

Hinduism

1 If required by relatives, inform the Hindu priest (Brahmin). If unavailable, relatives may wish to read from the *Bhagavad Gita* or make a request that staff read extracts during the last offices (see Chapters 2, 8 and 15 in *Bhagavad Gita*, edited by Jean Mascaro, Penguin, London, 1962).
2 The family may wish to stay with the patient during last offices. If possible, the eldest son should be present. Relatives of the same sex as the patient may wish to wash his or her body, but some prefer nursing staff to do this.
3 The patient's family may request that the patient be placed on the floor, and they may wish to burn incense.
4 Post-mortems are viewed as disrespectful to the deceased person, so are only carried out when strictly necessary.
5 For further information contact the nearest Hindu temple (see telephone directory). Alternatively, contact:

Bhavitiya Vidya Bhavan
4a Castletown Road
London W14 9HQ
Tel: 0171-381 3045

Jainism

1 The relatives of a Jainist patient may wish to contact their Brahman (priest) to recite prayers with the patient and family.
2 The family may wish to be present during the last offices, and also to assist with washing. Not all families will want to perform this task, however.
3 The family may ask for the patient to be clothed in a plain white gown or shroud with no pattern or ornament and then wrapped in a plain white sheet. They may provide the gown themselves.
4 Post-mortems may be seen as disrespectful, depending on the degree of orthodoxy of the patient.
5 Cremation is arranged whenever possible within 24 hours of death.
6 Orthodox Jains may have chosen the path of *Sallekhana*, that is, death by ritual fasting. This unusual

approach to death is permitted by the Jainist faith after permission has been granted by family and priests. This act is seen as the supreme path for fulfilling religious obligations.

7 For further information contact:

The Institute of Jainiology
81 Crundale Avenue
Kingsbury
London NW9 9BJ

Jehovah's Witness

1 Relatives may wish to be present during last offices, either to pray or to read from the Bible. The family will inform staff should there be any special requirements, which may vary according to the patient's country of origin.
2 Further information can be obtained from the nearest Kingdom Hall (see telephone directory).

Judaism

1 The family will contact their own community leader if they have one. If not, the hospital chaplaincy will advise. Prayers are recited by those present.
2 Eight minutes are required to elapse before the body is moved.
3 Usually close relatives will straighten the body, but nursing staff are permitted to perform any procedure for preserving dignity and honour. Nurses may:
   • Close the eyes;
   • Tie up the jaw;
   • Put the arms and hands straight by the side of the body;
   • Remove tubes and instruments (unless contraindicated).
   Patients must not be washed, but may be dressed in a plain shroud. The body will be washed by a nominated group, the Holy Assembly, which performs a ritual purification.
4 Watchers stay with the body until burial (normally completed within 24 hours of death). In the period before burial a separate non-denominational room is appreciated, where the body can be laid on the floor with its feet towards the door.
5 It is not possible for funerals to take place on the Sabbath (between sunset on Friday and sunset on Saturday).
6 Post-mortems are permitted only if required by law.
7 For further information, contact:

Orthodox:
The Office of the Chief Rabbi
Alder House
Tavistock Square
London WC1
Tel: 0171-387 1966

Reformed:
Reform Synagogues of Great Britain
80 East End Road
London N3 2SY
Tel: 0181-349 4731

Liberal and Progressive:
Union of Liberal and Progressive
Synagogues
109 Whitefield Street
London W1
Tel: 0171-580 1663

Guidelines: Requirements for people of different religious faiths (cont'd)

Mormon (Church of Jesus Christ of the Latter Day Saints)

1 There are no special requirements, but relatives may wish to be present during the last offices. Relatives will advise staff if the patient wears a one or two piece sacred undergarment. If this is the case, relatives will dress the patient in these items.
2 For further information contact the nearest Church of Jesus Christ of the Latter Day Saints (see telephone directory).

Muslim (Islam)

1 Family members will probably wish to stay with the dying patient and perform the last rites. If possible the patient's head (never the feet) should point towards Mecca, which in the UK is south east.
2 Ideally the body should be untouched by non-Muslims, but if it must be touched, gloves should be worn. If no family are present, close the patient's eyes and straighten the body. The head should be turned to the right shoulder, and the body covered with a plain white sheet. The body should not be washed.
3 The patient's body is normally either taken home or taken to a mosque as soon as possible to be washed by another Muslim of the same sex. A wife may wash her husband, but the reverse is not permitted.
4 Burial, never cremation, is preferred within 24 hours of death.
5 Post-mortems are only allowed if required by law, and organ donation is not encouraged.
6 For further information about Islamic groups, contact:

> **Ahmaddya:**
> London Mosque
> 16 Gressen Hall Road
> Putney
> London SW18
> Tel: 0181-870 8518
>
> **Ismaili:**
> Institute of Ismaili Studies
> 19 Portland Place
> London W1N 3AF
> Tel: 0171-436 1736
>
> **Shi'ite:**
> Iranian Embassy
> 16 Prince's Gate
> London SW7
> Tel: 0171-584 8101
>
> **Sunni:**
> London Central Mosque
> 146 Park Road
> London NW8
> Tel: 0171-742 3362

Rastafarian

1 Customary last offices are appropriate, although the patient's family may wish to be present during the preparation of the body to say prayers.
2 For further information contact:

> Rastafarian Advisory Centre
> 17a Netherwood Road

London W14
Tel: 0171-602 3767

Afro-Caribbean Community Association
Tel: 0181-985 0067

Sikhism

1 Family members (especially the eldest son) and friends will be present if they are able.
2 Usually the family takes responsibility for the last offices, but nursing staff may be asked to close the patient's eyes, straighten the body and wrap it in a plain white sheet.
3 The family will wash and dress the deceased person's body.
4 Post-mortems are only permitted if required by law.
5 Organ donation for transplant is not permitted.
6 For further information contact the nearest Sikh temple or Gurdwara (see telephone directory). Alternatively, contact:

Sikh Council for Inter Faith Relations
43 Dorset Road
Merton Park
London SW19 3EZ

Zoroastrian (Parsee)

1 Customary last offices are often acceptable to Zoroastrian patients.
2 The family may wish to be present during, or participate in, the preparation of the body.
3 Orthodox Parsees require a priest to be present, if possible.
4 After washing, the two sacred garments are required: the *Sadra* is placed next to the skin under the sheet, and the *Kusti* is replaced.
5 Relatives may cover the patient's head with a white cap or scarf.
6 It is important that the funeral takes place as soon as possible after death.
7 Post-mortems are forbidden unless required by law.
8 Organ donation is forbidden by religious law.
9 For further information contact:

The Zoroastrian Information Centre
88 Compayne Gardens
London NW6 3RV
Tel: 0171-328 6018

In addition to the addresses given above, further information is available from:

The Shap Working Party on World Religions in Education
The National Society's RE Centre
23 Kensington Square
London W8 5HN
Tel: 0171-937 7229

CHAPTER 25
Lumbar Puncture

Definition

Lumbar puncture is a medical procedure to withdraw cerebrospinal fluid by the insertion of a hollow spinal needle with a stylet into the lumbar subarachnoid space (Hickey, 1986).

Indications

Lumbar puncture is performed for the following purposes:

(1) Diagnosis.
(2) The introduction of contrast media for radiological examination.
(3) The introduction of chemotherapeutic agents, e.g. antibiotics or cytotoxics (Lindsay *et al.*, 1991).

Contraindications

The procedure should not be undertaken in the following circumstances

(1) Raised intracranial pressure. This could lead to herniation of the brainstorm (coning).
(2) Suspected cord compression.
(3) Local skin infection. Meningitis, a rare complication of lumbar puncture, could be potentiated if skin infection is present. The procedure should be delayed until the problem is resolved.
(4) Uncooperative patient. Maximum patient cooperation is essential to minimize the potential risks associated with the procedure.
(5) Severe degenerative spinal joint disease. In such cases difficulty will be experienced both in positioning the patient and in accessing between the vertebra (Hickey, 1986).

REFERENCE MATERIAL

Anatomy and physiology

The spinal cord lies within the spinal column (Fig. 25.1). It is encased and protected by the vertebrae and extends from the base of the brain to below the second lumbar vertebra where it continues as a fine thread – the filum terminale – which is attached internally to the coccyx. Like the brain the spinal cord is surrounded by three membranes known as the meninges; they are the dura, the arachnoid and the pia mater (Hickey, 1986).

The dura and arachnoid mater are separated by a potential space known as the subdural space. The arachnoid and pia mater are separated by the subarachnoid space which contains the cerebrospinal

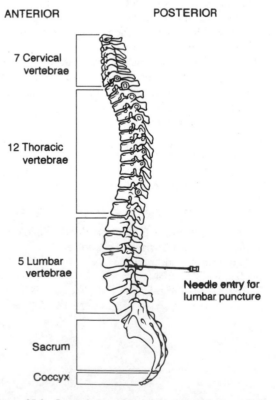

ANTERIOR   POSTERIOR

7 Cervical vertebrae

12 Thoracic vertebrae

5 Lumbar vertebrae

Needle entry for lumbar puncture

Sacrum

Coccyx

Figure 25.1 Lateral view of the spinal column and vertebrae, showing the needle entry site for lumbar puncture.

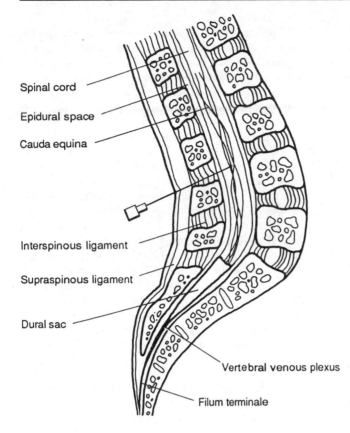

Spinal cord

Epidural space

Cauda equina

Interspinous ligament

Supraspinous ligament

Dural sac

Vertebral venous plexus

Filum terminale

Figure 25.2 Lumbar puncture. Saggital section through lumbosacral spine. The most common site for lumbar puncture is between L2 and L3. However the spaces between L3 and L4 and between L4 and L5 are also used if the patient's condition makes the choice necessary.

fluid (CSF). The space is fairly narrow until the first lumbar vertebra, where it widens as the spinal cord terminates (Draper, 1980). Below the first lumbar vertebra the subarachnoid space contains cerebrospinal fluid, the filum terminale and the cauda equinae (the anterior and posterior roots of the lumbar and sacral nerves). This anatomical site is used to obtain samples of cerebrospinal fluid by lumbar puncture as there is no danger of damage to the spinal cord (Fig. 25.2).

Cerebrospinal fluid is secreted by the choroid plexus which is situated in the ventricles of the brain. It is reabsorbed into the blood capillaries via the arachnoid villi and is returned to the circulating blood (Bowsher, 1979). Cerebrospinal fluid is clear, colourless and slightly alkaline with a specific gravity of 1005 (Draper, 1980). In an adult there are approximately 120–150 ml of cerebrospinal fluid present. Its constituents include:

- Water
- Mineral salts
- Glucose
- Protein – 20–30 mg per 100 ml (Keele *et al.*, 1983)
- Creatinine
- Urea (Lindsay *et al.*, 1991).

The functions of cerebrospinal fluid include:

- To act as a shock absorber.
- To carry nutrients to the brain.
- To remove metabolites from the brain.
- To support and protect the brain and spinal cord.
- To keep the brain and spinal cord moist (Hickey, 1986).

Sampling
Determined by the investigations required, approximately 5–10 ml of cerebrospinal fluid are withdrawn for laboratory analysis (Booth, 1983).

Abnormalities of cerebrospinal fluid
Reddening of the fluid is indicative of the presence of blood which is an abnormal finding. The presence of blood is diagnostic of either a traumatic lumbar puncture or a subarachnoid haemorrhage. If the cause of the blood presence is a traumatic spinal tap the blood will usually clot, and the fluid clear as the procedure continues. Alternatively, if the presence of blood is due to a subarachnoid haemorrhage no clotting will occur (Lindsay *et al.*, 1991). If the cerebrospinal fluid is cloudy

in appearance (turbidity) this is indicative of the presence of a large number of white cells, again an abnormal finding. The causes of such turbidity include infection or the secondary infiltration of the meninges with malignant disease, e.g. leukaemia or lymphoma. The presence of different types of blood cells in the cerebrospinal fluid can be diagnostic of a variety of neurological disorders. For example:

(1) *Erythrocytes* (red cells) are indicative of haemorrhage.
(2) *Polymorphonuclear leucocytes* are indicative of meningitis or cerebral abscess.
(3) *Monocytes* are indicatative of a viral or tubercular meningitis or encephalitis.
(4) *Lymphocytes* present in a number greater than five cells per mm^3 are indicative of viral meningitis or of infiltration of the meninges with malignant disease (Hickey, 1986).

Investigations

A number of tests can be performed on cerebrospinal fluid to aid diagnosis (Lindsay *et al.*, 1991):

(1) *Culture and sensitivity.* Identifying the presence of micro-organisms would confirm the diagnosis of bacterial/fungal meningitis or a cerebral abscess. The isolation of the causative organism would enable the initiation of appropriate antibiotic or antifungal therapy.
(2) *Virology screening.* The isolation of a causative virus would enable appropriate therapy to be initiated promptly.
(3) *Serology for syphilis.* Tests include: Wasserman test (WR), venereal disease research lab (VDRL) and *Treponema pallidum* immobilization test (TPI).
(4) *Protein.* The total amount of protein in cerebrospinal fluid should be 15.45 mg/dl (= 154.5 µg/ml). Proteins are large molecules which do not readily cross the blood–brain barrier. There is normally more albumin (80%) than globulin in cerebrospinal fluid as albumins are smaller molecules (Fischbach, 1984). Raised globulin levels are indicative of multiple sclerosis, neurosyphilis, degenerative cord or brain disease. However, raised levels of total protein can be indicative of meningitis, encephalitis, myelitis or the presence of a tumour.
(5) *Cytology.* Central nervous system tumours or secondary meningeal disease tend to shed cells into the cerebrospinal fluid, where they float freely. Examination of these cells morphologically after lumbar puncture will determine whether the tumour is malignant or benign (Fischbach, 1984).

Pressure

The pressure of cerebrospinal fluid can be measured at the time of lumbar puncture using a manometer. Normal cerebrospinal fluid pressure falls within the range of 60–180 mm H_2O (Hickey, 1986). Queckenstedt's test may be performed if indicated. This consists of applying pressure to the jugular vein. Normal response is a sharp rise in pressure followed by a sharp fall as pressure to the jugular vein is removed. Should the rise and fall in pressure be sluggish or absent, it would indicate blockage of the spinal canal. This test is potentially an extremely hazardous procedure. If both jugular veins are compressed at the same time, temporal lobe or brainstem herniation could occur (Draper, 1980).

Instillation of chemotherapy

A number of drugs do not cross the blood–brain barrier. Lumbar puncture is a method of introducing drugs into the central nervous system. Antibiotics can be instilled to treat specific infections such as bacterial meningitis; some cytotoxic drugs, e.g. methotrexate or cytosine arabinoside, can be instilled to treat malignant diseases such as leukaemia and can also be used as a prophylactically to prevent recurrence (Weinstein, 1993).

Complications associated with lumbar puncture

These are outlined by Hickey (1986) and include:

(1) Infection;
(2) Haemorrhage/localized bruising;
(3) Transtentorial or tonsillar herniation (if Queckenstedt's test is carried out in the presence of raised cerebrospinal fluid pressure);
(4) Headache;
(5) Backache;
(6) Leakage from puncture site.

References and further reading

Booth, J. A. (1983) *Handbook of Investigations*. Harper & Row, London.
Bowsher, D. (1979) *Introduction to the Anatomy and Physiology of the Nervous System*, 4th edn. Blackwell Scientific Publications, Oxford.
Draper, I. (1980) *Lecture Notes on Neurology*. Blackwell Scientific Publications, Oxford.
Fischbach, F. T. (1984) *A Manual of Laboratory Diagnostic Tests*, 2nd edn. J. B. Lippincott, Philadelphia.
Hickey, J. (1986) *The Clinical Practice of Neurological and Neurosurgical Nursing*, 2nd edn. J. B. Lippincott, Philadelphia.
Keele, C. A. *et al.* (1983) *Samson Wright's Applied Physiology*. Oxford Medical Publications, Oxford.
Lindsay, K. *et al.* (1991) *Neurology and Neurosurgery Illustrated*, 2nd edn. Churchill Livingstone, Edinburgh.
Weinstein, S. (1993) *Principles and Practice of Intravenous Therapy*, 5th edn. J. B. Lippincott, Philadelphia.

GUIDELINES: LUMBAR PUNCTURE

EQUIPMENT

1 Antiseptic skin-cleansing agents.
2 Selection of needles and syringes.
3 Local anaesthetic.
4 Sterile gloves.
5 Sterile dressing pack.
6 Lumbar puncture needles of assorted sizes.
7 Disposable manometer.
8 Three sterile specimen bottles. (These should be labelled 1, 2 and 3. The first specimen, which may be bloodstained due to needle trauma, should go into bottle 1. This will assist the laboratory to differentiate between blood due to procedure trauma and that due to subarachnoid haemorrhage.)
9 Plaster dressing or plastic dressing spray.

PROCEDURE

Action	Rationale
1 Explain and discuss the procedure with the patient.	To ensure that the patient understands the procedure and gives his/her valid consent.
2 Assist the patient into the required position on a firm surface:	
(a) Lying (Fig. 25.3): (i) One pillow under the patient's head. (ii) On side with knees drawn up to the abdomen and clasped by the hands.	To ensure maximum widening of the intervertebral spaces and thus easier access to the subarachnoid space.
(iii) Support patient in this position by holding him/her behind the knees and neck.	To avoid sudden movement by the patient which would produce trauma.
(b) Sitting: (i) Patient straddles a straight-backed chair so that his/her back is facing the doctor. (ii) Patient folds arms on the back of the chair and rests head on them.	This position may be used for those patients unable to maintain the lying position. It allows more accurate identification of the spinous processes and thus the intervertebral spaces.
3 Continue to support, encourage and observe the patient throughout the procedure.	To facilitate psychological and physical well-being. To monitor any physical or psychological changes.

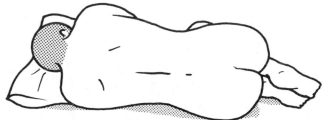

Figure 25.3 Position for lumbar puncture. Head is flexed onto chest and knees are drawn up.

Guidelines: Lumbar puncture (cont'd)

Action   **Rationale**

4 Assist the doctor as required. The doctor will
   proceed as follows:
   (a) Clean the skin with the antiseptic   To maintain asepsis throughout the procedure.
       cleansing agents.
   (b) Identify the area to be punctured and
       infiltrate the skin and subcutaneous layers
       with local anaesthetic.
   (c) Introduce a spinal puncture needle   This is below the level of the spinal cord but still
       between the second and third lumbar   within the subarachnoid space.
       vertebrae and into the subarachnoid
       space.
   (d) Ensure that the subarachnoid space has   To obtain a cerebrospinal fluid pressure reading
       been entered and attach the manometer   (normal pressure is 60–180 mm H_2O).
       to the spinal needle, if required.
   (e) Decide whether Queckenstedt's   To check for obstruction to cerebrospinal fluid flow
       manoeuvre may be performed (Fig. 25.4).   in the spinal column. (Usually obstruction is caused
                                                     by a tumour.)
   (f) The appropriate specimens of
       cerebrospinal fluid (about 10 ml in total)
       are obtained for analysis.
   (g) Once all specimens have been obtained
       and the appropriate pressure
       measurements made, the spinal needle is
       withdrawn.

5 When the needle is withdrawn, apply   To maintain asepsis and to stop blood and
   pressure over the lumbar puncture site using   cerebrospinal fluid flow.
a sterile topical swab.

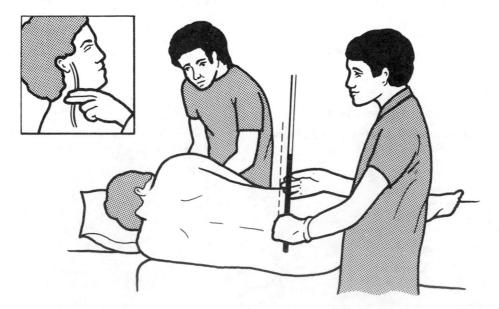

Figure 25.4 Queckenstedt's manoeuvre.

6 When all leakage from the puncture site has ceased, apply a plaster dressing or plastic dressing spray.

To prevent secondary infection.

7 Make the patient comfortable. He/she should lie flat or the head should be tilted slightly downwards for a period of up to 24 hours (according to the doctor's instructions).

To avoid headache and decrease the possibility of brainstem herniation (coning) due to a reduction in cerebrospinal fluid pressure.

8 Observe patient for the next 24 hours for the following:
(a) Leakage from the puncture site.

There may be a small amount of bloodstained oozing. The presence of clear fluid should be reported immediately to the doctor, especially if accompanied by fluctuation of other observations, as it may be a cerebrospinal fluid leak.

(b) Headache.

Not unusual following lumbar puncture. Usually relieved by lying flat and, if ordered by the doctor, a mild analgesic.

(c) Backache.

As above.

(d) Neurological observations/vital signs.

These may indicate signs of a change in intracranial pressure. (For further information on neurological observations and vital signs, see Chapter 28.)

9 Encourage a fluid intake of 2–3 litres in 24 hours.

To replace lost fluid and assist the patient to micturate, which may be difficult due to the supine position.

10 Remove equipment and dispose of as appropriate.

To prevent the spread of infection.

11 Record the procedure in the appropriate documents.

12 Ensure that specimens are labelled appropriately and sent with the correct forms to the laboratory.

NURSING CARE PLAN

Problem	Cause	Suggested action
Pain down one leg during the procedure.	A dorsal nerve root may have been touched by the spinal needle.	Inform the doctor, who will probably move the needle. Reassure the patient.
Headache following procedure (may persist for up to a week).	Removal of the sample of cerebrospinal fluid.	Reassure the patient that it is a transient symptom. Ensure that he/she lies flat for the specified period of time. Encourage a high fluid intake to replace fluid lost during the procedure. Administer on analgesic as ordered. If the headache is

Nursing care plan (cont'd)

Problem	Cause	Suggested action
		severe and increasing, inform a doctor – there is a possibility of rising intracranial pressure.
Backache following procedure.	(a) Removal of the sample of cerebrospinal fluid. (b) Position required for puncture.	Reassure the patient that it is usually a transient symptom. Ensure that he/she lies flat for the appropriate period of time. Administer an analgesic as ordered.
Fluctuation of neurological observations, i.e. level of consciousness, pulse, respirations, blood pressure or pupillary reaction.	Herniation (coning) of the brainstem due to the decrease of intracranial pressure. (Raised intracranial pressure is a contraindication to lumbar puncture.)	Observe the patient constantly for signs of alteration in intracranial pressure. The frequency may be decreased as the patient's condition allows. Report any fluctuations in these observations to a doctor immediately.
Leakage from the puncture site.	(a) Resolution of bleeding. (b) Leakage of cerebrospinal fluid.	(a) No further action required. (b) Report immediately to a doctor, especially if accompanied by fluctuation in neurological observations.

CHAPTER 26

Mouth Care

Definition

Mouth care (oral hygiene) is defined as the scientific care of the teeth and mouth (Thomas, 1981). The aims of oral care are to:

- Keep the mucosa clean, soft, moist and intact and to prevent infection.
- Keep the lips clean, soft, moist and intact.
- Remove food debris as well as dental plaque without damaging the gingiva.
- Alleviate pain and discomfort and enhance oral intake.
- Prevent halitosis and freshen the mouth.

(Daeffler, 1980.)

REFERENCE MATERIAL

Anatomy and physiology

The mouth is the oval cavity at the anterior end of the digestive tract (Mosby, 1994). It consists of the mouth cavity (cavum oris proprium) and the vestibule (vestibulum oris) which is bounded by the lips and cheeks, and the gums and teeth. The oral cavity is lined with moist stratified epithelium consisting of 15–20 layers of cells (Hinchliffe & Montague, 1988). It is an area of rapid replication designed to meet the constant demands of activities such as chewing and talking (Porter, 1994). The tongue forms the greater part of the floor of the oral cavity.

The mouth is lubricated by secretions from the salivary glands: parotid, submandibular and sublingual. Approximately 1.5 litres of saliva are produced each day (Torrance, 1990). The functions of saliva are both protective and digestive in nature.

The mouth has three main functions:

- Ingestion of food and water;
- Communication; and
- With the nasal cavity, breathing.

(Lippold & Winton, 1972.)

Predisposing factors to poor oral health are:

- Inability to take adequate fluids;
- Poor nutritional status;
- Insufficient saliva production;
- Major intervention altering oral status – surgery, radiotherapy or chemotherapy;
- Lack of knowledge or motivation towards maintaining oral hygiene.

(Trenter & Creason, 1986.)

Oral complications

Oral complications manifest as pain, ulcers, infection, bleeding, bone and dentition changes and functional disorders affecting verbal and non-verbal communication, chewing and swallowing, taste and respiration (Porter, 1994). Stomatitis (inflammation of the oral cavity) results from damage to the mucous membrane (Holmes, 1990). It may be induced by trauma, infection or by factors that decrease the proliferation rate of the cells (e.g. chemotherapy). Xerostomia is an alteration in the production of saliva. Salivary function can be reduced or even destroyed by radiation (Cherry & Glucksmann, 1959) as the salivary glands are highly sensitive to radiation (Carl, 1983).

The oral cavity harbours many varieties of bacteria which do not normally pose any problems (Clarke, 1993). However, treatment such as cytotoxic therapy and antifungal therapy may increase the pathogenicity of these organisms leading to local and systemic infection. Common organisms include *Pseudomonas*, *Klebsiella* and *Escherichia coli* (Goepfert & Toth, 1979) and *Candida* species (Martin *et al.*, 1981).

Mouth care

Mouth care involves oral assessment, the use of oral care tools, appropriate frequency of care and oral care agents.

Oral assessment

Oral assessment is required in planning effective care (Eilers *et al.*, 1988). Thorough assessment of the oral cavity is required to:

- provide baseline data
- monitor response to therapy
- identify new problems as they arise.

(Holmes & Mountain 1993.)

A number of oral assessment tools have been developed. Holmes & Mountain (1993) evaluated three oral assessment guides for reliability, validity and clinical usefulness. In their conclusion they showed a preference for the oral assessment guide developed by Eilers *et al.* (1988), but stressed that further work is required to develop a tool that is entirely satisfactory for use in clinical practice and future research.

Frequency of care

Ginsberg (1961) concluded that the incidence of oral complications was reduced by the frequency of care rather than the agents employed. However, since then there has been little research to indicate the most effective frequency. Studies have reported various suggested time intervals (Ginsberg, 1961; Howarth, 1977; Beck, 1979; Dudjak, 1987) and there is clearly a need for further research.

Oral care tools

A number of different oral care tools have been reported in the literature including toothbrush, foamstick, dental floss and gauze. The most appropriate tool should be determined by its efficacy together with its potential to damage the gingiva. The use of the toothbrush is well supported by the literature (Howarth, 1977; Carl, 1983; Trenter & Creason, 1986), however the foamstick has been cited as preferable when oral care is administered by the nurse (DeWalt, 1975) as it may cause less trauma. The foamstick, however, is much less effective than the toothbrush at removing debris from the teeth and gums.

Oral care agents

The choice of an oral care agent is dependent on the aim of care. The agent may be used to remove debris and plaque, prevent superimposed infection, alleviate pain, stop bleeding, provide lubrication or to treat specific problems (Porter, 1994). A wide variety of agents are available and should be determined by the individual needs of the patient together with a detailed nursing assessment. The agents described below comprise those included in *The Royal Marsden NHS Trust Prescribing Guidelines for Mouth Care.*

Maintaining good oral hygiene

- Clean teeth with toothpaste and toothbrush after meals.
- Chlorhexidine gluconate 0.2% 5 ml, four times a day

diluted in 100 ml of water retained in the mouth for at least 1 minute.

Oral candidiasis

Prophylaxis
Nystatin mouthwash 1 ml, four times a day rinsed around the mouth and retained for at least 1 minute. A time interval of 15–30 minutes should be allowed between administration of chlorhexidine and nystatin to ensure efficacy.

Treatment

- Surgical patients – First-line nystatin 5 ml four times a day. Second-line fluconazole 50 mg, daily for 7 days.

- Radiotherapy/chemotherapy – First-line patients fluconazole 50 mg orally, daily for 7 days. Use 100 mg IV daily if patients cannot tolerate oral therapy. Second-line fluconazole 200–400 mg IV, daily until able to tolerate oral therapy.

Painful mouth

- First-line   Aspirin mouthwash four times a day (1 to 2 × 300 mg soluble tablets) used as mouthwash for oral cavity or a gargle for the oropharynx, mixed with lemon mucilage to aid adherence of aspirin to the mucosa when treating the hypopharynx. Paracetamol is an alternative if aspirin is contraindicated
- Second-line   Lignocaine 2% gel applied four times a day for pain relief of mucositis or ulceration. For extensive mucositis use lignocaine spray.
or   Sucralfate suspension 5 ml, four times a day rinsed around the mouth and swallowed.
- Third-line   Low dose opiates by oral, subcutaneous or intravenous route.

Reduced salivary flow

Sodium fluoride (e.g. Fluorigard) mouthwash used in the morning after breakfast and subsequent cleaning of teeth and use of chlorhexidine mouthwash. No other mouthwash should be used for at least 1 hour after use. Fluoride gel (e.g. Gel-Kam) should be brushed on the teeth last thing at night.

Treatment of dry mouth
Artificial saliva (e.g. Glandosane or Luborant) two or three sprays up to four times daily or as often as necessary.

Chlorhexidine gluconate
Chlorhexidine is a compound with broad-spectrum antimicrobial activity that results in binding to and sustained release from mucosal surfaces (Ferretti et al., 1987). It has been shown to protect the patient from infection and to aid resolution of existing infections (Ferretti et al., 1987) and causes a reduction in soft tissue disease and oral microbial burden. It is effective against both anaerobes and aerobes as well as Candida (Walker, 1988; Mandel, 1988) and its efficacy is dose-related (Addy & Moran, 1991).

Fluconazole
Fluconazole is an orally absorbed antifungal azole which is soluble in water. It has been demonstrated to be effective in the treatment of candidosis of the oropharynx, oesophagous, urinary tract and a variety of deep tissue sites (Brammer, 1990).

Sucralfate
Barker et al. (1991) showed that consistent daily oral hygiene and use of a mouth-coating agent such as sucralfate in patients receiving radiotherapy results in less pain and may reduce weight loss and interruption of radiation therapy because of severe mucositis. Reduction in pain and increase in oral intake has also been shown in patients with chemotherapy induced ulcerating or erythematous mucositis taking oral sucralfate (Adams et al., 1686).

Nystatin
Nystatin is the best known and most commonly used antifungal agent (Campbell, 1995). It is an antifungal antibiotic that is used as an oral suspension (Daeffler, 1980). Barkvoll et al. (1989) showed in their in vitro study that combinations of nystatin and chlorhexidine digluconate were not effective against Candida albicans and recommended that the most efficient treatment plan must be restricted to the use of one of these drugs alone. Bristol-Myers Squibb Pharmaceuticals Ltd have suggested that it is logical to leave a time interval of 15–30 minutes between administration of each agent in such a combination to ensure adequate contact time.

Fluoride
Fluoride helps to prevent and arrest tooth decay, especially radiation caries, demineralization and decalcification. Following its use no diet or fluids should be taken for at least 30 minutes in order for it to work (Myers & Mitchell, 1988).

Artificial saliva
Saliva substitutes duplicate the properties of normal saliva (Kusler & Rambur, 1992). They buffer the acidity of the mouth and lubricate the mucous membranes (Heals, 1993).

References

Adams, S. C. et al. (1986) Evaluation of sucralfate as a compound oral suspension for the treatment of mucositis. In: Proceedings or the Annual Meeting of the American Society of Clinical Oncology, 5, 257.

Addy, M. & Moran, J. (1991) The effect of some chlorhexidine containing mouthrinses on salivary bacterial counts. Journal of Clinical Periodontology, 18, 90–93.

Barker, G. et al. (1991) The effects of sucralfate suspension and diphenhydramine syrup plus kaolin–pectin on radiotherapy-induced mucositis. Oral Surgery, Oral Medicine, Oral Pathology, 71(3), 288–93.

Barkvoll, P. et al. (1989) Effect of nystatin and chlorhexidine digluconate on Candida albicans. Oral Surgery, Oral Medicine, Oral Pathology, 279–81.

Beck, S. (1979) Impact of a systemic oral protocol on stomatitis after chemotherapy. Cancer Nursing, 2(S), 185–99.

Brammer, K. W. (1990) Management of fungal infection in neutropenic patients. Haematology and Blood Transfusion, 33, 546–50.

Campbell, S. (1995) Treating oral candidiasis. Nurse Prescriber, June, 12–13.

Carl, W. (1983) Oral complications in cancer patients. American Family Physician, 27, 161–70.

Cherry, C. P. & Glucksmann, A. (1959) Injury and repair following irradiation of salivary glands in male rats. British Journal of Radiology, 32, 596–608.

Clarke G. (1993) Mouth care in the hospitalized patient. British Journal of Nursing, 2(4), 221–7.

Daeffler, P. (1990) Oral hygiene measures for patients with cancer, part 1. Cancer Nursing, 3(5), 347–56.

Daeffler, R. (1980) Oral hygiene measures for patients with cancer. II. Cancer Nursing, December, 427–31.

Dewalt, E. M. (1975) Effect of timed hygienic measures on oral mucosa in a group of elderly subjects. Nursing Research, 24, 104–8.

Dudjak, L. (1987) Mouth care for mucositis due to radiation therapy. Cancer Nursing, 10, 131–40.

Eilers, J. et al. (1988) Development, testing and application of the oral assessment guide. Oncology Nursing Forum, 15(3), 325–30.

Ferretti, G. et al. (1987) Chlorhexidine for prophylaxis against oral infections and associated complications in patients receiving bone marrow transplants. Journal of the American Dental Association, 114(4), 461–7.

Ginsberg, M. (1961) A study of oral hygiene nursing care. *American Journal of Nursing*, 61, 67–9.

Goepfert, H. & Toth, B. B. (1979) Head and neck complications of cancer chemotherapy. *The Laryngoscope*, 89, 315–19.

Heals, D. (1993) A key to wellbeing: oral hygiene in patients with advanced cancer. *Professional Nurse*, March, 391–8.

Hinchliffe, S. & Montague, S. (1988) *Physiology for Nursing Practice*. Ballière Tindall, London.

Holmes, S. (1990) *Cancer Chemotherapy. Lisa Sainsbury Foundation*, pp. 180–81. Austen Cornish, London.

Holmes, S. & Mountain, E. (1993) Assessment of oral status: evaluation of three oral assessment guides. *Journal of Clinical Nursing*, 2, 35–40.

Howarth, H. (1977) Mouth care procedures for the very ill. *Nursing Times*, 73, 354–5.

Kusler, D. L. & Rambur, B. A. (1992) Treatment for radiation-induced xerostomia: an innovative remedy. *Cancer Nursing*, 15(3), 191–5.

Lippold, A. J. C. & Winton, F. R. (1972) *Hearing and Speech Human Physiology*, pp. 443–64. Churchill Livingstone, Edinburgh.

Mandel, I. (1988) Chemotherapeutic agents for controlling plaque and gingivitis. *Journal of Clinical Periodontology*, 15, 488–98.

Martin, U. V. *et al.* (1981) Yeast flora of the mouth and skin during and after irradiation for oral and laryngeal cancer. *Journal of Medical Microbiology*, 14, 457–67.

Mosby (1994) *Mosby's Medical, Nursing and Allied Health Dictionary*, 4th edn. C. V. Mosby, Missouri.

Myers, R. E. & Mitchell, L. D. (1988) Fluoride for the head and neck radiation patient. *Military Medicine*, 153(8), 411.

Porter, H. J. (1994) Mouth care in cancer. *Nursing Times*, 90(14), 27–9.

Thomas, C. L. (1981) *Taber's Cyclopedic Medical Dictionary*, 14th edn. F. A. Davis, Philadelphia.

Torrance, C. (1990) Oral hygiene. *Surgical Nurse*. The Medicine Group (UK) Ltd.

Trenter, P. & Creason, N. S. (1986) Nurse administered oral hygiene: is there a scientific basis? *Journal of Advanced Nursing*, 11, 323–31.

Walker, C. (1988) Microbial effects of mouthrinses containing antimicrobials. *Journal of Clinical Periodontology*, 15, 499–505.

GUIDELINES: MOUTH CARE

EQUIPMENT

1 Clinically clean tray.
2 Plastic cups.
3 Mouthwash or clean solutions.
4 Appropriate equipment for cleaning.
5 Clean receiver or bowl.
6 Paper tissues.
7 Wooden spatula.
8 Small-headed, soft toothbrush.
9 Toothpaste.
10 Disposable gloves.
11 Denture pot.

All the above items may be left on the patient's locker when appropriate, and should be cleaned, renewed or replenished daily.

12 Small torch.

PROCEDURE

Action	Rationale
 1 Explain and discuss the procedure with the patient.	To ensure that the patient understands the procedure and gives his/her valid consent.
2 Wash hands with bactericidal soap and water or with bactericidal alcohol hand rub and dry with paper towel.	To reduce the risk of cross-infection.

| 3 | Prepare solutions required. | Solutions must always be prepared immediately before use to maximize their efficacy and minimize the risk of microbial contamination. |

4   Remove the patient's dentures if necessary, using paper tissues or topical swabs, and place them in a denture pot.

Removal of dentures is necessary for cleaning of underlying tissues. A tissue or topical swab provides a firmer grip of the dentures and prevents contact with patient's saliva.

5   Inspect the patient's mouth with the aid of a torch and spatula.

The mouth is examined for changes in condition with respect to moisture, cleanliness, infected or bleeding areas, ulcers, etc.

6   Using a small toothbrush and toothpaste, brush the patient's natural teeth, gums and tongue.

To remove adherent materials from the teeth, tongue and gum surfaces. Brushing stimulates gingival tissues to maintain tone and prevent circulatory stasis.

7   Brush the inner and outer aspects of the teeth with firm, individual strokes directed outwards from the gums.

Brushing loosens and removes debris trapped on and between the teeth and gums. This reduces growth medium for pathogenic organisms and minimizes the risk of plaque formulation and dental caries. Foam sticks are ineffective for this.

8   Give a beaker of water or mouthwash to the patient. Encourage patient to rinse the mouth vigorously then void contents into a receiver. Paper tissues should be to hand.

Rinsing removes loosened debris and toothpaste and makes the mouth taste fresher. The glycerine content of toothpaste will have a drying effect if left in the mouth.

9   If the patient is unable to rinse and void, use a rinsed toothbrush to clean the teeth and moistened foam sticks to wipe the gums and oral mucosa. Foam sticks should be used with a rotating action so that most of the surface is utilized.

10   Apply artificial saliva to the tongue if appropriate and/or suitable lubricant to dry lips.

To increase the patient's feeling of comfort and well-being and prevent further tissue damage.

11   Clean the patient's dentures on all surfaces with a denture brush or toothbrush. Rinse them well and return them to the patient.

Cleaning dentures removes accumulated food debris which could be broken down by salivary enzymes to products which irritate and cause inflammation of the adjacent mucosal tissue. Some commercial denture cleaners may have an abrasive effect on the denture surface. This then attracts plaque and encourages bacterial growth.

12   Dentures should be soaked in chlorhexidine for ten minutes if oral *Candida* species are present.

Soaking in chlorhexidine reduces the risk of reinfecting the mouth with infected dentures.

13   Discard remaining mouthwash solutions.

To prevent the risk of contamination.

14   Wash hands with soap and water or alcohol hand rub and dry with paper towel.

To reduce the risk of cross-infection.

NURSING CARE PLAN

Problem	Cause	Suggested action
Dry mouth.	Inadequate hydration.	Monitor the fluid balance and increase the fluid intake where necessary.
	Impaired production of saliva, e.g. as a consequence of radiotherapy or chemotherapy.	Apply artificial saliva to the oral cavity as required. Give the patient ice cubes to suck.
	Presence of specific stressors, e.g. mouth breathing, oxygen therapy, no oral intake, intermittent oral suction.	Inspect the mouth frequently, e.g. half-hourly. Swab mucosa with water.
Dry lips.	As above.	Smear a thin layer of appropriate lubricant.
Thick mucus.	Postoperative closure of a tracheostomy. Radiotherapy. Poor swallowing mechanism.	Use sodium bicarbonate solution in the mouth care procedure. Rinse the mouth afterwards with water or saline.
Patient unable to tolerate toothbrush.	Pain, e.g. post-operatively; stomatitis.	Use foam sticks to clean the patient's gums and mucosa. Saline is advisable. For severe pain use an anaesthetic mouth spray or mouthwash before giving mouth care.
Toothbrush inappropriate or ineffective.	Infected stomatitis. Accumulation of dried mucus, blood or debris.	Take a swab of any new lesions for culture before giving mouth care.

CHAPTER 27

Moving and Handling Patients

Manual handling operations are defined as:

'any transporting or supporting of a load including the lifting, putting down, pushing, pulling, carrying or moving thereof by hand or bodily force' (Health and Safety Executive, 1992).

Lifting has wrongly become a generic term used to describe many of the manual handling tasks undertaken by nurses in the clinical situation. However, the Royal College of Nursing defines a lift as taking the patient's full weight:

'. . . upwards or vertically, at least initially whilst being supported before being moved downwards or horizontally' (Royal College of Nursing, 1992).

For any manual handling operation to be considered successful it must meet two prime objectives. The handler needs to employ minimal effort, while the patient experiences minimal discomfort. These objectives can be achieved and the risk of injury reduced by undertaking a comprehensive assessment of the task's requirements.

REFERENCE MATERIAL

Potential hazards

Manual handling procedures involve both hazards and risks, factors which exist to a greater or lesser extent in any operation which involves the manual handling of a load. A hazard can be defined as something which has the potential to cause harm, whilst risk is an expression of probability of injury, in relation to the severity of the hazard. Hazards and risks are present for both nurses and patients involved in manual handling, particularly if an unsuitable system or method is employed. The experience of being moved physically by others can be unpleasant and frightening, especially if no prior explanation of the manoeuvre has been given.

It is well known that nursing is one of the occupational groups most likely to suffer from back pain. Stubbs *et al.*

(1983, 1984) provide a comprehensive account of this, and demonstrate that there is a significant incidence of back problems amongst nurses, which is a big factor in nurse wastage (Stubbs *et al.*, 1986). This is supported by the Confederation of Health Service Employees who estimate that each year 3650 nurses leave the profession permanently as a result of back injury, and 1 in 4 nurses experience back pain in the course of a working day (COSHE, 1992). Approximately 40% of back injuries go unreported for fear of job loss (Cole, 1994). The cost of back injuries is not only counted in terms of the suffering of individual nurses. It is estimated that 1 500 000 working days are lost annually in the NHS because of back pain, at a cost of £140 million (Simon & The National Back Pain Association, 1992).

The Manual Handling of Loads Regulations 1992 came into effect on 1 January 1993 under the terms of the Health and Safety at Work Act 1974, thereby implementing European Directive 90/269/EEC. As a result employers and employees acquired greater responsibilities for the design, development and maintenance of safe systems of practice. The regulations state that all hazardous manual handling tasks must if reasonably practical, be eliminated. If this is not possible then a 'suitable and sufficient' written assessment of the risk must be undertaken by the employer (or someone designated by the employer). In order for assessments to be considered as suitable and sufficient they must consider the task, the weight and size of the load, the working environment and individual capability. Employers are required to provide suitable mechanical handling aids if the handling operation can not be avoided, and training for employees in the use of equipment to maintain a safe working environment. Employees are obliged to make use of safe systems of work implemented by their employers, and to report to an appropriate person any hazards identified, as well as changes in their own ability to undertake manual handling tasks safely (e.g. pregnancy, back injury or deterioration in health status).

In addition employees are obliged:

'generally to make use of appropriate equipment provided for them in accordance with their training and the instructions, this would include machinery and other aids provided for the safe handling of loads' (Health and Safety Executive, 1992).

The risk of injury to both handler and patient can be reduced by fully assessing the task and identifying the best system for completing the procedure. However, assessment of the task and training are not sufficient on their own to minimize the risk or the incidence of back pain (Pheasant & Stubbs, 1991). It is important that nurses understand how ergonomic principles contribute to providing and maintaining a safe environment for the handling of patients, and they must develop the ability to change their practices. Manual handling of any patient makes considerable demands upon the handler; the application of skill rather than strength alone can reduce the strain considerably (Gonnet & Kryzwon, 1991; McCall, 1991).

The Royal College of Nursing through the Advisory Panel of Back Pain in Nurses has published a Code of Practice for the Handling of Patients (Royal College of Nursing, 1996). The Code advocates that no nurse should be expected to move a patient where he/she bears most or all of the patient's weight and a hoist, sliding or other appropriate handling aid should always be used. The panel has always believed that the profession has no option but to work towards the elimination of manual lifting from nursing practice. This can be achieved by the introduction of sliding devices and mechanical hoists in all areas where non independent patients are cared for, along with the required and associated education and training.

Biomechanics of load management

Because of its gentle 'S' shape the spine is able to withstand considerable compressive forces being applied to it. This can be ten times more than it could withstand if it were a straight structure. Despite this it can become easily damaged if those forces become torsional, twisting or sheering, affecting the surface of intravertebral discs.

When a person stands erect, most of the forces applied to the spine are the result of gravity acting upon the head and trunk. These forces are applied directly down through the spinal column, and very little muscular activity is required to maintain a stable upright position, However when the trunk begins to move forward, away from the erect position the nature and direction of the forces being applied to the spinal structure can change. In erect and near erect position the forces upon the spine are compressive; in the stooped position, forces can acquire harmful, sheering characteristics (Fig. 27.1) (Pheasant, 1991).

Compression forces are cause by the greater effort exerted by the erector spinae muscles to maintain a counter balance to the forward weight of the trunk and to the weight of any load being moved. They increase in direct proportion to the distance the load is held away from the operator's body (Pheasant, 1991). Rotational or jerking movements can increase sheering forces by up to 400% (Nachemson, 1981). It is always safer to move any load with the natural curves of the spine maintained and the object or patient as close to the body as possible with the weight of the load symmetrically spread through both arms. This makes use of the large, strong muscles of the hip and thigh to provide the momentum for the movement of the load, reducing the sheering forces produced in the back. This is not only safer but is also more mechanically efficient. Mechanical efficiency is further improved by always using sliding sheets and mechanical lifting devices, thus eliminating the need to physically lift any patient (Ortengren et al., 1981).

Figure 27.1 illustrates the direction of forces being applied to the lumbosacral region in a person who is standing upright and bending forward to the horizontal. Figure 27.2 gives a model for the calculation of the magnitude of these forces, assuming the subject to be a man weighing 70 kg; the distance between the back (erector spinae) muscle and the centre of motion (d) = 0.05 m; the horizontal distance between the line of gravity along which the weight of the upper body acts and the L4/5 disc (x) = 0.3 m and the weight of the upper body (W) = 40 kg (equivalent to a force of 400 N).

The force (F) applied to the spine when bent forward to the horizontal position, measured in Newtons, is equivalent to:

$$\frac{W \left(\text{weight of upper body}\right) \times x \left(\text{horizontal distance from line of gravity of L4/5}\right)}{d \left(\text{erector spinae muscle to centre of motion}\right)}$$

$$= \frac{400\,N \times 0.3\,m}{0.05\,m}$$

$$= 2400\,N \left(240\,kg\right)$$

If the man in this position lifted a load of 30 kg (300 N) the force (F) applied to the spine would now be equivalent to:

$$\frac{\left(400\,N + 300\,N\right) \times 0.3\,m}{0.05\,m} = 4200\,N \left(420\,kg\right)$$

In the near erect position where x is reduced to 0.1 m, the force without extra loading would be equivalent to:

$$\frac{400\,N \times 0.1\,m}{0.05\,m} = 800\,N \left(80\,kg\right)$$

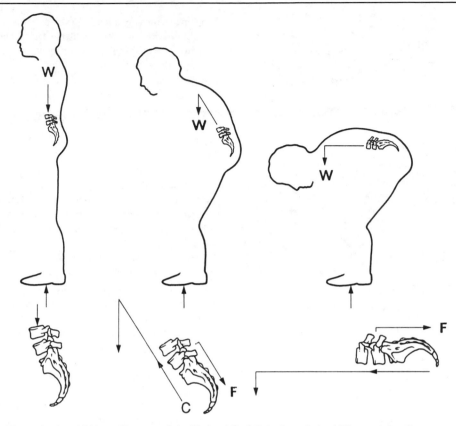

Figure 27.1 Biomechanics of lifting. (Coutesy of the National Back Pain Association.) W = weight of upper part of body; F = tension in back muscles; C = equal and opposite reaction to compressing dics.

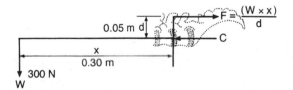

W = weight of upper part of body as newtons (N): 1 kg = 10 N

x = horizontal distance between line of gravity along which 'W' acts and the L4/5 disc (this decreases with less forward flexion)

d = distance between back muscle and centre of motion (metres)

F = tension in back muscles as newtons (N)

C = equal and opposite reaction to 'F' compressing disc

Figure 27.2 A model for the calculation of the magnitude of forces applied to the lumbosacral region. (Courtesy of the National Back Pain Association.)

and with the same 30 kg weight, the force would be calculated thus:

$$\frac{\left(400\,\text{N} + 300\,\text{N}\right) \times 0.1\,\text{m}}{0.05\,\text{m}} = 1400\,\text{N}\left(140\,\text{kg}\right)$$

The force applied to the spine, therefore, is significantly reduced the closer the upper body is kept to an upright position.

Factors affecting spinal stress during load handling

Changes in intra-abdominal pressure (IAP) during manual handling procedures can be measured using a pressure-sensitive radio pill. It has been shown that there is a close, positive correlation between a load acting upon the spine and the increase in IAP (Davis, 1981; Ortengren *et al.*, 1981). Intra-abdominal pressure can exert a supporting and stabilizing effect upon the spine during load handling by relieving some of the inter-vertebral compression (Fig. 27.3). This effect is most pronounced when the handler adopts a symmetrical position (Schultz *et al.*, 1982). It is however only

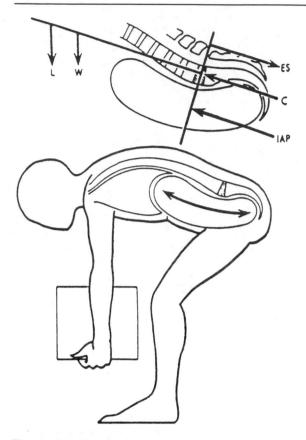

Figure 27.3 Diagram showing spine, thoracic and abdominal cavities during lifting, together with a force diagram showing how the increases in intra-abdominal pressure (IAP) may relieve the intervertebral compresion (C) which is equal and opposite to the tensile force in erector spinae (ES) required to raise the load (L) and the upper part of the body (W). (Courtesy of *Physiotherapy Journal*.)

temporary, and ceases when the handler inhales (Troup, 1979).

Pressures within the intervertebral discs, as well as rises in IAP, give an indication of loading on the spine (Nachemson & Morris, 1964; Nachemson & Elfstrom, 1970). Figure 27.4 shows percentage change in disc pressure in subjects in a variety of static positions: the heavier the load, the greater the stress on the spinal structures. Confused, paralysed or uncooperative patients make handling unpredictable and the use of a pre-arranged technique difficult, producing higher pressures and a greater potential for injury while moving them (Hyde, 1980).

Moving patients

Stresses exerted on the spine during manual handling tasks are largely the result of the technique used when handling or moving a load (Leskinen *et al.*, 1983). Indeed the elimination of manual lifting tasks would result in very little extra spinal stress being experienced (Gonnet & Kryzwon, 1991; McCall, 1991). The ideal is that wherever patients who require assisted mobility are cared for, then hoists, sliding aids and handling slings should be provided. Employers who do not make this kind of provision are in conflict with the law, as are carers who choose not to use such equipment and systems of practice, which have been implemented for their own safety and protection (DoH, 1993). The use of such equipment *must always* be the first considered option and the manual lifting of the patient should only be considered (following suitable assessment, Fig. 27.5) if the use of handling equipment is contraindicated. This is rarely likely to be the case.

Many patients are able to assist nurses while being moved, and should be encouraged to help in ways that are comparable with their capabilities or health status. This would have become apparent during the assessment period. It may be necessary to give the patients some education about how they can best move. They may well be able to use small aids such as 'monkey poles', rope ladders or hand blocks (Fig. 27.6), which might allow the patient to be independent of the nurse while moving in bed.

Awareness of the existence and training in the use of these aids is unfortunately not widespread (Royal Col-

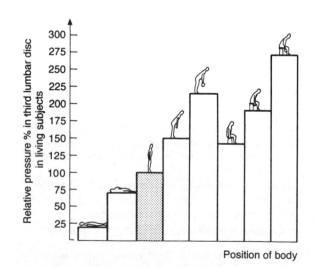

Figure 27.4 Relative increase and decrease in intradiscal pressure in different supine, standing and sitting postures compared to the pressure in upright standing (100%). (Source: Nachemson, A. (1976) *Spine*, 1, 59–71. J. B. Lippincott, Philadelphia.)

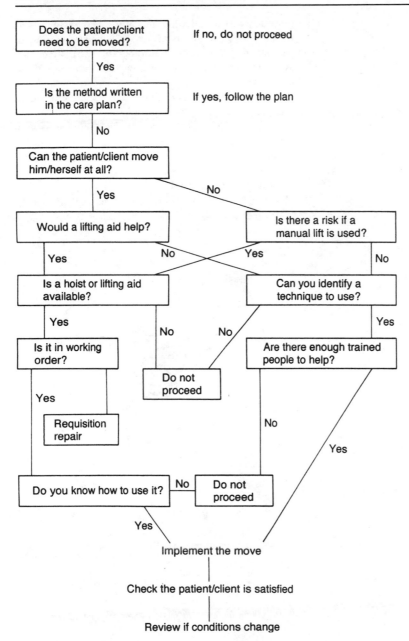

Figure 27.5 Guidelines for moving a patient/client. (Courtesy of *Trainer's Manual for Prevention of 'Back Injury'*, K. L. Barker, R. E. Bell, W. H. Green & J. Klaber-Moffett).

lege of Nursing, 1990). Currently some 60 different hoists and 150 small aids are available to assist with the moving and handling of patients within a care setting (Disabled Living Foundation, 1994). Arguably, such a wide range of aids and devices means that there is little reason to undertake hazardous manual handling tasks (lifting).

As the skills of the handler develop, their techniques in the use of these aids become more effective although it must be recognized that even with the use of mechanical hoists there is still an element of manual handling to be done (once a patient is in the hoist the hoist will still need to be moved, by pushing or pulling). Therefore it is always essential for nurses to recognize in advance whether this task will exceed their capabilities, and be assertive enough to refuse unless they have suitable and sufficient extra assistance. It is important to remember that even when using aids, prior assessment of the task and the environment is essential to make the operation as safe as possible.

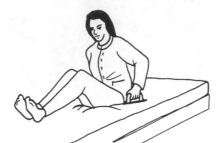

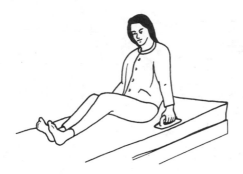

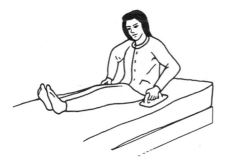

Figure 27.6 Patient using hand blocks. (Adapted from the Disabled Living Foundation *Handling People* pack.)

Equipment

Sliding devices (e.g. the Mini–Slide or the Phil-E-Slide) are simple but effective in moving someone up or down a bed. The traditional poles and canvas method of transferring a patient from bed to bed or bed to trolley can be replaced by more effective lateral transfer aids such as roller boards or Patslide (Fig. 27.7). The effort required to carry out a log roll where the patient's condition requires either the maintenance of spinal alignment or the abduction of the hip joint can be drastically reduced by the use of a turning frame (Fig. 27.8), while 'banana boards' and hoists do away with the need to lift even the

most dependant patient in and out of bed or chair. The use of low friction sheets makes the lateral positioning of patients much easier. A number of these items are available (e.g. Easi-slide turning slide; the carelet or multicover).

It must be remembered that the use of any equipment must be in line with the manufacturer's guidelines and instructions, and that the use of such equipment is kept under review for new information and developments in its use.

Moving techniques

Slide one (Fig. 27.9) is indicated for moving patients up or down the bed.

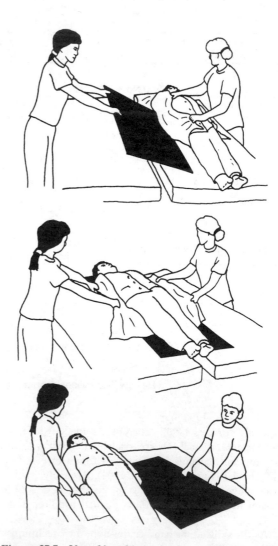

Figure 27.7 Use of low friction boards. (Adapted from the Disabled Living Foundation *Handling People* pack.)

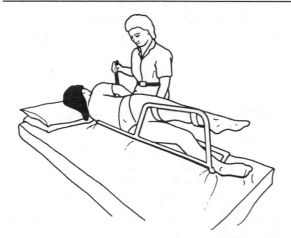

Figure 27.8 One nurse using turning frame to log roll a patient. (Adapted from the Disabled Living Foundation *Handling Patients* pack.)

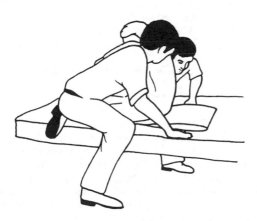

Figure 27.9 Slide one.

Contraindications

- Patients who are unable to sit up unsupported.
- Confused patients.
- Patients with stiff or injured shoulders or injuries to the chest or upper back.
- Following hip surgery where there may be a risk of dislocation.
- Patients who have no control of their neck and head.

Procedure

(1) The bed height should be set just above the knee (if the handlers are of different height, the shorter of the two dictates bed height whilst the taller compensates by adjusting their position).

(2) The sliding device is placed under the patient following manufacturer's instructions and a handling sling is placed under the patient's thighs in close proximity to their buttocks.

(3) The patient is assisted into a sitting position.

(4) Both handlers face the opposite direction to the patient.

(5) The handlers place their inside knee on the bed as close to the patient as possible and level with the patient's buttocks. The outside foot is placed flat on the floor, as close to the bed as possible and parallel to the inside knee. The knee of the outside leg is therefore slightly bent.

(6) Each handler's inside shoulder is then placed below the patient's axilla in the side of the chest, supporting him/her in an upright position, while the patient's arms rest on the handler's back.

(7) The handler's inside hand takes hold of the handling sling.

(8) The handler's outside hand rests on the bed behind the patient as a supporting strut.

(9) The handlers ensure that the natural curves of the spine are maintained and their shoulders and hips are parallel to each other and at right angles to the bed.

(10) Upon the agreed command the handlers kneel up, simultaneously straightening the outside elbow and knee, thus causing the patient to slide along the sliding device into the required position.

Slide two (Fig. 27.10) is indicated for moving patients up or down the bed.

Contraindications

- Following hip surgery where there is a risk of dislocation.

Procedure

(1) As with slide one, the bed height is adjusted according to the height of the shorter handler with the taller making adjustments to his/her position.

(2) The sliding device is placed beneath the patient following the manufacturer's instructions (the Phil-E-Slide does not require the use of a handling sling).

(3) The handlers face the same direction as the patient.

(4) Their inside knees are placed on the bed as close to the patient as possible and level with the patient's hip joint.

(5) The outside leg is placed close to the bed but slightly posterior to the inside knee.

(6) The handler's outside hand takes hold of the patient's hand or arm in a manner which is mutually comfortable. This is to offer support only.

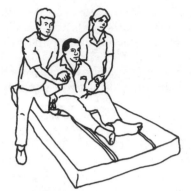

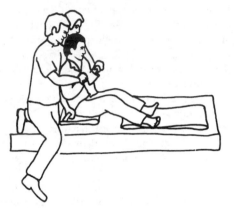

Figure 27.10   Slide two. (Courtesy of ERGO-IKE Associate-makers of Phil-E-Slide).

(7) The inside hand takes hold of the handles on the sliding device (or the handling sling if required by the type of aid).

(8) Upon the agreed command, the handlers sit back on their heels, causing the patient to be moved into the required position on the sliding device.

Drag can be further reduced by using a second sliding sheet under the patient's feet, eliminating the majority of friction between the feet and the bed.

Turning the patient

Turning patients on to their side can be easily achieved by using the patient's own body weight. With the bed at waist height the patient's furthest arm is placed across his/her chest, the furthest knee is then bent up (if possible) and gentle but firm pressure is applied to this knee, at the same time as supporting the patient's furthest shoulder. The patient will easily turn on to their side. If this is performed with a sliding/turning sheet *in situ* the patient can then be positioned in the bed once the turn has been completed.

References and further reading

Asquwith, B. (1995) *Manual Handling and Lifting; Croner's Health Service Manager, M31–M36.* Croner Publications, London.

COHSE (1992) *Back Breaking Work.* Confederation of Health Service Employees, Banstead.

Cole, A. (1994) Staff hide back pain for fear of dismissal. *Nursing Times*, 90(16), 9.

Davis, P. R. (1981) The use of intra abdominal pressure in evaluating stresses on the lumbar spine. *Spine*, 6(1), 90–92.

Department of Health (1993) *Risk Management in the NHS.* Department of Health, London.

Disabled Living Foundation (1994) *Handling People: Equipment, Advice and Information.* The Disabled Living Foundation, London.

Gonnet, L. & Kryzwon, A. (1991) Preventing back pain through education, *Nursing Standard*, 5(24), 25–7.

Health and Safety Executive (1992) *Manual Handling: Guidance on Regulations.* HMSO, London.

Hyde, N. J. (1980) *A comparative analysis of a lifting method commonly used by nurses versus a recommended method of lifting patients, using pressure-sensitive radio pill methodology.* BSc thesis, Leeds Polytechnic.

Leskinen, T. P. J. *et al.* (1983) A dynamic analysis of spinal compression with different lifting techniques. *Ergonomics*, 26, 595–604.

McCall, J. (1991) Watch your back. *Nursing Standard*, 5(24), 50–51.

Nachemson, A. (1981) Disc pressure measurement. *Spine*, 6(1), 93–7.

Nachemson, A. & Elfstrom, G. (1970) Intravital dynamic pressure measurements in lumbar discs. A study of common movements, manoeuvres and exercises. *Scandinavian Journal of Rehabilitation Medicine*, Supplement, 1–40.

Nachemson, A. & Morris, J. M. (1964) *In vivo* measurement of intra discal pressures. Discometry – a method for the determination of pressure in the lower lumbar discs. *Journal of Bone and Joint Surgery*, 46A, 1077–92.

Ortengren, R. *et al.* (1981) Studies of relationships between lumbar disc pressure myoelectric back muscle activity and intra-abdominal (intergastric) pressure. *Spine*, 6(1), 98–103.

Pheasant, S. T. (1986) *Bodyspace – Anthropometry, Ergonomics and Design.* Taylor and Francis, London.

Pheasant, S. (1991) *Ergonomics: Work and Health.* Macmillan Academic and Professional, Basingstoke.

Pheasant, S. & Stubbs, D. (1991) *Lifting and Handling – An Ergonomic Approach.* The National Back Pain Association with Thorn EMI UK Rental, London.

Royal College of Nursing (1990) Equipment to save your back. *Nursing Standard*, 4(34), 26–9.

Royal College of Nursing (1992) *Advisory Panel for Back Pain in Nurses: Code of Practice for the Handling of Patients.* Royal College of Nursing, London.

Royal College of Nursing (1996) *Advisory Panel for Back Pain in Nurses: Code of Pracice for the Handling of Patients Revised.* Royal College of Nursing, London.

Schultz, A. *et al.* (1982) Loads on the lumbar spine. Validation of a biomechanical analysis by measurements of intradiscal pressures and myoelectric signals. *Journal of Bone and Joint Surgery of America*, 64(5), 713–20.

Simon, P. & The National Back Pain Association (1992) In the hidden scandal. *Nursing Times*, 88(41), 24–6.

Stubbs, D. & Buckle, P. (1984) The epidemiology of back pain in nursing. *Nursing*, 2(32), 935–7.

Stubbs, D. A. *et al.* (1983) Back pain in the nursing profession 1. Epidemiology and pilot methodology. *Ergonomics*, 26(8), 755–65.

Stubbs, D. *et al.* (1986) Backing out; nurse wastage associated with back pain. *International Journal of Nursing Studies*, 23(4), 325–36.

Troup, J. D. G. (1979) Biomechanics of the vertebral column. *Physiotherapy*, 65(8), 238–44.

GUIDELINES: MOVING AND HANDLING OF PATIENTS

PROCEDURE

Action	Rationale
1 Assess the needs of the patient, the environment and necessity for the procedure (Fig. 27.5).	To ensure that action is in the patient's best interests. To ascertain whether there is sufficient space and appropriate equipment to perform procedure.
2 Inform all participating staff of the results of the assessment and confirm that details have been understood.	All staff participating in the procedure understand the plan of action in order to coordinate their actions correctly.
3 Prepare area by moving away any unwanted furnishings or equipment	To provide an ergonomic workspace with sufficient space to manoeuvre and perform the required task.
4 Select appropriate equipment as specified in the hospital training programme and the assessments.	To ensure the patient is moved with the minimum of effort, safely, and experiences as little discomfort as is possible.
5 Assist the patient into the desired position, with one handler acting as leader and coordinator for the procedure.	To ensure that effort is exerted at the same time by the handlers to prevent unequal strain on the handlers.
6 Check that the patient is comfortable following the manoeuvre and store equipment correctly and in line with safe practice	To evaluate the methods used and maintain a safe working environment.

Note: The use of handling aids must be considered before physical handling in all cases. Should anything go wrong when moving a patient and they appear to be falling *do not* attempt to prevent it from happening. It is safest to allow the patient to fall in a controlled fashion to the floor or bed.

Should a patient be found on the floor, they should be made comfortable but no attempt to move them should be made without proper assessment by a medical practitioner for indications of other injuries. A hoist should always be used to get patients up from the floor unless they can get up themselves or there are extremely exceptional medical contraindications for its use.

CHAPTER 28
Neurological Observations

Definition
Neurological observations relate to the evaluation of the integrity of an individual's nervous system.

Indications
Neurological observations are required to monitor and evaluate changes in the nervous system by indicating trends, thus aiding diagnosis and treatment, which in turn may affect prognosis and rehabilitation (Abelson, 1982; Jennett & Teasdale, 1984).

The frequency of neurological observations will depend upon the patient's condition and the rapidity with which changes are occurring or expected to occur.

REFERENCE MATERIAL
The main emphasis is on observing five critical areas:

(1) Level of consciousness.
(2) Pupillary activity.
(3) Motor function.
(4) Sensory function.
(5) Vital signs.

Level of consciousness
Level of consciousness is the single most important indicator of a patient's brain function (derived from Abelson (1982), Nikas (1982) and Allen (1986)). It ranges, on a continuum, from alert wakefulness to deep coma with no apparent responsiveness. Categories of impaired consciousness include the following:

(1) *Full consciousness*: the patient is aware of self and environment and this is reflected in the ability of the patient to be aroused, perceive internal or external stimuli and respond appropriately on a cognitive or motor level. Responses may be altered by focal, sensory and/or motor deficits.
(2) *Lethargy/drowsiness*: the patient is inactive and indifferent, responds slowly or unpurposefully to stimuli and may not respond verbally. The patient may be described as drowsy but rousable (Abelson, 1982).
(3) *Coma*: the patient has total absence of awareness of self and environment. Response to arousal from painful stimulus may be absent.

Specific diseases and injuries can impair level of consciousness since they may depress or destroy the reticular activating system (RAS) (Fig. 28.1). The RAS in the brainstem maintains normal consciousness. Processes that disturb its function will lead to altered consciousness (Fuller, 1993)(refer to Chapter 44).

Arousability
This depends on the integrity of the RAS. This core of nuclei extend from the brainstem to the thalamic nuclei in the cerebral hemispheres. Thus cognitive ability depends on the ability of the cerebral cortex to permit reciprocal stimulation and conscious behaviour.

Awareness
This requires an intact cerebral cortex to interpret sensory input and respond accordingly. This is the content of the consciousness (Nikas, 1982; Scherer, 1986).

Levels of consciousness may vary and are dependent on the location and extent of any neurological damage. Previous and/or co-existing problems should be heeded when noting levels of consciousness, e.g. deafness.

Assessment of level of consciousness
This involves three phases:

(1) Eye opening.
(2) Evaluation of verbal responses.
(3) Evaluation of motor response.

There is no universally accepted method for recording neurological assessment. The Glasgow Coma Scale has been found to be reliable and easy to use to measure conscious level, since it gives an instant graphic representation of the conscious state. It avoids making divi-

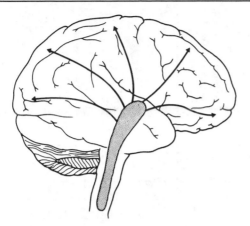

Figure 28.1 Reticular activating system.

Table 28.1 The Glasgow Coma Scale (taken from Sherman, 1990).

(1) *Eye opening:*
Score 4 Spontaneously
3 In response to voice
2 In response to pain
1 No response

(2) *Best verbal response:*
Score 5 Orientated
4 Confused
3 Inappropriate speech
2 Incomprehensible speech
1 No response

(3) *Best motor response:*
Score 6 Obeys commands
5 Localizes pain
4 Flexes and withdraws from pain
3 Assumes flexor posturing in response to pain
2 Assumes extensor posturing in response to pain
1 No response

Lowest score could be 3; highest score, 15, indicates full consciousness.

sions between consciousness and unconsciousness, which are times on a continuum (Jennett & Teasdale, 1984) (Fig. 28.2).

The Glasgow Coma Scale gives an objective measure of level of consciousness and eliminates the need for potentially ambiguous terms such as 'obtunded'. Possible scores range from 3 to 15 (Sherman, 1990) (Table 28.1). The score (according to Allen, 1984) is of little practical use and was developed as a statistical research tool. It is not used universally.

Eye opening

This indicates that the arousal mechanism in the brain is active. Eye opening may be: spontaneous; to speech, e.g. spoken name; to painful stimulus; none at all.

It must be remembered that swollen or permanently closed eyes (e.g. after tarsorrhaphy) will not open and do not necessarily indicate a falling conscious level.

Evaluation of verbal response

This may be:

(1) Orientated; the patient is aware of self and environment.
(2) Confused; the patient's responses to questions are incorrect and patient is unaware of self or environment.
(3) Incomprehensible; the patient may moan and groan without recognisable words.
(4) None; the patient does not speak or make sounds at all.

The absence of speech may not always indicate a falling level of consciousness. The patient may not speak English, may have a tracheostomy or may be dysphasic.

Evaluation of motor response

This is the best response from the patient; it is important and should be recorded. The patient should be asked to obey commands, e.g. 'squeeze my hands' (both sides). The nurse should note power in the hands. If movement is spontaneous, the nurse should note which limbs move, and how, e.g. purposefully or not.

Response to painful stimulus may be:

(1) Localized; the patient moves the other hand to the site of the stimulus.
(2) Flexor; the patient's limb flexes away from pain.
(3) Extensor; the patient's limb extends from pain.
(4) Flaccid – no motor response at all.

Use of the terms 'decerebrate' and 'decorticate' should be avoided as they carry anatomical implications (Abelson, 1982; Scherer, 1986).

Painful stimuli

Painful stimuli should be employed only if the patient does not respond to firm, clear commands. Use the least amount of pressure to elicit a response. (For suggested methods see below.) As the ability to localize pain is lost, various responses may be observed when painful stimuli are applied (Hudak *et al.*, 1982).

Painful stimuli can be applied in the following way:

(1) Place the patient's finger between the thumb and a pencil or pen.
(2) Pressure is gradually increased over a few seconds until the slightest response is seen.

The Royal Marsden NHS Trust

NEUROLOGICAL OBSERVATION CHART

NAME

RECORD No.

DATE

TIME

C O M A	Eyes open	Spontaneously
		To speech
		To pain
		None
		Eyes closed by swelling = C
S C A L E	Best verbal response	Orientated
		Confused
		Inappropriate Words
		Incomprehensible Sounds
		None
		Endotracheal tube or tracheostomy = T
	Best motor response	Obey commands
		Localise pain
		Flexion to pain
		Extension to pain
		None
		Usually record the best arm response
		Muscle relaxant = M

240
230
220
210
200
190
180
170

Temperature °C

40
39
38
37
36
35
34

1
2
3
4

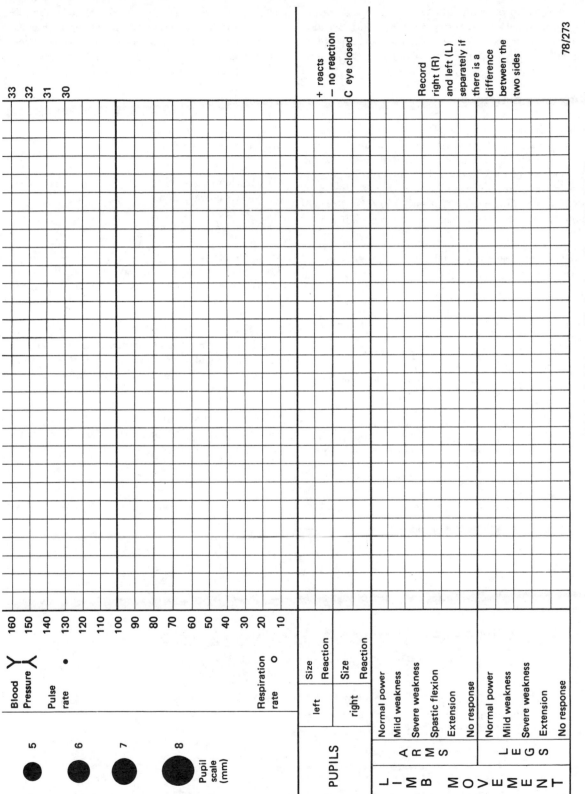

Figure 28.2 Glasgow Coma Scale. (Reproduced with permission of Institute of Neurological Sciences, The Southern General Hospital, Glasgow.)

Any finger can be used, although the third and fourth fingers are often most sensitive (Frawley, 1990). Because of the risk of bruising, pressure should not be applied to the nail bed or sternum. Do not stick pins in the patient (Nikas, 1982).

Pupillary activity

Careful examination of the reactions of the pupils to light is an important part of neurological assessment (Table 28.2). Note the size, shape, equality and reaction to light (both direct and consensual responses). Check the position of the eyes. Are they deviated upwards or downwards? Are both eyes looking in the same direction or are they disconjugate (Stolarik, 1985)? Impaired pupillary accommodation signifies that the midbrain it-

self may be suffering from pressure exerted by a swelling mass in the brain (or inside the cranium). (Pupillary constriction and dilation are controlled by cranial nerve III (oculomotor). Any changes may indicate pressure on this nerve, or brain stem damage) (Fig. 28.3).

Motor function

Damage to any part of the motor nervous system can affect the ability to move. Motor function assessment involves an evaluation of the following:

(1) Muscle strength.
(2) Muscle tone.
(3) Muscle coordination.
(4) Reflexes.
(5) Abnormal movements.

Muscle strength

This involves testing the patient's muscle strength against one's own muscle resistance and then against the pull of gravity.

Muscle tone

This involves flexing and extending the patient's limbs on both sides and noting how well such movements are resisted. Increased resistance would denote increased muscle tone and vice versa.

Muscle co-ordination

Any disease or injury that involves the cerebellum or basal ganglia will affect coordination. Assessment of

Table 28.2 Examination of the pupils (taken from Fuller, 1993).

What you find	Pupil size	Pupil reactiveness	Indication
Pupils equal	Pinpoint		Opiates or pontine lesion
	Small	Reactive	Metabolic encephalopathy
	Mid-sized	Fixed	Midbrain lesion
		Reactive	Metabolic lesion
Pupils unequal	Dilated	Unreactive	IIIrd palsy
	Small	Reactive	Horner's syndrome

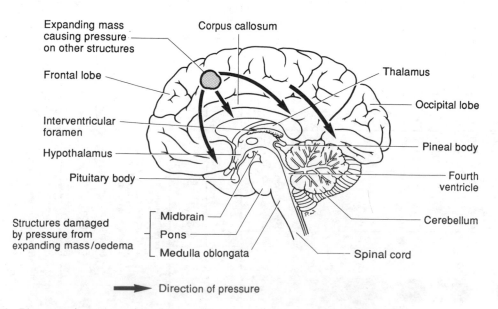

Figure 28.3 Diagrammatic representation of pressure from expanding mass and/or cerebral oedema.

hand and arm and leg coordination can be achieved by testing the rapidity and rhythm of alternating movements and of point-to-point movements. Nikas (1982) and Hudak *et al.* (1982) describe cerebellar function tests in detail.

Reflexes

Among the most important reflexes are: blink, gag and swallow, oculocephalic and plantar.

(1) *Blink*: is a protective reflex and can be affected by the Vth nerve (trigeminal) and the VIIth nerve (facial) involvement (Hudak *et al.*, 1982).
(2) *Gag and swallow*: also protective reflexes. Involvement of the IXth nerve (glosso-pharyngeal) and Xth nerve (vagus) may impair these reflexes (Hudak *et al.*, 1982).
(3) *Oculocephalic*: this reflex is an ocular movement that occurs only in patients with a severely decreased level of consciousness. When the reflex is present, the patient's eyes will move in the opposite direction from the side to which the head is turned. If the reflex is impaired, the eyes may not move at all, or only one eye may move (Hudak *et al.*, 1982; Scherer, 1986). This is known as the 'doll's eye' reflex.
(4) *Plantar*: movement of the foot at the ankle joint is plantar flexion (Tortora & Anagnostakos, 1992): this reflex helps to locate the anatomical site of the lesion (Nikas, 1982).

Abnormal movements

When carrying out neurological observations, any abnormal movements such as seizures, tics and tremors must be noted.

Sensory functions

Constant sensory input enables an individual to alter responses and behaviour to suit the environment. When disease or injury damages the sensory pathways, the sensory responses are always affected. Any assessment of sensory function should include an evaluation of the following:

(1) Central and peripheral vision.
(2) Hearing and ability to understand verbal communication.
(3) Superficial sensations (light touch, pain) and deep sensations (muscle and joint pain, muscle and joint position) (Hudak *et al.*, 1982; Fuller, 1993).

Vital signs

It is recommended that assessments of vital signs should be made in the following order:

(1) Respirations.
(2) Temperature.
(3) Blood pressure.
(4) Pulse.

(See also Chapter 30, Observations.)

Respirations

Of these four vital signs, respiratory patterns give the clearest indication of how the brain is functioning since respirations are controlled by different areas of the brain. Any disease or injury that affects these areas may produce respiratory changes. The rate, character and pattern of a patient's respiration must be noted. Abnormal respiratory patterns are listed in Table 28.3.

Table 28.3   Abnormal respiratory patterns.

Type	Pattern	Significance
Cheyne–Stokes	Rhythmic waxing and waning of both rate and depth of respirations, alternating regularly with briefer periods of apnoea	May indicate deep cerebral or cerebellar lesions, usually bilateral; may occur with upper brainstem involvement
Central neurogenic hyperventilation	Sustained, regular, rapid respirations, with forced inspiration and expiration	May indicate a lesion of the low midbrain or upper pons areas of the brainstem
Apnoeustic	Prolonged inspiration with a pause at full inspiration; there may also be expiratory pauses	May indicate a lesion of the low pons or upper medulla, or hypoglycaemia, or drug-induced respiratory depression
Cluster breathing	Clusters of irregular respirations alternating with longer periods of apnoea	May indicate a lesion of low pons or upper medulla
Ataxic breathing	A completely irregular pattern with random deep and shallow respirations; irregular pauses may also appear	May indicate a lesion of the medulla

Table 28.4 Visual pathways (taken from Fuller, 1993).

Defect	Implication
Monocular field defects	Lesion anterior to optic chiasm
Bitemporal field defects	Lesion at the optic chiasm
Homonymous field defects	Lesion behind the optic chiasm
Congruous homonymous field defects	Lesion behind lateral geniculate bodies

Temperature

Damage to the hypothalamus, the temperature-regulating centre, may result in grossly fluctuating temperatures (Nikas, 1982).

Blood pressure, pulse and respirations

Observations of blood pressure, pulse and respirations will provide evidence of increased intracranial pressure. When intracranial pressure is greater than 33 mm Hg for even a short time cerebral blood flow is significantly reduced. The resulting ischaemia stimulates the vasomotor centre, causing systemic blood pressure to rise. The patient becomes bradycardic and the respiratory rate falls. Abnormalities of blood pressure and pulse usually occur late, after the patient's level of consciousness has begun to deteriorate. This change in the blood pressure was first described by Cushing and is known as the Cushing reflex (Nikas, 1982).

General points

The initial assessment of a patient should include a history (taken from relatives or friends if appropriate) including noting changes in: mood, intellect, memory and personality, since these may be indicators of a longstanding problem, e.g. brain tumour (Barker, 1990).

Visual acuity

May be tested using Snellen's chart or newspaper prints, with and without glasses if worn.

Visual fields

Plotting may indicate a lesion in the retina, optic nerve, optic tract, temporal lobe, parietal lobe or occipital lobe (Table 28.4). Nikas (1982) and Hudak (1982) discuss visual field defects in detail.

References and further reading

Abelson, N. M. (1982) Observation of the neurosurgical patient. *Curiatonis*, 5(3), 32–7.

Allen, D. (1984) Glasgow Coma Scale. *Nursing Mirror*, 158(2), 32.

Allen, D. (1986) Nursing the unconscious patient. *Professional Nurse*, 2(1), 15–17.

Barker, E. (1990) Brain tumour: frightening diagnosis, nursing challenge. *Registered Nurse*, 53(9), 46–56.

Barr, M. L. & Kiernan, J. A. (1983) *The Human Nervous System*, 4th edn. Harper & Rowe, Philadelphia.

Frawley, P. (1990) Neurological observations. *Nursing Times*, 86(35), 29–34.

Fuller, G. (1993) *Neurological Examinations Made Easy*. Churchill Livingstone, Edinburgh.

Hickey, J. V. (1986) *The Clinical Practice of Neurological and Neurosurgical Nursing*, 2nd edn. Lippincott, Philadelphia.

Hinkle, J. L. (1986) Treating traumatic coma. *American Journal of Nursing*, 86(5), 550–6.

Hudak, C. M. *et al.* (1982) Nervous system (B. Fuller) pp. 321–34; Pathophysiology of CNS, pp. 335–48; Management modalities, pp. 349–78; Assessment skills, pp. 379–89. In: *Critical Care Nursing*, 3rd edn. Lippincott, NJ.

Jennett, B. & Teasdale (1984) *An Introduction to Neurosurgery*, 4th edn., pp. 23–9. William Heinemann Medical Books, London.

Lindsay, K. W. *et al.* (1991) *Neurology and Neurosurgery Illustrated*, 2nd edn. Churchill Livingstone, Edinburgh.

Netter, F. H. (1975) *IHL Printing of CIBA Collection of Medical Illustrations, Volume 1, Nervous System*, pp. 58–9. CIBA, Summit, NJ.

Nikas, D. (ed.) (1982) *The Critically Ill Neurosurgical Patient*, pp. 1–27, 77–80, 100–3. Churchill Livingstone, New York, Edinburgh, London and Melbourne.

Scherer, P. (1986) The logic of coma. *American Journal of Nursing*, pp. 542–9.

Sherman, D. W. (1990) Managing an acute head injury. *Nursing*, April, 20(4), 47–51.

Stolarik, A. (1985) What the comatose patient can tell you. *Registered Nurse*, April, 48(4), 26–33.

Tortora, G. J. & Anagnostakos (1992) *Principles of Anatomy and Physiology*, 7th edn., pp. 579–83. Harper Collins, London.

Vernberg, K. *et al.* (1983) The Glasgow Coma Scale: How do you rate? *Nurse Educator*, 8(3), 33–7.

GUIDELINES: NEUROLOGICAL OBSERVATIONS AND ASSESSMENT

Note: The following describes a full neurological assessment. It may be inappropriate, unnecessary or impossible for the nurse to carry out all of the procedures every time the patient is observed.

EQUIPMENT

1 Pencil torch.
2 Thermometer.
3 Sphygmomanometer.
4 Tongue depressor.
5 Cotton wool balls.
6 Patella hammer.
7 Sterile needle.
8 Two test tubes.

PROCEDURE

Action

1 Inform the patient, whether conscious or not, and explain and discuss the observations

2 Talk to the patient. Note whether he/she is alert and is giving full attention or whether he/she is restless or lethargic and drowsy. Ask the patient who he/she is, the correct day, month and year, where he/she is, and to give details about family.

3 Ask the patient to squeeze and release your fingers (include both sides of the body) and then to stick out the tongue.

4 If the patient does not respond, apply painful stimuli. Suggested methods have been discussed earlier.

5 Record, precisely, the findings. Write exactly what stimulus was used, where it was applied, how much pressure was needed to elicit a response, and how the patient responded.

6 Hold the eyelids open and note the size, shape and equality of the pupils.

7 Darken the room, if necessary, or shield the patient's eyes with your hands.

8 Hold each eyelid open in turn. Move torch towards the patient from the side. Shine it directly into the eye. This should cause the pupil to constrict promptly.

9 Hold both eyelids open but shine the light into one eye only. The pupil into which the

Rationale

Sense of hearing is frequently unimpaired even in unconscious patients. To ensure, as far as is possible, that the patient understands the procedure and gives his/her valid consent.

To establish whether the patient's level of consciousness is deteriorating. If the patient is becoming disorientated, changes will occur in this order:
(a) Disorientation as to time.
(b) Disorientation as to place.
(c) Disorientation as to person.

To evaluate motor responses.

Responses grow less purposeful as the patient's level of consciousness deteriorates. As the condition worsens, the patient may no longer localize pain and respond to it in a purposeful way (Vernberg et al., 1983).

Vague terms can be easily misinterpreted. Record the patient's best response (Allen, 1984).

To assess the size, shape and equality of the pupils as an indication of brain damage. Normal pupils are spherical, usually at mid-position and have a diameter ranging from 1.5 to 6mm (Nikas, 1982).

To enable a better view of the eye.

To assess the reaction of the pupils to light. A normal reaction indicates no lesions in the area of the brainstem regulating pupil constriction.

To assess consensual light reflex. Prompt constriction indicates intact connections between the

Guidelines: Neurological observations and assessment (cont'd)

Action	Rationale

light is not shone should also constrict.

brainstem areas regulating pupil constriction (Scherer, 1986)

10 Record unusual eye movements.

To assess cranial nerve damage.

11 Extend your hands and ask the patient to squeeze your fingers as hard as possible. Compare grip and strength.

To test grip and ascertain strength.

12 Ask the patient to close the eyes and hold the arms straight out in front, with palms upwards, for 20–30 seconds. The weaker limb will 'fall away'.

To show weakness in limbs.

13 Stand in front of the patient and extend your hands. Ask the patient to push and pull against your hands. Ask the patient to lie on his/ her back in bed. Place the patient's leg with knee flexed and foot resting on the bed. Instruct the patient to keep the foot down as you attempt to extend the leg. Flex the knee and place your hand in the flexion. Instruct the patient to straighten the leg while you offer resistance.
Note: if a patient cannot follow the instruction due to a language barrier or unconsciousness, observe spontaneous movements and note how strong they appear. Then, if necessary, apply painful stimuli.

To test arm strength. If one arm drifts downwards or turns inwards, it may indicate hemiparesis. To test flexion and extension strength in the patient's extremities by having patient push and pull against your resistance.

14 Flex and extend all the patient's limbs. Note how well the movements are resisted.

To test muscle tone.

15 Ask the patient to pat the thigh as fast as possible. Note whether the movements seem slow or clumsy. Ask the patient to turn the hand over and back several times in succession. Evaluate coordination. Ask the patient to touch the back of the fingers with the thumb in sequence rapidly.

To assess hand and arm coordination. The dominant hand should perform better.

16 Extend one of your hands towards the patient. Ask the patient to touch your index finger, then his/her nose, several times in succession. Repeat the test with the patient's eyes closed.

To assess hand and arm coordination.

17 Ask the patient to place a heel on the opposite knee and slide it down the shin to the foot. Check each leg separately.

To assess leg coordination.

18 Ask the patient to look up or hold the eyelid open. With your hand, approach the eye unexpectedly or touch the eyelashes.

To test the blink reflex.

19 Ask the patient to open the mouth, and hold down the tongue with a tongue depressor. Touch the back of the pharynx, on each side, with a cotton wool swab.

To test the gag reflex.

20 Ask the patient to lie on his/her back in bed. Place your hand under the knee, raise and flex it. Tap the patellar tendon. Note whether the leg responds.

To assess the deep tendon reflex.

21 Stroke the lateral aspect of the sole of the patient's foot. If the response is abnormal (Babinski's response), the big toe will dorsiflex and the remaining toes will fan out.

To assess for upper motor neurone lesion.

22 Ask the patient to read something aloud. Check each eye separately. If vision is so poor that the patient is unable to read, ask the patient to count your upraised fingers or distinguish light from dark.

To test the visual acuity.

23 Occlude the ear with a cotton wool swab. Stand a short way from the patient. Whisper numbers into the open ear. Ask for feedback. Repeat for both ears.

To test hearing and comprehension.

24 Ask the patient to close the eyes. Using the point of a sterile needle, stroke the skin. Use the blunt end occasionally. Ask patient to tell you what is felt. See if the patient can distinguish between sharp and dull sensations.

To test superficial sensations to pain.

25 Ask the patient to close the eyes. Fill two test tubes with water: one warm, one cold. Touch the patient's skin with each test tube and ask patient to distinguish between them.

To test superficial sensations to temperature.

26 Stroke a cotton wool swab lightly over the patient's skin. Ask the patient to say what he/she feels.

To test superficial sensations to touch.

27 Ask the patient to close the eyes. Hold the tip of one of the patient's fingers between your thumb and index finger. Move it up and down and ask the patient to say in which direction it is moving. Repeat with the other hand. For the legs, hold the big toe.

To test proprioception (Netter, 1975; Tortora & Anagnostakos, 1992).
Definition of proprioception: the receipt of information from muscles and tendons to the labyrinth that enables the brain to determine movements and the position of the body.

28 Note the rate, character and pattern of the patient's respirations.

Respirations are controlled by different areas of the brain. When disease or injury affects these areas, respiratory changes may occur.

29 Take and record the patient's temperature at specified intervals.

Damage to the hypothalamus, the temperature-regulating centre in the brain, will be reflected in grossly abnormal temperatures.

30 Take and record the patient's blood pressure and pulse at specified intervals.

To monitor signs of increased intracranial pressure. Hypertension and bradycardia usually occur late, after the patient's level of consciousness has begun to deteriorate. Call for medical assistance as soon as it is evident that there is a deterioration in the patient's level of consciousness (Scherer, 1986; Tortora & Anagnostakos, 1992).

NURSING CARE PLAN

Category

All patients diagnosed as suffering from neurological or neurosurgical conditions.

Unconscious patients (including ventilated and anaesthetized patients).

Frequency

At least 4-hourly, affected by the patient's condition.

Frequency indicated by patient's condition.

Rationale

To monitor the condition of the patient so that any necessary action can be instigated.

To monitor the condition closely and to detect trends so that appropriate action may be taken.

CHAPTER 29
Nutritional Support

Definition

Nutritional support refers to any method of giving nutrients which encourages an optimal nutritional status. It includes modifying the types of foods eaten, dietary supplementation, enteral tube feeding and parenteral nutrition.

Indications

Nutritional support should be considered for anybody unable to maintain their nutritional status by taking their usual diet.

(1) Patients unable to eat their usual diet (e.g. because of anorexia, mucositis, taste changes or dysphagia, see Nursing care plan) should be given advice on modifying their diet.
(2) Patients unable to meet their nutritional requirements, despite dietary modifications, should take dietary supplements.
(3) Patients unable to take sufficient food and dietary supplements to meet their nutritional requirements should be considered for an enteral tube feed.
(4) Patients unable to eat at all should have an enteral tube feed. Reasons for complete inability to eat include carcinoma of the head and neck area or oesophagus, surgery to the head or oesophagus, radiotherapy treatment to the head or neck, fistulae of the oral cavity or oesophagus.
(5) Total parenteral nutrition (TPN) may be indicated in patients with a non-functioning or inaccessible gastrointestinal (GI) tract who are likely to be 'nil by mouth' for 5 days or longer. Reasons for a non-functioning or inaccessible GI tract include bowel obstruction, short bowel syndrome, gut toxicity following bone marrow transplantation or chemotherapy, major abdominal surgery, uncontrolled vomiting or enterocutaneous fistulae.

Patients in any group may have an increased requirement for nutrients due to an increased metabolic rate, as found in patients with burns, major sepsis, trauma or cancer cachexia (Thomas, 1994, pp. 80–92; Kinney, 1995).

REFERENCE MATERIAL

Assessment of nutritional status

Before the initiation of nutritional support the patient must be assessed. The purpose of assessment is to identify whether a patient is undernourished, the reasons why this may have occurred and to provide baseline data for planning and evaluating nutritional support (Pichard & Jeejeebhoy, 1993). It is useful to use more than one method of assessing nutritional status. For example, a dietary history may be used to assess the adequacy of a person's diet but does not reflect actual nutritional status, whereas percentage weight loss does give an indication of nutritional status. However, percentage weight loss taken in isolation gives no idea of dietary intake and likelihood of improvement or deterioration in nutritional status (Sitges-Serra & Franch-Arcas, 1995).

Diet history

This is a valuable method of assessing nutritional status (Ralph, 1993). A 24-hour recall may be used to assess appetite, food habits and preferences and the presence of any eating difficulty, and provides an estimate of recent nutritional intake (Burke, 1974).

Body weight and weight loss

Accurate weighing scales are necessary for measurement of body weight. Comparison of the patient's weight with charts of ideal body weight for height are not a good indicator of whether the patient is at risk nutritionally, as an apparently normal weight can mask severe muscle wasting. Of greater use is the comparison of current weight with the patient's usual weight. Percentage weight loss is a useful measure of the risk of malnutrition:

% weight loss

$$= \frac{\text{usual weight} - \text{actual weight}}{\text{usual weight}} \times 100$$

An unintentional weight loss over 6 months of 10% represents malnutrition and a loss of 20%, severe malnutrition (Jensen et al., 1983). Obesity and oedema may make interpretation of body weight difficult; both may mask loss of lean body mass and potential malnutrition (Bistrain, 1981).

Skinfold thickness
Skinfold thickness measurements can be used to assess stores of body fat. They are rarely used in routine nutritional assessment due to the insensitivity of the technique and the variation between measurements made by different observers. They are more appropriate for long-term assessments or research purposes. Calipers are used to measure the thickness of subcutaneous fat at four sites: the triceps, biceps, subscapular and supra-iliac. The measurements can be used to determine the percentage of body fat of a person (Durnin & Wolmersley, 1974). Percentage charts for skinfold thickness measurements may be used to assess nutritional status (Thomas, 1994, Appendix 3).

Clinical examination
General nutritional depletion may be seen on clinical examination (Golder, 1993). Specific nutritional deficiencies may be identifiable in some patients by a trained observer or clinician; such deficiencies may include polyneuropathy, cardiac enlargement and oedema in thiamin deficiency, or swollen, bleeding gums and poor wound healing in vitamin C (ascorbic acid) deficiency (Thomas, 1994, pp. 52–7).

Biochemical investigations
Biochemical tests carried out on blood may give information on the patient's nutritional status. The most commonly used are:

(1) Plasma proteins. Low levels of plasma proteins may reflect malnutrition. Changes in plasma albumin may arise due to physical stress, changes in circulating volume, hepatic and renal function, shock conditions and septicaemia. The long half-life of albumin (20 days) makes it an insensitive marker of nutritional status. Pre-albumin and retinol binding protein have much shorter half-lives (2 days and 10 hours, respectively), and are therefore more sensitive indicators of nutritional depletion (Jensen et al., 1983). It may be useful to review serum albumin concentrations in conjunction with C-reactive protein (CRP) which is an acute phase protein produced by the body in response to injury or trauma. CRP greater than 10 mg/l and serum albumin less than 30 g/l suggests 'illness'. CRP less than 10 mg/l and serum albumin less than 30 g/l suggests protein depletion (Thomas, 1994, pp. 52–7). Pre-albumin, retinol binding proteins and CRP are rarely measured routinely.

(2) Haemoglobin. This is often below haematological reference values in malnourished patients (men: 13.5–17.5 g/dl; women: 11.5–15.5 g/dl). This can be due to a number of reasons, such as loss of blood from circulation, increased destruction of red blood cells or reduced production of erythrocytes and haemoglobin, e.g. due to dietary deficiency of iron or folate (Chanarin, 1993).

(3) Serum vitamin and mineral levels. Clinical examination of the patient may suggest a vitamin or mineral deficiency. For example, gingivitis may be due to a deficiency of vitamin C, vitamin A, niacin or riboflavin. Goitre is associated with iodine deficiency, and tremors, convulsions and behavioral disturbances may be caused by magnesium deficiency (Thomas, 1994, pp. 52–7). Serum vitamin and mineral levels are rarely measured routinely, as they are expensive and often cannot be performed by hospital laboratories.

(4) Immunological competence. Total lymphocyte count may reflect nutritional status although levels may also be depleted with malignancy, chemotherapy, zinc deficiency, age and non-specific stress (Thomas, 1994, pp. 52–7).

If a patient is considered to be malnourished by one or more of the above methods of assessment then a referral to a dietitian should be made immediately (Burnham, 1995).

Calculation of nutritional requirements
Energy requirements may be calculated using equations such as those derived by Schofield (1985), which take into account height, weight, age, sex and injury. However, an easier method is to use body weight and allowances based on the patient's clinical condition (Table 29.1).

Fluid and nitrogen (or protein) requirements can be calculated in a similar way. If additional nitrogen is being given in situations where losses are increased, for example due to trauma, gastrointestinal losses or major sepsis, then additional energy intake is required to assist in promoting a positive nitrogen balance. Additional fluid of 500–750 ml is necessary for every one degree C rise in temperature in pyrexial patients (Elwyn, 1980).

Vitamin and mineral requirements calculated as detailed in the Committee on Medical Aspects of Food

Table 29.1 Guidelines for estimation of patient's daily protein and energy requirements

	Normal	*Intermediate (moderate infection, postoperative patients, most cancer patients)*	*Severely hypermetabolic (multiple injuries, severe infection, severe burns)*
Energy per kg body weight	30 kcal	35–40 kcal	40–60 kcal
Nitrogen per kg body weight	0.16 g	0.2–0.3 g	0.3–0.5 g
Protein per kg body weight	1 g	1.3–1.9 g	1.9–3.1 g
Fluid per kg body weight	30–35 ml	30–35 ml	30–35 ml + 500–700 ml additional fluid for every 1°C rise in temperature in pyrexial patients

Policy (COMA) Report 41 on dietary reference values (Department of Health, 1991) apply to groups of healthy people and are not necessarily appropriate for those who are ill. Some conditions may improve with the use of additional vitamins and minerals, for example somebody with poor wound healing may benefit from an increased intake of vitamin C and zinc (Hallböök & Lanner, 1972; Taylor *et al.*, 1974).

Planning nutritional support

Factors which may influence future food intake (e.g. surgery, chemotherapy or radiotherapy) also need to be considered when planning nutritional support, as clinical experience shows these may exert a deleterious effect on appetite and the ability to maintain an adequate nutritional intake (Feitkau, 1991).

Modification of diet

Timing and frequency of food and drink
Patients unable to eat their usual portions, e.g. patients who have undergone gastrectomy or who have ascites or anorexia, may benefit from small frequent snacks.

Altering food consistency
Patients may benefit from very soft foods or even liquids alone if they have a sore mouth or throat, find it difficult to chew or have dysphagia.

Altering food choice
A sore mouth or throat may be exacerbated by certain flavours or foods, such as salt, spices, vinegar, citrus fruits. Foods and drinks containing these items should be avoided.

Taste changes may mean foods previously liked are disliked and those previously disliked now enjoyed. Taste blindness may result in the patient feeling that food and drinks are lacking in taste.

Nausea and vomiting may be exacerbated by the smell of hot food and drinks, by fatty and spicy foods and by large quantities of food on a plate. Cold food and drinks, fizzy drinks and small frequent snacks high in carbohydrates (e.g. biscuits and toast) may help reduce nausea and vomiting.

Fortifying food
Food may be fortified with energy and protein for those patients unable to eat and drink sufficient amounts.

Practical information on modification of diet can be found in The Royal Marsden NHS Trust Patient Information Series No 9, *Overcoming Eating Difficulties*, 1994 (Thomas, 1994, pp. 590–593).

Dietary supplements
These may be used to improve an inadequate diet or may be used as a sole source of nutrition if taken in sufficient quantity.

Sip feeds
These come in a range of flavours, both sweet and savoury, and are presented as a powder in a packet or ready prepared in a can or Tetrapak. Sip feeds contain whole protein, hydrolysed fat and carbohydrates. Most are called 'complete feeds' since they provide all protein, vitamins, minerals and trace elements to meet requirements if 2000 ml are taken (Thomas, 1994, pp. 65–75).

Energy supplements

Carbohydrates
Glucose polymers in powder or liquid form contain approximately 350 kcal per 100 g and 187–299 kcal per 100 ml respectively. Powdered glucose polymer is virtually tasteless and may be added to anything in which it will dissolve, e.g. milk and other drinks, soup, cereals and milk pudding; liquid glucose polymers may be fruit flavoured or neutral (Thomas, 1994, pp. 696–709).

Fat
Fat may be in the form of long chain triglycerides (LCT) or medium chain triglycerides (MCT) and comes as a liquid which can be added to food and drinks. These oils

provide 416–772 kcal per 100 ml – the oils with a lower energy value are presented in the form of an emulsion and those with a higher energy value are presented as pure oil (Thomas, 1994, pp. 696–709).

Mixed fat and glucose polymer solutions and powders are available and provide 150 kcal per 100 ml or 486 kcal per 100 g, depending on the relative proportion of fat and carbohydrates in the product.

Products containing MCT are used in preference to those containing LCT where a patient suffers from gastrointestinal impairment causing malabsorption.

Always check with the manufacturer for the exact energy content of products.

Note: products containing a glucose polymer are unsuitable for patients with diabetes mellitus.

Protein supplements

These come in the form of a powder and provide 55–90 g protein per 100 g. Protein supplement powders may be added to any food or drink in which they will dissolve, e.g. milk, fruit juice, soup, milk pudding.

Energy and protein supplements are not used in isolation as these would not provide an adequate nutritional intake. They are used in conjunction with sip feeds and a modified diet. The detailed nutritional compositions of dietary supplements are available from the manufacturers (Silk, 1995).

Enteral tube feeding

Nasogastric feeding is the most commonly used enteral tube feed and is suitable for short-term use. A gastrostomy or jejunostomy may be more appropriate where long-term feeding is anticipated or if the patient feels that a nasogastric tube is unacceptable for cosmetic reasons, or there is an obstruction in the upper gastrointestinal tract which restricts the passage of a nasogastric tube (Moran, 1994).

If a patient cannot be endoscoped for insertion of a percutaneous endoscopic gastrostomy (PEG) tube, then a surgically placed gastrostomy or jejunostomy may be a more suitable feeding route. For a patient with pyloric obstruction a jejunostomy, placed below the level of the obstruction, would be most appropriate (Thomas, 1994, pp. 65–75).

Types of enteral feed tubes

Nasogastric/nasoduodenal

Fine-bore feeding tubes should be used whenever possible as these are more comfortable for the patient than wide-bore tubes. They are less likely to interfere with swallowing or cause oesophageal irritation (Passmore & Eastwood, 1986). Polyurethane or silicone tubes are preferable to PVC as they withstand gastric acid and can stay in position longer than the 10–14 day lifespan of the PVC tube.

Nasogastric tubes may either have a tungsten-weighted tip or be unweighted. A wire introducer is provided with many of the tubes to aid intubation if necessary. The weighted tip of a tube may facilitate the passage of the tube towards the soft palate and pharynx after insertion into the nasal passage. Weighted tubes may also be used to facilitate duodenal intubation; this may be useful for patients with abnormal gastric function where there is risk of aspiration (Thomas, 1994, pp. 65–75).

Gastrostomy

Percutaneous endoscopically-guided gastrostomy (PEG) tubes are the gastrostomy tube of choice. They are made from polyurethane or silicone and are therefore suitable for short- or long-term feeding. A flange or inflated balloon holds the tube in position. The use of conventional balloon urinary catheters is now outdated, particularly as these are at risk of allowing gastric acid to leak at the tube entry site. However, gastrostomy tubes held in place with an inflatable balloon are available. Such tubes have the benefit over urinary catheters of being less likely to leak and are also made from polyurethane or silicone rather than from PVC. Clinical trials have shown that complications with PEG tubes, such as leakage, are rare (Ruppin & Lux, 1986). For long-term feeding, (i.e. longer than 1 month), a gastrostomy tube may be replaced with a button which is made from silicone. The entry site for feeding is flush with the skin, making it neat and less obvious than a gastrostomy tube. The button is held in place by a balloon or dome inside the stomach (Thomas, 1994, pp. 590–593).

PEG tubes may be placed while the patient is sedated, thereby avoiding the risks associated with general anaesthesia.

Jejunostomy

Fine-bore feeding jejunostomy tubes may be inserted with the use of a jejunostomy kit, which consists of a needle-fine catheter. The use of needles and an introducer wire allows a fine-bore polyurethane catheter to be inserted into a loop of jejunum. Alternatively, some gastrostomy tubes allow the passage of a fine-bore tube into the jejunum. A jejunostomy is preferable to a gastrostomy if a patient has undergone gastric surgery or in cases of severely delayed gastric emptying.

Enteral feeding equipment

The administration of enteral feeds may be via gravity drip or pump-assisted. There are many enteral feeding pumps available which vary in their range of flow rate from 1 ml to 300 ml per hour. The following systems may be used for feeding via a pump or gravity-drip:

(1) Plastic bottles into which the feed is decanted before connection to a giving set. This system may cut down wastage compared with a system which delivers a set amount of feed.
(2) A PVC bag into which the feed is decanted. The giving set may be an integral part of the bag and some bags may have a rigid neck to assist filling.
(3) A glass or plastic bottle containing feed which is attached directly to the giving set. This gives less flexibility in choice of feed or additional liquids than the plastic bottle or bag, but is quick and easy for the patient on a standard feed (Payne-James, 1995).

Enteral feeds

Commercially prepared feeds should be used for nasogastric, gastrostomy or jejunostomy feeding. Available in liquid or powder form, they have the advantage of being of known composition and are sterile when packaged.

(1) Whole protein/polymeric feeds contain protein, hydrolysed fat and carbohydrate and so require digestion. These may provide 1 kcal/ml or 1.5 kcal/ml (see manufacturer's specifications). As the energy density of the feed increases so does the osmolarity. Hyperosmolar feeds tend to draw water into the lumen of the gut and can contribute to diarrhoea if given too rapidly. The majority of feeds are low residue, although some contain dietary fibre.
(2) Feeds containing medium-chain triglycerides (MCT). In some whole protein feeds a proportion of the fat or long-chain triglycerides may be replaced with medium-chain triglycerides. The feed often has a lower osmolarity, and is therefore less likely to draw fluid from the plasma into the gut lumen. MCT is transported via the portal vein rather than the lymphatic system. These feeds are suitable for patients with mildly impaired gastrointestinal function (Thomas, 1994).
(3) Chemically defined/elemental feeds. These contain free amino acids, short-chain peptides or a combination of both as the nitrogen source. They are often low in fat or may contain some fat as MCT. Glucose polymers provide the main energy source. These feeds require little or no digestion and are suitable for those patients with impaired gastrointestinal function (O'Morain *et al.*, 1984). They are hyperosmolar and low in residue.
(4) Modular feeds. The feed is made up by mixing separate fat, protein and carbohydrate sources in a combination to suit the individual.
(5) Special application feeds. Low protein and mineral feeds may be used for patients with liver or renal failure.

High fat, low carbohydrate feeds may be used for ventilated patients because less carbon dioxide is produced per calorie intake compared with a low fat, high carbohydrate feed.

Very high energy and protein feeds may be used where nutritional requirements are exceptionally high, e.g. burns, severe sepsis. These feeds contain approximately double the amount of energy and protein compared to standard whole protein feeds.

Glutamine and arginine enriched feeds are available and may be used in cases of impaired gastrointestinal function. These feeds are chemically defined/elemental (predigested) and those containing glutamine present as powder which is made up with water when the feed is required.

Up-to-date information on the exact composition of dietary supplements and enteral feeds can be obtained from the manufacturers (Pichard & Jeejeebhoy, 1993; Silk, 1995).

Total parenteral nutrition

Total parenteral nutrition is the direct infusion into a vein of solutions containing the essential nutrients in quantities to meet all the daily needs of the patient.

TPN solution

The basic components of a TPN regime are provided by solutions of:

(1) Amino acids (nitrogen source). Commercially available solutions provide both essential amino acids, usually in proportions to meet requirements, and non-essential amino acids, such as alanine and glycine.
(2) Glucose (carbohydrate energy source). Glucose is the carbohydrate source of choice. It provides 3.75 kcal/g.
(3) Fat emulsion (fat energy source). Fat generates 9 kcal/g and its inclusion in TPN is necessary to provide essential fatty acids. Fat usually provides 30–50% of non-nitrogen energy. Nitrogen:non-nitrogen energy is usually provided in the ratio of 1:150–200. An insufficient energy supply from carbohydrate and fat will encourage the use of nitrogen for energy.
(4) Electrolytes, e.g. sodium, potassium.
(5) Vitamins: both water-soluble and fat-soluble are required.
(6) Trace elements, e.g. zinc, copper, chromium, selenium.

(Pichard & Jeejeebhoy, 1993.)

Table 29.2   An example of a TPN regime for a patient of body weight over 60 kg

Components		Nutritional composition	
Intralipid 20%	500 ml	Fat	1000 kcal
Glucose anhydrous	300 g	Glucose	1200 kcal
Amino acids	85 g	Non protein energy	2200 kcal
Water to	2580 ml	Total nitrogen	14 g
		N/Kcal ratio	1:157
Trace elements,	10 ml	Total volume	2580 ml
e.g. Additrace (Pharmacia)		Sodium	80 mmol
		Potassium	60 mmol
Fat soluble vitamins,	10 ml	Calcium	5 mmol
e.g. Vitlipid N (Pharmacia)		Magnesium	5 mmol
		Phosphate	28 mmol
Water soluble vitamins,	1 vial	Chloride	80 mmol
e.g. Solivito N (Pharmacia)		Zinc	100 micromol
		Iron	20 micromol

Choice of a TPN regime

TPN is usually administered from a single infusion container in which all the requirements for a 24-hour feed are premixed. Such infusions are prepared either by the hospital pharmacy or are purchased. (See Chapter 11, Central Venous Catheterization for details of administration sets, and maintaining control of the rate of infusion.)

The regime for a particular patient may be formulated according to the patient's needs for energy and nitrogen (see calculation of nutritional requirements, Table 29.1). The majority of commercial vitamin and mineral preparations aim to meet both short- and long-term requirements.

Standard TPN regimes may be suitable for some patients who require short-term nutritional support and do not appear to have excessively altered nutritional requirements (Table 29.2).

The choice of such regimes depends on the patient's body weight. To allow for the possible need to vary the constituents of the infusion in response to changes in the patient's electrolyte or nutritional requirements, TPN solutions should be ordered daily. An exception to this may be at weekends or public holidays when it is necessary to order and prepare them in advance on Fridays, or the last working day before the holiday.

Monitoring of TPN

During intravenous feeding monitoring is necessary to detect and minimize complications:

- Daily:
  TPR–BP
  body weight
  urinalysis (glucose and protein)

  urea and creatinine
  electrolyes
  blood glucose
  fluid balance
- Prior to commencing TPN and a minimum of twice weekly:
  full blood count
  calcium
  phosphate
  alkaline phosphatase
  alanine transaminase
  bilirubin

Once feeding is established and the patient is biochemically stable then the frequency of monitoring may be reduced if the clinical condition of the patient permits. It may be appropriate to reduce the frequency of daily monitoring to twice weekly (Nordenström, 1995).

- Weekly:
  Serum magnesium.

This may be measured more often if the patient is on magnesium-losing drugs, e.g. cyclosporin and cisplatin. Additional patient monitoring such as 24-hour urine collection for urinary urea, nitrogen, serum zinc may be carried out where indicated, e.g. in severe malnutrition, poor wound healing.

Metabolic complications of TPN

Metabolic complications should be detected by appropriate monitoring. Some more common complications are:

(1) *Fluid overload.* This may occur when other blood products and fluids are given concurrently. It may be possible to reduce the volume of a 24-hour bag of

TPN whilst maintaining the nutritional content. Pharmacy can advise on the feasibility of making such regimes.

(2) *Hyperglycaemia*. This may occur due to stress-induced insulin resistance or carbohydrate overload. A simultaneous sliding scale insulin infusion may be required. Failure to recognize hyperglycaemia may result in osmotic diuresis.

(3) *Hypoglycaemia*. Abrupt cessation of TPN may result in a rebound hypoglycaemia. A reduction in infusion rate to half the rate prior to stopping the infusion may help prevent this occurring.

(4) *Azotaemia*. Raised plasma urea may indicate renal dysfunction or dehydration. Alterations in the non-protein energy content of the TPN may be required or an increase in fluid input (Nordenström, 1995).

Other complications such as metabolic acidosis, electrolyte disturbances, hyperammonaemia, hypernatraemia and hypokalaemia may require a review of the TPN solution, rate of administration, additional fluids, blood products and drugs.

Termination of TPN

Total parenteral nutrition should not be terminated until oral or enteral tube feeding is well established. The patient needs to be taking a minimum of 50% of their nutritional requirements via the enteral route. It is important that all members of the multidisciplinary team are involved in the decision to terminate TPN.

The final unit of TPN can be given as two halves, each one being administered over 24 hours. This may provide the opportunity for enteral intake to be established whilst continuing to provide nutritional support.

Elective removal of catheter

See Chapter 11, Central Venous Catheterization.

Home TPN

There are few indications for home TPN. It may be necessary in patients who have complete intestinal failure, e.g. short bowel syndrome due to Crohn's disease or radiation enteritis. The cost of home parenteral feeding is high and requires first class training with an efficient and comprehensive back-up service. It is recommended that only hospitals which have the appropriate facilities to train patients and provide the necessary care in case of an emergency should be involved in home TPN (Lennard-Jones, 1992; BAPEN, 1994a).

Multidisciplinary team

It is important that all members of the multidisciplinary team, including dietitian, nurse, doctor, pharmacist, catering department and community services, are involved in the patient's nutritional care to ensure a thorough and coordinated approach to nutritional management (BAPEN, 1994b).

References and further reading

Bistrain, B. (1981) Assessment of protein energy malnutrition in surgical patients. In: *Nutrition and the Surgical Patient* (ed. C. L. Hill), pp. 39–57. Churchill Livingstone, Edinburgh.

British Association for Parenteral and Enteral Nutrition (BAPEN) (1994a) *Enteral and Parenteral Nutrition in the Community*, (ed. M. Elia). BAPEN, Maidenhead.

British Association for Parenteral and Enteral Nutrition (BAPEN) (1994b) *Organisation of Nutritional Support in Hospitals*, (ed. D. B. A. Silk). BAPEN, Maidenhead.

Burke, B. S. (1974) The dietary history as a tool in research. *Journal of the American Dietetic Association*, 23, 1041–6.

Burnham, W. R. (1995) The role of the nutrition support team. In: *Artificial Nutrition Support in Clinical Practice*, (eds J. Payne-James, G. Grimble & D. Silk), 1st edn., pp. 175–86. Edward Arnold, London.

Chanarin, I. (1993) Nutritional management of diseases of the blood. In: *Human Nutrition and Dietetics*, (eds J. S. Garrow & W. P. T. James), 9th edn., pp. 584–96. Churchill Livingstone, Edinburgh.

Department of Health (1991) *Dietary Reference Values for Food Energy and Nutrients for the United Kingdom*. COMA Report 41. HMSO, London.

Durnin, J. B. & Wolmersley, J. (1974) Body fat assessed from total body density and its estimation from skinfold thickness: measurements on 481 men and women aged from 16 to 72 years. *British Journal of Nutrition*, 32, 77–9.

Elwyn, D. H. (1980) Nutritional requirements of adult surgical patients. *Critical Care Medicine*, 8, 9–20.

Feitkau, R. (1991) Percutaneous endoscopically guided gastrostomy in patients with head and neck cancer. *Recent Results in Cancer Research*, 121, 268–82.

Golder, B. E. (1993) Primary protein – energy malnutrition. In: *Human Nutrition and Dietetics*, (eds J. S. Garrow & WPT James), 9th edn., pp. 440–55. Churchill Livingstone, Edinburgh.

Grant, A. & Todd, E. (1987) *Enteral and Parenteral Nutrition*. Blackwell Scientific Publications, Oxford.

Hallböök, T. & Lanner, E. (1972) Serum zinc and healing of venous leg ulcers. *Lancet*, 14, 780–82.

Jensen, T. G. *et al.* (1983) *Nutritional Assessment – A Manual for Practitioners*. Prentice-Hall, London.

Kinney, J. M. (1995) Metabolic response to starvation, injury and sepsis. In: *Artificial Nutrition Support in Clinical Practice*, (eds J. Payne-James, G. Grimble & D. Silk), 1st edn., pp. 1–11. Edward Arnold, London.

Lennard-Jones, J. E. (1992) *A Positive Approach to Nutrition as Treatment*. King's Fund Centre, London.

Moran, B. J. (1994) Access methods in nutritional support. *Proceedings of the Nutrition Society*, 53, 465–71.

Nordenström, J. (1995) Metabolic complications of parenteral nutrition. In: *Artificial Nutrition Support in Clinical Practice*, (eds J. Payne-James, G. Grimble & D. Silk), 1st edn., pp. 333–342. Edward Arnold, London.

O'Morain, C. *et al.* (1984) Elemental diet as a primary treatment of acute Crohn's Disease: a controlled trial. *British Medical Journal*, 288, 1859–62.

Passwood, R. & Eastwood, M. A. (eds) (1986) Special feeding methods. In: *Human Nutrition and Dietetics*, pp. 490–501. Churchill Livingstone, Edinburgh.

The Royal Marsden NHS Trust (1994) *Patient Information Series No 9. Overcoming Eating Difficulties*. Haigh & Hochland Publications.

Payne-James, J. (1995) Enteral nutrition: tubes and techniques of delivery. In: *Artificial Nutrition Support in Clinical Practice*, (eds J. Payne-James, G. Grimble & D. Silk), 1st edn., pp. 197–213. Edward Arnold, London.

Pichard, C. & Jeejeebhoy, K. N. (1993) Nutritional management of clinical undernutrition. In: *Human Nutrition and Dietetics*, (eds J. S. Garrow & W. P. T. James), 9th edn., pp. 421–39. Churchill Livingstone, Edinburgh.

Ralph, A. (1993) Methods for dietary assessment. In: *Human Nutrition and Dietetics*, (eds J. S. Garrow & W. P. T. James), 9th edn., pp. 777–81. Churchill Livingstone, Edinburgh.

Ruppin, H. & Lux, G. (1986) Percutaneous endoscopic gastrotomy in patients with head and neck cancer. *Endoscopy*, 18, 149–52.

Schofield, W. N. (1985) Predicting basal metabolic rate. New standards and review of previous work. *Human Nutrition and Clinical Nutrition*, 39C, Supplement 15, 41.

Silk, D. B. A. (1995) Enteral diet choices and formulations. In: *Artificial Nutrition Support in Clinical Practice*, (eds J. Payne-James, G. Grimble & D. Silk), 1st edn., pp. 215–45. Edward Arnold, London.

Sitges-Serra, A. & Franch-Arcas, G. (1995) Nutrition assessment. In: *Artificial Nutrition Support in Clinical Practice*, (eds J. Payne-James, G. Grimble & D. Silk), 1st edn., pp. 127–36. Edward Arnold, London.

Taylor, T. V. *et al.* (1974) Ascorbic acid supplementation in the treatment of pressure sores. *Lancet*, 7, 544–6.

Thomas, B. (1994) *Manual of Dietetic Practice*, 2nd edn. Blackwell Science, Oxford.

GUIDELINES: NASOGASTRIC INTUBATION WITH TUBES USING AN INTRODUCER

EQUIPMENT

1 Clinically clean tray.
2 Fine-bore nasogastric tube.
3 Introducer for tube.
4 Sterile receiver.
5 Sterile water.
6 10 ml syringe.
7 Hypoallergenic tape.
8 Adhesive patch if available.
9 Glass of water.
10 Lubricating jelly.

PROCEDURE

Action	Rationale
1 Explain and discuss the procedure with the patient.	To ensure that the patient understands the procedure and gives his/her valid consent.
2 Arrange a signal by which the patient can communicate if he/she wants the nurse to stop, e.g. by raising his/her hand.	The patient is often less frightened if he/she feels able to have some control over the procedure.
3 Assist the patient to sit in a semi-upright position in the bed or chair. Support the patient's head with pillows
Note: The head should not be tilted backwards or forwards.	To allow for easy passage of the tube. This position enables easy swallowing and ensures that the epiglottis is not obstructing the oesophagus.

4 Select the appropriate distance mark on the tube by measuring the distance on the tube from the patient's ear lobe to the bridge of the nose plus the distance from the bridge of the nose to the bottom of the xiphisternum.

To ensure that the appropriate length of tube is passed into the stomach.

5 Wash hands with bactericidal soap and water or bactericidal alcohol hand rub, and assemble the equipment required.

To minimize cross-infection.

6 Inject 10 ml sterile water down the tube before inserting introducer. Lubricate proximal end of tube with jelly.

Contact with water activates coating inside tube and on the tip. This lubricates the tube assisting its passage through the nasopharynx and allowing easy withdrawal of the introducer.

7 Check that the nostrils are patent by asking the patient to sniff with one nostril closed. Repeat with the other nostril.

To identify any obstructions liable to prevent intubation.

8 Insert the rounded end of the tube into the clearest nostril and slide it backwards and inwards along the floor of the nose to the nasopharynx. If any obstruction is felt, withdraw the tube and try again in a slightly different direction or use the other nostril.

To facilitate the passage of the tube by following the natural anatomy of the nose.

9 As the tube passes down into the nasopharynx, ask the patient to start swallowing and sipping water.

To focus the patient's attention on something other than the tube. A swallowing action closes the glottis, enabling the tube to pass into the oesophagus.

10 Advance the tube through the pharynx, as the patient swallows until the predetermined mark has been reached. If the patient shows signs of distress, e.g. gasping or cyanosis, remove the tube immediately.

The tube may have accidently been passed down the trachea instead of the pharynx. Distress may indicate that the tube is in the bronchus.

11 Remove the introducer by using gentle traction. If it is difficult to remove, then remove the tube as well.

If the introducer sticks in the tube, it may be indicative that the tube is in the bronchus.

12 Check the position of the tube to confirm that it is in the stomach by:
  (a) Taking an X-ray of chest and upper abdomen;
  (b) Aspirating 2 ml of stomach contents and testing with litmus paper;
  (c) Introducing 5 ml of air into the stomach via the tube and checking for a bubbling sound using a stethoscope placed over the epigastrium.

To confirm placement of radio-opaque NG tube.

Paper turns pink to confirm stomach contents.

Air can be detected by a bubbling sound when entering the stomach.

X-ray of radio-opaque tubes is the most accurate confirmation of position.

13 Secure the tube to the nostril with hypoallergenic tape and to the cheek with an adhesive patch (if available).

To hold the tube in place. To ensure patient comfort. Feeding via the tube must not begin until the correct position of the tube has been confirmed by X-ray.

GUIDELINES: NASOGASTRIC INTUBATION WITH TUBES WITHOUT USING AN INTRODUCER, E.G. A RYLE'S TUBE

EQUIPMENT

1 Clinically clean tray.
2 Nasogastric tube that has been stored in a deep freeze for at least half an hour before the procedure is to begin, to ensure a rigid tube that will allow for easy passage.
3 Topical gauze.
4 Lubricating jelly.
5 Hypoallergenic tape.
6 20 ml syringe.
7 Blue litmus paper.
8 Receiver.
9 Spigot.
10 Glass of water
11 Stethoscope.

PROCEDURE

Action	Rationale
1 Explain and discuss the procedure with the patient.	To ensure that the patient understands the procedure and gives his/her valid consent.
2 Arrange a signal by which the patient can communicate if he/she wants the nurse to stop, e.g. by raising his/her hand.	The patient is often less frightened if he/she feels able to have some control over the procedure.
3 Assist the patient to sit in a semi-upright position in the bed or chair. Support the patient's head with pillows.	To allow for easy passage of the tube. This position enables easy swallowing and ensures that the epiglottis is not obstructing the oesophagus.
4 Mark the distance which the tube is to be passed by measuring the distance on the tube from the patient's ear lobe to the bridge of the nose plus the distance from the bridge of the nose to the bottom of the xiphisternum.	To indicate the length of tube required for entry into the stomach.
5 Wash hands with bactericidal soap and water or bactericidal alcohol hand rub, and assemble the equipment required.	To minimize cross infection.
6 Check the patient's nostrils are patent by asking him/her to sniff with one nostril closed. Repeat with the other nostril.	To identify any obstructions liable to prevent intubation.
7 Lubricate about 15–20 cm of the tube with a thin coat of lubricating jelly that has been placed on a topical swab.	To reduce the friction between the mucous membranes and the tube.
8 Insert the proximal end of the tube into the clearest nostril and slide it backwards and inwards along the floor of the nose to the nasopharynx. If an obstruction is felt, withdraw the tube and try again in a slightly different direction or use the other nostril.	To facilitate the passage of the tube by following the natural anatomy of the nose.

9 As the tube passes down into the nasopharynx, ask the patient to start swallowing and sipping water.	To focus the patient's attention on something other than the tube. The swallowing action closes the glottis, enabling the tube to pass into the oesophagus.
10 Advance the tube through the pharynx as the patient swallows until the tape-marked tube reaches the point of entry into the external nares. If the patient shows signs of distress, e.g. gasping or cyanosis, remove the tube immediately.	Distress may indicate that the tube is in the bronchus.
11 Check the position of the tube to confirm that it is in the stomach by:	
(a) Taking an X-ray of chest and upper abdomen;	To confirm placement of radio-opaque NG tube.
(b) Aspirating 2 ml of stomach contents and testing with litmus paper;	Paper turns pink to confirm stomach contents.
(c) Introducing 5 ml of air into the stomach via the tube and checking for a bubbling sound using a stethoscope placed over the epigastrium.	Air can be detected by a bubbling sound when entering the stomach.
	X-ray of radio-opaque tubes is the most accurate confirmation of position.
12 Secure the tube to the nostril with hypoallergenic tape and to the cheek with an adhesive patch (if available).	To hold the tube in place. To ensure patient comfort.

NURSING CARE PLAN

Supervision of patients with swallowing difficulties is important and in some cases patients may require support at meal times, or when drinking, to carry out the recommended strategies. It is important for nurses to participate in educational programmes for patients and carers in order to encourage awareness of the implications of dysphagia. Anxieties associated with dysphagia should be allayed and confidence to undertake safe eating and drinking techniques built up. Patients may experience one or a number of the following problems.

Problem	Cause	Prevention	Suggested action
Patient experiencing difficulties with drinking and or eating (which may lead to dehydration, insufficient nutritional intake, and compromised airway).	(a) Mechanical. Patients who have undergone surgery and/or radiotherapy to the oral cavity, pharynx, larynx, or trachea (including temporary or permanent tracheostomy) are likely to experience swallowing difficulties of a temporary or more persistent nature (Fig. 29.1)		Refer to specialist speech and language therapist for full assessment and management plan. Refer to dietitian for nutritional assessment and management plan.

Nursing care plan (cont'd)

Problem	Cause	Prevention	Suggested action
	(b) Neurological. Patients who have tumours which affect the brain stem area and thus the cranial nerves will present with symptoms of dysphagia. These symptoms will continue as long as the disease and/or treatment effects are evident.		
	(c) Oesophageal obstruction or dysfunction. Patients who have tumours of the upper gastrointestinal tract may well experience discomfort and difficulty with the oesophageal phase of the swallow. The only way to alleviate oesophageal difficulties is through medical or surgical management. Swallowing therapy		

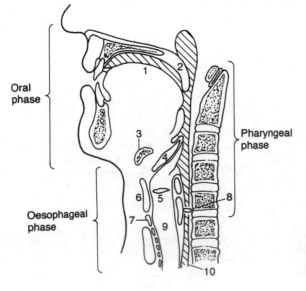

Oral phase

Pharyngeal phase

Oesophageal phase

Figure 29.1 The normal swallow.
(1 tongue; 2 soft palate; 3 hyoid bone; 4 epiglottis; 5 vocal cords; 6 thyroid cartilage; 7 cricoid cartilage; 8 pharyngoesophageal sphincter; 9 trachea; 10 oesophagus.) The oral, pharyngeal and oesophageal phases are separate but highly coordinated.

is not indicated in these circumstances, although the specialist speech and language therapist may be able to offer advice to mininize difficulties experienced by the patient.

Dehydration and/or difficulty in maintaining adequate hydration.	Thin liquids (e.g. water) are difficult for the patent with dysphagia to manage. Watery liquids do not retain their cohesion in the mouth and therefore pass swiftly into the pharynx. Patients may avoid liquids of this consistency and become dehydrated.	Identify patients who are at risk.	Seek medical advice on the appropriateness of intravenous hydration.
Difficulty in maintaining a clear airway (may be severe enough to block airway in tracheostomy patients).	Inability to manage secretions, indicated by drooling and/or gurgly voice. Tracheostomy patients may feel breathing is laboured.	Monitor patient's progress carefully and regularly and liaise with the speech and language therapist about any changes noted.	Following assessment by specialist speech and language therapist, adjusting the patient's position may help (e.g. sitting posture and head position before and after swallowing). Oral suction may be required. See Chapter 41, Tracheostomy Care and Laryngectomy Voice Rehabilitation.
Patient requires nutritional support and/or alternative feeding method.	Dysphagia and/or disease process leading to inadequate nutrition.	All patients with dysphagia should be fully assessed by a dietitian to ensure current nutritional requirements are met by nutritional support, alternative feeding method, normal diet, or a combination of these.	Nutritional support and/or alternative feeding method may be indicated following discussion with members of the multidisciplinary team. Following assessment by a specialist speech and language therapist recommendations may be made about sitting posture, head position, and consistency of food and drink. These will be individually tailored to the patient's needs.

Nursing care plan (cont'd)

Problem	Cause	Prevention	Suggested action
			Nursing staff should monitor progress carefully, noting changes and reporting them to the appropriate professional.
Dysphagia in oral and/or pharyngeal stages of swallowing, related to head position and or structural or neurological deficits.	Patients with tumours of the upper gastrointestinal tract may experience difficulty with the oesophageal phase of the swallow; patients with tumours affecting the brain stem/cranial nerves will experience dysphagia.		Proceed as advised by the specialist speech and language therapist: modified head positions, e.g. turned to the affected or unaffected side, tilted to the unaffected side, or chin flexed may be appropriate. Do *not* attempt these manoeuvres without prior assessment and advice from a specialist speech and language therapist.
Selecting suitable food and/or drink.	Not all members of the multidisciplinary team and/or catering and other staff may be aware of the extent of the patient's swallowing difficulties.	Liaise with specialist speech and language therapist and dietitian.	Provide food and drink of a consistency which will not exacerbate the patient's problems. This might include soft foods, thickened liquids, or purees. Food and drink must be individually tailored to suit the patient.

(Logemann, 1983; Groher, 1992.)

References and further reading

Appleton, J. & Machin, J. (1995) *Working with Oral Cancer.* Winslow, Bicester.

Groher, M. (1992) *Dysphagia: Diagnosis and Management.* Butterworth & Heinemann, Boston.

Logemann, J. (1983) *The Evaluation and Treatment of Swallowing Disorders.* College Hill Press, San Diego.

CHAPTER 30

Observations

PULSE

Definition
The pulse is a pressure wave of blood caused by the alternating expansion and recoil of elastic arteries during each cardiac cycle.

Indications
The pulse is taken for the following reasons:

(1) To determine the individual's pulse on admission as a base for comparing future measurements.
(2) To monitor fluctuations in pulse.

BODY SITES WHERE THE PULSE IS MOST EASILY PALPATED

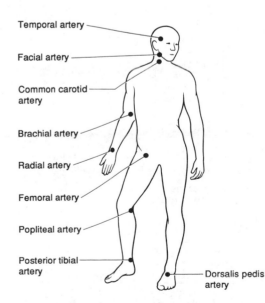

Temporal artery

Facial artery

Common carotid artery

Brachial artery

Radial artery

Femoral artery

Popliteal artery

Posterior tibial artery

Dorsalis pedis artery

Figure 30.1 The pulse can be felt in arteries lying close to the body surface.

(3) To gather information on the heart rate, pattern of beats (rhythm) and amplitude (strength) of pulse.

REFERENCE MATERIAL
The arterial pulse rate reflects the heart rate and is influenced by activity, postural changes and emotion (Marieb, 1995). Each time the heart beats, it propels blood through the arteries. This pumping action of the heart causes the walls of the arteries to expand and distend. The effect can be felt with the fingers as a wave-like sensation felt as the pulse (Timby, 1989). The pulse can be felt in any arteries lying close to the body surface (Fig. 30.1) by lightly compressing the artery against firm tissue and by recording the number of beats (Timby, 1989).

The pulse is palpated to note the following:

(1) Rate
(2) Rhythm
(3) Amplitude.

Rate
The normal pulse rate varies in different client groups as age related changes affect the pulse rate. The approximate range is illustrated in Table 30.1 (Timby, 1989).

The pulse may vary depending on the posture of an individual. For example, the pulse of a healthy man may

Table 30.1 Normal pulse rates per minute at various ages.

Age	Approximate range	Average
Newborn	120–160	140
1–12 months	80–140	120
12 months–2 years	80–130	110
2 years–6 years	75–120	100
6 years–12 years	75–110	95
Adolescent	60–100	80
Adult	60–100	80

be around 66 beats per minute when he is lying down; this increases to 70 when sitting up, and 80 when he stands suddenly (Marieb, 1995).

The rate of the pulse of an individual with a healthy heart tends to be relatively constant. However, when blood volume drops suddenly or when the heart has been weakened by disease, the stroke volume declines and cardiac output is maintained only by increasing the rate of heart beat.

Cardiac output is the amount of blood pumped out by each heart ventricle in one minute, while the stroke volume is the amount of blood pumped out by a ventricle with each contraction. The relationship between these and the heart rate is expressed in the following equation:

Cardiac output = heart rate × stroke volume

The heart rate and hence pulse rate are influenced by various factors acting through neural, chemical and physically induced homeostatic mechanisms (Fig. 30.2):

(1) Neural changes in heart rate are caused by the activation of the sympathetic nervous system which increases heart rate, while parasympathetic activation decreases heart rate (Ganong, 1995).
(2) Chemical regulation of the heart is affected by hor-

mones (adrenaline and thyroxine) and electrolytes (sodium, potassium and calcium) (Ganong, 1995). Imbalances of electrolytes may excite or depress heart muscle, posing a danger to health (Brunner & Suddarth, 1989).

(3) Physical factors that influence heart rate are age, sex, exercise and body temperature (Marieb, 1995).

Tachycardia is defined as an abnormally fast heart rate, over 100 beats per minute in adults, which may result from a raised body temperature, stress, certain drugs or heart disease (Marieb, 1995).

Bradycardia is a heart rate slower than 60 beats per minute. It may be the result of a low body temperature, certain drugs or parasympathetic nervous system activation. It is also found in fit athletes when physical and cardiovascular conditioning occurs. This results in hypertrophy of the heart with an increase in its stroke volume. These heart changes result in a lower resting heart rate but with the same cardiac output (Marieb, 1995). If persistent bradycardia occurs in an individual as a result of ill health, this may result in inadequate blood circulation to body tissues. Bradycardia is a sign of brain oedema after head trauma or surgery (Hickey, 1986).

THE INFLUENCE OF NEURAL, CHEMICAL AND PHYSICAL FACTORS ON CARDIAC OUTPUT AND HENCE PULSE

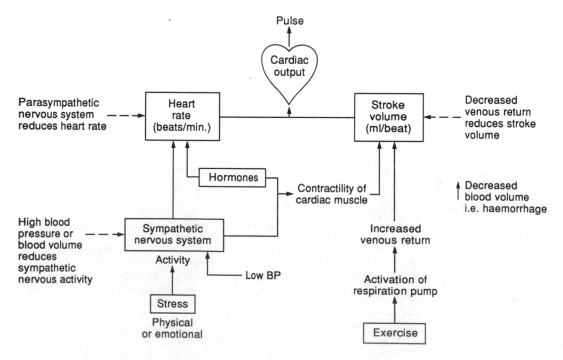

Figure 30.2   Factors affecting cardiac output and pulse.

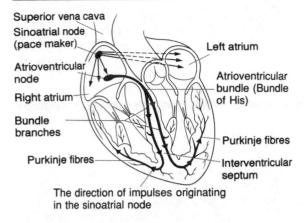

Figure 30.3 Intrinsic conduction system of the heart.

Rhythm

The pulse rhythm is the sequence of beats. In health, these are regular. The coordinated action of the muscles of the heart in producing a regular heart rhythm is due to the ability of cardiac muscle to contract inherently without nervous control (Marieb, 1995). The coordinated action of the muscles in the heart results from two physiological factors:

(1) Gap junctions in the cardiac muscles which form interconnections between adjacent cardiac muscles and allow transmission of nervous impulses from cell to cell (Marieb, 1995).
(2) Specialized nerve-like cardiac cells that form the nodal system. These initiate and distribute impulses throughout the heart, so that the heart beats as one unit (Marieb, 1995). These are the sinoatrial node, atrioventricular node, atrioventricular bundle and the Purkinje fibres.

The sinoatrial node is the pacemaker, initiating each wave of contraction. This sets the rhythm for the heart as a whole (Fig. 30.3). Its characteristic rhythm is called *sinus rhythm*.

Defects in the conduction system of the heart can cause irregular heart rhythms, or arrhythmias, resulting in uncoordinated contraction of the heart.

Fibrillation is a condition of rapid and irregular contractions. A fibrillating heart is ineffective as a pump (Marieb, 1995). *Atrial fibrillation* is a disruption of rhythm in the atrial areas of the heart occurring at extremely rapid and uncoordinated intervals. The rapid impulses result in the ventricles not being able to respond to every atrial beat and, therefore, the ventricles contract irregularly. The cause of this condition is usually ischaemic heart disease (Brunner & Suddarth, 1989).

Ventricular fibrillation is an irregular heart rhythm characterized by chaotic contraction of the ventricles at very rapid rates. Ventricular fibrillation can cause death in minutes if it is not reversed rapidly. The cause of this condition is often myocardial infarction, electrical shock, acidosis and electrolyte disturbances (Brunner & Suddarth, 1989).

Because body fluids are good conductors of electricity it is possible through electrocardiography to observe how the currents generated are transmitted through the heart. The electrocardiograph provides a graphic representation and record (electrocardiogram) of electrical activity as the heart beats. The electrocardiogram (ECG) makes it possible to identify abnormalities in electrical conduction within the heart. The normal ECG consists of a series of three distinct areas called deflection waves. The first of these is the P wave, which results from an electrical impulse in the sinoatrial node. The large QRS complex results from ventricular depolarisation, and takes place prior to contraction of the heart muscles. The T wave is caused by ventricular repolarisation. In a healthy heart, the size and rhythm of the deflection waves tend to remain constant (Fig. 30.4). Changes in the pattern or timing of the ECG may indicate problems with the heart's conduction system, such as those caused by myocardial infarction (Marieb, 1995). Examples of conduction abnormalities are shown in Fig. 30.5.

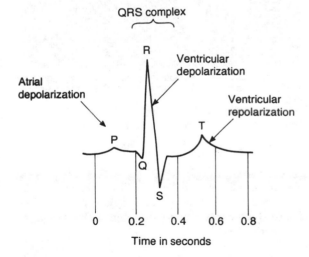

Figure 30.4 An ECG tracing illustrating the normal deflection waves.

Amplitude

Amplitude is a reflection of pulse strength and the elasticity of the arterial wall. The flexibility of the artery of the young adult feels very different from the hard artery of the patient suffering from arteriosclerosis. A full,

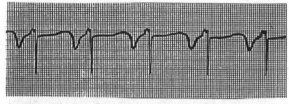

Normal sinus rhythm

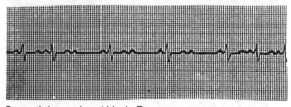

Junctional rhythm. Sinoatrial node is non-functional, P waves are absent and heart rate is paced by the AV node

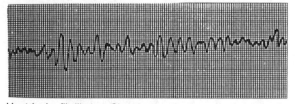

Second degree heart block. P waves are not conducted through the AV node

Ventricular fibrillation. Chaotic electrical conduction, grossly irregular. This is seen in an acute heart attack and electrical shock

Figure 30.5 Normal and abnormal ECG tracings.

throbbing pulse may indicate such conditions as complete heart block, anaemia or heart failure. Anxiety, alcohol or exercise may produce the same result (Brunner & Suddarth, 1989).

Assessing gross pulse irregularity

Paradoxical pulse is a pulse that markedly decreases in size during inspiration (Brunner & Suddarth, 1989). On inspiration, more blood is pooled in the lungs and so decreases the return to the left side of the heart; this affects the consequent stroke volume. A paradoxical pulse is usually regarded as normal, although in conjunction with such features as hypotension and dyspnoea, it may indicate cardiac tamponade.

When there is a gross pulse irregularity, it may be useful to use a stethoscope to assess the apical heart beat. This is done by placing the bell of the stethoscope over the apex of the heart and counting the beats for 60 seconds. A second nurse should record the radial pulse at the same time. The deficit between the two should be noted using, for example, different colours on the patient's chart to indicate the apex and radial rates.

Conditions where a patient's pulse may need careful monitoring are described below:

(1) Post-operative and critically ill patients require monitoring of the pulse to assess for cardiovascular stability. The patient's pulse should be recorded pre-operatively in order to be able to make comparisons. Hypovolaemic shock post surgery from the loss of plasma or whole blood results in a decrease in circulatory blood volume. The resulting acceleration in heart rate causes a tachycardia that can be felt in the pulse. A large volume deficit of 1800–2500 ml results in a thready as well as a tachycardic pulse (Brunner & Suddarth, 1989).

(2) Blood transfusions require the careful monitoring of the pulse as an incompatible blood transfusion may lead to a rise in pulse rate (Cluroe, 1989) (see Chapter 43, Transfusion of Blood and Blood Products).

(3) Patients receiving intravenous infusions require the monitoring of pulse to observe for bacteraemia. Contamination of equipment or solutions may cause a sudden rise in pulse rate (Brunner & Suddarth, 1989).

(4) Patients with local or systemic infections or neutropenia require monitoring of their pulse to detect septicaemic shock. This is characterized by a decrease in the circulatory blood volume with a resulting rise in pulse rate (Brunner & Suddarth, 1989).

(5) Patients with cardiovascular conditions require monitoring of the pulse to evaluate their condition and the effectiveness of medications.

References and further reading
Birdsall, C. (1985) How do you interpret pulses? *American Journal of Nursing*, 85(7), 785–6.

Brunner, L. S. & Suddarth, D. S. (1989) *The Lippincott Manual of Medical-Surgical Nursing*, Vol. 2. Harper & Row, London.

Cluroe, S. (1989) Blood transfusions. *Nursing*, 3(40), 8–11.

Ganong, W. F. (1995) *Review of Medical Physiology*, 17th edn. Appelton & Lange, Norwalk, Connecticut.

Jarvis, C. M. (1980) Vital signs: a preview of problems. In: *Assessing Vital Functions Accurately*. Intermed Communications.

Hickey, J. V. (1986) *The Clinical Practice of Neurological and Neurosurgical Nursing*, 2nd edn. J. B. Lippincott, Philadelphia.

Marieb, E. M. (1995) *Human Anatomy and Physiology*, 3rd edn.
   Benjamin Cummings, California.
Timby, B. (1989) *Clinical Nursing Procedure*. J. B. Lippincott,
Philadelphia.
Wieck, L. *et al.* (1986) *Illustrated Manual of Nursing Techniques*,
   3rd edn. J. B. Lippincott, Philadelphia.

GUIDELINES: PULSE

PROCEDURE

Action	Rationale
1 Explain and discuss the procedure with the patient.	To ensure that the patient understands the procedure and gives his/her valid consent.
2 Measure where possible the pulse under the same conditions each time. Ensure that the patient is comfortable.	To ensure continuity and consistency in recording. To ensure that the patient is comfortable.
3 Press gently against the peripheral artery being used to record the pulse.	The radial artery is usually used as it is often the most readily accessible.
4 Place the second or third fingers along the appropriate artery and press gently.	The fingertips are sensitive to touch. The thumb and forefinger have pulses of their own that may be mistaken for the patient's pulse.
5 The pulse should be counted for 60 seconds.	Sufficient time is required to detect irregularities or other defects.
6 Record the pulse rate.	To monitor differences and detect trends, any irregularities should be brought to the attention of the appropriate personnel.

Note: in children under two years of age, the pulse should not be taken in this way; the rapid pulse rate and small area for palpation can lead to inaccurate data. The heart rate should be assessed by utilizing a stethoscope and listening to the apical heart beat (Brunner & Suddarth, 1989).

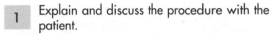

12 LEAD ELECTROCARDIOGRAM (ECG)

Definition
A 12 lead ECG is a non-invasive procedure that is used to ascertain information about the electrophysiology of the heart. It is performed electively prior to various interventions such as surgery and anti-cancer chemotherapy. ECGs are also an important investigation during an acute situation, particularly in the presence of chest pain, haemodynamic disturbance or cardiac rhythm changes.

GUIDELINES: 12 LEAD ECG

EQUIPMENT

1 ECG machine.
2 Disposable electrodes.
3 Swabs saturated with 70% isopropyl alcohol.
4 ECG conducting gel (optional).

Guidelines: 12 lead ECG (cont'd)

PROCEDURE

Action

1 Explain to the patient that the ECG is to be taken.

Rationale

To ensure that the patient understands the procedure and gives his/her valid consent.

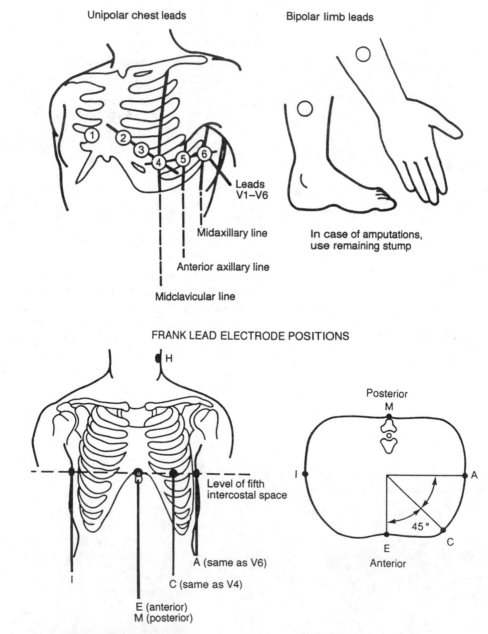

STANDARD 12-LEAD ELECTRODE POSITIONS

Unipolar chest leads

Bipolar limb leads

Leads V1–V6

Midaxillary line

Anterior axillary line

Midclavicular line

In case of amputations, use remaining stump

FRANK LEAD ELECTRODE POSITIONS

H

Posterior
M

Level of fifth intercostal space

I

A

45°

E

C

Anterior

A (same as V6)

C (same as V4)

I

E (anterior)
M (posterior)

Lead F on left leg (not shown)
Lead RL on right leg (not shown)

Figure 30.6 12 lead ECG. (Courtesy of Hewlett–Packard Ltd.)

2	Ensure that the patient is comfortably positioned either lying or sitting.	To ensure optimal recording.
3	Clean limb and chest electrode sites (Fig. 30.6). If necessary prepare skin by clipping hairs.	To ensure good contact between skin and electrode and therefore less electrical artefact.
4	Apply the ten electrodes as described in Fig. 30.6.	To obtain the ECG recording from vertical and horizontal planes.
5	Attach the ten leads from the ECG machine to the electrodes.	To obtain the ECG recording.
6	Check that the leads are connected correctly and to the relevant electrode.	To ensure the correct polarity in the ECG recording.
7	Ensure that the leads are not pulling on the electrodes or lying over each other.	To reduce electrical artefact.
8	Ask patient to relax and refrain from movement.	To obtain the optimal recording by the reduction of artefact from muscular movement.
9	Check that calibration is 10 mm/mv.	To ensure standard recording to aid interpretation.
10	Commence 12 lead recording.	To obtain ECG.
11	In the case of artefact or poor recording check electrodes and connections.	To ensure optimal recording.

PATIENT CABLE CONNECTIONS

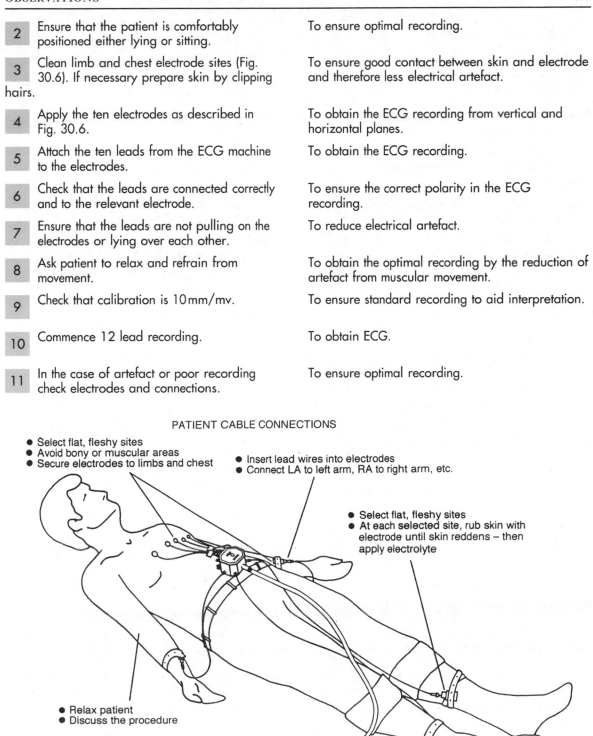

- Select flat, fleshy sites
- Avoid bony or muscular areas
- Secure electrodes to limbs and chest

- Insert lead wires into electrodes
- Connect LA to left arm, RA to right arm, etc.

- Select flat, fleshy sites
- At each selected site, rub skin with electrode until skin reddens – then apply electrolyte

- Relax patient
- Discuss the procedure

- Connect patient cable to cardiograph

- Locate patient and patient cable away from all power cords

Figure 30.6 Continued.

Guidelines: 12 lead ECG (cont'd)

Action	Rationale
12 If necessary record a rhythm strip utilizing leads II and V1.	To assist with interpretation if there have been any acute rhythm disturbances.
13 Detach ECG printout and label with patient's name, hospital number, date and time.	To ensure that the ECG is labelled with the correct patient and date and time.
14 Inform patient that the procedure is now finished and help to remove the electrodes.	To ensure that the patient can relax and that the electrodes are removed.
15 Mount the ECG recording in the appropriate documentation.	To ensure that the recording does not get lost.
16 Inform medical staff that ECG has been completed and its location.	To enable relevant medical staff to use the ECG data in their care planning.

BLOOD PRESSURE

Definition

Blood pressure may be defined as the force exerted by blood against the walls of the vessels in which it is contained. Differences in blood pressure between different areas of the circulation provide the driving force that keeps the blood moving through the body (Marieb, 1995). Blood pressure is usually expressed in terms of millimetres of mercury (mm Hg).

Indications

Blood pressure is measured for one of two reasons:

(1) To determine the patient's blood pressure on admission as a baseline for comparision with future measurements.
(2) To monitor fluctuations in blood pressure.

REFERENCE MATERIAL

Blood flow is defined as the volume of blood flowing through a vessel at a given time from the heart. Blood flow is equivalent to cardiac output. Resistance to the cardiac output is opposite to flow and is a measure of the friction the blood encounters as it passes through the differently sized vessels (Marieb, 1995). There are three important sources of resistance: blood viscosity, vessel length and vessel diameter (Fig. 30.7).

Viscosity is the internal resistance to flow and may be thought of as the 'stickiness' of a fluid. Blood is more viscous than water due to the elements of plasma proteins and cells that form its constituent parts, and consequently blood moves more slowly. The longer the vessel length, the greater the resistance encountered. The relationship between vessel length and viscosity is often con-

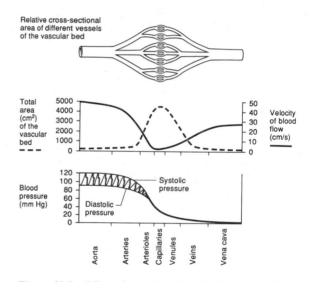

Figure 30.7 Effect of vessel length and diameter on blood pressure and blood flow.

stant; however, blood vessel diameter changes frequently and is an important factor in altering peripheral resistance. Increased peripheral resistance occurs by altering the fluid flow. In a small blood vessel more of the fluid is in contact with the vessel walls which results in increased friction. Arterioles are the major determinants of peripheral resistance because they are small diameter blood vessels which can expand in response to neural and chemical controls (Ganong, 1995).

Normal blood pressure is maintained by neural, chemical and renal controls. The neural controls operate via reflex arcs (Marieb, 1995) derived from stretch receptors found in the wall of the proximal arterial tree, especially in the region of the aortic arch and carotid sinuses. When arterial pressure rises, there is increased stimulation of these nerve endings. The increased number of impulses along the vagus and glosso-pharyngeal nerves leads to reflex vagal slowing of the heart and reflex release of vasoconstrictor tone in the peripheral blood vessels. The resulting fall in cardiac output and the reduction of peripheral resistance tend to restore the blood pressure to the normal value. A fall in the arterial pressure decreases the stimulation of the arterial stretch receptors. The reflex tachycardia and vasoconstriction that ensue tend to raise the blood pressure to its normal value forming a continuous homeostatic process (Ganong, 1995). When the oxygen content of the blood drops sharply, chemoreceptors in the aortic arch transmit impulses to the vasomotor centre and reflex constriction occurs. The rise in blood pressure that follows helps to increase blood return to the heart and lungs (Marieb, 1995). Renal regulation provides a major long-term mechanism of influencing blood pressure. When there is a fall in arterial pressure this results in chemical changes which lead to the release of the enzyme renin. Renin triggers a series of enzymatic reactions that result in the formation of angiotensin, a powerful vasoconstrictor chemical. Angiotensin also stimulates the adrenal cortex to release aldosterone, a hormone that increases renal reabsorption of sodium. The sodium, in turn, increases the volume of water reabsorbed by the kidneys; such retention of fluid and vasoconstriction of blood vessels raises arterial pressure (Marieb, 1995).

Blood pressure varies not only from moment to moment but also in the distribution between various organs and areas of the body. It is lowest in neonates and increases with age, weight gain, with stress and anxiety (Brunner & Suddarth, 1989). Shock, myocardial infarction and haemorrhage are factors which cause a fall in blood pressure as they reduce cardiac output and peripheral vessel resistance or they diminish venous return after fluid loss (Fig. 30.8).

Normal blood pressure

Normal blood pressure generally ranges from 100/60 to 140/90 mm Hg. Blood pressure can fluctuate within a wide range and still be normal. Table 30.2 provides a guide for average normal and upper limits of normal blood pressure measurements for people of various ages.

Systolic pressure

The systolic pressure is the maximum pressure of the blood against the wall of the vessel following ventricular

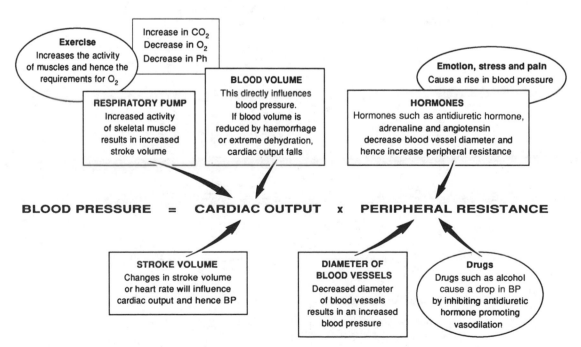

Figure 30.8 Factors affecting changes in blood pressure.

Table 30.2 Average and upper limits of blood pressure according to age (Timby, 1989).

Age	Average normal blood pressure	Upper limits of normal blood pressure
1 year	95/65	Undetermined
6–9 years	100/65	119/79
10–13 years	110/65	124/84
14–17 years	120/80	134/89
18+ years	120/80	139/89

contraction and is taken as an indication of the integrity of the heart, arteries and arterioles (Marieb, 1995).

Diastolic pressure

The diastolic pressure is the minimum pressure of the blood against the wall of the vessel following closure of the aortic valve and is taken as a direct indication of blood vessel resistance (Marieb, 1995).

Hypotension or low blood pressure is generally defined in adults as a systolic blood pressure below 100 mmHg (Marieb, 1995). In many cases, hypotension simply reflects individual variations; however, it may indicate orthostatic hypotension, i.e. postural changes that result

in a lack of normal reflex response leading to a low blood pressure.

Hypertension is defined as an elevation of systolic blood pressure. This may be a temporary response to fever, physical exertion or stress. Persistent hypertension is a common disease and approximately 30% of people over the age of 50 years are hypertensive (Marieb, 1995). Persistent hypertension is diagnosed in an individual when the average of three or more blood pressure readings taken at rest, several days apart, exceeds the upper limits illustrated in Table 30.2.

Mean arterial pressure

The mean arterial pressure is the average pressure required to push blood through the circulatory system. This can be determined electronically or mathematically as well as by using an intra-arterial catheter (see Chapter 3) and mercury manometer.

Mathematically, for example:

$$\text{mean arterial pressure} = \frac{1}{3}\text{ systolic pressure}$$
$$+ \frac{2}{3}\text{ diastolic pressure}$$

A blood pressure of 130/85 mmHg gives a mean arterial pressure of 100 mmHg.

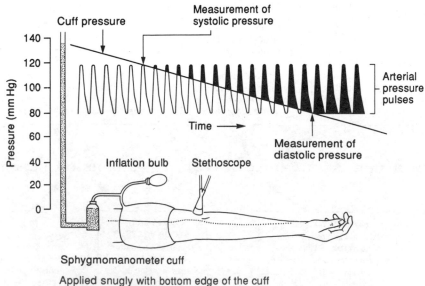

PRINCIPLES OF SPHYGMOMANOMETER AND THE
APPEARANCE AND DISAPPEARANCE OF KOROTKOFF'S SOUNDS

Figure 30.9 Using a sphygmomanometer.

Factors affecting blood pressure

The main factors that regulate blood pressure by altering peripheral resistance and blood volume are shown in Fig. 30.8.

Methods of recording and equipment

There are two main methods for recording the blood pressure: direct and indirect.

Direct methods are more accurate than indirect methods. The ideal method of measuring blood pressure involves the insertion of a minute pressure transducer unit into an artery for transmission of a waveform or digital display on a monitor. The most commonly used techniques involve placing a cannula in an artery and attaching a pressure-sensitive device to the external end (see Chapter 3, Arterial Lines).

The *indirect* method is the auscultatory method. This procedure is used to measure blood pressure in the brachial artery of the arm.

The sphygmomanometer

The sphygmomanometer (Fig. 30.9) consists of a compression bag enclosed in an unyielding cuff, and inflating bulb, pump or other device by which the pressure is increased, a manometer from which the applied pressure is read, and a control valve to deflate the system.

Manometer

Mercury sphygmomanometers are reliable, on the whole, and easily maintained. Care should be taken to avoid loss of mercury. Substantial errors may occur if the manometer is not kept vertical during the measurement. The air vent at the top of the manometer must be kept patent. Aneroid sphygmomanometers are generally less accurate than mercury ones (Campbell *et al.*, 1990).

Cuff

The cuff is an inelastic cloth that encircles the arm and encloses the inflatable rubber bladder. It is secured around the arm or leg by wrapping its tapering end to the encircling material, by Velcro surfaces or by hooks.

Croft & Cruikshank (1990) in studying adults found that in terms of precision there is no basis for using two different cuff sizes. Readings from large cuffs came close to intra-arterial pressures in large arms and were also accurate for small arms. They recommend the use of large cuffs only.

Inflatable bladder

A bladder that is too short and/or too narrow will give falsely high pressures. The British Hypertension Society recommended in 1986 that the bladder length should be 80% of the arm circumference and the width at least 40%.

Control valve, pump and rubber tubing

The control valve is a common source of error. It should allow the passage of air without excessive pressure needing to be applied on the pump. When the valve is closed it should hold the mercury at a constant level and, when released, it should allow a controlled fall in the level of mercury. The rubber tubing should be long (approximately 80 cm) and with airtight connections that can easily be separated.

Campbell *et al.* (1990), in reviewing the methods for sphygmomanometer inaccuracies, found that errors in technique and equipment malfunction accounted for differences in readings of more than 15 mm Hg.

It is essential that the sphygmomanometer be kept in good working order. Conceicao *et al.* (1976) and North (1979) have shown that as many as 50% of the sphygmomanometers used in the hospitals they studied were inaccurate.

The stethoscope

Using the stethoscope it is possible to identify a series of five phases as blood pressure falls from the systolic to the diastolic. These phases are known as Korotkoff's sounds (Fig. 30.10).

When the cuff pressure has fallen to just below the systolic pressure, a clear but often faint tapping sound

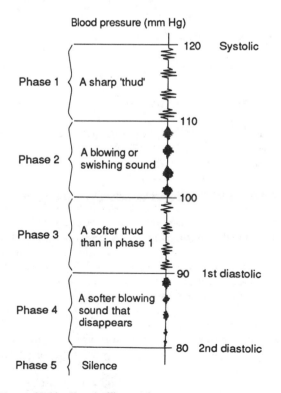

Figure 30.10 Korotkoff's sounds.

suddenly appears in phase with each cardiac contraction. The sound is produced by the transient and turbulent blood flowing through the brachial artery during the peak of each systole.

As the pressure in the cuff is reduced further, the sound becomes louder, but when the artery is no longer constricted and the blood flows freely, the sounds become muffled and then can no longer be heard. The diastolic pressure is usually defined as the cuff pressure at which 'muffling' and not disappearance occurs. However, if there is an obvious difference between these, both values are reported (Fig. 30.10) (Brunner & Suddarth, 1989).

The stethoscope's bell should be placed lightly over the brachial artery (Frohlich et al., 1988). The bell is designed to amplify low frequency sounds such as Korotkoff's sounds (Hill & Grim, 1991). Excessive pressure on the stethoscope's bell may partially occlude the brachial artery and delay the occurrence of Korotkoff's sounds.

Korotkoff's sounds form five phases:

(1) The appearance of faint, clear tapping sounds which gradually increase in intensity.
(2) The softening of sounds, which may become swishing.
(3) The return of sharper sounds which become crisper but never fully regain the intensity of the phase 1 sounds.
(4) The distinct muffling sound which becomes soft and blowing.
(5) The point at which all sound ceases.

Additional information

Much recent research has focused on the faulty techniques employed when blood pressures are taken (Campbell et al., 1990). Blood pressure readings are altered by various factors that influence the patient, the techniques used and the accuracy of the sphygmomanometer. The variability of any readings can be reduced by an improved technique and by taking several readings (Campbell et al., 1990). Maxwell (1982) has shown that the number of patients diagnosed as hypertensive may be grossly overestimated due to the use of undersized cuffs. Thompson (1981) discusses the methodology of blood pressure recording and identifies poor technique and observer bias as possible sources of error. He concludes that many nurses are inadequately trained in blood pressure measurement and that more attention needs to be paid to this area, particularly as responsibility for recording vital signs increasingly falls to nursing staff.

These conclusions are supported by studies by Mancia et al. (1987) and Feher & Harris St John (1992).

Poor technique can cause marked variation in the accuracy of measurements and can lead to inappropriate treatment decisions (Kemp et al., 1994).

Ambulatory blood pressure is increasingly regarded as superior to individual blood pressure readings (National High Blood Pressure Education Programme Coordinating Committee, 1990; Perloff et al., 1993). Ambulatory blood pressure monitoring is expensive, time-consuming and has some risks as it can cause phlebitis (Creery et al., 1985). Although ambulatory blood pressure monitoring is considered more accurate, manual measurement remains the most common method (Veerman & van Monfrans, 1993).

Variations in the procedure and frequency of taking blood pressure may be required in different patient groups with differing conditions. With a child it is important that the correctly sized cuff is used and that the average of repeated measurements is recorded. Low diastolic pressures are common in children and thus the pressure at muffling (Korotkoff phase 4) may be difficult to determine. Hill & Grim (1991) suggest recording the onset of muffling sounds as well as that of no sounds (Korotkoff phase 5) and record it as, for example, 96/54/46 mm Hg. Low diastolic pressures are common in elderly patients who may have atherosclerosis, and in patients with an increased cardiac output, i.e. as a result of pregnancy, exercise or hypothyroidism. These patients may need to have their blood pressure recorded in a similar way to children.

In pregnancy, changes in blood pressure may indicate pregnancy-induced hypertension. An increase of 30 mm Hg or more systolic pressure and 15 mm Hg diastolic pressure over the previous readings may be indicative of this condition (Ferris, 1990).

Patients with lines or shunts for dialysis in their arms may be unsuitable for upper arm measurements of blood pressure; however, the blood pressure may be measured in the leg or forearm. For this procedure the patient lies prone and a thigh or large cuff is applied to the lower third of the thigh. The cuff is wrapped securely with its lower edge above the knee and its bladder centred over the posterior popliteal artery. The stethoscope bell should be applied on the artery below the cuff. Systolic blood pressure is normally 20–30 mm Hg higher in the leg than in the arm. The right sized cuff should be used for obtaining the blood pressure using the forearm, and the bladder should be centred over the radial artery below the elbow, and the cuff wrapped in a similar manner to the normal procedure. The stethoscope bell should be positioned over the radial artery about 2.5 cm above the wrist. Forearm blood pressure measurements may vary significantly from an upper arm measurement, and therefore it is important to document cuff size and location (Hill & Grim, 1991) .

Conditions where a patient's blood pressure may need careful monitoring are described below:

(1) Hypertension is never diagnosed on a single blood pressure reading. The blood pressure is monitored to evaluate the condition of the patient and the effectiveness of medication (Marieb, 1995).

(2) Post-operative and critically ill patients require monitoring of blood pressure to assess for cardiovascular stability. The patient's blood pressure should be recorded pre-operatively in order to make significant comparisons. The reduction in cardiac diastole after surgery may result in a decreased coronary perfusion and therefore reduced cardiac output and vasoconstriction. Report immediately a falling systolic pressure as this may be an indication of hypovolaemic shock (Brunner & Suddarth, 1989). Haemorrhage may be primary at the time of operation or intermediary in the first few hours after surgery. The blood pressure returns to the patient's normal levels and causes loosening of poorly tied vessels and the flushing out of clots. The resulting blood loss causes a decrease in cardiac output and hypotension. Secondary haemorrhage can occur some time after surgery and is due to infection. This also results in a fall in blood pressure (Brunner & Suddarth, 1989) (see Chapter 32, Peri-operative Care).

(3) Blood transfusions require careful monitoring of the blood pressure for several reasons. An incompatible blood transfusion may lead to agglutination and a resulting fall in the blood pressure. Circulatory overload may lead to a rise in blood pressure, while the infusion of large quantities of blood may alter clotting factors and result in bleeding, causing a fall in blood pressure (Cluroe, 1989).

(4) Patients receiving intravenous infusions require blood pressure monitoring to observe for circulatory overload (this occurs more frequently in elderly patients). The resulting increase in blood volume causes a rise in blood pressure (Brunner & Suddarth, 1989).

(5) Patients with local or systemic infections or neutropenia require monitoring of their blood pressure in order to detect septicaemic shock. This is characterized by a change in the capillary epithelium, permitting loss of blood and plasma through capillary walls into surrounding tissues. The decrease in the circulating volume of blood results in impaired tissue perfusion culminating in cellular hypoxia (Ganong, 1995).

References and further reading

Brunner, L. S. & Suddarth, D. S. (1989) *The Lippincott Manual of Medical-Surgical Nursing*, Vol. 2. Harper & Row, London.

Campbell, N. R. *et al.* (1990) Accurate, reproducible measurement of blood pressure. *Canadian Medical Association Journal*, 143(1), 19–24.

Cluroe, S. (1989) Blood transfusions. *Nursing*, 3(40), 8–11.

Conceicao, S. *et al.* (1976) Defects in sphygmomanometers. *British Medical Journal*, 2, 886–8.

Creery, T. C. *et al.* (1985) Phlebitis associated with non-invasive 24 hour ambulatory blood pressure monitor. *JAMA*, 254, 2411.

Croft, P. R. & Cruikshank, J. K. (1990) Blood pressure measurement in adults: large cuffs for all. *Journal of Epidemiology and Community Health*, 44, 107–73.

Feher, M. & Harris St John, K. (1992) Blood pressure measurement by junior hospital doctors: a gap in medical education? *Health Trends*, 24(2), 59–61.

Ferris, T. F. (1990) Hypertension in pregnancy. *The Kidney*, 23(1), 1–5.

Frohlich, E. D. *et al.* (1988) Recommendations for human blood pressure determination by sphygmomanometers. Report of a special task force appointed by the steering committee, American Heart Association. *Hypertension*, 11, 210a–21a.

Ganong, W. F. (1995) *Review of Medical Physiology*, 17th edn. Appelton & Lange, Norwalk, Connecticut.

Geddes, L. A. & Whistler, S. J. (1978) The error in indirect blood pressure measurement with the incorrect size of cuff. *American Heart Journal*, 96(1), 4–8.

Hill, M. N. & Grim, C. M. (1991) How to take a precise blood pressure. *American Journal of Nursing*, 91 (2), 38–42.

Jamieson, M. (1990) The measurement of blood pressure, sitting or supine, once or twice? *Journal of Hypertension*, 8, 635–40.

Jarvis, C. M. (1980) Vital signs: a preview of problems. In: *Assessing Vital Functions Accurately*. Intermed Communications.

Kemp, F. *et al.* (1994) How effective is training for blood pressure measurement? *Professional Nurse*, 9(8), 521–4.

Kilgour, D. & Speedie, G. (1985) Taking the pressure off. *Nursing Mirror*, 160(9), 39–40.

Londe, S. & Klitzner, T. (1984) Auscultatory blood pressure measurement: effect of pressure on the head of stethoscope. *Western Journal of Medicine*, 141(2), 193–5.

Mancia, G. *et al.* (1987) Alerting reaction and rise in blood pressure during measurement by physician and nurse. *Hypertension*, 9, 209–15.

Marieb, E. M. (1995) *Human Anatomy and Physiology*, 3rd edn. Benjamin Cummings, California.

Maxwell, M. H. (1982) Error in blood pressure measurement due to incorrect cuff size in obese patients. *Lancet*, 2, 33–6.

National High Blood Pressure Education Programme Coordinating Committee (1990) Report on ambulatory blood pressure monitoring. *Archives of Internal Medicine*, 150, 2270–80.

North, L. W. (1979) Accuracy of sphygmomanometers. *Association of Operating Room Nurses Journal*, 30, 996–1000.

Padfield, D. *et al.* (1990) Problems in the measurement of blood pressure. *Journal of Human Hypertension*, 4 (Supplement 2), 3–7.

Perloff, D. *et al.* (1993) The prognostic value of ambulatory blood pressures. *JAMA*, 249, 2792–8.

Petrie, J. C. *et al.* (1986) Recommendations on blood pressure measurement. *British Medical Journal*, 293, 611–15.

Rebenson-Piano, M. *et al.* (1987) An examination of the differences that occur between direct and indirect blood pressure measurement. *Heart and Lung*, 16(3), 285–94.

Thompson, D. R. (1981) Recording patients' blood pressure: a review. *Journal of Advanced Nursing*, 6(4), 283–90.

Timby, B. (1989) *Clinical Nursing Procedure*. J. B. Lippincott, Philadelphia.

Veerman, D. P. & van Monfrans, G. A. (1993) Nurse measured or ambulatory blood pressure in routine hypertension care? *Journal of Hypertension*, 11, 287–92.

Webster, J. *et al.* (1984) Influence of arm position on measurement of blood pressure. *British Medical Journal*, 288, 1574–5.

Wells, D. (1990) A case for accuracy – monitoring blood pressure. *Professional Nurse*, 6(1). 30–2.

GUIDELINES: BLOOD PRESSURE

EQUIPMENT

1 Sphygmomanometer.
2 Stethoscope.

PROCEDURE

Action	Rationale
1 Explain to the patient that blood pressure is to be taken and discuss the procedure.	To ensure that the patient understands the procedure and gives his/her valid consent.
2 Measure where possible the blood pressure under the same conditions each time.	To ensure continuity and consistency in recording.
3 Ensure that the patient is in the desired position: lying, standing or sitting. Also ensure that the sphygmomanometer is positioned at heart level, with the palm of the hand facing upwards, regardless of whether the patient is standing or sitting (Frohlich *et al.*, 1988).	To obtain an accurate reading. Measurements made with the arm dangling by the hip can be 11–12 mm Hg higher than those made with the arm supported and the cuff at heart level. Measurements with the arm raised can be falsely high (Webster *et al.*, 1984).
4 Use a large cuff size (Croft & Cruikshank, 1990).	To obtain the correct reading.
5 Apply the cuff of the sphygmomanometer snugly around the arm, 2.5 cm above the antecubital fossa (Timby, 1989). If the patient is sitting or standing, the blood pressure cuff must be placed at the level of the patient's heart. If the patient is supine, rest arm next to patient on a flat surface with the cuff in line with the midaxilla (Hill & Grim, 1991).	Measurement made with the cuff in the wrong position may give false results. For every cm that the cuff sits above or below the heart level, the blood pressure varies by 0.8 mm Hg (Hill & Grim, 1991).
6 Inflate cuff until radial pulse can no longer be felt. This provides an estimation of systolic pressure. Deflate the cuff completely and wait 15–30 seconds before continuing to measure (Hill & Grim, 1991).	A low systolic pressure may be reported in patients who have an auscultatory gap. This is when Korotkoff's sounds disappear shortly after what corresponds to the systolic pressure is heard, and resume well above what corresponds to the diastolic pressure. About 5% of the population have an auscultatory gap and it is commonest in those with hypertension (Hill & Grim, 1991). This error can be avoided if the systolic pressure is first estimated by palpation.

7	The cuff is then inflated to a pressure 30 mm Hg higher than the estimated systolic pressure (Timby, 1989).	Pressure exerted by the inflated cuff prevents blood from flowing through the artery.
8	Place the bell of the stethoscope over the brachial artery.	Apply just enough pressure on the stethoscope to keep it in its place over the brachial artery. Excessive pressure can distort sounds or make them persist for longer than normal (Londe & Klitzner, 1984).
9	Deflate the cuff at 2–3 mm Hg per second.	At a slower rate of deflation, venous congestion and arm pain can develop, resulting in a falsely low reading. At faster rates of deflation the mercury may fall too quickly, resulting in an imprecise reading (Hill & Grim, 1991).
10	Record the systolic and diastolic pressures and compare the present reading with previous readings. It may be necessary to record both phases 4 and 5 of Korotkoff's sounds if they are indistinct. Any irregularities should be brought to the attention of the appropriate personnel.	The average of two or more blood pressure readings are often taken to represent a patient's normal blood pressure. Taking more than one measurement reduces the influence of anxiety and may provide a more accurate record (Hill & Grim, 1991).
11	Remove the equipment and clean after use.	To prevent the spread of infection.

RESPIRATIONS

Definition
The function of the respiratory system is to supply the body with oxygen and remove carbon dioxide. This is achieved by the diffusion of gases between the air in the alveoli of the lungs and the blood in the alveolar capillaries (Marieb, 1995).

Indications
The respiration rate is evaluated:

(1) To determine the per minute rate on admission as a base for comparing future measurements.
(2) To monitor fluctuations in respiration.
(3) To evaluate the patient's response to medications or treatments that affect the respiratory system.

REFERENCE MATERIAL
The body cells require a continuous supply of oxygen to carry out their vital functions and this is provided by respiration (Marieb, 1995).

To accomplish respiration, four distinct events must occur:

(1) Ventilation is where air is moved into and out of the lungs so that gas in the air sacs is replenished.
(2) Gaseous exchange between the blood and the alveoli.
(3) Oxygen and carbon dioxide are transported to and from the lungs by the cardiovascular system. This is called respiratory transportation.
(4) Internal respiration is the cellular respiration that occurs in the cell where oxygen is utilized and carbon dioxide produced.

Ventilation
Ventilation results from pressure changes transmitted from the thoracic cavity to the lungs (Fig. 30.11). Inspiration is initiated by contraction of the diaphragm and external intercostal muscles. This results in the rib cage rising up, and the thrusting forward of the sternum. The ribs also swing outwards expanding their diameter and hence the volume of the thorax (Marieb, 1995). Because the lungs adhere tightly to the thoracic wall, attached by the layers of parietal and visceral pleura, this increases the intrapulmonary volume (Marieb, 1995). Gases travel from an area of high pressure to areas of low pressure. The increased intrapulmonary volume results in a negative pressure of 1–3 mm Hg less than the atmospheric pressure (Marieb, 1995). The resulting pressure gradient causes air to rush into the lungs (Fig. 30.12).

Expiration is largely passive, occurring as the inspiratory muscles relax, the lungs recoil as a result of their elastic properties (Marieb, 1995). When intrapulmonary pressure exceeds atmospheric pressure this compresses the microscopic air sacs (alveoli) and an expiration of gases occurs.

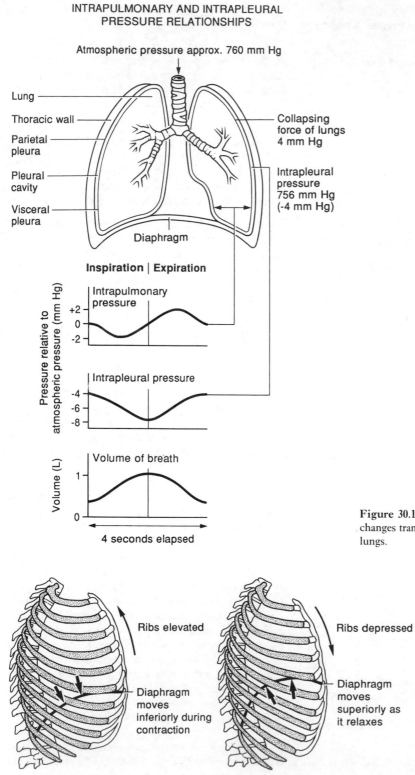

INTRAPULMONARY AND INTRAPLEURAL
PRESSURE RELATIONSHIPS

Atmospheric pressure approx. 760 mm Hg

Lung

Thoracic wall

Parietal
pleura

Pleural
cavity

Visceral
pleura

Collapsing
force of lungs
4 mm Hg

Intrapleural
pressure
756 mm Hg
(-4 mm Hg)

Diaphragm

Inspiration | Expiration

Intrapulmonary
pressure

Pressure relative to
atmospheric pressure (mm Hg)

+2
0
-2

Intrapleural pressure

-4
-6
-8

Volume of breath

Volume (L)

1

0

4 seconds elapsed

Figure 30.11 Ventilation occurs due to pressure
changes transmitted from the thoracic cavity to the
lungs.

Ribs elevated

Ribs depressed

Diaphragm
moves
inferiorly during
contraction

Diaphragm
moves
superiorly as
it relaxes

INSPIRATION

EXPIRATION

Figure 30.12 Changes in thoracic
volume during breathing.

Disease that effects the pleura of the individual may influence ventilation. Pleurisy, inflammation of the pleura where secretion of pleural fluid declines, causes a stabbing pain with each inspiration. Alternatively an excessive increase in pleural secretions may hinder breathing (Marieb, 1995). Air in the pleural space results in lung collapse (atelectasis). This affects the intrapulmonary pressure and hence ventilation. A chest wound or rupture of the visceral pleura may allow air to enter the pleural space from the respiratory tract. The presence of air in the intrapleural space is referred to as a pneumothorax.

The degree to which the lungs stretch and fill during inspiration and return to normal during expiration is due to the compliance and elasticity of lung tissue.

Lung compliance depends on the elasticity of lung tissue and the flexibility of the thorax (Marieb, 1995). When this is impaired expiration becomes an active process, requiring the use of energy. Emphysema is an example of a disease that influences the elasticity of the lung walls (Marieb, 1995). In emphysema the lungs become progressively less elastic and more fibrous which hinders both inspiration and expiration. The increased muscular activity results in greater energy required to breath.

Compliance is diminished by any factor that:

(1) Reduces the natural resilience of the lungs.
(2) Blocks the bronchi or respiratory passageways.
(3) Impairs the flexibility of the thoracic cage.

Friction in the air passageways causes resistance and affects ventilation (Ganong, 1995). Normally, airway resistance is reduced so that minimal opposition to airflow occurs. However, any factor that amplifies airway resistance such as the presence of mucus, tumour or infected material in the airways demands that breathing movements become more strenuous (Marieb, 1995).

Respiratory volumes and capacity tests

The amount of air that is breathed varies depending on the condition of inspiration and expiration. Information about a patient's respiratory status can be gained by measuring various lung capacities, which consist of the sum of different respiratory volumes.

The respiratory volumes shown in Fig. 30.13 represent normal values for a healthy 20-year-old male weighing about 70 kg (Marieb, 1995).

Tidal volume (TV)

The tidal volume is the amount of air inhaled or exhaled with each breath under resting conditions (about 500 ml).

Inspiratory reserve volume (IRV)

The amount of air that can be inhaled forcibly after a normal tidal volume inhalation (about 3100 ml).

Expiratory reserve volume (ERV)

The expiratory reserve volume is the maximum amount that can be exhaled forcibly after a normal tidal volume exhalation (about 1200 ml).

Residual volume (RV)

The residual volume is the amount of air remaining in the lungs after a forced expiration (about 1200 ml).

Respiratory capacities

These values are measured for diagnostic purposes. They consist of two or more respiratory lung volumes.

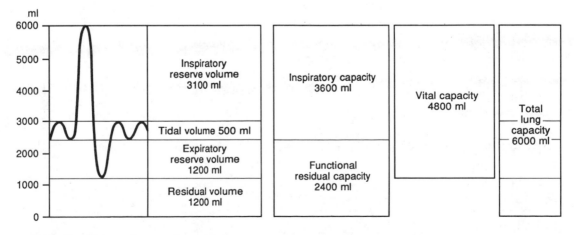

Figure 30.13 Respiratory volumes and capacities.

Total lung capacity (TLC)

The total long capacity is the amount of air in the lungs at the end of a maximum inspiration.

$$TLC = TV + IRV + ERV + RV \ (6000\,ml)$$

Vital capacity (VC)

The vital capacity is the maximum amount of air that can be expired after a maximum inspiration.

$$VC = TV + IRV + ERV \ (4800\,ml)$$

Inspiratory capacity (IC)

The inspiratory capacity is the maximum amount of air that can be inspired after a normal expiration.

$$IC = TV + IVR \ (3600\,ml)$$

Functional residual capacity (FRC)

This describes the amount of air remaining in the lungs after a normal tidal volume expiration.

$$FRC = ERV + RV \ (2400\,ml)$$

Dead space

Some of the inspired air fills the respiratory passageways and does not contribute to gaseous exchange. This is termed the anatomical dead space.

Gaseous exchange

Oxygen in the inspired air enters while carbon dioxide leaves the blood in the lungs in the process of ventilation. These gases move in opposite directions in the alveoli by the mechanism of diffusion (Marieb, 1995). Adjacent to the alveoli is a dense vascular network. Oxygen moves

TRANSPORT AND EXCHANGE OF CARBON DIOXIDE AND OXYGEN

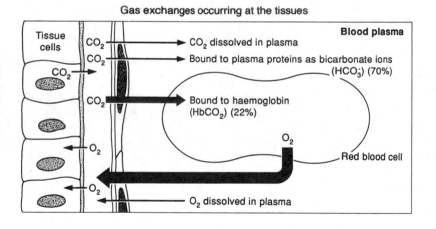

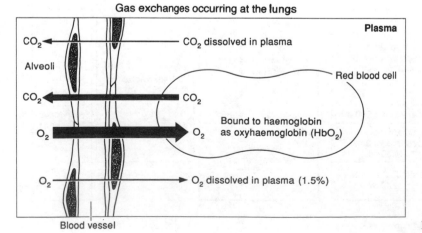

Figure 30.14   Gaseous exchange.

Table 30.3 Composition of gas in the atmosphere and alveoli.

	Atmosphere inspired (%)	Alveoli (%)
Oxygen	20.9	13.7
Carbon dioxide	0.04	5.2
Nitrogen	78.6	74.9
Water	0.46	6.2

into the alveolar capillaries and carbon dioxide moves out (Fig. 30.14). This process is called gaseous exchange. Factors influencing this process include the partial pressure gradients, the thickness of the respiratory membrane and the surface area available.

The gaseous composition of the atmosphere and alveoli is demonstrated in Table 30.3. The atmosphere consists almost entirely of oxygen and nitrogen, the alveoli contain more carbon dioxide and water vapour and considerably less oxygen. These different figures reflect the following processes:

(1) Gaseous exchange in the lungs.
(2) Humidification of air by the respiratory passageways.
(3) The mixing of alveolar gas that occurs with each breath.

Respiratory transportation

Oxygen is carried in the blood in two ways, bound to the haemoglobin within the red blood cells and dissolved in plasma. Haemoglobin carries 98.5% of the oxygen from the lungs and the tissues. The amount of oxygen bound to haemoglobin depends on several factors:

(1) The partial pressure of oxygen (PO_2) and the partial pressure of carbon dioxide (PCO_2) in the blood. The gradient of partial pressure influences the rates of diffusion, the oxygen gradient being steeper than that of carbon dioxide. Carbon dioxide is transported from the tissue primarily as bicarbonate ions in the plasma (70%), whereas only small amounts are transported by haemoglobin in the red blood cells (22%).
(2) The blood pH influences the affinity of haemoglobin for oxygen: as the pH decreases, as in acidosis, the amount of oxygen unloaded in the tissues increases.
(3) As body temperature rises above normal levels, the affinity of haemoglobin for oxygen declines, and therefore oxygen unloading is enhanced. This effect is seen in localized temperature changes such as inflammation.

Diseases that reduce the oxygen-carrying ability of the blood whatever the cause are termed anaemia. This is characterized by oxygen blood levels that are inadequate to support normal metabolism (Marieb, 1995). Common causes of anaemia include:

(1) Insufficient number of red cells, including destruction of red cells, haemorrhage and bone marrow failure.
(2) Decreases in haemoglobin content, including iron deficiency anaemia and pernicious anaemia.
(3) Abnormal haemoglobin, including thalassaemia and sickle cell anaemia (Marieb, 1995).

Internal respiration

Internal respiration is the exchange of gases that occurs within the tissues between the capillaries and the cells. Carbon dioxide enters the blood and oxygen moves into the cells (Fig. 30.14).

Hypoxia is the result of an inadequate amount of oxygen delivered to body tissues. The blue coloration of tissues and mucosal membranes is termed cyanosis.

Control of respiration

Respiratory centre

The respiratory centre generates the basic pattern of breathing. It is located in the brain and is made up of groups of nerve cells in the reticular formation of the medulla oblongata. Regular impulses are sent by these cells to the motor neurones in the anterior horn of the spinal cord which supply the intercostal muscles and the diaphragm (Ganong, 1995). When the motor neurones are stimulated, the muscles contract and inspiration occurs. When the neurones are inhibited, the muscles relax and expiration follows.

Although the respiratory centre generates the basic rhythm, the depth and rate of breathing can be altered in response to the body's changing needs. The most important factors are those of nervous and chemical control (Fig. 30.15).

Nervous control

Lung tissue is stretched on inspiration and this stimulates afferent fibres in the vagus nerve. These impulses cause inspiration to cease and expiration occurs. Emotion, pain and anxiety also cause an increased respiratory rate (Marieb, 1995).

Chemical control

An increase in the amount of carbon dioxide in the blood supplying the respiratory centre stimulates the respiratory centre and breathing becomes faster and deeper.

During exercise, carbon dioxide is produced in the muscles by the oxidation of carbohydrate. The amount of carbon dioxide in the blood increases and this stimu-

FACTORS INFLUENCING THE RATE AND DEPTH OF BREATHING

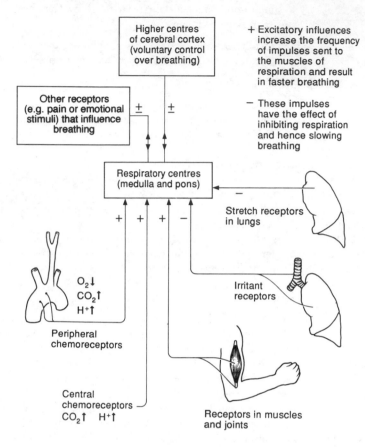

Figure 30.15   Control of respiration.

lates the respiratory centre, producing an increase in depth and rate of respiration. More oxygen is made available in the alveoli for the blood to transport to the muscles, at the same time eliminating more carbon dioxide.

Any substance which, like carbon dioxide, lowers the pH of the blood will stimulate the respiratory centre. Figure 30.15 illustrates the factors influencing the rate and depth of breathing.

Patients with respiratory disease, e.g. emphysema and chronic bronchitis, who maintain high levels of carbon dioxide, will have arterial oxygen levels below 60 mm Hg. This is termed the 'hypoxic drive'. This chronic elevation of the partial pressure of carbon dioxide results in the chemoreceptors becoming unresponsive to this chemical stimulus. The change in respiratory drive results in respiration being stimulated by decreases in oxygen levels rather than levels of carbon dioxide (Marieb, 1995). This may be detrimental to the patient's respiration if oxygen is administered therapeutically at high levels.

Lung defence mechanisms

The upper airway is designed to warm, humidify and filter inspired air. The nasal passages absorb noxious gases and trap inhaled particles. Smaller particles are removed by the cough reflex.

Observation of respiration

Respirations in an individual should be observed for rate, depth and pattern of breathing.

Rate

Rate and depth determine the type of respiration. The normal rate at rest is approximately 14–18 breaths per minute in adults and is faster in infants and children (Table 30.4). The ratio of pulse rate to respiration rate is approximately 5 : 1.

Changes in the rate of ventilation may be defined as follows. *Tachypnoea* is an increased respiratory rate, seen in fever, for example, as the body tries to rid itself of excess heat. Respirations increase by about seven breaths a minute for every 1°C rise in temperature above normal.

Table 30.4 Respiratory rates (Timby, 1989).

Age	Average range/minute
Newborn	30–80
Early childhood	20–40
Late childhood	15–25
Adulthood – male	14–18
Adulthood – female	16–20

They also increase with pneumonia, other obstructive airway diseases, respiratory insufficiency and lesions in the pons of the brainstem (Brunner & Suddarth, 1989).

Bradypnoea is a decreased but regular respiratory rate, such as that caused by the depression of the respiratory centre in the medulla by opiate narcotics, or by a brain tumour.

Depth

The depth of respiration is the volume of air moving in and out with each respiration. This tidal volume is normally about 500 ml in an adult and should be constant with each breath. A spirometer is used to measure the precise amount (see respiratory capacities). Normal, relaxed breathing is effortless, automatic, regular and almost silent.

Dyspnoea is undue breathlessness and an awareness of discomfort with breathing. There are several types of dyspnoea:

(1) Exertional dyspnoea is shortness of breath on exercise and is seen with heart failure.
(2) Orthopnoea is a shortness of breath on lying down which is relieved by the patient sitting upright. This is often caused by left ventricular failure of the heart.
(3) Paroxysmal, nocturnal dyspnoea is a sudden breathlessness that occurs at night when the patient is lying down and is often caused by pulmonary oedema and left ventricular failure (Brunner & Suddarth, 1989).

Pattern

Changes in the pattern of respiration are often found in disorders of the respiratory control centre (Brunner & Suddarth, 1989). Examples of changes in respiratory pattern follow:

Hyperventilation is an increase in both the rate and depth of respiration. This follows extreme exertion, fear and anxiety, fever, hepatic coma, midbrain lesions of the brainstem, and acid-base imbalance such as diabetic ketoacidosis (Kussmaul's respiration) or salicylate overdose (in both of these situations the body compensates

for the metabolic acidosis by increased respiration), as well as an alteration in blood gas concentration (either increased carbon dioxide or decreased oxygen). The breathing pattern is normally regular and consists of inspiration, pause, longer expiration and another pause. But this may be altered by some defects and diseases. In adults, more than 20 breaths per minute is considered moderate, more than 30 is severe.

Apnoeustic respiration is a pattern of prolonged, gasping inspiration, followed by extremely short, inefficient expiration, seen in lesions of the pons in the midbrain.

Cheyne–Stokes respiration is periodic breathing, characterized by a gradual increase in depth of respiration followed by a decrease in respiration, resulting in apnoea (Brunner & Suddarth, 1989).

Biot's respiration is an interrupted breathing pattern, like Cheyne–Stokes respiration, except that each breath is of the same depth. It may be seen with spiral meningitis or other central nervous system conditions.

Conditions where a patient's respirations may need careful monitoring are described below:

(1) Patients with conditions that affect respiration, such as those described in the text, require monitoring of respiration to evaluate their condition and the effectiveness of medication.
(2) Postoperative and critically ill patients require monitoring of respiration. The patient's respiration should be recorded pre-operatively in order to make significant comparisons. The breathing is observed to assess for the return to normal respiratory function.
(3) Patients receiving oxygen inhalation therapy or receiving artificial respiration require monitoring of breathing to assess respiratory function.

References and further reading

Bell, G. H. *et al.* (1980) *Textbook of Physiology and Biochemistry*, 10th edn. Churchill Livingstone, Edinburgh.

Boylan, A. & Brown, P. (1985) Respirations. *Nursing Times*, 81, 35–8.

Brunner, L. S. & Suddarth, D. S. (1989) *The Lippincott Manual of Medical-Surgical Nursing*, Vol. 2. Harper & Row, London.

Ganong, W. F. (1995) *Review of Medical Physiology*, 17th edn. Appelton & Lange, New York.

Glennister, T. W. A. & Ross, R. W. (1980) *Anatomy and Physiology for Nurses*, 3rd edn. William Heinemann Medical Books, London.

Jarvis, C. M. (1980) Vital signs: a preview of problems. In: *Assessing Vital Functions Accurately*. Intermed Communications.

Kertson, L. D. (1989) *Comprehensive Respiratory Nursing: A Decision-making Approach*. W. B. Saunders, Philadelphia.

Marieb, E. M. (1995) *Human Anatomy and Physiology*, 3rd edn. Benjamin Cummings, California.

Roberts, A. (1980) Systems and signs. Respiration 1, 2. *Nursing Times*, 76, *Systems of Life*, Nos 71, 72, p. 8.

Rokosky, J. S. (1981) Assessment of the individual with altered respiratory function. *Nursing Clinics of North America*, 16(2), 195–9.

Timby, B. (1989) *Clinical Nursing Procedure*. J. B. Lippincott, Philadelphia.

TEMPERATURE

Definition

Body temperature represents the balance between heat gain and heat loss.

Indications

Measurement of body temperature is carried out for two reasons:

(1) To determine the patient's temperature on admission as a baseline for comparison with future measurements.
(2) To monitor fluctuations in temperature.

REFERENCE MATERIAL

All tissues produce heat as a result of cell metabolism, and this is increased by exercise and activity (Marieb, 1995). Body temperature is usually maintained between 36°C and 37.5°C regardless of the environmental temperature (Sims-Williams, 1976). Man is described as homoeothermal, that is, having a core temperature that remains constant in spite of environmental changes. The body core generally has the highest temperature while the skin is the coolest (Fig. 30.16). Core temperature reflects the heat of arterial blood and represents the balance between the heat generated by body tissues in metabolic activity and that lost through various mechanisms.

A relatively constant temperature is maintained by homeostasis, which is a constant process of heat gain and heat loss. The body requires stability of its temperature to produce an optimum environment for biochemical and enzyme reactions to maintain cellular function. A body temperature above or below this normal range affects total body function (Boore *et al.*, 1987). A temperature above 41°C can cause convulsions and a temperature of 43°C renders life unsustainable.

The hypothalamus within the brain acts as the body's thermostat, controlling the body's temperature by various physiological mechanisms (Fig. 30.17). Heat is gained through metabolic activity of the body, especially of the muscles and liver. Heat loss is achieved through the skin by the processes of radiation, convection, conduction and evaporation.

There are various factors that cause fluctuations of temperature:

(1) The body's circadian rhythms cause daily fluctuations. The body temperature is higher in the evening than in the morning (Brown, 1990). Minor & Waterhouse (1981) in a research study recorded a difference of 0.5–1.5°C between morning and evening measurements.
(2) Ovulation results in a fluctuation of temperature.
(3) Exercise and eating cause an elevation in temperature (Boylan & Brown, 1985).
(4) Extremes of age affect a person's response to environmental change. The young or elderly are unable to maintain an efficient equilibrium. Thermoregulation is inadequate in the newborn and especially in low birth weight babies. In old people there is an increased sensitivity to cold, and a lower body temperature generally (Howell, 1972).

Hypothermia is where body temperature drops and mechanisms to increase heat production are ineffective. This causes a decline in the metabolic rate and a resulting decrease in all bodily functions (Boore *et al.*, 1987). Hypothermia can be classified according to the severity and the length of time of the condition. Hypothermia is

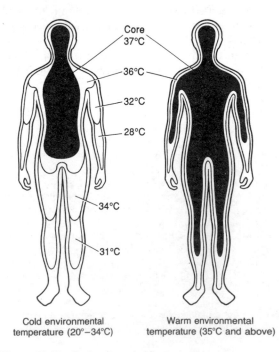

Core
37°C
36°C
32°C
28°C
34°C
31°C

Cold environmental
temperature (20°–34°C)

Warm environmental
temperature (35°C and above)

Figure 30.16   Body core and skin temperatures.

MECHANISMS OF BODY TEMPERATURE REGULATION

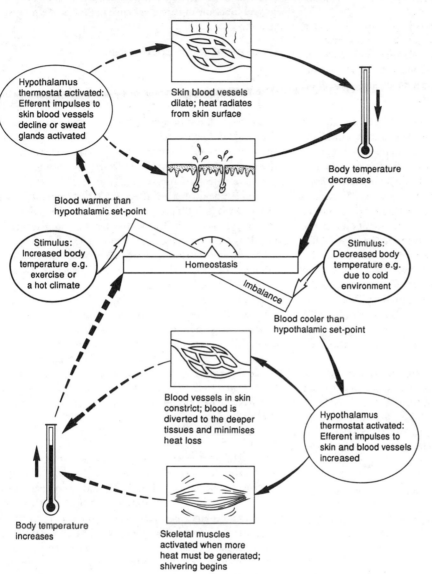

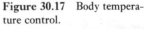

Figure 30.17 Body temperature control.

recognized at temperature recordings of below 35°C (Sims-Williams, 1976).

Pyrexia is defined as a significant rise in body temperature. *Fever* caused by pyrexia is the result of the internal thermostat resetting to higher levels. This resetting of the thermostat results from the action of pyrogens on the thermoregulatory centre of the hypothalamus. The endogenous pyrogens involved are released mainly from leucocytes as a result of cell damage (Hensel, 1981). The exact mechanisms of their influence on the hypothalamus are not understood but it has been suggested that prostaglandins, chemicals produced in

inflammatory responses, are involved (Boore *et al.*, 1987).

Rigor is a condition that results from the rapid rise in body temperature. In a rigor, shivering is marked and the patient complains of feeling cold. The temperature quickly rises as a result of the normal physiological response to cold. This results in the following physiological changes:

(1) Thermoreceptors in the skin are stimulated resulting in vasoconstriction. This decreases heat loss through conduction and convection.

(2) Sweat gland activity is reduced to minimize evaporation.

(3) Shivering occurs, muscles contract and relax out of sequence with each other, thus generating heat.

(4) The body increases catecholamine and thyroxine levels, elevating the metabolic rate in an attempt to increase temperature (Boore *et al.*, 1987; Damanhouri & Tayeb, 1992).

All of these changes contribute to a rise in metabolism with an increase in carbon dioxide excretion and the need for oxygen. This leads to an increased respiratory rate. When the body temperature reaches its new 'set-point' the patient no longer complains of feeling cold, shivering ceases and sweating commences. High temperatures may also be the result of heat exhaustion or heat stroke from hot environmental conditions or the loss of the normal body mechanisms for heat loss. Heat exhaustion occurs predominantly in individuals as a result of sodium depletion. Heat stroke may develop from heat exhaustion but, more commonly, appears to develop rapidly in those exposed to high temperatures who are not yet acclimatised to heat (Boore *et al.*, 1987; Damanhouri & Tayeb, 1992).

There are several grades of pyrexia, and these are described in Table 30.5.

There are different methods for lowering body temperature. Antipyretics such as drugs like aspirin can cause a marked fall in temperature (Vane, 1978). It is thought that these drugs inhibit the inflammatory action of prostaglandins, affecting the hypothalamus by temporarily resetting the thermostat to normal levels. Treatment with aspirin is effective for approximately 2 hours.

Fanning is of benefit for moderate to high pyrexias. Fanning is not recommended while the patient's temperature is still rising as this will only make the patient feel colder and increase shivering (Krikler, 1990).

Table 30.5   Grades of pyrexia.

Low-grade pyrexia	Normal to 38°C	Indicative of an inflammatory response due to a mild infection, allergy, disturbance of body tissue by trauma, surgery, malignancy or thrombosis
Moderate to high-grade pyrexia	38–40°C	This may be caused by wound, respiratory or urinary tract infections
Hyperpyrexia	40°C and above	A pyrexia in this range may arise because of bacteraemia, damage to the hypothalamus or high environmental temperatures

Recordings of body temperature are an index of biological function and are a valuable indicator of a patient's health.

Temperature recording site

Oral

The most common means of measuring body temperature is the oral method (Brown, 1990). Temperature is measured in the sublingual pocket of tissue at the base of the tongue. This area is in close proximity to the thermoreceptors which respond rapidly to changes in the core temperature, hence changes in core temperatures are reflected quickly here (Blainey, 1974).

Oral temperatures are affected by the temperatures of ingested foods and fluids and by the muscular activity of chewing. Smoking will also affect the thermometer reading. It is recommended that the nurse waits 15 minutes following any of these activities before inserting the thermometer to allow the temperature to return to baseline level (Kozier & Erb, 1982).

It is important that the thermometer is placed in the sublingual pocket and not in the area under the front of the tongue as there may be a temperature difference of up to 1.7°C between these areas. This temperature difference is due to the sublingual pockets being more protected from the air currents which cool the frontal areas (Neff *et al.*, 1989). Oxygen therapy has been shown not to affect the oral temperature reading (Hasler & Cohen, 1982; Lim-Levy, 1982).

Rectal

The rectal temperature is often higher than the oral temperature because this site is more sheltered from the external environment. Rectal thermometry has been demonstrated in clinical trials to be more accurate than oral thermometry. The researchers (Jensen *et al.*, 1994) conclude that rectal thermometry is the more accurate route for daily measurements, but is more invasive and time consuming. Although this method is more precise, fever can still be detected by oral screening. If greater accuracy is required the rectal method offers greater precision. The presence of soft stool may separate the thermometer from the bowel wall and give a false reading, especially if the central temperature is changing rapidly. In infants this method is not recommended as it provides a risk of rectal ulceration or perforation.

A rectal thermometer should be inserted at least 4 cm in an adult to obtain the most accurate reading.

Axilla

The axilla is considered less desirable than the other sites since it is not close to major vessels, and skin surface temperatures vary more with changes in temperature of the environment. It is a convenient site for patients who are unsuitable for, or who cannot tolerate, oral thermometers, e.g. after general anaesthetic or those patients with mouth injuries.

To take an axillary temperature reading the thermometer should be placed in the centre of the armpit, with the patient's arm firmly against the side of the chest. It is important that the same arm is used for each measurement as there is often a variation in temperature between left and right (Howell, 1972).

Whichever route is used for temperature measurement, it is important that this is then used consistently, as switching between sites can produce a record that is misleading or difficult to interpret. The assumption that the rectal temperature is about 0.5°C higher, and axillary recordings 0.5°C lower, than oral temperatures is not supported by research findings (Boore et al., 1987).

Time for recording temperatures

The average person experiences circadian rhythms which make their highest body temperature occur in the late afternoon or early evening, i.e. between 4 PM and 8 PM The most sensitive time for detecting pyrexias appears to be between 7 PM and 8 PM (Angerami, 1980). This should be considered when interpreting variations in 4-hourly or 6-hourly observations, and when taking once-daily temperatures.

The time required to record an accurate temperature has been the subject of much research. Nichols et al. (1972) have studied this area extensively and suggest that, with a glass thermometer, oral or axillary temperatures should be taken for 1–12 minutes, and rectal temperatures for 1–9 minutes. The commonly used 3-minute timing led to marked inaccuracy. It was recommended that the thermometer should be left in position for 7–8 minutes in the mouth, 9 minutes in the axilla or 2 minutes in the rectum. The use of the appropriate timings was found to give 90% accuracy for recording the patient's temperature. Takacs & Valenti (1981) observed nurses' temperature taking practice and found that the timing of thermometer placement varied from 42 seconds to 9.5 minutes, and that this time was determined by the other nursing tasks being carried out. Electronic thermometers take only approximately 30 seconds to record temperatures accurately (Boore et al., 1987).

Types of thermometer

A variety of thermometers are now available, from clinical glass thermometers with oral or rectal bulbs to the electronic sensor thermometer. The glass thermometer is the most extensively used. Moorat (1976) compared the cost-effectiveness of the different methods of taking temperatures. He used three types of thermometer, the heat-sensitive strip, the glass thermometer and the electronic sensor thermometer. The electronic thermometer proved to be the most cost-effective, reducing costs by

300%. This was largely because of the amount of time saved. Stronge (1980) costed the difference between the use of a glass thermometer (using a 2-minute placement) and that of the electronic sensor, and found that the electronic thermometer saved a substantial amount of time and was therefore more cost-effective.

Conditions where a patient's temperature requires careful monitoring are described below:

(1) Patients with conditions that affect basal metabolic rate, such as disorders of the thyroid gland require monitoring of body temperature. Hypothyroidism is a condition where an inadequate secretion of hormones from the thyroid gland results in a slowing of physical and metabolic activity, thus the individual has a decrease in body temperature. Hyperthyroidism is excessive activity of the thyroid gland; a hypermetabolic condition results, with an increase in all metabolic processes. The patient complains of a low heat tolerance. Thyrotoxic crisis is a sudden increase in thyroid hormones and can cause a hyperpyrexia (Brunner & Suddarth, 1989; Mize et al., 1993).

(2) Post-operative and critically ill patients require monitoring of temperature. The patient's temperature should be observed pre-operatively in order to make any significant comparisons. In the post-operative period the nurse should observe the patient for hyperthermia or hypothermia as a reaction to the surgical procedures (Brunner & Suddarth, 1989; Mize et al., 1993).

(3) Patients with a susceptibility to infection, for example those with a low white blood cell count (less than 1000 cells/mm^3), or those undergoing radiotherapy, chemotherapy or steroid treatment, will require a more frequent observation of temperature. The fluctuation in temperature is influenced by the body's response to pyrogens. Immunocompromised patients are less able to respond to infection. Bacteraemia means a bacterial invasion of the blood stream. Septic shock is a circulatory collapse as a result of severe infection. Pyrexia may be absent in those who are immunosupressed or in the elderly.

(4) Patients with a systemic or local infection require monitoring of temperature to assess development or regression of infection.

(5) Patients receiving a blood transfusion require careful monitoring of temperature for incompatible blood reactions. Reaction to a blood transfusion is most likely to occur in the early stages and a rise in the patient's temperature is indicative of a reaction. Cluroe (1989) suggests frequent recordings of temperature in the first 15 minutes of a blood transfusion as well as general observation of the patient. Pyrexia can occur throughout a blood transfusion,

and results from a reaction by recipient antibodies. This may be as little as one to one-and-a-half hours after the start of blood transfusion (Cluroe, 1989).

References and further reading

Abbey, J. C. *et al.* (1978) How long is that thermometer accurate? *American Journal of Nursing*, 78, 1375–6.

Angerami, E. L. S. (1980) Epidemiological study of body temperature in patients in a teaching hospital. *International Journal of Nursing Studies*, 17, 91–9.

Blainey, C. G. (1974) Site selection in taking body temperatures. *American Journal of Nursing*, 74, 1859–61.

Boore, J. *et al.* (1987) Disturbances of temperature control. In: *Nursing the Physically Ill Adult. A Textbook of Medical Surgical Nursing.* Churchill Livingstone, Edinburgh.

Boylan, A. & Brown, P. (1985) Temperature. *Nursing Times*, 81(16), 36–40.

Brown, S. (1990) Temperature taking – getting it right. *Nursing Standard*, 5(12), 4–5.

Campbell, K. (1983) Taking temperature. *Nursing Times*, 79(32), 63–5.

Cluroe, S. (1989) Blood transfusions. *Nursing*, 3(40), 8–11.

Damanhouri, Z. & Tayeb, O. S. (1992) Animal models for heat stroke studies. *Journal of Pharmacological and Toxicological Methods*, 28, 119–27.

Davies, S. P. *et al.* (1986) A comparison of mercury and digital clinical thermometers. *Journal of Advanced Nursing* 11(5), 273–4.

Erikson, R. (1980) Oral temperature differences in relation to thermometer and technique. *Nursing Research*, 29(3), 157–64.

Gooch, J. (1986) Taking temperature. *Professional Nurse*, 1(10), 273–4.

Hasler, M. & Cohen, J. (1982) The effect of oxygen administration on oral temperature assessment. *Nursing Research*, 31, 265–8.

Hensel, H. (1981) *Thermoreception and Temperature Regulation.* Academic Press, London.

Howell, T. (1972) Axillary temperature in aged women. *Age and Ageing*, 1, 250–4.

Jensen, B. N. *et al.* (1994) The superiority of rectal thermometry to oral thermometry with regard to accuracy. *Journal of Advanced Nursing*, 20, 660–65.

Kozier, B. & Erb, G. (1982) *Foundations of Nursing: Concepts and Procedures.* Addison Wesley, London.

Krikler, S. (1990) Pyrexia: what to do about temperatures. *Nursing Standard*, 4(25), 37–8.

Litsky, B. Y. (1976) A study of temperature-taking systems. *Supervisor Nurse*, 7(5), 48–53.

Lim-Levy, F. (1982) The effect of oxygen inhalation on oral temperature. *Nursing Research*, 31, 150–2.

Marieb, E. M. (1995) *Human Anatomy and Physiology*, 3rd edn. Benjamin Cummings, California.

Minor, D. G. & Waterhouse, J. M. (1981) *Circadian Rhythms and the Human.* Wright, Bristol.

Mize, J. *et al.* (1993) The forgotten vital sign: temperature patterns and associations in 642 trauma patients at an urban level 1 trauma centre. *Journal of Emergency Nursing*, 19, 303–5.

Moorat, D. S. (1976) The cost of taking temperatures. *Nursing Times*, 72(20), 767–70.

Neff, J. *et al.* (1989) Effect of respiratory rate, respiratory depth, and open versus closed mouth breathing on sublingual temperature. *Research in Nursing and Health*, 12, 195–202.

Nichols, G. A. et al. (1972) Time analysis of afebrile and febrile temperature readings. *Nursing Research*, 21, 463–4.

Samples, J. F. et al. (1985) Circadian rhythms: basis for screening fever. *Nursing Research*, 34(6), 377–9.

Sims-Williams, A. (1976) Temperature-taking with glass thermometers: a review. *Journal of Advanced Nursing*, 1(6), 481–93.

Stronge, J. L. (1980) Electronic thermometers: a costly rise in efficiency? *Nursing Mirror*, 151(8).

Takacs, K. & Valenti, W. (1981) Temperature measurement in a clinical setting. *Nursing Research*, 31(6), 368–70.

Vane, J. R. (1978) In: *Pharmacology of the Hypothalamus*, (eds Cox *et al.*). Macmillan, London.

GUIDELINES: TEMPERATURE

EQUIPMENT

1 Electronic thermometer and oral probe.
2 Disposable probe covers.

PROCEDURE

Action	Rationale
1 Explain and discuss the procedure with the patient.	To ensure that the patient understands the procedure and gives his/her valid consent.
2 Remove the probe from the stored position in the thermometer and check that the reading is 34°C.	If the readout does not register the machine is faulty and should not be used.

| 3 | Push the probe firmly into the probe cover. | The probe cover protects the tip of the probe and is necessary for the functioning of the instrument. |

| 4 | Ask the patient to open the mouth and insert the probe under the tongue into the 'heat pocket' at the posterior base of the tongue. | The highest oral temperature reading is at the posterior base of the tongue, which is least affected by environmental conditions. |

| 5 | Ask the patient to close the mouth. | To increase the patient's comfort and to keep the probe in place. |

| 6 | Hold the thermometer in place until an audible tone is heard and the machine signals the correct temperature. | Tissue contact must be maintained for an accurate reading to be obtained. |

| 7 | If figures on the display stop rising without an audible tone, tissue contact has been lost. Regain tissue contact and continue. | The probe must be supported outside the mouth as its top-heavy shape tends to move the sensitive tip out of the heat pocket. |

| 8 | Remove the probe from the patient's mouth when signalled by the machine and note the temperature displayed. | An audible tone indicates that the reading is complete. |

| 9 | Discard the probe cover into a waste bag by pressing the probe from the thumb. | Probe covers are for single use only. The discard mechanism prevents transfer of the patient's saliva to the nurse's hands. |

| 10 | Return the probe to its storage position in the thermometer, cancelling the temperature reading. | The probe is best protected from damage in this storage position. |

URINALYSIS

Definition

Urinalysis is the testing of the physical characteristics and composition of freshly voided urine.

Indications

The composition of urine can change dramatically as a result of disease processes. It may contain red blood cells, glucose, proteins, white blood cells, or bile (Marieb, 1995). The presence of such abnormalities in urine is an important warning sign of illness and may be helpful in clinical assessment in the following ways:

(1) To determine the individual's urine status on admission as a baseline for comparisons with future assessments.
(2) To monitor changes in urinary constituents as a response to medication.
(3) To be used as a screening test to gather information about physical status.

REFERENCE MATERIAL

Urine is formed in the kidneys which process approximately 180 litres of blood-derived fluid a day. Approxi-

mately 1.5% of this total actually leaves the body. Urine formation and the simultaneous adjustment of blood composition involves three processes (Marieb, 1995) (Fig. 30.18):

(1) Glomerular filtration
(2) Tubular reabsorption
(3) Tubular secretion.

Glomerular filtration occurs in the glomeruli of the kidney which act as non-selective filters. Filtration occurs as a result of increased glomerular blood pressure caused by the difference in diameter between afferent and efferent arterioles. The effect is a simple mechanical filter that permits substances smaller than plasma proteins to pass from the glomeruli to the glomerular capsule (Marieb, 1995).

Tubular reabsorption then occurs, removing necessary substances from the filtrate and returning them to the peritubular capillaries. Tubular reabsorption is an active process that requires protein carriers and energy. Substances reabsorbed include nutrients and most ions. It is also a passive process, however, driven by eletrochemical gradients. Substances reabsorbed in this way include sodium ions and water. Creatinine and the metabolites of drugs are not reabsorbed either because of their size, insolubility, or a lack of carriers. Most of the nutrients,

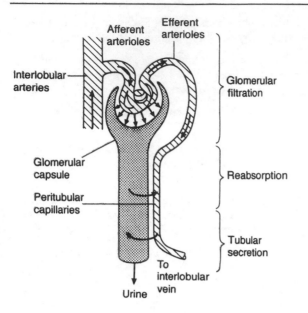

Figure 30.18 The nephron depicted diagramatically to show the three major mechanisms by which urine is produced:
(1) Glomerular filtration.
(2) Tubular reabsorption.
(3) Tubular secretion.

80% of the water and sodium ions, and the majority of actively transported ions are reabsorbed in the proximal convoluted tubules (Marieb, 1995).

Reabsorption is controlled by hormones. Aldosterone increases the reabsorption of sodium (and hence also water), and antidiuretic hormone (ADH) enhances the reabsorption of water in the collecting tubules (Marieb, 1995).

Tubular secretion is both an active and a passive process in which the tubules excrete drugs, urea, excess ions and other substances into the filtrate. It plays an important part in maintaining the acid–base balance of the blood (Marieb, 1995).

Regulation of urine concentration and volume occurs in the loop of Henle where the osmolarity of the filtrate is controlled. As the filtrate flows through the tubules the permeability of the walls controls how dilute or concentrated the resulting urine will be. In the absence of ADH dilute urine is formed because the filtrate is not reabsorbed as it passes through the kidneys. As levels of ADH increase, the collecting tubules become more permeable and water moves out of the filtrate back into the blood. Consequently, smaller amounts of more concentrated urine are produced (Marieb, 1995).

Characteristics of urine

Urine is typically clear pale to deep yellow in colour and slightly acidic (pH6), though pH can change as a result of metabolic processes or diet. Vomiting and bacterial infection of the urinary tract can cause urine to become alkaline. Urinary specific gravity ranges from 1.001 to 1.035, according to how concentrated the urine is (Marieb, 1995).

The colour of urine is due to a pigment called urochrome which is derived from the body's destruction of haemoglobin. The more concentrated urine is, the deeper yellow it becomes. Changes in colour may reflect diet (e.g. beetroot or rhubarb), or may be due to blood or bile in the urine. If fresh urine is turbid (cloudy), the cause may be an infection of the urinary tract. The urinary tract is the most common site of bacterial infection. It is thought to affect 10–20% of the female population (Mims *et al.*, 1993). There are many predisposing factors (Fig. 30.19), the most common of which is instrumentation, that is, cystoscopy and urinary catheterization (Johnson, 1986).

Bacteriuria is defined as the presence of bacteria in the urine. Because urine specimens can become contaminated with periurethral flora during collection, infection is distinguished by counting the number of bacteria. Significant bacteriuria is defined as a presence of more than 10^5 organisms per ml of urine in the presence of clinical symptoms (Fig. 30.20). Covert bacteriuria is the presence of more than 10^5 organisms per ml of urine without clinical symptoms. Distinguishing between counts of 10^3 and 10^5 can be difficult, making it important that urine is collected carefully and transported rapidly to the laboratory (Mims *et al.*, 1993).

Fresh urine smells slightly aromatic. This can change as a result of disease processes such as diabetes mellitus, when acetone is present in the urine, giving it a fruity smell. The composition of urine can change dramatically as a result of disease, and abnormal substances may be

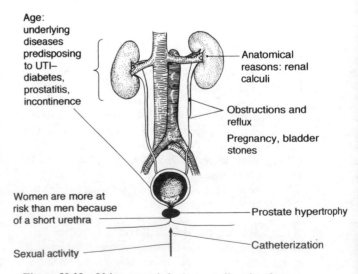

Figure 30.19 Urinary tract infections: predisposing factors.

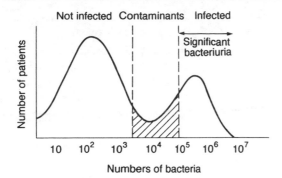

Figure 30.20 Significant bacteriuria. Specimens of urine are rarely sterile. A cut-off point is identified to distinguish true infection (significant bacteriuria) from the effects of contamination from surrounding tissues.

present. Urinalysis can identify many of these substances, and should be part of every physical assessment (Stevens, 1989).

Changes to composition of urine and their possible causes

Substance	Name of condition	Possible causes
Glucose	Glycosuria	Diabetes mellitus
Proteins	Proteinuria	May be seen in pregnancy and high protein diets; heart failure; severe hypertension; infection; asymptomatic renal disease
Ketone bodies	Ketonuria	Starvation; untreated diabetes mellitus
Haemoglobin	Haemoglobinaemia	Transfusion reaction; haemolytic anaemia; severe burns
Bile pigments	Bilirubinaemia	Liver disease, or obstruction of the bile ducts
Erythrocytes	Haematuria	Bleeding in urinary tract: kidney stones, infection, or trauma
Leucocytes	Pyuria	Urinary tract infection

Renal clearance is the rate at which the kidneys clear a particular chemical from the plasma. Studies of renal clearance provide information about renal function or the course of renal disease. There is no single test of renal function.

References and further reading

Bonnardeux, A. *et al.* (1994) Study of the reliability of dipstick urinalysis. *Clinical Nephrology*, 41(3), 167–72.

Cooper, C. (1993) What colour is that urine specimen? *American Journal of Nursing*, 93(8), 37.

Flanagan, P. G. *et al.* (1989) Evaluation of four screening tests for bacteriuria in elderly people. *Lancet*, 1(8647), 1117–19.

Hiscoke, C. *et al.* (1990) Validation of a method for the rapid diagnosis of urinary tract infection suitable for use in general practice. *British Journal of General Practice*, 40, 403–5.

Hurlbut, T. A. & Littenberg, B. (1991) The diagnostic accuracy of rapid dipstick tests to predict urinary tract infection. *American Journal of Clinical Pathology*, 96, 582–8.

Johnson, A. (1986) Urinary tract infection. *Nursing*, 3, 102–5.

Keeler, L. L. (1994) Tests to detect asymptomatic urinary tract infections. *Journal of the American Medical Association*, 271(18), 1399–400.

Kunin, C. M. (1979) *Detection, Prevention, and Management of Urinary Tract Infections*. Henry Kimpton, London.

Lowe, P. (1986) Chemical screening and prediction of bacteriuria – a new approach. *Medical Laboratory Sciences*, 43, 28–33.

Marieb, E. M. (1995) *Human Anatomy and Physiology*. Benjamin Cummings, California.

Mills, S. J. *et al.* (1992) Screening for bacteriuria in urological patients using reagent strips. *British Journal of Urology*, 70, 314–17.

Mims, C. A. *et al.* (1993) *Medical Microbiology*, C. V. Mosby, London.

Ravichandra, D. *et al.* (1994) Urine testing for acute lower abdominal pain in adults. *British Journal of Surgery*, 81, 1459–60.

Stevens, M. (1989) Screening urines for bacteriuria. *Medical Laboratory Science*, 46, 194–206.

Woodward, M. N. & Griffiths, D. M. (1993) Use of dipsticks for routine analysis of urine from children with acute abdominal pain. *British Medial Journal*, 306, 1512.

Dipstick (reagent) tests

Strips that have been impregnated with chemicals are dipped quickly in urine and read as a means of testing urine. When dipped in urine, the chemicals react with abnormal substances and change colour. Although dipstick reagents have been primarily used as screening tools for protein or glucose in the urine, more sophisticated reagents are now available. These reagents test for nitrites and leucocyte esterase as indicators of bacterial infection. Leucocyte esterase is an enzyme from neutrophils not normally found in urine and is a marker of infection. Nitrites are produced in urine by the bacterial breakdown of dietary nitrates (Woodward & Griffiths, 1993). Screening for bacteriuria can have significant cost savings for departments that routinely screen for urinary tract infection by sending samples of midstream urine (MSU) from all patients. Lowe (1986) found that by using dipstick reagents to screen for infection, it was possible to reduce by 40% microbiology workload with subsequent cost savings. This has been substantiated in further studies by Flanagan et al. (1989) and Hiscocke (1990).

The routine use of urine dipsticks for testing for infection is not widespread in the UK (Woodward & Griffiths, 1993). This is mainly due to concern about the sensitivity of these sticks. Several studies have recently looked at the accuracy of using these dipstick reagents for screening for urinary tract infections (Hurlbut & Littenberg, 1991). Flanagan et al. (1989) in a study found that the sticks had a 96.1% sensitivity to infection while Mills et al. (1991) in a study of surgical patients found 91% sensitivity pre-operatively, but that sensitivity fell to 71% post-surgery. They concluded that dipstick reagents are a useful screening tool. However, specimens still need to be microbiologically examined to determine the nature and sensitivity of the infection for treatment. Overall there is a good correlation between these biochemical tests and microscopic analysis with reagent sticks costing approximately 18 pence in comparison with £13 for microbiological analysis (Ravichandra et al., 1994). When interpreting the results of reagent sticks it is important to remember the limitations of the test as false negatives are possible.

There are many drugs which may influence urine tests.

How drugs may influence the results of reagent sticks

Drug	Reagent test	Effect on the results
Ascorbic acid	Glucose, blood, nitrite	High concentrations may diminish colour
L-dopa	Glucose	High concentrations may give a false negative reaction
	Ketones	Atypical colour
Nalidixic acid Probenacid	Urobilinogen	Atypical colour
Phenazopyridine (pyridium)	Protein	May give atypical colour
	Ketones	Coloured metabolites may mask a small reaction
	Urobilinogen, bilirubin	May mimic a positive reaction
	Nitrite	
Rifampicin	Bilirubin	Coloured metabolites may mask a small reaction
Salicylates (aspirin)	Glucose	High doses may give a false negative reaction

It is therefore important to assess the patient's medication when considering the results of dipstick urinalysis. The wide range of urine tests available and the ease with which they can be used have established the use of reagent sticks throughout clinical practice. It is important to be aware, however, that they do have limitations and that manufacturers' instructions should be followed carefully as results, especially tests for glucose and protein, can influence treatment and care decisions.

GUIDELINES: REAGENT STICKS

PROCEDURE

Action	Rationale
1 Store reagent sticks in accordance with manufacturer's instructions. This often includes any dark place or in a refrigerator.	Tests may depend on enzymatic reaction. To ensure reliable results.

2	Explain and discuss the procedure with the patient.	To ensure that the patient understands the procedure and gives his/her valid consent.
3	Obtain clean specimen of fresh urine from patient.	Urine that has been stored deteriorates rapidly and can give false results.
4	Dip the reagent strip into the urine. The strip should be completely immersed in the urine and then removed immediately and tapped against the side of the container.	To remove any excess urine.
5	Hold the stick at an angle.	Urine reagent strips should not be held upright when reading them because urine may run from square to square mixing various reagents.
6	Wait the required time interval before reading the strip against the colour chart.	The strips must be read at exactly the time interval specified, or the reagents will not have time to react, or may be inaccurate.

GUIDELINES: MID-STREAM SPECIMEN OF URINE

A clean catch mid-stream specimen of urine is the most effective method of obtaining a voided specimen of urine for laboratory analysis.

EQUIPMENT

1 Sterile specimen container.

PROCEDURE

Action

Rationale

1	Explain and discuss the procedure with the patient.	To ensure that the patient understands the procedure and gives his/her valid consent.
2	Ask the patient to carefully clean the labia or glans with soap and water (not antiseptic).	This cleansing is to reduce the amount of contamination from surrounding tissues. Antiseptics can influence the result of the urinalysis (Mims et al., 1993).
3	Allow the first part of the urine stream to be voided and then catch the rest.	This helps wash out any contaminants that may be present in the urethra.
4	Specimens should be clearly labelled and sent immediately to the laboratory.	Delay allows the specimen to deteriorate, leading to inaccurate results. If it is not possible to send the specimen immediately, it should be refrigerated.

CHAPTER 31

Pain Assessment

Definition

Pain is not a simple sensation but a complex phenomenon having both a cognitive (physical) and an affective (emotional) component. Because pain is subjective the favoured definition for use in clinical practice, proposed originally by McCaffery (1968), is: 'Pain is whatever the experiencing person says it is, existing whenever the experiencing person says it does.' The aim of pain assessment, therefore, is to identify *all* the factors – physical and non-physical – which affect the patient's perception of pain.

REFERENCE MATERIAL

There are several ways to categorize the types of pain that occur in patients with cancer, but it is important to recognize that cancer patients may experience both acute and chronic pain. Foley (cited by Doyle *et al.*, 1993) describes the following types of pain, which are also recognized by McCaffery & Beebe (1989).

Acute pain

The characteristics of acute pain are:

- It is usually of brief duration.
- It is normally associated with injury or disease and is expected to subside when the injury or disease process has resolved, i.e. it has a predictable end.

Acute pain may be either sudden or slow in onset and may be of any intensity ranging from mild to severe.

Chronic pain

- Chronic pain is usually prolonged and defined as pain that persists for more than 3 months.
- Chronic pain is associated with major changes in personality, lifestyle and functional ability.

In addition to the above it is essential to mention episodic, incident and breakthrough pains, which are all terms referring to 'a transitory exacerbation of pain experienced by the patient who has relatively stable and adequately controlled baseline pain' (Hanks, 1983). The breakthrough pain experienced by the patient is when the regular opioid regimen used for baseline pain fails to provide adequate analgesic cover. During pain assessment it is essential that nurses include exploration of this type of pain.

Factors affecting pain assessment

Patients with chronic, particularly cancer-related, pain rarely present with this one symptom. For example, approximately two-thirds of advanced cancer patients will also complain of anorexia, one half will have a symptomatic dry mouth and constipation, and one-third will suffer nausea, vomiting, insomnia, dyspnoea, cough or oedema (Hanks, 1983). It will be clear from those figures that pain assessment cannot be seen in isolation; identification of all related symptoms is of equal importance as they will contribute to a lowered pain threshold (the least stimulus intensity at which a person perceives pain) and impaired pain tolerance (the greatest stimulus intensity causing pain that a person is prepared to tolerate).

Furthermore, cancer pain is often multifocal. Less than 20% of advanced cancer patients will have a single site of pain, and approximately 50% of patients will have three or more individual pains (Twycross & Fairfield, 1982).

A diagnosis of cancer does not necessarily mean that the malignant process is the cause of the pain. Pain in cancer may be:

(1) Caused by the cancer itself.
(2) Caused by treatment.
(3) Associated with debilitating disease, such as a pressure ulcer.
(4) Unrelated to either the disease or the treatment, such as headache.

The cause of *each* pain should therefore be identified carefully; many pains unrelated to the cancer will respond to specific treatment. If the pain is due to the cancer, then it is important to determine the precise

Table 31.1 Factors affecting pain sensitivity

Sensitivity increased:
Discomfort
Insomnia
Fatigue
Anxiety
Fear
Anger
Sadness
Depression
Boredom

Sensitivity lowered:
Relief of symptoms
Sleep
Rest
Sympathy
Understanding
Companionship
Diversional activity
Reduction in anxiety
Elevation of mood

mechanism of pain because treatment will vary accordingly.

The perception of painful stimuli will always be modulated by the emotional response to that perception. Changes in mood may alter considerably the experience of pain (McCaffery & Beebe, 1989). Pain assessment needs to acknowledge this fact, and particular attention must be paid to factors which will modulate pain sensitivity (Table 31.1).

Need for assessment tools

Accurate pain assessment is a prerequisite of effective control and is an essential component of nursing care. In the assessment process, the nurse gathers information from the patient that allows an understanding of the patient's experience and its effect on the patient's life. The information obtained guides the nurse in planning and evaluating strategies for care. Pain is rarely static; therefore its assessment is not a one-time process but is ongoing.

Pain assessment is difficult to achieve. For example, the tendency suggested by both research and clinical practice is for the patient not to report any pain or to do so inadequately or inaccurately, minimizing the pain experience (McCaffery, 1983; McCaffery & Beebe, 1989). Hunt *et al.* (1977) found that nurses tended to overestimate the pain relief obtained from analgesia and underestimate the level of the patient's pain.

Pain charts have been considered as useful tools for assisting nurses to assess pain and plan nursing care. Raiman (1986) found that the use of a chart improved communication between staff and patients. Walker *et al.* (1987) found that the specific advantages of using a chart lie in promoting both the initial assessment of pain and its monitoring. It was also found that the involvement of many patients in their pain management helped to increase their confidence in it.

Introduction to the use of assessment tools

There are numerous methods of assessing pain, and the published literature indicates that pain assessment charts can be used successfully to assess and monitor pain (McCaffery & Beebe, 1989). Some degree of caution, however, must be exercised in their use. The nurse must be careful to select the tool which is most appropriate for a particular type of pain experience. For example, it would not be appropriate to use a pain assessment chart which had been designed for use with patients with chronic pain, to assess postoperative pain. Furthermore, pain charts should not be used totally indiscriminately. Walker *et al.* (1987) found that charts appeared to have little value in cases of unresolved or intractable pain.

The Royal Marsden NHS Trust Pain Assessment Chart

A study was carried out at The Royal Marsden NHS Trust in order to design a chart for use with patients with chronic cancer pain and to evaluate its effectiveness (Walker *et al.*, 1987). The study indicated that the chart (Fig. 31.1) was a valuable tool for pain assessment in 98% of cases. The following guidelines are written with reference to The Royal Marsden NHS Trust pain chart, but it is recognized that nurses may modify the chart to meet the needs of their own particular branch of nursing.

References and further reading

Cherny, N. I. & Portency, R. K. (1993) Cancer pain management current strategy. *Cancer*, Supplement 72(11).

Dicks, B. (1990) Programmed instruction, cancer pain. *Cancer Nursing*, 13(4), 256–61.

Doyle, D. *et al.* (1993) *Oxford Textbook of Palliative Medicine*. Oxford University Press, Oxford.

Foley, K. M. (1989) Controversies in cancer pain. Medical perspectives. *Cancer*, Supplement 63, 2259–65.

Hanks, G. W. (1983) Management of symptoms in advanced cancer. *Update*, 26, 1691–702.

Hoskin, P. J. & Dicks, B. (1988) Symptom Control. In: *Oncology for Nurses and Health Care Professionals*, (eds R. Tiffany & P. Webb), vol. 2, 2nd edn. Harper & Row, London.

Hunt, J. M. *et al.* (1977) Patients with protracted pain; a survey conducted at the London Hospital. *Journal of Medical Ethics*, 3(2), 61–73.

McCaffery, M. (1968) *Nursing practice theories related to cognition, bodily pain, and man–environment interactions.* University of California, Los Angeles.

The Royal Marsden NHS Trust

Pain Assessment Chart

Surname: *Hospital no.*

First name: *Date*:

Initial Assessment

Patient's own description of the pain(s):

What helps relieve the pain?

What makes the pain worse?

Do you have pain

1 *At night*?   Yes/No   (comment if required).

2 *At rest*?   Yes/No   (comment if required).

3 *On movement*?   Yes/No   (comment if required).

Pain sites
Please draw on the body outlines below to show where you feel pain. Label each site of pain with a letter A.B.C. etc.

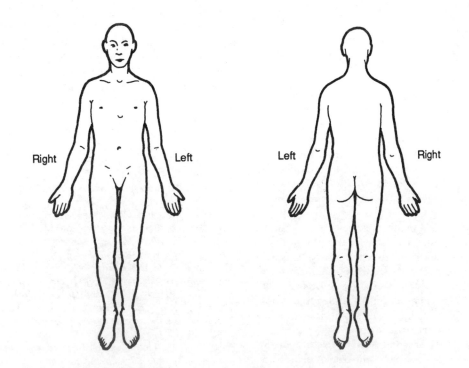

Figure 31.1   The Royal Marsden NHS Trust Pain Assessment Chart.

Pain Assessment Chart

Continuation no: _____

Key to pain intensity:

0 = no pain	4 = very severe pain
1 = mild pain	5 = intolerable/overwhelming pain
2 = moderate pain	
3 = severe pain	s = sleeping

It may be easier to determine the intensity of pain by looking at the pain scale below.

no pain   0 — 1 — 2 — 3 — 4 — 5   intolerable/overwhelming pain

mild pain   moderate pain   severe pain   very severe pain

Date	Times	Pain sites								Analgesia name, route & dose	Patient activity and comments
		A	B	C	D	E	F	G	H		

Figure 31.1 *Continued.*

McCaffery, M. (1983) *Nursing the Patient in Pain*. Harper & Row, London.

McCaffery, M. & Beebe, A. (1989) *Pain: Clinical Manual for Nursing Practice*. Mosby, USA.

Melzac, R. & Dennis, S. G. (1980) Phylogenetic evolution of pain expression in animals. In: *Pain and Society*, (eds H. W. Kosterlitz & L. Y. Teranius). Chomie, New York.

Raiman, J. (1986) Pain relief – a two way process. *Nursing Times*, 82(15), 24–8.

Schofield, P. (1995) Using assessment tools to help patients in pain. *Professional Nurse*, 10(11), 703–6.

Twycross, R. G. & Fairfield, S. (1982) Pain in far advanced cancer. *Pain*, 14, 303–10.

Walker, V. S. *et al.* (1987) Pain assessment charts in the management of chronic cancer pain. *Palliative Medicine*, 1, 111–16.

World Health Organization (1990) *Cancer Pain Relief and Palliative Care*. WHO, Geneva.

GUIDELINES: INITIAL ASSESSMENT

Action

1 Explain the purpose of using the chart to the patient.

2 Where appropriate, encourage the patient to complete the pain chart himself/herself.

3 Where the nurse completes chart, record the patient's *own* description of his/her pain.

4 (a) Record any factors which influence the intensity of the pain, e.g. activities or interventions which reduce or increase the pain such as distractions or a heat pad.
(b) Record whether or not the patient is pain free at night, at rest or on movement.

Rationale

To ensure that the patient understands the procedure and gives his/her valid consent and cooperation.

To encourage patient participation.

To reduce the risk of misrepresentation.

Ascertaining how and when the patient experiences pain enables the nurse to plan realistic goals. For example, relieving the patient's pain during the night and while he/she is at rest is usually easier to achieve than relief from pain on movement.

GUIDELINES: PAIN SITES

Action

1 Encourage the patient, where appropriate, to identify pain himself/herself.

2 Index each site (A to H) (see Fig. 31.1) in whatever way seems most appropriate, e.g. shading or colouring of areas or arrows to indicate shooting pains.

Rationale

The body outline (Fig. 31.1) is ideally a vehicle for the patient to describe own pain experience.

This enables individual pain sites to be located.

GUIDELINES: MONITORING PAIN INTENSITY

Action

1 Give each pain site a numerical value according to the key to pain intensity or the pain scale and note time recorded.

Rationale

To indicate the intensity of the pain at each site.

| 2 | Record any analgesia given and note route and dose. | To monitor efficacy of prescribed analgesia. |
| 3 | Record any significant activities which are likely to influence the patient's pain. | Extra pharmacological or non-pharmacological interventions might be indicated. |

Note: Fixed times for reviewing the pain have been omitted intentionally to allow for flexibility. It is suggested that, initially, the patient's pain be reviewed every 4 hours. When a patient's level of pain has stabilized, recordings may be made less frequently, e.g. 12-hourly or daily. The chart should be discontinued if a patient's pain becomes totally controlled.

CHAPTER 32
Peri-Operative Care

PRE-OPERATIVE CARE

Definition

Pre-operative care is the preparation and assessment, physical and psychological, of a patient before surgery.

Pre-operative objectives

Physical

(1) To minimize postoperative complications, e.g. by teaching the patient deep breathing exercises and the relevance after surgery to wellbeing.
(2) To assess the physical condition of the patient so that potential problems can be anticipated and prevented.
(3) To ensure that the patient is in an optimum physical condition before surgery.

Psychological

(1) To ensure that the patient understands the nature of the surgery to be undergone.
(2) To teach the patient what to expect post-operatively, e.g. about any drains, catheters and so on that may be necessary afterwards.
(3) To assess areas of anxiety that the patient may have and discuss them, using nursing interventions if appropriate.

REFERENCE MATERIAL

Patient education and post-operative pain

Much research and discussion has been devoted to the subject of post-operative pain and the ways in which pre-operative patient education can influence the pain experience. Since pain and anaesthesia are often the patient's greatest fears (Carnevali, 1966) it is necessary to address this cause of anxiety in the pre-operative period.

Reducing patient anxiety by giving pre-operative in-formation has been shown to reduce post-operative pain (Hayward, 1975; Bray, 1986). It also results in the patient requiring less analgesia. The reduction of anxiety and promoting post-operative recovery can be achieved in several ways. The fragmentation of nursing care could account for some patient anxiety (Copp, 1988), and pre-operative visiting by nurses from theatres is being undertaken in many hospitals. It has been found that this can 'help the patient to manage his anxiety, not least by providing a continuity of care in collaboration with other members of the surgical teams' (Leonard & Kalideen, 1985). Copp (1988) also found that teaching patients recovery exercises decreased their feelings of helplessness and, therefore, reduced anxiety, and that the use of cognitive coping methods is an effective way of reducing anxiety.

Further research (Balfour, 1989) has shown that 'patients continue to suffer unrelieved pain following abdomen surgery' and that 'nurses continue to under-administer prescribed analgesics'. Jackson (1995) suggested that 50% of patients have pain for most of the 72 hours after surgery. Post-operative analgesia is often administered on a *pro re nata* (as required) basis so that patients request it when they are in pain. One strategy is to use methods to maintain a constant drug concentration in the blood via a continuous infusion. This often reduces side-effects, such as nausea, while providing good analgesic cover. Use of patient-controlled analgesia (PCA) gives the patient a sense of autonomy which may decrease anxiety, and which will in turn influence the patient's pain perception (Carr, 1989).

Skin preparation

Before surgery the patient is required to have a bath or shower. The aim of a pre-operative bath or shower is to reduce the risk of post-operative wound infection.

Research into the use of antiseptic preparations to be used in the pre-operative bath or shower is contradictory. Wells *et al.* (1983) found a single bath using chlorhexidine did not reduce post-operative infections in patients undergoing open heart surgery. This is supported by Leigh *et al.* (1983), who found that a single chlorhexidine bath eliminated the skin carriage of *Staphylococcus aureus* but did not reduce post-operative wound infection rates.

Hayek *et al.* (1987) studied the effects of two pre-operative baths comparing the use of chlorhexidine against ordinary soap and a placebo. The findings indicated that the two pre-operative chlorhexidine showers reduced the post-operative infection rate in 'clean' surgery. In the clean group, chlorhexidine use reduced the incidence of *Staphylococcus* by 50%; in the clean/contaminated surgery group there was some reduction of staphylococcal infections. Although chlorhexidine caused a reduction of overall infection in the contaminated wounds, it was not statistically significant.

Shaving is also a common pre-operative procedure. Studies suggest that there is a direct relationship between wound infection and hair removal, with the lowest wound infection rates obtained in cases where no hair was removed and the highest infection rate occurring when a razor was used (Alexander *et al.*, 1983; Willford, 1983).

One alternative method is to use a depilatory cream, which has demonstrated lower post-operative infection rates when the absence of hair from the operation site is required (*Lancet*, 1983). Winfield (1986) found that although depilatory cream is more expensive than shaving, it can save nursing time as most patients can apply the cream themselves. Similarly, although skin irritation can occur (in 9% of cases), it compares favourably with skin irritation from razors (13%), including grazes and small cuts.

Pre-operative fasting

Any patient presenting for anaesthesia may have undigested food in the stomach. For elective surgery the patient is usually 'nil by mouth' for long enough to allow the stomach to empty. Research by Thomas (1987) has revealed that patients often did not know why they were fasting, and that they were often deprived of food and drink for longer than the recommended time of 6 hours. Patients on an afternoon theatre list were less likely to be starved for as long as those on the morning list, who were frequently starved from midnight.

Stomach emptying on average takes 6 hours for solid food and 4 hours for fluids (Carrie & Simpson, 1988). However, gastric emptying may be delayed by anxiety or the action of some drugs, e.g. opiates. Atropine and hyoscine are sometimes prescribed as part of the patient's premedication, primarily to reduce saliva production. However, they also have a blocking action on the parasympathetic nervous system, which reduces motility of the digestive tract and therefore reduces the likelihood of vomiting (Green, 1986).

Anti-embolic stockings

Deep vein thrombosis, if it occurs, is usually diagnosed 3–14 days post-operatively. The incidence is highest in middle-aged and elderly patients, those on prolonged bedrest, and after major surgery of the lower abdomen, pelvis or hip joints. Patients with a history of coronary artery disease are also at risk (Carrie & Simpson, 1988). Once high-risk patients have been identified, prophylactic treatment can begin.

One such treatment is the use of anti-embolic stockings (Allen *et al.*, 1983). These stockings work by promoting venous flow and reducing stasis. They increase the velocity of flow, not only in the legs, but also in the pelvic veins and inferior vena cava (Drinkwater, 1989).

During surgery the use of heel supports which reduce the pressure on the calves on the operating table will also encourage venous return. The use of intermittent calf compression air boots which promote venous flow during surgery have also been reported to be effective (Pierce, 1994). Good pain control will encourage patients to mobilize early and carry out postoperative exercises, which are also important in preventing serious postoperative complications.

References and further reading

Alexander *et al.* (1983) The influence of hair removal methods on wound infections. *Archives of Surgery*, 118, 347–52.

Allen *et al.* (1983) The use of graduated compression stockings in the prevention of deep vein thrombosis. *British Journal of Surgery*, 10, 172–4.

Balfour, S. E. (1989) Will I be in pain? Patient and nurse attitudes to pain after abdominal surgery. *Professional Nurse*, 1(5), 28–33.

Biley, F. C. (1989) Nurse perception of stress in pre-operative surgical patients. *Journal of Advanced Nursing*, 14, 575–81.

Bray, C. A. (1986) Post-operative pain. Altering the patient's experience through education. *AORN Journal*, 43(3), 679–83.

Brown, S. A. (1983) Venous thrombosis: another complication of cancer (care plan). *Oncology Nursing Forum*, 10(2), 41–7.

Carnevali, D. L. (1966) Pre-operative anxiety. *American Journal of Nursing*, 66(7), 1536–8.

Carr, F. (1989) Waking up to post-operative pain. *Nursing Times*, 85(3), 38–9.

Carrie, L. E. S. & Simpson, P. J. (1988) *Understanding Anaesthesia*. William Heinemann, London.

Clarke, J. (1983) The effectiveness of surgical skin preparations. *Nursing Times, Theatre Nursing Supplement*, 28 September, 79(39), 8–17.

Copp, G. (1988) Intra-operative information and pre-operative visiting. *Surgical Nurse*, 1(2), 27–8.

Davis, P. S. (1988) Changing nursing practice for more

effective control of post-operative pain through a staff-initiated educational programme. *Nurse Education Today*, 8, 325–31.

Drinkwater, K. (1989) Management of deep vein thrombosis. *Surgical Nurse*, 2(1), 24–6.

Gooch, J. (1989) Who should manage pain – patient or nurse? *Professional Nurse*, 4(6), 295–6.

Green, J. H. (1986) *Basic Clinical Physiology*, 3rd edn. Oxford University Press, Oxford.

Hayek, L. J. *et al.* (1987) A placebo-controlled trial of the effect of pre-operative baths or showers with chlorhexidine detergent on postoperative wound infection rates. *Journal of Hospital Infection*, 10(2), 165–72.

Hayward, J. (1975) *Information: A Prescription Against Pain.* Royal College of Nursing (Research Series), London.

Jackson, J. (1995) Acute pain: its physiology and the pharmacology of analgesia. *Nursing Times*, 91(16), 27–8.

Johnson, A. (1989) Preparing for elective surgery. *Nursing Standard*, 3(23), 22–4.

Lancet (1983) Pre-operative depilation. *Lancet*, 1(8337), 1311.

Leigh, D. A. *et al.* (1983) Total body bathing with 'Hibiscrub'

(chlorhexidine) in surgical patients. A controlled trial. *Journal of Hospital Infection*, 4(3), 229–35.

Leonard, M. D. & Kalideen, P. (1985) 'So you're going to have an operation.' *National Association of Theatre Nurses News*, 22(2), 12–21.

Lore, C. (1990) Deep vein thrombosis: threat to recovery. Part 1, *Nursing Times*, 86(5), 40–3.

McConnell, E. A. (1990) Clinical do's and don'ts: applying antiembolism stockings (pictoral, protocol). *Nursing*, 20(10), 92.

Pierce, L. A. (1994) Patient positioning during surgical procedures. *Plastic Surgery Nursing*, 14(4), 242–3.

Thomas, A. E. (1987) Pre-operative fasting – a question of routine? *Nursing Times*, 83(49), 46–7.

Wells, F. C. *et al.* (1983) Wound infection in cardiothoracic surgery. *Lancet* 1, 1209–10.

Willford, P. S. (1983) Hair removal – shave, preps, depilation, and other pre-operative considerations. Are they really necessary? *Journal of Operating Room Research Institute*, 3(3) 26–8.

Winfield, V. (1986) Too close a shave? *Nursing Times, Journal of Infection Control Nursing*, 82(10), 64–8.

GUIDELINES: PRE-OPERATIVE CARE

EQUIPMENT

1 Theatre gown.
2 Labelled denture container if necessary.
3 Hypo-allergenic tape to cover wedding rings.
4 Any equipment and documents required by law and hospital policy if a pre-medication has been prescribed.

PROCEDURE

Action	Rationale
1 Ensure the patient is wearing an identification bracelet with the correct information.	To ensure correct identification and prevent possible problems.
2 Assess the pre-operative education received by the patient and ensure that it is complete and understood.	To ensure that the patient understands the nature and outcome of the surgery and reduce anxiety and possible post-operative complications.
3 Record the patient's pulse, blood pressure, respirations, temperature and weight.	To provide data for comparison post-operatively. The weight is recorded so that the anaesthetist can calculate the dose of drugs to be used.
4 Check that the patient has undergone relevant procedures, e.g. X-ray, ECG, blood tests and that these results are included with the patient's notes.	To ensure all relevant information is available to the nurses, anaesthetists and surgeons. Absence of results may delay or cause cancellation of an operation .
5 Instruct the patient on showering or bathing.	To minimise risk of post-operative wound infection.

6 Assist the patient to change into a theatre gown.

7 Long hair should be held back with, for example, a non-metallic tie.

8 Ensure that patients undergoing major surgery or abdominal/pelvic surgery, the elderly frail or bedbound patients or those with a previous history of emboli or other high-risk factors have antiembolic stockings applied correctly. The use of intermittent calf compression boots should be considered.

To reduce the risk of post-operative deep vein thrombosis or pulmonary emboli.

9 Complete the pre-operative check list by asking the patient and checking records and notes before giving any pre-medication.

Note: questioning pre-medicated patients is not a reliable source of checking information as the patient may be drowsy and/or disorientated.

    (a) Check when patient last had food or drink and ensure that it was at least 6 hours before.

To reduce the risk of regurgitation and inhalation of stomach contents on induction of anaesthetic.

    (b) Check whether patient micturated before pre-medication.

To prevent urinary incontinence and embarrassment. To allow better access to abdominal cavity for abdomen or pelvic surgery if a catheter is not to be used.

    (c) Note whether the patient has dental crowns, bridge work or loose teeth.

The anaesthetist needs to be informed to prevent accidental damage. Loose teeth or a dental prosthesis could be inhaled by the patient when an endotracheal tube is inserted.

    (d) Ensure prostheses, dentures and contact lenses are removed.

To prevent trauma to the patient.

    (e) Spectacles may be retained until the patient is in the anaesthetic room. Hearing aids may be retained until the patient has been anaesthetized. (These may be left in position if a local anaesthetic is being used.) Any prosthesis should then be labelled clearly and retained in the recovery room.

To allow patient to see and hear, thus reducing anxiety and enabling the patient to understand any procedures carried out.

    (f) All jewellery (apart from wedding ring), cosmetics, nail varnish and clothing, other than the theatre gown, are to be removed.

Metal jewellery may be accidentally lost or may be cause of harm to patient, e.g. – diathermy burns. Facial cosmetics can make the patient's colour difficult to assess. Nail varnish makes the use of the pulse oximeter, used to monitor the patient's pulse and oxygen saturation levels, impossible and masks peripheral cyanosis.

10 Valuables should be placed in the hospital's custody and recorded according to the hospital policy.

To prevent loss of valuables.

11 Check the consent form is correctly completed, signed and dated.

To comply with legal requirements and hospital policy.

12 Check the operation site is marked correctly.

To ensure the patient undergoes the correct surgery for which he/she has consented.

13 Check that the patient has undergone pre-anaesthetic assessment by the anaesthetist.

To ensure that the patient can be given the most suitable anaesthetic.

Guidelines: Pre-operative care (cont'd)

Action

14 Give the pre-medication, if prescribed, in accordance with the anaesthetist's instructions and conforming to legal requirements and hospital policy.

15 Advise the patient to remain in bed once the pre-medication has been given and to use the nurse call system if assistance is needed.

16 Ensure the patient is supported fully on the canvas, especially the head, when transferred from the ward bed to the trolley.

17 Ensure that all relevant information, e.g. X-rays, notes, blood results, accompany the patient to the operating theatre.

18 The patient should be accompanied to the theatre by a ward nurse who remains until the patient is anaesthetized.

19 The ward nurse should give a full handover to the anaesthetic nurse or operating department assistant on arrival of the patient at the anaesthetic room.

Rationale

Different drugs may be prescribed to complement the anaesthetic to be given, e.g. temazepam to reduce patient anxiety by inducing sleep and relaxation.

To prevent accidental patient injury as the pre-medication may make the patient drowsy and disorientated .

To prevent injury to the neck, etc. during transfer from the ward to the operating theatre.

To prevent delays which can increase the patient's anxiety, and to ensure that the anaesthetist and surgeon have all the information they require for the safe treatment of the patient.

To reduce the patient's anxiety.

To ensure the patient has the correct operation. To ensure continuity of care by exchanging all relevant information.

INTRA-OPERATIVE CARE

Definition
Intra-operative care is the physical and psychological care given to the patient in the anaesthetic room and theatre until transferral to the recovery room.

Objectives
(1) To ensure that the patient understands what is happening at all times in order to minimize anxiety.
(2) To ensure that the patient has the surgery for which the consent form was signed.
(3) To ensure patient safety at all times and minimize postoperative complications by:
  (a) Giving the required care for the unconscious patient.
  (b) Ensuring no injury is sustained from hazards associated with the use of swabs, needles, instruments, diathermy and power tools.
  (c) Minimizing post-operative problems associated with patient positioning, such as nerve or tissue damage.
  (d) Maintaining asepsis during surgical procedures to reduce the risk of post-operative wound infection in accordance with hospital policies on infection control.

REFERENCE MATERIAL

Diathermy
Diathermy is used routinely during many operations to control haemorrhage by cauterizing blood vessels or cutting or fulgerizing body tissues. Diathermy is potentially hazardous to the patient if used incorrectly. It is important that all theatre nurses know how to test and use all diathermy equipment in their department to prevent patient injury (3M, 1986; Theatre Safeguards, 1988).

The main risk when using diathermy is of thermo-electrical burns. The most common cause is incorrect application of the patient plate or a break in the connecting lead (Moakes, 1991). If this occurs when using an isolated diathermy machine then the current output will stop. However, if a grounded diathermy machine is used then the electrical current will find an alternative route back to the diathermy machine (Wainwright, 1988). If the patient is in contact with any metal, e.g. on the operating table (3M, 1986, p. 4), then loss of plate contact using a grounded unit could result in a serious burn.

Other causes of burns include skin preparation solutions or other liquids pooling around the plate site. With alcohol-based skin preparations especially, the skin should be allowed to dry before diathermy is used, as the alcohol can ignite (Wainwright, 1988). If the patient's position is changed during the operation the patient plate should be rechecked to ensure that it is still in contact and that the connecting clamp or lead is not causing pressure in the new position.

Use of diathermy and the plate position should be noted on the nursing care plan, and the patient's skin condition should be checked post-operatively.

Patient positioning

The position of the patient on the operating table must be such as to facilitate access to the operation site(s) by the surgeon, taking into account the patient's airway, monitoring equipment or intravenous lines. Nor should it compromise the patient's circulation, respiratory system or nerves (*American Operating Room Nursing Journal*, 1990). Pre-operative assessment will identify patients with particular needs which may be influenced by factors such as weight, nutritional state, age, skin condition and pre-existing disease. All these factors may indicate the need for extra precautions during positioning. Consideration by and the cooperation of all theatre personnel can help prevent many of the pre-operative complications related to intra-operative positioning.

All equipment that may be needed to support the patient during surgery, e.g. the table, arm supports, lithotomy poles and securing straps, should be checked to ensure that they are in working order, clean and free from sharp edges. Metal parts that may come into contact with the patient should be covered as there is an increased risk of burns if diathermy is used (Wainwright, 1988). Padding should be placed at the patient's elbows and heels, and pillows positioned between the legs if the patient is lying in a lateral position. Special consideration should also be given to areas such as the back of the head and ears. The use of a warm air mattress on the operating table can also help to reduce pressure on vulnerable areas such as the hips or sacrum, as well as reducing the risk of hypothermia (Atkinson & Kohn, 1986).

When a patient is transferred between the trolley or bed and operating table, adequate personnel should be present to ensure patient and staff safety (*American Operating Room Nursing Journal*, 1990). It is recommended that an approved rolling or sliding device is used to transfer patients from trolley to operating table, in compliance with legislation on manual handling. Safe manual handling and the safety of the patient depends on the participation of the correct number of staff in the specified handling manoeuvre.

All movements of the limbs of the unconscious patient should take into account the anatomy and natural planes of movement of that limb to avoid stretching and pressure on the related nerve planes (Theatre Safeguards, 1988). Hyperabduction of the arm when placed on a board, for example, could stretch the brachial plexus causing some post-operative loss of sensation and reduced movement of the forearm, wrist and fingers. The ulnar and radial nerves may be affected by direct pressure as a result of insufficient padding on arm supports or lack of care when inserting poles into the canvas and hitting the elbows.

Pre-existing conditions such as backache or sciatica can be exacerbated, particularly if the patient is in the lithotomy position as the sciatic nerve can be compressed against the poles (Underwood & Jameson, 1990). Most postoperative palsies are due to improper positioning of the patient on the operating table (Nightingale, 1985).

Control of infection and asepsis in operating theatres

The term asepsis means the absence of any infectious agents. The aseptic technique is the foundation on which contemporary surgery is built (Gruendemann & Meeker, 1983). The aim of operating theatres is to provide an area free from infectious agents. Large quantities of bacteria are present in the nose, mouth, on the skin, hair and on the attire of personnel, therefore people entering the operating theatres wear clean scrub suits and lint-free surgical hats to eliminate the possibility of these bacteria, hair or dandruff being shed (Hambraeus & Laurell, 1980). Sterile gowns and gloves are worn to prevent cross infection. It is recommended that waterproof footwear are worn by staff (Ayliff *et al.*, 1992). Face masks are worn to prevent droplets falling from the mouth into the operating field. A new mask should be worn for each operation, and masks that become damp must be replaced. The extent to which face masks are capable of preventing droplet spread is disputed. Orr (1981) found no increase in the infection rate when masks were not worn during general surgery. It is, however, accepted that masks offer protection to the wearer from blood splashes and for safety reasons should be worn by the scrub team.

The scrubbing procedure is essential to the maintenance of asepsis in the operating theatre. An antiseptic soap or detergent preparation (such as 4% chlorhexidine solution, e.g. Hibiscrub or povidone-iodine (e.g. Betadine, Disadine)) should be used. A 2 minute scrub is recommended, and any visible dirt or blood must be removed from the skin and from under fingernails (Ayliffe *et al.*, 1992). The closed method of donning sterile surgical gloves is preferred.

Universal precautions should be taken in theatres to minimize the risk of infection from blood and body fluids. These include the wearing of gloves, masks, barrier gowns and aprons. Protective eyewear or face shields should be worn during procedures likely to cause splashes or droplets of blood or generate bone chips. (Ayliffe *et al.*, 1992). Instruments must be handled carefully, and needle holders and forceps used to manipulate sutures to minimize the risk of needlestick or sharps injury.

Laparoscopic surgery

Laparoscopy has evolved from a diagnostic modality into a widespread surgical technique. Advantages for the patient include: a shorter stay in hospital, reduced postoperative pain and a shorter recovery period (Hulka, 1985). Laparoscopic surgery is now common in operating departments, and it is important that potential complications are identified and steps taken to minimize risk to the patient, both during surgery and in the recovery period. Patients should be prepared psychologically and physically for an open procedure, which may be undertaken under certain circumstances. Instruments and supplies for an open procedure must be readily available in the operating theatre.

Laparoscopy involves insufflation of the abdomen with carbon dioxide (CO_2). Prolonged insufflation can cause hypothermia, as thermal loss due to CO_2 is known to occur at the rate of 0.3°C per 40–50 litres of gas (Williams & Murr, 1993). Holzman *et al.* (1992) refer to the increased risk of hypercarbia and surgical emphysema during insufflation with CO_2. Careful monitoring and recording of the patient's vital signs, including oxygen saturation and expiratory gas levels, is therefore essential during laparoscopy.

Haemorrhage can occur during the procedure and may be difficult to detect because surgeons have a limited view of the area being operated upon. Electrosurgical injuries to organs may occur as a result of capacitive coupling (Tucker *et al.*, 1992) (capacative coupling is the transfer of electrical currents from the active electrode through coupling of stray currents into other conductive surgical equipment). Theatre staff must be aware of potential complications and ensure that equipment is used safely and according to the manufacturer's instructions.

The equipment used for laparoscopic surgery is very specialised and can be daunting for theatre staff. The Association of Operating Room Nurses (1994) recommends that all equipment is regularly and competently maintained and a maintenance record kept in a log. Policies and procedures should be developed for the checking procedure, and all staff thoroughly instructed in the operation of laparoscopic equipment.

References and further reading

American Operating Room Nursing Journal (1990) Proposed recommended practices; positioning the surgical patient. *AORN Journal*, 51(1), 216–22.

Association of Operating Room Nurses (1994) Proposed recommended practices: endoscopic minimal access surgery. *AORN Journal*, 59(2), 507–14.

Atkinson, L. J. & Kohn, M. L. (1986) *Berry and Kohn's Introduction to Operating Room Technique*. McGraw Hill, New York.

Ayliffe, G. *et al.* (1992) *Control of Hospital Infection: A Practical Handbook*, 3rd edn. Chapman & Hall, London.

Gillette, M. K. & Cansico, C. C. (1989) Intra-operative tissue injury, major causes and preventative measures (study). *AORN Journal*, 50(1), 66–8.

Gruendemann, B. & Meeker, H. M. (1983) *Alexander's Care of the Patient in Surgery*, 7th edn. Mosby, St Louis.

Hambraeus, A. & Laurell, G. (1980) Protection of the patient in the operating suite. *Journal of Hospital Infection*, 1, 5.

Holzman, M. *et al.* (1992) Hypercarbia during carbon dioxide gas insufflation for therapeutic laparoscopy: a note of caution. *Surgical Laparoscopy and Endoscopy*, 2(1), 11–14.

Hulka, J. F. (1985) *Textbook of Laparoscopy*. Gruene & Stratton, Orlando.

Joint Memorandum by Medical Defence Union and Royal College of Nursing (1978) *Safeguards Against Failure to Remove Swabs and Instruments From Patients*.

Lamp (cover story) (1990) There's more in the wash than dirty linen! *Lamp*, 47(3), 12.

3M (1986) *Safety in Diathermy*. 3M Health Care Ltd., Loughborough.

Moakes, E. (1991) Electrosurgical unit safety. *AORN Journal*, 53(3), 744–52.

Nightingale, K. (1985) Hazards to patients during surgery. *National Association of Theatre Nurses News*, January, 13–16.

Orr, N. (1981) Is a mask necessary in the operating theatre? *Annals of the Royal College of Surgeons of England*, 63, 390.

Theatre Safeguards (1988) MDU, RCN, NATN.

Tucker, R. D. *et al.* (1992) Capacitive coupled stray currents during laparoscopic and endoscopic electrosurgical procedures. *Biomedical Instrumentation and Technology*, 26(4), 303–11.

Underwood, M. J. & Jameson, J. (1990) Preventing nerve injuries. *Technic*, 83, 11–13.

Wainwright, D. (1988) Diathermy – How safe is it? *National Association of Theatre Nurses News*, 25(1), 7–8.

Williams, M. D. & Murr, P. C. (1993) Laparoscopic insufflation of the abdomen depresses cardiopulmonary function. *Surgical Endoscopy*, 7, 12–16.

GUIDELINES: INTRA-OPERATIVE CARE

Action	Rationale
1 Greet the patient by name. Confirm with the ward nurse that it is the correct patient for the scheduled operation.	To make the patient feel welcome. To ensure that the patient is safeguarded against problems related to misidentity.
2 Identify the patient by checking the name bracelet and number against the patient's notes and the operating list.	To question the pre-medicated patient can be unreliable (Theatre Safeguards, 1988).
3 Examine the pre-operative checklist (Fig. 32.1).	To ensure that all of the listed measures have been completed and that any additional information has been recorded.
4 Check that the blood results, X-rays, etc. are present in the patient's notes.	To ensure that all of the required results are available for the medical team's use
5 Maintain a calm, quiet environment and explain all the procedures to patient.	To reduce anxiety and enhance the smooth induction of anaesthesia.
6 When the patient is anaesthetized ensure that the eyes are closed and hypoallergenic tape is applied.	To prevent corneal damage due to drying or accidental abrasion.
7 Ensure that there are adequate staff to transfer the patient to the operating table. Ensure the brakes on the trolley and operating table have been applied. Ensure the patient's head and limbs are supported when transferring to the operating table.	To ensure that the patient receives no injury during the transfer.
8 Check with anaesthetist before moving patient.	To ensure airway is protected.
9 Ensure all limbs are supported and secure on the table. Ensure adequate padding and cushioning of bony prominences. The patient's position will be dictated by the nature of the surgery but must take into account the requirements of the anaesthetist and the physical, psychological and social needs of the patient.	If the patient is unconscious and unable to maintain a safe environment, support is necessary to prevent injury. The patient is especially at risk from damage due to pressure and stretching, so measures to maintain the skin's integrity are vital. Nerve damage due to compression or stretching must be prevented.
10 Ensure the patient is covered by the gown or blanket. These items should only be removed immediately before surgery.	To maintain the patient's dignity. To help prevent a reduction in body temperature or accidental hypothermia.
11 Use a warm air mattress on the operating table. Ensure all fluids used are warmed if possible.	To help maintain the patient's body temperature and prevent postoperative complications due to hypothermia.
12 Ensure all the equipment to be used is checked and in working order before the operating list commences, including suction, the anaesthetic machine, medical gases, monitoring equipment, diathermy and operating table.	To prevent accidental injury due to faulty equipment and to ensure all equipment necessary to the patient's treatment is present.

Guidelines: Intra-operative care (cont'd)

Action	Rationale
13 Ensure diathermy patient plate is attached securely in accordance with the manufacturer's instructions and hospital policy.	To ensure that no injury is sustained from the use of diathermy during surgery.

THE ROYAL MARSDEN NHS TRUST

Date ....Patient Name ....Hospital No. ....

Consultant .... Ward ....

PRE-OPERATIVE ASSESSMENT
(Relevant information to include potential medical/physical and communication problems e.g. Diabetes, Blindness/Deafness, Language differences etc.)

PATIENT WEIGHT:

T.P.R. B/P

ALLERGIES:

PRE-OPERATIVE CHECKLIST

	YES/NO	INITIAL
SECTION A – To be checked by observing/asking patient		
Identiband present and correct	....	....
Time food or drink last taken	....	....
Urine passed prior to pre-medication	....	....
Dental crowns /bridge work / loose teeth	....	....
Dentures removed (with patient)	....	....
Hearing Aid (with patient)	....	....
Contact lenses removed	....	....
Patient correctly prepared for theatre –		
e.g. shaved if necessary	....	....
Jewellery removed (rings taped)	....	....
Cosmetic and clothing removed	....	....
Valuables placed in hospital custody	....	....
SECTION B – To be checked from nursing/medical notes		
Consent to anaesthetic/operation form signed	....	....
Operation site marked if appropriate	....	....
Patient has undergone pre-anaesthetic examination	....	....
Pre-medication given at	(time)......................	....
Case notes accompany patient –	....	....
X-rays accompany patient –	....	....

TIME IN ANAESTHETIC ROOM ....SIGNATURE WARD NURSE ....

SIGNATURE OF CHECKING ODA / NURSE ....

Figure 32.1 The Royal Marsden NHS Trust theatre care document.

DOCUMENTATION OF CARE

TIME IN THEATRE.....................	TEMP (18 - 21C)	YES/NO
PATIENT CARE	HUMIDITY (30% - 50%)	YES/NO
identification / consent YES/NO	EQUIPMENT CHECKED	YES/NO

POSITION OF PATIENT: Supine   Prone   Lateral   Lithotomy   Trendelenburg

Other (please specify) ....

Apparatus used for safe positioning of patient:

Arm supports   Heel support   Gamgee   Arm Boards   Head Ring

Other (please specify) ....

Hot air mattress   Yes/No   TED Stockings/Venous stimulators

Position of Diathermy Plate ....

Catheter (size/type/balloon size) ....

Skin preparation   Iodine – Aqueous / Alcoholic

Chlorhexidine – Aqueous / Alcoholic

Other (please specify) ....

Throat pack ....

Tourniquet times   on.....................off ....

SURGEON(S)...

SCRUB PERSON(S) ....CIRCULATING PERSON(S)...

....

ANAESTHETIST.. ODA/NURSE ....
LA   /   GA

PROCEDURE PERFORMED ....

....

Swab / Needle / Instrument Count ....

Condition of patient's skin at end of surgery ....

Diathermy site checked (Initial) ....

Skin Closure : Sutures (Interrupted / Continuous) – Type ....

Staples Other (please specify) ....

Drains :   Vacuum   Silicone   Yeates / Corrugated   Other (specify) ....

Dressings: ....   Packs   vaginal / nasal ....

Specimens – Histology (Formalin / Fresh / Frozen Section) Microbiology Cytology

Signature of Scrub Person ....

Figure 32.1 *Continued.*

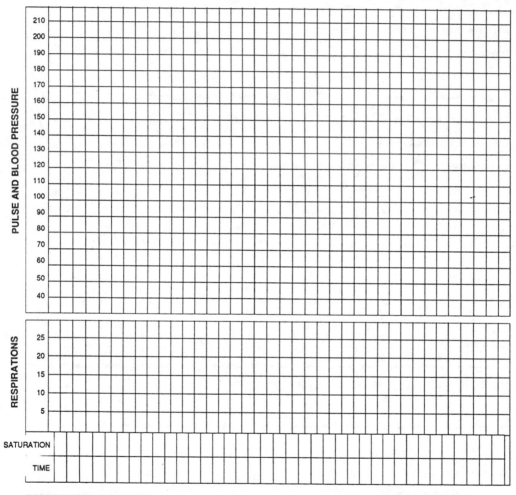

THEATRE RECOVERY

TIME IN ....

RESPIRATORY FUNCTION –

ACTION & EVALUATION

AIRWAY – observe, assess and ensure patency

BREATHING – record respiratory rate, observe chest movement

Give O_2 as prescribed

Record O_2 saturation

Figure 32.1   *Continued.*

CARDIOVASCULAR FUNCTION

Record Pulse & Blood Pressure

Observe skin/ mucosa for temperature and
perfusion

Observe wound sites, dressings and
drains

LEVEL OF CONSCIOUSNESS
Observe responsiveness,
orientation & mobility

FLUID BALANCE
Observe and record all input/drainage from
IVIs, catheters, NG tubes etc.

MEDICATION
Record all drugs given, time of administration
and effect

COMMENTS AND INSTRUCTIONS SPECIFIC TO PATIENT

ACTION & EVALUATION

....

SIGNATURE OF RECOVERY NURSE

Figure 32.1 *Continued.*

Guidelines: Intra-operative care (cont'd)

Action	Rationale
14 Follow hospital policy for the checking of swabs, needles and instruments.	To ensure that swabs, needles and instruments are accounted for at the end of the operation (Joint Memorandum by MDU and RCN, 1978).
15 Follow hospital policy for the disposal of sharps and clinical waste.	To prevent risk of injury to the patient and staff.
16 Ensure the surgeon is informed that the number of swabs, needles and instruments is correct.	It is the responsibility of the nurse and surgeon to check that nothing is accidentally left inside the patient on completion of surgery.
17 The scrub nurse accompanies the patient with the anaesthetist to the recovery area. A handover is given that includes:	To ensure continuity of care of the patient.
(a) What procedure was performed.	
(b) The presence, position and nature of any drains, infusions or intravenous or arterial lines.	To ensure that the recovery nurse has all the information required to assess the patient's recovery needs.
(c) Information including allergies or pre-existing medical conditions, such as diabetes mellitus.	To assist the recovery nurse in the assessment of post-operative problems with which the patient may present.
(d) The patient's cardiovascular state and pattern of anaesthesia used.	
(e) Specific instructions from the anaesthetist for post-operative care.	
(f) Information about any anxieties of the patient expressed before surgery such as a fear of not waking after anaesthesia or fear about coping with pain.	To ensure appropriate action can be taken as the patient regains consciousness and to enable an assessment of the efficacy of nursing interventions used.
(g) All information is to be recorded on the theatre nursing care plan.	To provide a written record of nursing intervention for use by recovery staff and ward nursing staff.

POST-ANAESTHETIC RECOVERY

Definition
Post-anaesthetic recovery involves the short-term critical care required by patients during their immediate postoperative period until they are stable, conscious and orientated.

Indication
All patients undergoing surgery and anaesthesia.

REFERENCE MATERIAL
The post-anaesthetic recovery room is an area within the operating department specifically designed, equipped and staffed for the support, monitoring and assessment of patients through the reversing stages of anaesthesia.

The recovery period is potentially hazardous. 'About 20% of the deaths associated with anaesthesia occur during the first 30 minutes after operation', and 'almost half the deaths occurring in the immediate postoperative period are due to inadequate nursing' (Atkinson *et al.*, 1982). While the majority of patients can be expected to achieve an uneventful recovery, they are vulnerable to many complications, notably respiratory and circulatory ones. One in 5.5 patients develop one or more complications during their time in the recovery room (Farman, 1978). Continuous individual nursing is required until patients are able to maintain their own airway (Association of Anaesthetists of Great Britain and Ireland, 1985). Obstruction of the upper airway is the commonest respiratory complication in the immediate post-operative period. Close observation and appropriate action can prevent the sequence of respiratory obstruction resulting in hypoxia leading to cardiac arrest (Campbell & Spence, 1990).

Guedel's classification of general anaesthesia

Guedel first published his systemization of the signs of inhalation anaesthesia, based on the description of patients under open-drop ether anaesthesia in 1920. Current practice does not depend on the use of a single agent administered in this way and the effects of opiates and muscle relaxants will affect the signs of the stages of anaesthesia as formulated in his classification. However, the system can still be used as a framework within which to assess the progress of post-anaesthetic recovery as long as other factors influencing the return of consciousness are taken into consideration (Table 32.1). With modern anaesthetic agents particulary propofol (Diprivan), rapid and symptom-free recovery from anaesthesia is seen and the frequency of nausea and vomiting, headaches and confusion/restlessness has been shown to be reduced (Grant & Mackenzie, 1985). This type of anaesthetic is commonly used in day surgery.

Table 32.1 Guedel's classification of general anaesthesia (Guedel, 1937; Lunn, 1982)

Classification

Stage I	Analgesia or the stage of disorientation from induction of anaesthesia to loss of consciousness
Stage II	Excitement: reflexes remain and coughing, vomiting and struggling may occur, respiration can be irregular with breath holding
Stage III	Surgical anaesthesia, divided into four planes:
	Plane I – eyelid reflex lost, swallowing reflex disappears, marked eyeball movement but loss of conjunctival reflex
	Plane II – eyeball movement ceases, laryngeal reflex lost although inflammation of the upper respiratory tract increases reflex irritability, corneal reflex disappears, secretion of tears increases, respiration automatic and regular, movement and deep breathing as a response to skin stimulation disappears
	Plane III – diaphragmatic respiration, progressive intercostal paralysis, pupils dilated and light reflex abolished. The laryngeal reflex lost in plane II can still be initiated by stimuli arising in the anus or cervix
	Plane IV – complete intercostal paralysis to diaphragmatic paralysis
Stage IV	Medullary paralysis with respiratory arrest and vasomotor collapse as a result of anaesthetic overdose

Assessment for discharge

The length of any patient's stay in the recovery room is dependent on the patient's condition and the rate at which that patient returns to a physical, mental and emotional state where he or she can be left unattended between routine observations.

Minimum criteria for discharge are:

(1) The patient is conscious and orientated and all protective reflexes have returned to normal.
(2) Respiratory function is adequate and good oxygenation is being maintained.
(3) Pulse and blood pressure are within normal pre-operative limits on consecutive observation.
(4) There is no persistent or excessive bleeding from wound or drainage sites.
(5) Patients with urinary catheters have passed adequate amounts of urine (more than 0.5 ml/kg/h) (Eltringham et al., 1989).
(6) Satisfactory analgesia has been provided for the patient, prescribed by the anaesthetist.

Wherever possible, a prior knowledge of patients gained from pre-operative contact is of great value in assessing their return to a normal state. It also has the advantage of helping their orientation to time and place, as familiarity generates a degree of security and confidence.

Local and regional anaesthesia

Patients having surgical procedures performed under local or spinal anaesthesia, whether intra- or extra-(epi-) dural, will require a period of post-operative observation, although the priorities of their care will be geared towards different considerations.

Layout of equipment

While a greater part of the nursing procedures carried out in the recovery room will of necessity be of a routine and repetitive nature, the reason for their performance is for the detection of potential as well as actual complications and the initiation of appropriate intervention. The need for speed, efficiency and economy of movement is essential when time becomes a critical factor in the ultimate safety of the patient. Thus the basic equipment for monitoring, airway maintenance and assisted ventilation must be available at the patient's head in each recovery bay. Equipment must be arranged for ease of access and always be clean and in full working order. Further support equipment should be available centrally, whenever possible being stored on trolleys for ease of transportation.

Summary

Post-anaesthetic care can best be described and understood as a series of many nursing procedures performed in sequence and simultaneously on patients who are in an artificially induced and traumatised condition. These patients will display varying degrees of responsiveness and physical and emotional states. It is important to establish a rapport with each individual to prevent the feeling of 'conveyor-belt processing' and gain the patient's confidence and co-operation. It is also necessary to understand that when emerging from the final stage of anaesthesia, some patients can behave in an emotional and disinhibited fashion, at variance with their normal behaviour (Lambrechts & Parkhouse, 1961). These displays are always transient and fortunately patients seldom have any recollection of them. While most patients can be expected to achieve an uneventful recovery, the duration and extent of surgery and anaesthesia are indicators of the pattern of recovery from the procedure and it can be judged to be uneventful only from hindsight. Physical and psychological recovery can be unpredictable at times.

References and further reading

Andrews, S. J. (1979) The recovery room as a nursing service. *Journal of the Royal Society of Medicine*, 72, 275–7.

Atkinson, R. S. *et al.* (1982) *A Synopsis of Anaesthesia*, 9th edn. John Wright, Bristol.

Asbury, A.J. (1981) Problems of the immediate post-anaesthesia period. *British Journal of Hospital Medicine*, 25, 159–63.

Association of Anaesthetists of Great Britain and Ireland (1985) *Post-Anaesthetic Recovery Facilities – Working Party Recommendations*.

Bales, R. (1988) Hypothermia, a postoperative problem that's easy to miss. *Registered Nurse*, 51(4), 42–3.

Bowers Feldman, M. E. (1988) Inadvertent hypothermia, a threat to homeostasis in the postanaesthetic patient. *Journal of Postanaesthetic Nursing*, 3(2), 82–7.

Campbell, D. & Spence, A. A. (1990) *Norris and Campbell's Anaesthetics, Resuscitation and Intensive Care*, 7th edn. Churchill Livingstone, Edinburgh.

Crayne, H. E. *et al.* (1988) Thermoresuscitation for postoperative hypothermia using reflective blankets. *AORN Journal*, 47(1), 222–3, 226–7.

Drummond, G. B. (1991) Keep a clear airway. *British Journal of Anaesthesia*, 66, 153–66.

Eltringham, R. (1979) Complications in the recovery room. *Journal of the Royal Society of Medicine*, 72, 278–80.

Eltringham, R. *et al.* (1989) *Post-Anaesthetic Recovery: A Practical Approach*, 2nd edn. Springer-Verlag, Berlin.

Fallacaro, M. *et al.* (1986) Inadvertent hypothermia – etiology, effects and preparation. *AORN Journal*, 44(1), 54–61.

Farman, J. V. (1978) The work of the recovery room. *British Journal of Hospital Medicine*, 19, 606–16.

Farman, J. V. (1979) Do we need recovery rooms? *Journal of the Royal Society of Medicine*, 72, 270–2.

Grant, J.S. & Mackenzie, N. (1985) Recovery following propofol ('Diprivan') anaesthesia. A review of three different anaesthetic techniques. *Postgraduate Medical Journal*, 61(3), 133–7.

Guedel, A. E. (1937) *Inhalation Anaesthesia: A Fundamental Guide*. Macmillan, New York.

Hudson, R. B. S. (1979) Pattern of work in the recovery room. *Journal of the Royal Society of Medicine*, 72, 273–5.

Lambrechts, W. & Parkhouse, J. (1961) *British Journal of Anaesthesia*, 33, 397.

Levinson, B. W. (1965) *British Journal of Anaesthesia*, 37, 544.

Lunn, J. N. (1982) *Lecture Notes on Anaesthetics*, 2nd edn. Blackwell Scientific Publications, Oxford.

Mallett, J. (1990) Communication between nurses and post-anaesthetic patients. *Intensive Care Nursing*, 6, 45–53.

Nimmo, W. S. *et al.* (eds) (1994) *Anaesthesia*, 2nd edn. Blackwell Science, Oxford.

White, H. E. *et al.* (1987) Body temperature in elderly surgical patients. *Research in Nursing and Health*, 10(5), 317–21.

GUIDELINES: POST-ANAESTHETIC RECOVERY

EQUIPMENT

1 Theatre trolley bed, which must incorporate the following features:
   (a) Oxygen supply.
   (b) Trendelenburg tilt mechanism.
   (c) Adjustable cot sides.
   (d) Adjustable back rest.
   (e) Brakes.
   (f) Radio translucency.
2 Basic equipment required for each patient:
   (a) Oxygen supply, preferably wall mounted with tubing, facemasks (with both fixed and variable settings), a T-piece system and full range of oropharyngeal and nasopharyngeal airways.
   (b) Suction – regulatable with tubing, and a range of nozzles and catheters.

Note: spare oxygen cylinders with flowmeters and an electrically powered portable suction machine should always be available in case of pipeline failure.

   (c) Sphygmomanometer and stethoscope. Automatic blood pressure recorders are a valuable means of saving time and of minimizing disturbance to patients, especially those in pain or disorientated, and leaving the nurse's hands free to attend to other needs. However, such equipment can be nonfunctioning in certain cases, e.g. shivering or profoundly bradycardic patients, and is subject to electrical and mechanical failure.

(d) Pulse oximeter, whenever possible.

(e) Miscellaneous items: receivers, tissues, disposable gloves, sharps container and waste receptacle.

3 Essential equipment centrally available for respiratory and cardiovascular support:

(a) Self-inflating resuscitator bag, e.g. Ambu bag and/or Mapleson C circuit with facemask.

(b) Full intubation equipment: laryngoscopes with spare bulbs and batteries, range of endotracheal tubes, bougies and Magill's forceps, syringe and catheter mount.

(c) Anaesthetic machine and ventilator.

(d) Wright respirometer.

(e) Cricothyroid puncture set.

(f) Range of tracheotomy tubes and tracheal dilator.

(g) Intravenous infusion sets and cannulae, range of intravenous fluids.

(h) Central venous cannulae and manometer.

(i) Emergency drug box – contents in accordance with current hospital policy.

(j) Defibrillator.

4 Standard equipment for routine nursing procedures.

PROCEDURE

The following recommended actions are not necessarily listed in order of priority. Many will be carried out simultaneously and much will depend on the patient's condition, surgery and level of consciousness. All actions must be accompanied by commentary and explanation regardless of the apparent responsiveness as the sense of hearing returns before the patient's ability to respond (Lambrechts & Parkhouse, 1961; Levinson, 1965).

Action	Rationale
1 Assess the patency of the airway by feeling for movement of expired air.	To determine the presence of any respiratory depression or neuromuscular blockade. Observe chest and abdominal movement, respiratory rate, depth and pattern (Drummond, 1991).
(a) Listen for inspiration and expiration. Apply suction if indicated. Observe any use of accessory muscles of respiration and check for tracheal tug.	To ensure absence of material in the airway, i.e. blood, mucus, vomitus. To ascertain absence of laryngeal spasm.
(b) If indicated, support the chin with the neck extended.	In the unconscious patient the tongue is liable to fall back and obstruct the airway and protective reflexes are absent.
(c) Apply a facemask and administer oxygen at the rate prescribed by the anaesthetist. If an endotracheal tube or laryngeal mask is in position, check whether the cuff or mask is inflated and administer oxygen by means of a T-piece system.	To maintain adequate oxygenation. Oxygen should be administered to all patients in the recovery room (Nimmo et al., 1994).
(d) Observe skin colour and temperature. Check the colour of lips and conjunctiva, then peripheral colour and perfusion.	Central cyanosis indicates impaired gaseous exchange between the alveoli and pulmonary capillaries. Peripheral cyanosis indicates low cardiac output (Nimmo et al., 1994).
2 Feel the pulse. The patient's position will probably mean that the head, carotid, facial or temporal arteries will offer the easiest access. Note the rate, rhythm and volume and record.	To assess cardiovascular function and establish a postoperative baseline for future observations.
3 Obtain full information about anaesthetic technique, potential problems and the patient's general medical condition.	To plan subsequent treatment.

Guidelines: Post-anaesthetic recovery (cont'd)

Action

4 Obtain full information about the surgical procedure and any drains, packs, blood loss and specific postoperative instructions.

Rationale

To ensure intervention is based on informed observation.

Note: the information gained from points 3 and 4 will be recorded on the anaesthetic chart and the nursing care document (Fig. 32.1), but an initial verbal handover will ensure that there is no delay in providing care that may be needed before all relevant information can be gathered from documentation.

5 Take and record blood pressure on reception and at a minimum of 5-minute intervals. Record the pulse and respiratory rate at the same interval unless patient's condition dictates otherwise.

To enable any fluctuations or gross abnormalities in observations to be established quickly. Accurate records are of medico-legal importance in the event of an enquiry.

6 Hypothermia. Check the temperature of the patient, especially those who are at high risk of hypothermia, e.g. the elderly, children, those who have undergone long surgery or where large amounts of blood or fluid replacement therapy have been used. Check patients who are shivering, restless, confused or with respiratory depression (hypothermia interferes with the effective reversal of muscle relaxants: Bowers Feldman, 1988). Use 'space' (reflective) blankets and warm blankets to warm the patient.

More than 90% of patients undergoing surgery experience some degree of postoperative hypothermia (Fallaccaro *et al.*, 1986; White *et al.*, 1987).
The symptoms of hypothermia can mimic those of other postoperative complications, which may result in inappropriate treatment. Some of the symptoms such as shivering, put an increased demand on cardiopulmonary systems as oxygen consumption is increased (Bowers Feldman, 1988). Other complications such as arrhythmias or myocardial infarct can result (Bales, 1988), and the longer the duration of the postoperative hypothermia, the greater the patient mortality (Crayne *et al.*, 1988).

7 Check wound site(s) and observe dressings and any drains. Note and record drainage.

To be aware of any changes or bleeding and take appropriate action, e.g. inform the surgeon.

8 Ensure any intravenous infusions are running at the prescribed rate. Check the prescription chart for any medications prescribed for administration during the immediate postoperative period.

To ensure correct treatment given.

9 Remain with the patient at all times. Assess level of consciousness during reversing stages of anaesthesia, observing for returning reflexes, i.e. swallowing, tear secretion and eyelash and lid reflexes and response to stimuli – both physical (*not* painful) and verbal (do not shout).

To ascertain progress towards normal function.

10 Orientate the patient to time and place as frequently as is necessary.

To alleviate anxiety, provide reassurance, gain the patient's confidence and cooperation. Pre-medication and anaesthesia can induce a degree of amnesia and disorientation.

11 Suction of the upper airway is indicated if gurgling sounds are present on respiration and if blood secretions or vomitus are evident or suspected, and the patient is unable to swallow or

Foreign matter can obstruct the airway or cause laryngeal spasm in light planes of anaesthesia. It can also be inhaled when protective laryngeal reflexes are absent. Vagal stimulation can induce

cough either at all or adequately. Suction must be applied with care to avoid damage to mucosal surfaces and further irritation or initiation of a gag reflex or laryngeal spasm.

bradycardia in susceptible patients (Atkinson *et al.*, 1982, p. 819).

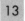 **12** Endotracheal suction is performed following the same procedure as that for suction of tracheostomy tubes. (For further information see the procedure on mouth care, Chapter 26).

To maintain the patency of the tube and remove secretions.

13 Give mouth care. (For further information, see Guidelines: Mouth care, Chapter 26.)

Pre-operative fasting, drying gases and manipulation of lips, etc. leave mucosa vulnerable, sore and foul tasting.

14 After regional and/or spinal anaesthesia, assess the return of sensation and mobility of limbs. Check that the limbs are anatomically aligned.

To prevent inadvertent injury following sensory loss.

NURSING CARE PLAN

Note: no observation of cardiovascular function is informative when taken in isolation. Full assessment must be made of respiratory function in conjunction with observations of pulse, blood pressure, emotional state and significant medical history.

Problem	Cause	Suggested action
Airway obstruction.	Tongue occluding the airway.	Support chin forward from the angle of the jaw. If necessary insert a Guedel airway. Use a nasopharyngeal airway if the teeth are clenched or crowned. Apply suction.
	Foreign material, blood, secretions, vomitus.	Always check for the presence of throat pack.
	Laryngeal spasm	Increase the rate of oxygen. Assist ventilation with an Ambu bag and facemask. If there is no improvement inform anaesthetist and have intubation equipment ready. Offer the patient reassurance.
Hypoventilation.	Respiratory depression from opiates, inhalations, agents, barbiturates.	Inform the anaesthetist and have available naloxone (opiate antagonist and doxapram) (respiratory stimulant) *Note*: if naxolone is given it can reverse the analgesic effects of opiates and has a duration of action of only 20–30 minutes. The patient must be observed for signs of returning

Nursing care plan (cont'd)

Problem	Cause	Suggested action
		hypoventilation (Nimmo *et al.*, 1994).
	Decreased respiratory drive from a low partial pressure of carbon dioxide ($PaCO_2$), loss of hypoxic drive in patients with chronic pulmonary disease.	With chronic pulmonary disease, give oxygen using, e.g., a Venturi mask with graded low concentrations (Atkinson *et al.*, 1982).
	Neuromuscular blockade from continued action of non-depolarizing muscle relaxants, potentiation of relaxants caused by electrolyte imbalance, imparied excretion with renal or liver disease.	Inform the anaesthetist, have available neostigmine and glycopyrolate, or atropine potassium chloride and 10% calcium chloride.
		Often the degree of blockade is mild and will wear off in minutes without treatment, but it is extremely frightening and patients will need continuous reassurance that their condition is not unnoticed and is resolving and that they will not be left alone.
Hypotension.	Hypovolaemia.	Take central venous pressure (CVP) readings if catheter is in place. Give oxygen. Lower the head of the trolley unless contraindicated, e.g. hiatus hernia, gross obesity. Check the record of anaesthetic agents used which might cause hypotension, e.g. enflurane, halothane, beta-blockers, nitroprusside, opiates, droperidol, sympathetic blockade following spinal anaesthesia. Check the peripheral perfusion. If the CVP is low increase intravenous infusion unless contraindicated, e.g. congestive cardiac failure. Check drains and dressings for visible bleeding and haematomata. Inform the anaesthetist or surgeon.
Hypertension.	Pain, carbon dioxide retention.	Treat pain with prescribed analgesia. Pain from certain operation sites can also be alleviated by changing the patient's position.

	Distended bladder. Some anaesthetic drugs.	Offer a bedpan or urinal. Check the prescription chart for those patients on regular antihypertensive therapy. If the situation is not resolved inform the anaesthetist.
Bradycardia.	Very fit patient, opiates, reversal agents, beta-blockers, pain, vagal stimulation, hypoxaemia from respiratory depression.	Check the prescription chart and anaesthetic sheet. Connect the patient to the ECG monitor to exclude heart block. Inform the anaesthetist.
Tachycardia.	Pain, hypovolaemia, some anaesthetic drugs, septicaemia, fear, fluid overload.	Provide analgesia. Check the anaesthetic chart. Connect the patient to the ECG monitor to exclude ventricular tachycardia.
Pain.	Surgical trauma, worsened by fear, anxiety and restlessness.	Provide prescribed analgesia and assess its efficacy. Reassure and orientate the patients who can be unaware that surgery has been performed, in which case their pain is more frightening. Try positional changes where feasible, e.g. experience has shown that after breast surgery some relief can be obtained from raising the back support by 20–40°; patients with abdominal or gynaecological surgery can be more comfortable lying on their side; elevate limbs to reduce swelling where appropriate. Unless significant relief is obtained, inform the anaesthetist.
Nausea and vomiting.	Opiates, hypotension, abdominal surgery, pain; some patients are prone to vomiting.	Offer anti-emetics if the patient is conscious. Encourage slow, regular breathing. If the patient is unconscious, turn onto the side, tip the head down and suck out pharynx, give oxygen. Note: have wire-cutters available if the jaws are wired.
Hypothermia.	Depression of the heat-regulating centre, vasodilatation, following abdominal surgery, large infusions of blood and fluids.	Use extra blankets or a 'space blanket'. Monitor the patient's temperature.
Shivering.	Some inhalational anaesthetics, especially halothane, hypothermia.	Give oxygen, reassure the patient and take patient's temperature.

Nursing care plan (cont'd)

Problem	Cause	Suggested action
Hyperthermia.	Infection, blood transfusion reaction. Malignant hyperpyrexia.	Give oxygen, use a fan or tepid sponging if this is warranted. Medical assessment of antibiotic therapy. Malignant hyperpyrexia is a medical emergency and a malignant hyperpyrexia pack with the necessary drugs should be readily available.
Oliguria.	Mechanical obstruction of catheter, e.g. clots, kinking. Inadequate renal perfusion, e.g. hypotension, systolic pressures under 60 mm Hg, hypovolaemia, dehydration. Renal damage, e.g. from blood transfusion, infection, drugs, surgical damage to the ureters.	Check the patency of the catheter. Take blood pressure and CVP if available. Increase intravenous fluids. Inform the anaesthetist. Refer to the anaesthetist or surgeon.

GUIDELINES: POST-OPERATIVE RECOVERY

PROCEDURE

After discharge from the recovery room to the ward, the nursing care given during the post-operative period is directed towards the prevention of those potential complications resulting from surgery and anaesthesia which might be anticipated to develop over a longer period of time.

Consideration of the psychological and emotional aspects of recovery will of necessity be altered by the changed state of consciousness, awareness and knowledge of patients and their differing responses to surgery, diagnosis and treatment.

Potential respiratory complications

Action	Rationale
1 Observe respirations, noting rate and depth and any presence of dyspnoea or orthopnoea. (a) Observe chest movement for equal, bilateral expansion. (b) Observe colour and perfusion. (c) Position the patient to facilitate optimum lung expansion and reinforce pre-operative teaching of deep breathing exercises and coughing.	Respiratory function post-operatively can be influenced by a number of factors: increased bronchial secretions from inhalation anaesthesia; decreased respiratory effort from opiate medication; pain or anticipation of pain from surgical wounds; surgical trauma to the phrenic nerve; pneumothorax as a result of surgical or anaesthetic procedures. All factors limiting the adequate expansion of the lung and the ejection of bronchial secretions will encourage the development of atelectasis and consolidation of the affected lung tissue.
2 Change position of patients on bedrest every 2–3 hours.	

3 Provide adequate prescribed analgesia.

Patients in pain are more likely to be disorientated and show signs of high blood pressure and tachycardia (Nimmo *et al.*, 1993).

4 Record temperature and pulse. If sputum produced observe nature and quantity for culture.

If infection follows there may be a rise in temperature, pulse and respiratory rate.

Potential circulatory problems

Deep venous thrombosis and pulmonary embolus

Action

1 Encourage early mobilization where patient's condition allows. For patients on bedrest, encourage deep breathing and exercises of the leg – flexion/extension and rotation of the ankles.

Rationale

Patients are at increased risk of developing deep venous thrombosis as a result of muscular inactivity, postoperative respiratory and circulatory depression, abdominal and pelvic surgery, prolonged pressure on calves from lithotomy poles, etc., increased production of thromboplastin as a result of surgical trauma, pre-existing coronary artery disease.

2 Where worn, ensure that antiembolic stockings are of the correct size and fit smoothly.

3 Advise against crossing of legs or ankles.

4 Record temperature.

5 Report any complaints of calf of thigh pain to medical staff.

6 Observe for any dyspnoea, chest pain or signs of shock.

Haemorrhage

Action

1 Observe dressings, drains and wound sites; and quantity and nature of drainage. Observe pulse, blood pressure, respirations and colour.

2 Observe wound for redness, tenderness and increased temperature.

Rationale

Early haemorrhage may occur as the patient's blood pressure rises. Record post-operatively re-establishing blood flow or blood as a result of the slipping of a ligature or the dislodging of a clot.

Secondary haemorrhage may occur after a period of days as a result of infection and sloughing.

Potential fluid and electrolyte imbalance and malnutrition

Action

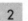
1 Maintain accurate records of intravenous infusions, oral fluids, wound and stoma drainage, nasogastric drainage, vomitus, urine and urological irrigation.

Rationale

Pre-operative fasting and dehydration, increased secretion of antidiuretic hormone, blood loss and paralytic ileus all contribute to potential fluid and electrolyte imbalance.

Guidelines: Post-operative recovery (cont'd)

Action	Rationale
	Vomiting and stasis of intestinal fluid may lead to potassium depletion.
2 Observe nature and quantity of all drainage, aspirate, faeces, etc.	
3 Give prescribed antiemetics if nausea or vomiting occur.	
4 Observe state of mouth for coating, furring and dryness.	
5 Encourage oral fluids as soon the patient is able to take them unless the nature of the surgery contraindicates this.	
6 Encourage early resumption of diet.	Return to an adequate nutritional state is necessary for wound healing (see Chapter 48, Wound Management); it is particularly important that diabetic patients should return to their pre-operative insulin/diet regime to avoid increased risk of metabolic disturbance.

Potential problem of pain

Action	Rationale
1 Observe the patient, noting physiological signs indicative of pain, e.g. sweating, tachycardia, hypotension, pallor or flushed appearance.	
2 Note restlessness, immobility and facial expressions.	Continuous severe pain can cause restlessness, anxiety, insomnia and anorexia, and may thus interfere with recovery by impeding deep breathing, mobilization and nutrition.
3 Listen to the patient and ascertain the location and nature of the pain.	Communication skills are necessary for the effective assessment and alleviation of pain as there may be multiple contributory factors, both physical and emotional in origin.
4 Administer prescribed analgesia and observe effect.	
5 Try changing position of patient. Give attention, information and reassurance; assist with relaxation exercises.	

CHAPTER 33

Peritoneal Dialysis and Continuous Venovenous Haemodiafiltration

Definition

Dialytic therapies are procedures used for patients with inadequate renal function who are unable to rid the body of waste products such as urea. To effect dialysis an alternative membrane or filter is used. In the case of peritoneal dialysis it is the peritoneal membrane itself that is used. In all other forms of dialysis an artificial filter is used. Dialytic therapies may be instituted when there is an acute problem with renal function and can also be used in the chronic situation if renal transplantation is not possible.

Dialysis is possible because of the properties of substances which permit diffusion, osmosis and convection. Diffusion is the force acting on gaseous, solid or liquid molecules to spread them from a region of high concentration to a region of lower concentration. Osmosis is the passage of a solvent through a semi-permeable membrane that separates solutions of different concentrations. The force that causes this movement of solvents is osmotic pressure and this varies directly with the concentration of the solution. As the solvent moves across the membrane, it tends to pull certain amounts of solute with it. This is known as the solvent drag effect. Equilibration is the achievement of equalization of solute and solvent concentrations on both sides of the membrane. As equilibration is achieved, dialysis ceases and solvents and solutes can be absorbed back into the bloodstream (Fig. 33.1).

Convection is the use of hydrostatic pressure to force water and solutes through a semi-permeable membrane.

Types of dialytic therapies

There are several dialytic therapies available:

- Haemodialysis;
- Peritoneal dialysis;
- Continuous venovenous haemodiafiltration;
- Ultrafiltration.

The choice of procedure is determined by patient suitability, resources and manpower implications.

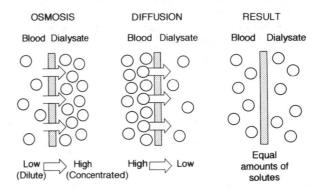

Figure 33.1 The process of osmosis and diffusion. (From *Nursing Times*, 22 April 1987, p. 41, with permission.)

If the patient has chronic renal failure the optimum procedure is haemodialysis. This is usually performed 2–3 times a week either in the patient's home or in the chronic dialysis unit. Many patients and their families learn this technique. Haemodialysis is also used in the acute setting if patients are hypercatabolic and other therapies are not appropriate (Ahmad *et al.*, 1988).

Peritoneal dialysis and the continuous slow filtration therapies are both performed outside specialist renal centres and will therefore be discussed in greater detail.

PERITONEAL DIALYSIS (PD)

Indications

Peritoneal dialysis may be selected for the following reasons (Oh, 1995):

(1) Widespread availability;
(2) Technical simplicity;
(3) Patients may remain ambulant;
(4) Low maintenance costs.

REFERENCE MATERIAL

In 1926 Rosenak, basing his work on that of Ganter, conceived the possibility of using the peritoneum of humans as a dialysing membrane (Blumenkrantz & Roberts, 1979). The use of peritoneal dialysis reached a peak in 1959 with the introduction of commercial dialysis solutions and tubing. In the 1960s advances in peritoneal dialysis were being made by Tenckhoff (Warren, 1989), and long-term access now became a reality. At this time the technique of haemodialysis was introduced and the two treatments are now used widely (Warren, 1989).

Anatomy and physiology

The peritoneum is the largest serous membrane of the body. In adults it has a surface area of approximately 2.2 m². It is a closed unit consisting of two parts:

(1) The parietal peritoneum that lines the inside of the abdominal wall.
(2) The visceral peritoneum that is reflected over the viscera.

The space between the two parts is the peritoneal cavity. This cavity is normally a potential space containing only a small amount of serous fluid. The serous fluid lubricates the viscera and allows them to move freely upon one another and the parietal peritoneum (Marieb, 1989).

The visceral peritoneum consists of five layers of fibrous and elastic connective tissue and a sixth layer called the mesothelium. Blood and lymphatic capillaries are found only in the deepest layer of tissue in adults. A substance that passes from the bloodstream into the peritoneal cavity must pass through the capillary endothelium, the mesothelium and the five layers of the visceral peritoneum. The mesothelium represents the major barrier to mass transfer for most substances (Marieb, 1989).

For peritoneal dialysis to achieve maximum effectiveness, fresh solutions must be instilled at the point of equilibration to prevent reabsorption of water and uraemic toxins (Smith, 1980). It should be noted that solvent drag enhances the efficiency of peritoneal dialysis.

Solution concentrations

The osmotic pressure of dextrose is utilized in peritoneal dialysis to remove water and solids from the patient. The composition of most commercially available peritoneal dialysis solutions falls into the following three groups:

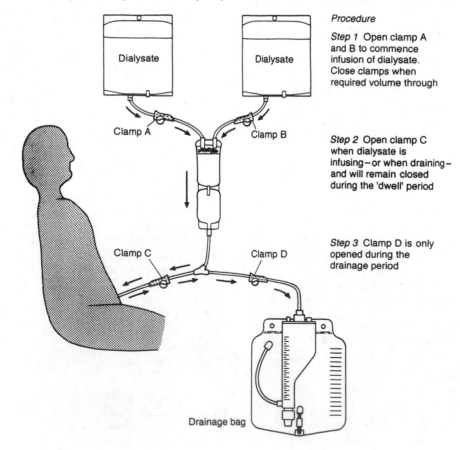

Procedure

Step 1 Open clamp A and B to commence infusion of dialysate. Close clamps when required volume through

Step 2 Open clamp C when dialysate is infusing – or when draining – and will remain closed during the 'dwell' period

Step 3 Clamp D is only opened during the drainage period

Figure 33.2   Using the Y-type administration set.

(1) The solution's electrolyte composition approximates normal extracellular fluid, i.e. its potassium concentration is 4 mmol/l and its glucose concentration is 1.3–1.5%.
(2) As solution 1, but contains no potassium.
(3) Hypertonic solution with a glucose concentration of 6.3% and the same potassium concentration as solution 1.

The choice of dialysate solution will depend on the primary aim of dialysis and the patient's baseline plasma electrolyte levels (Bloe, 1990).

Dialysis cycle
Normally, a cycle consists of three stages (Fig. 33.2).

Stage 1 (inflow)
The dialysis solution at body temperature is infused into the peritoneal cavity to initiate the dialysis. The fluid infuses by gravity and its rate can be controlled by raising or lowering the container in relation to the patient's abdomen or by releasing or compressing the occluding clamp on the tubing.

Stage 2 (dwell time)
The dwell time is the time that the fluid remains in the peritoneal cavity to allow for equilibration. Different dwell times may be established to remove substances of differing molecular weights. The dwell time is relevant to the type of solute and the amount of solute removed.

Stage 3 (drainage)
The drainage stage is that of emptying the equilibrated solution from the peritoneal cavity to complete dialysis or to prepare for the infusion of fresh solution. Drainage is also dependent on gravity.

Types of peritoneal dialysis

Intermittent
For peritoneal dialysis used in the acute situation, a manual system is usually used to effect a quick and gentle dialysis (Fig. 33.3). Optimal dialysis is achieved with short dialysis cycles of about one hour each, with a dwell time of 30 minutes and drainage time of 20 minutes. Specific numbers of exchanges are prescribed and dialysis is then discontinued temporarily, with initiation recurring as uraemia increases (Bloe, 1990).

Continuous ambulatory peritoneal dialysis (CAPD)
The CAPD technique was first introduced in 1975. It is a closed, continuous system of peritoneal dialysis and allows the patient the independence of a life free from dialysis machines. The regime practised is usually four

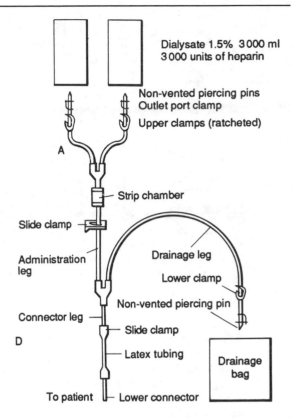

Figure 33.3 Peritoneal dialysis system set-up (courtesy of Abbott Renal Care).

exchanges per day with the last staying in the peritoneal cavity overnight. Many devices have been developed to assist patients in their own homes to cope with the treatment while remaining free from the danger of infection and peritonitis (Warren, 1989).

Clear outlines of CAPD can be found in Ainge (1981), Arenz (1982), Sorrels (1981), Stansfield (1985) and Zappacosta & Perras (1984).

CONTINUOUS FILTRATION METHODS

Definition
These methods mimic the filtration that would occur in the glomerulus of the kidney. Water and solutes are forcibly moved from the plasma through a semipermeable membrane. Membranes are synthetic and vary in terms of the size of molecular solutes they filter out. Selection of the filter depends on the clinical situation. Continuous filtration therapies involve the production of large volumes of filtrate (300–800 ml/hour). This output must be balanced by the administration of electrolyte solutions (Oh, 1995).

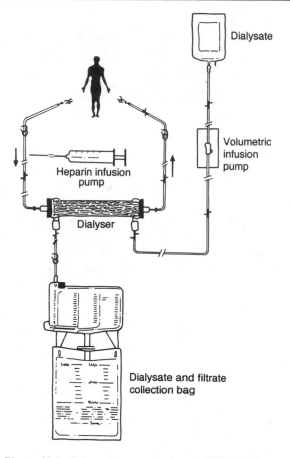

Figure 33.4 Schematic representation of CVVHD. (Reproduced by permission of Fresenius Haemodialysis Systems.)

REFERENCE MATERIAL

The use of continuous filtration methods has increased significantly since the late 1980s with advances in technology and the training of critical care nurses. These methods are used in particular in high dependency or intensive therapy settings because of their ability to provide excellent clearance of solutes and fluid whilst avoiding haemodynamic instability that can result from conventional haemodialysis (Tinker & Zapol, 1992). Several methods are available, including:

- Ultrafiltration (UF);
- Slow continuous ultrafiltration (SCUF);
- Continuous arterio–venous ultrafiltration (CAVH);
- Continuous venovenous haemodiafiltration (CVVHD).

CVVHD is the therapy with the widest application to a variety of clinical situations and is therefore examined in greater detail here.

CVVHD

Continuous venovenous haemodiafiltration combines convection and diffusion. The convection of ultrafiltration utilizes a large hydrostatic pressure gradient which means that up to 2 litres of water an hour can be removed from the plasma via the filter (Hakim & Lazarus, 1986). Diffusion of the solutes (i.e. urea, creatinine and potassium) is achieved by blood flow through the filter whilst dialysate is administered in a counter current using an infusion device.

In CVVHD the 'artificial kidney' used ensures effective clearance of solutes with small and middle-sized molecular weights (Hakim & Lazarus, 1986). Because blood flows through an extra-corporeal circuit and over a filter there is a danger of blood clots forming in the patient circuit. An anticoagulant is therefore administered continuously. For a diagrammatic representation of the circuit, see Fig. 33.4.

References and further reading

Ahmad, S. *et al.* (1988) Center and home chronic hemodialysis. In: *Diseases of the Kidney*, (eds R. W. Scrier & C. W. Gottschalk). Little, Brown & Co, Boston.

Ainge, T. M. (1981) Continuous ambulatory peritoneal dialysis. *Nursing Times*, 77, 1636–8.

Arenz, R. (1982) Continuous ambulatory peritoneal dialysis. *AORN Journal*, 35(5), 946, 948, 950, 952, 954.

Bloe, C. G. (1990) Peritoneal dialysis. *Professional Nurse*, April, 5(7), 345–9.

Blumenkrantz, M. J. & Roberts, M. (1979) Progress in peritoneal dialysis: an historical prospective. *Contrib. Nephrology*, 17, 101–10.

Brunner, L. S. & Suddarth, D. S. (1982) *The Lippincott Manual of Medical–Surgical Nursing*, Vol. 3, pp. 253–8. Harper & Row, London.

Hakim, R. M. & Lazarus, J. M. (1986) Medical aspects of hemodialysis. In: *The Kidney*, (eds B. M. Brenner & F. C. Rector). W. B. Saunders, Philadelphia.

Marieb, E. N. (1989) *Human Anatomy and Physiology*, Benjamin Cummings, California.

Nursing (US) (1982) Fear of floating to a renal unit: nurses guide to peritoneal dialysis complications. *Nursing*, 12, 42–3.

Oh, T. E. (1995) *Intensive Care Manual*. Butterworth, Sydney.

Smith, K. (1980) *Fluids and Electrolytes: A Conceptual Approach*. Churchill Livingstone, Edinburgh.

Sorrels, A. J. (1981) Peritoneal dialysis: a rediscovery. *Nursing Clinics of North America*, 16(3), 515–29.

Stansfield, G. (1985) Coping with CAPD. *Nursing Mirror*, 161(14), 28–9.

Tinker, J. & Zapol, W. (1992) *Care of the Critically Ill Patient*. Springer Verlag, London.

Warren, H. (1989) Changes in peritoneal dialysis nursing. *ANNA Journal*, 16(3), 237–41.

Zappacosta, A. & Perras, S. (1984) *CAPD*. J. B. Lippincott, Philadelphia.

GUIDELINES: PERITONEAL DIALYSIS

EQUIPMENT

1 Dialysis Y type administration set and drainage bag.
2 Sterile peritoneal set containing forceps, blade and holder, topical swabs, towels, suturing equipment.
3 Sterile gown, gloves.
4 Peritoneal catheter stylet or trocar and drainage bag.
5 Local anaesthetic – 1 to 2% lignocaine hydrochloride.
6 Syringe, needle.
7 Chlorhexidine in 70% isopropyl alcohol.
8 Supplementary drugs as prescribed.
9 Peritoneal dialysis fluid, as prescribed, warmed to 37°C.

PROCEDURE

Action	Rationale

1 Explain and discuss the procedure with the patient. An acutely ill patient may be confused and restless but every effort should be made to inform patient of what is about to happen.

To ensure that the patient understands the procedure and gives his/her valid consent. Some hospitals require a patient to sign a consent form before the procedure can be carried out.

2 Ask the patient to micturate and defaecate before the procedure begins.

To avoid perforation of the bladder and/or rectum when the trocar is introduced into the peritoneum.

3 Record the patient's vital signs before the procedure begins.

To assess physical/psychological state and to monitor changes.

4 Weigh the patient before the procedure begins and then daily.

To assess hydration and to monitor any fluid losses.

5 Assist the patient to lie in the semi-recumbent position.

To ensure that the patient is in the best position for the procedure's requirements.

6 Continue to observe and reassure the patient throughout the procedure.

To assess and monitor any physical/psychological changes.

7 Assist the doctor as required.

To facilitate a smooth and effective procedure for the patient.

Insertion of catheter

Action	Rationale

1 Using aseptic technique, the doctor prepares the abdomen surgically and injects the skin and subcutaneous tissues with a local anaesthetic.

To reduce the risk of contamination and infection. To minimize the pain of the incision.

2 A small incision is made in the abdominal wall 3 to 5 cm below the umbilicus. The trocar is inserted through the incision. The patient is asked to raise the head from the pillow after the trocar is introduced.

This tightens the abdominal muscles and permits easier penetration of the trocar without danger of injury to the internal organs.

3 When the peritoneum is punctured, the trocar is directed to the left side of the pelvis. The

To prevent the omentum from adhering to the catheter or occluding its opening.

Guidelines: Peritoneal dialysis (cont'd)

Action	Rationale
stylet is removed and the catheter is inserted through the trocar and gently manoeuvred into position.	
 4 Once the trocar is removed, the skin may be sutured and a sterile dressing placed around the catheter.	To prevent the loss of the catheter in the abdomen. To prevent leakage of peritoneal fluid onto the surrounding skin.
5 The tubing is flushed with the dialysis fluid.	To prevent air from entering the peritoneal cavity.

Preparation of dialysis fluid

Action	Rationale
1 Wash hands with bactericidal soap and water or bactericidal alcohol hand rub. Proceed using aseptic technique.	To reduce risk of infection.
2 The dialysis fluid should have been warmed to body temperature (37°C).	For the patient's comfort. To prevent abdominal pain. Heating causes dilation of the peritoneal vessels and increases clearance of urea. Cold fluid would decrease rate of removal of large molecular solutes and can cause abdominal cramp pain.
3 Add any drugs, e.g. heparin, to the dialysis fluid if prescribed.	Heparin prevents fibrin clots from occluding the catheter.
4 Attach the dialysis fluid to the giving set via luer lock connections.	
5 Attach the catheter connector to the giving set.	
6 Allow the dialysis fluid to flow freely into the peritoneal cavity. (This normally takes from 5–10 minutes.)	To ascertain whether the catheter is in the required position. The flow should be steady and brisk. If not, the tip of the catheter may be buried in the omentum or it may have been occluded by a blood clot.
7 Allow fluid to remain in the peritoneal cavity for the prescribed time. Prepare the next exchange while the first container of fluid is in the peritoneal cavity.	The fluid must remain in the peritoneal cavity for the prescribed dwell time so that potassium, urea and other waste products may be removed. The solution is most effective over the first 5–10 minutes when the concentration gradient is at its greatest (Tinker & Zapol, 1992).
8 Unclamp the drainage tube. Drainage time will vary with each patient but, on average, should be completed in 10 minutes.	To rid the body of the required products. The abdomen is drained by a siphon effect through the closed system. Drainage is normally straw coloured.
9 Clamp off the drainage tube when outflow ceases and begin infusing the next exchange, again using aseptic technique.	To enable the next cycle to begin. To reduce the risk of local and/or systemic infection.

10 Record the following:
(a) Time of commencement and completion of each exchange and the start and finish of the drainage stage
(b) Amount of fluid infused and recovered
(c) Fluid balance after each complete exchange
(d) Any medication added to the dialysis fluid.

To detect and monitor trends and fluctuations and to identify any outflow obstruction.

11 Take and record the vital signs:
(a) Blood pressure and pulse every 15 minutes during the first exchange and hourly thereafter, depending on the patient's condition.

Hypotension may be indicative of excessive fluid loss due to the glucose concentration of the dialysis fluid. Changes in pulse may indicate impending shock or overhydration.

(b) Temperature every 4 hours, or more frequently if condition demands.

To monitor for any signs of infection. Infection is more likely to become evident after dialysis has been discontinued.

12 Record fluid balance accurately.

To prevent complications such as circulatory overload and hypertension that may occur if most of the fluid is not recovered during the drainage stage. The fluid balance should be about even or show slight fluid loss, unless the reason for treatment was to remove excess fluid.

13 Dialysis is usually continued until blood chemistry levels are satisfactory.

The duration of dialysis is related to the severity of the condition and the size and weight of the patient. The usual time is about 12–36 hours, giving between 24 and 28 exchanges.

14 Ensure that the patient is comfortable during dialysis by attending to pressure area care and altering the patient's position as required. Assist the patient to sit in a chair for short periods as the condition allows.

The period of dialysis is lengthy and often exhausts the patient.

15 Send a daily specimen of peritoneal fluid for microscopy and culture.

To monitor for any infections, etc.

NURSING CARE PLAN

Problem	Cause	Suggested action
Peritonitis, indicated by fever, persistent abdominal pain and cramping, abdominal fullness, abdominal rigidity, slow dialysis drainage, cloudy and offensive smelling drainage, swelling and tenderness around the catheter and increased white blood cell count.	Poor aseptic technique during catheter insertion or dialysis.	If peritonitis is suspected, notify the doctor immediately. Send a peritoneal fluid sample to the laboratory for fluid analysis, culture and sensitivity testing, Gram staining and cell count. Antibiotics may be prescribed by the doctor either locally or systemically in severe cases.

Nursing care plan (cont'd)

Problem	Cause	Suggested action
		Monitor vital signs; careful pain control is required.
Infection at the site of entry, indicated by redness, swelling, rigidity, tenderness and purulent drainage around the catheter.	Poor aseptic technique during catheter insertion or dialysis, or incomplete healing around the site of entry.	Notify a doctor. Obtain a specimen of the drainage fluid and send it to the laboratory. Antibiotics and pain control may be prescribed as above. Monitor vital signs.
Subcutaneous tunnel infection with cuffed catheter indicated by redness, rigidity and tenderness over subcutaneous tunnel.	Poor aseptic technique during catheter insertion or dialysis, or incomplete healing in subcutaneous tunnel.	Notify a doctor. Antibiotics may be prescribed as above. Monitor vital signs.
Perforation of the bladder or the bowel, indicated by signs and symptoms of peritonitis, bright yellow dialysis fluid drainage (if bladder is perforated) or faeces in drainage (if bowel is perforated).	Catheter inserted when the patient had a full bladder or bowel.	If perforation is suspected, stop dialysis and notify a doctor immediately. Monitor vital signs. Only minimal oral fluids should be given in case surgery is required.
Bleeding through the catheter.	Minor trauma to the abdomen or minor trauma to the subcutaneous tunnel (with a cuffed catheter) or perforation of a major abdominal blood vessel during surgery.	Bleeding usually stops spontaneously. If it does not, notify the doctor, who may order blood transfusions. One-litre hourly dialysis exchanges may be ordered until the drainage fluid is clear.
Dialysis fluid leaking around the catheter.	Excessive instillation of dialysis fluid or incomplete healing. Incomplete healing around the cuff of the catheter. Catheter obstruction. Catheter dislodged or positioned improperly.	Instil less dialysis fluid at exchanges. Drain the patient's abdomen completely during outflow. Use small volumes of dialysis fluid in exchanges through a new catheter. Irrigate the catheter with sterile 0.9% sodium chloride solution. Inform a doctor, who will replace the catheter or revise its position surgically.
Kinking of the cuffed catheter.	Subcutaneous tunnel too short or scarring in the subcutaneous tunnel.	Inform a doctor, who will remove the catheter and implant a new one.
Lower back pain.	Pressure and weight of dialysis fluid in the abdomen (particularly so in continuous ambulatory peritoneal dialysis (CAPD) patients).	Doctor may order analgesics. Exercises to strengthen the patient's muscles and improve posture may also be ordered.

Abdominal or rectal pain (with possible referred pain in shoulder).	Improperly positioned catheter tip causing irritation.	Catheter position to be revised surgically.
	Dialysis fluid accumulating under the diaphragm. Dialysis fluid not at 37°C. With 2 litres of 6.36% solution, severe shoulder pain can occur.	Drain the abdomen completely during outflow. Ensure that the fluid is infused at the correct temperature. If hypertonic dialysis fluid is used, only one container should be used per cycle.
	If air enters the peritoneal cavity, pain may occur.	Maintain a closed system.
Paralytic ileus indicated by sharp pain in abdomen, constipation, abdominal distension, nausea and vomiting, and diarrhoea.	Catheter manipulated excessively during insertion.	Notify the doctor immediately as signs and symptoms may indicate peritonitis. A nasogastric tube to suction the stomach may be ordered. Cholinergic medication, such as neostigmine, may be prescribed. Administer fluids and electrolytes as prescribed. If general condition allows, encourage patient to walk, unless advised otherwise by the doctor. Prepare the patient for surgery, as advised by the doctor. The condition may disappear spontaneously after 12 hours.
Cramping.	Dialysis fluid warmer or cooler than 37°C.	Adjust the temperature of the dialysis fluid to 37°C before infusion.
	Too rapid infusion or drainage.	Decrease the infusion or drainage rate to a regime the patient can tolerate.
	Pressure from excess dialysis fluid in the abdomen.	Infuse less dialysis fluid at exchanges to a total volume that the patient can tolerate.
	Chemical irritation.	Use a dialysis fluid with a dextrose concentration lower than 7%.
	Air in the abdomen.	Clamp off the dialysis tubing before the dialysis fluid empties completely into the abdomen.
Excessive fluid loss.	Use of dialysis fluid with too great a dextrose concentration for the patient or inadequate sodium intake or inadequate fluid intake.	Monitor the patient's weight and blood pressure. Ensure that the patient is receiving dialysis fluid with the correct dextrose concentration. The doctor may prescribe a reduced dextrose concentration.
Fluid overload.	Use of dialysis fluid with an osmotic pressure that is too low	Monitor the patient's weight and blood pressure. The doctor will

Nursing care plan (cont'd)

Problem	Cause	Suggested action
	for the patient or excessive sodium intake or excessive fluid intake.	order a reduced fluid and sodium intake. The doctor may also order increased use of dialysis fluid with a 4.25% dextrose concentration.
Metabolic disturbance usually affects plasma levels of glucose, potassium or sodium.	Continued use of inappropriate dialysate fluid.	Monitor relevant plasma levels pre- and post-dialysis. If patient has pre-existing diabetes mellitus or insulin deficiency, insulin dosage should be titrated carefully.
Respiratory difficulties.	Pressure from the fluid in the peritoneal cavity and upward displacement of the diaphragm or 'splinting' of the diaphragm, resulting in shallow breathing.	Elevate the head of the bed. Encourage breathing exercises and coughing. Involve the physiotherapist to establish respiratory care.

GUIDELINES: PREPARATION OF EQUIPMENT FOR CONTINUOUS VENOVENOUS HAEMODIAFILTRATION (CVVHD) UTILIZING A GAMBRO MACHINE

When using the CVVHD method of filtration, the patient access is gained by a single double-lumen catheter. This will be inserted into a central vein, usually the internal jugular, sub-clavian or femoral vein. The catheter will then be flushed with a heparinized solution and capped off ready to commence CVVHD.

EQUIPMENT

1 Fluid warming infusion device.
2 Volumetric pumps ×2.
3 CVVHD machine (Gambro).
4 Artificial kidney/filter.
5 Set of dialysate lines: 1 red, 1 blue.
6 Intravenous infusion lines ×2.
7 Y connector.
8 Fluid warming insert.
9 20-ml luer lock syringe.
10 10-ml luer lock syringe.
11 Plastic clamps ×5.
12 Gloves.
13 Chlorhexidine in 70% spirit.
14 Low-linting gauze swabs.

PROCEDURE

Action	Rationale
1 Discuss patient's condition with the multidisciplinary team and establish treatment plan.	To ensure all medical and nursing teams are aware of patient's biochemistry and haematological profiles and the plan for treatment.

2	Collect all equipment together as above.	To ensure that all the equipment is available before commencing the procedure.
3	Instill 2000 units of heparin into each litre of 0.9% sodium chloride.	To anti-coagulate lines and the filter to provide prophylactic cover against clotting in the extracorporeal circuit.
4	Lace up the machine with the two lines: one red and one blue.	To form the CVVHD circuit.
5	Connect the spiked end of the red line to one of the heparinised litres of saline and apply a plastic clamp to the line.	To be ready to commence priming the filter lines. To stop fluid infusion until the circuit is ready.
6	Attach the bell shaped end of the blue marked tubing to the nozzle on the machine situated just below the housing for bubble trap – this is the venous pressure manometer.	To ensure the venous pressure is accurately monitored.
7	Attach a 20 ml luer lock syringe to the open end of the blue line next to the bubble trap.	This will be used to draw air out or push air in to the bubble trap thus maintaining the fluid at the correct level in the bubble trap.
8	Undo the clamp on the red line that is attached to the litre of heparinized saline.	To have everything ready to commence priming the lines.
9	Turn on the blood pump to a speed of 75–100 ml per hour.	To commence circulation of heparinized saline.
10	As the fluid circulates and enters the bubble trap draw air gently out of the trap until fluid is at a level with the mark an inch below the top of the trap.	This is to ensure that there is enough fluid to allow trapping of bubbles in the circulating fluid.
11	Continue circulating fluid until there are only about 200 ml left in the litre bag. Clamp the line and stop the pump.	The circulation of the first litre will have primed the tubing and started to fill the filter and expand the fibres. The pump needs to be stopped before the end of the litre to ensure that no further air enters the circuit.
12	Attach the second heparinized litre to red spike. Undo the clamp and start the pump at a speed of 75–100 ml per hour.	To further prime the line and completely saturate the fibres in the filter.
13	As the second litre is running gently rotate the filter.	To ensure good filling and flow throughout the filter.
14	When there are about 200 ml left in the litre bag clamp the line and stop the pump. Turn off the machine.	The priming is now complete and stopping the pump before the bag is completed prevents air entering the circuit.
15	Disconnect the red spiked end from the litre bag and attach to the small blue patient end of the dialysate lines.	To prepare the patient circuit.
16	Attach the dialysate fluid via the fluid warmer to the now free port on the filter.	To provide access for the warmed dialysate fluid into the filter to achieve movement of solutes.
17	Decide on anti-coagulant regime and if appropriate attach anticoagulant syringe to the free line on the red side and feed through the dedicated heparin pump.	To ensure delivery of anticoagulant as prophylaxis against the circuit or filter clotting and blocking.

Guidelines: Preparation of equipment for CVVHD utilizing a Gambro machine (cont'd)

Action   **Rationale**

18 The system is now ready to use.

GUIDELINES: COMMENCEMENT OF CVVHD

PROCEDURE

Action   **Rationale**

1   Explain and discuss the procedure with the   To ensure that the patient understands the
    patient and his/her family.   procedure and gives his/her valid consent.

2   Ensure that all information concerning   To have a baseline from which to work and to
    patient's blood biochemistry, full blood count monitor any change in the patient.
    and clotting profile are available.

3   Ensure that the patient's mean arterial   During the first 2 hours of CVVHD there is usually
    pressure is above 60 mmHg or that   a large fluid drainage which can result in a sudden
    physician's guidelines have been provided.   drop in the blood pressure.

4   Ensure that baseline recordings of weight,   To have a baseline from which to work and to
    temperature, heart rate, blood pressure,   monitor any change in the patient.
    respiratory rate, tissue oxygen saturation (SaO_2)
    and central venous pressure (CVP) have been
    recorded.

5   Ensure that the patient is attached to a   CVVHD can cause cardiac instability although this
    haemodynamic monitor.   is rare (Oh, 1995).

6   Ensure that a treatment programme has been   To ensure that the plan for cycling and the total
    agreed with the multidisciplinary team.   fluid removal has been discussed.

7   Prepare the appropriate fluid replacement.   There is a rapid fluid loss with CVVHD and
                                                    patients often require replacement of this loss.

8   Prepare a sterile field and apply gloves.   To reduce the risk of infection and provide
                                                    protection for the nurse.

9   Whilst keeping the patient catheter clamped   To reduce the risk of infection and to prevent
    remove the bungs from both lumens and   haemorrhage.
    clean with chlorhexidine in 70% spirit.

10 Flush each lumen with heparinized saline.   To ensure that the patient catheter is patent.

11 Apply plastic clamps to the patient ends of   To prevent air entering the lines and to reduce the
    the red and blue lines and separate from   risk of infection.
    each other. Clean with chlorhexidine in 70% spirit.

12 Connect red line to the red lumen of the   To complete patient circuit.
    catheter and blue line to the blue lumen of
    the catheter.

13 Undo catheter clamps and plastic clamp on   To ensure free flow.
    line.

14	Ensure that there are no clamps left on and that all connections are secure.	To ensure that there is no obstruction to flow and no risk of fluid leakage.
15	Turn on machine and start blood pump at 75–100 ml per hour.	To commence CVVHD at a gentle speed.
16	Observe patient, monitors and dialysis circuit carefully.	To ensure that any alteration in patient condition is noted immediately.
17	As blood circulates ensure bubble trap fluid level stays constant.	To ensure trapping of bubbles.
18	If everything is stable increase speed to appropriate level, probably between 100 and 150 ml per hour.	To ensure good filtration.
19	Observe fluid drainage. Once the colour changes from clear to straw empty the drainage bag.	To ensure correct fluid balancing.
20	Commence dialysate fluid infusion at appropriate rate usually between 1 and 2 litres per hour.	To provide the counter-current and achieve movement of solutes.
21	Continue monitoring patient – hourly heart rate, rhythm, BP, CVP, SaO_2 and respiratory rate or more frequently if required.	To ensure any change in patient condition is noted immediately and dealt with as appropriate.
22	Maintain accurate fluid balancing.	To ensure patient is protected from large positive or negative fluid shifts.
23	Send regular blood samples for biochemical analysis.	To adjust dialysate fluid and electrolyte replacement therapy as appropriate.
24	Send regular blood samples for clotting profile.	To provide appropriate anticoagulant therapy.
25	Ensure patient lines and circuit easily visible and free from obstruction.	To protect patient from sudden disconnection or obstruction to lines.
26	Review patient's condition regularly with multidisciplinary team.	To ensure optimum patient monitoring and evaluation of care to enable appropriate treatment.
27	Ensure optimum recording in documentation of venous pressure, pump speeds and drainage.	To ensure information exchange between members of nursing team.

CHAPTER 34

Personal Hygiene

Definition

The science of hygiene can be described as 'a condition or practice, such as cleanliness, that is conducive to the preservation of health' (Weller & Wells, 1990). The aspect of personal hygiene refers to 'individual measures taken to preserve one's own health' (Weller & Wells, 1990), which pertains to the person taking responsibility to meet this fundamental need. The prevention of infection is also pertinent and will be referred to within the text (see Chapter 5, Barrier Nursing).

REFERENCE MATERIAL

'Cleanliness is not a luxury in a highly developed country it is . . . a basic human right' (Young, 1991). When an individual becomes ill they may depend on others to perform this elementary intervention. If this occurs, it is important that the nurse is able to appropriately observe and assess the patient.

Hygiene is a personal entity and everyone will have their own individual requirements and standards of cleanliness. In this way 'nurses must take care not to impose their own norms on patients and clients and should respect their autonomy in decisions concerning care' (Spiller, 1992). When assessing personal considerations the patient's religious and cultural beliefs should be taken into account. Various examples of this will be given throughout the text.

In Western culture privacy is of the utmost importance and considered to be a basic human right. In some cultures modesty is crucial, e.g. for Moslems, and can cause problems in the hospital setting (Neuberger, 1987). Patients will feel a great deal of embarrassment having to depend on another person to help/assist them with this extremely private act and consideration should be given to their personal needs (Wagnild & Manning, 1985; Spiller, 1992). It is therefore surprising to find that such little reference is made to these elements in the literature. The nurse's role is 'the maintenance of an acceptable level of cleanliness' (Young, 1991) which promotes 'comfort, safety and well-being' (Heath, 1995) for the patient. Frequently the time taken to attend to personal hygiene will provide ample opportunity for communication. Wilson (1986) states

'a bedbath facilitates listening and enables the nurse to pick up cues to a patient's anxieties and fears. It provides the time and opportunity for the nurse to offer support and encouragement when difficult situations have to be confronted, solutions sought and decisions made'.

Nursing models, which provide a conceptual framework for practice, all make some reference to meeting the patient's hygiene needs. Roper *et al*. (1981) adapted Henderson's original concept of nursing (Henderson, 1966) to develop a model reflecting the activities of daily living. This model has generally been adopted for the purpose of student nurse training because of the 12 basic elements (Pearson & Vaughan, 1988). They refer to the hygiene component as 'personal cleansing and dressing'.

Another example was given by Orem (1980) who focused on the ability of the patient to self-care and refers to the universal self-care requisites of the 'condition of the skin, nails and hair' and the 'usual patterns of hygiene'. The assessment process will show if there is a 'deficit' and then an appropriate nursing intervention can result.

The assessment should allow the nurse to carry out the appropriate intervention(s) and evaluate the effectiveness of care given.

Areas of care

Skin

Maintaining the skin's integrity is essential to the prevention of infection and the promotion of health. The skin has several functions:

- Maintenance of temperature
- Protection

- Excretion and
- Sensation.

It is made up of three layers: the epidermis, dermis and the deep subcutaneous layer.

The *epidermis* is the outer coating of the skin and contains no blood vessels or nerve endings. The cells on the surface are continually being rubbed off and replaced by new cells which have arisen from deeper layers. The epidermis has hairs, sweat glands and the ducts of sebaceous glands passing through it.

The *dermis* is the thicker layer which contains blood vessels, nerve fibres, sweat and sebaceous glands and lymph vessels. It is made up of white fibrous tissue and yellow elastic fibres which given the skin its toughness and elasticity.

The *subcutaneous layer* contains the deep fat cells (areolar and adipose tissue) and provides the heat regulation factor for the body. It is also the support structure for the outer layers of the skin (Ross & Wilson, 1982).

The skin will go through many changes in the course of development, e.g. temperature, texture, elasticity, and has a great ability to adapt to changes in the environment and stimuli. Its integrity, continuity and cleanliness are essential to maintain its physiological functions.

Care of the skin

An initial assessment using observational skills is essential to ascertain the skin's general condition. Several factors may influence the appearance of the tissue.

(1) Hydration state – dehydration will cause loss of elasticity and drying of the skin. Oedema will cause stretching and thinning of the skin.
(2) The individual's age, health and mobility status (Gooch, 1989), e.g. presence of pressure ulcers (see Chapter 48, Wound Management).
(3) Treatment therapies e.g. radiotherapy (skin may become moist and cracked), chemotherapy (some cytotoxic agents such as methotrexate can cause erythematous rashes (Tierney, 1987), steroids (skin may become papery and fragile) (see Chapter 37, Sealed and Unsealed Radioactive Source Therapy and Chapter 13, Cytotoxic Drugs: Handling and Administration).
(4) Any concurrent skin conditions, e.g. eczema, psoriasis.

Frailty and the presence of pressure ulcers, redness, abrasions, cuts, papery skin and open wounds should prompt the nurse to take extra care in the bathing procedure. Involving the patient in their care plan ensures that correct and/or preferred lotions are used. For example, some people prefer not to apply soap to the facial area and others will need to use a particular soap which does not contain perfumes. Persistent use of some soaps can alter the pH of the skin, leading to drying and cracking (Gooch, 1989). In addition, patients may like to use moisturizers and this should be respected and applied accordingly. Care should be taken with skin folds and crevices, paying particular attention to thorough drying of the areas and observing for any breaks in the skin.

Frequently patients may have intravenous lines and wound drains inserted as part of their therapy and these should be handled with caution to prevent the hazards of introducing infection or of 'pulling' the tubes.

Each patient will require assessment of their individual needs (Heath, 1995) and encouragement to promote rehabilitation as appropriate. If a full blanket bath is needed then the nurse must respect the patient's privacy and comfort. A refreshing change to the original version of the bed bath was researched by Lisa Wright, a ward sister at Sheffield Hospital. After obtaining a bursary to enable her to visit the USA she was able to observe the nurses performing a towel bath which consisted of using a large bath towel and a no-rinse skin-cleansing product. This alternative practice ensured the patient's privacy and comfort and was well evaluated by staff and patients (Wright, 1990).

Patients who require minimal assistance may be able to have a bath or shower depending on the level of dependence, e.g. equipment they may be attached to and particular preferences. Attention should be given to religious and cultural needs, for example European and Asian people prefer to sit under running water as opposed to sitting in a bath. Other patients may need a full blanket bath.

Perineal/perianal care

Perineal care is probably the area most likely to produce embarrassment and humiliation (Heath, 1995). It is, however, important to be meticulous with this area, especially for those people who may be more prone to infection, e.g. patients with indwelling urinary catheters (see Chapter 45, Urinary Catheterization).

Problems arising from treatment therapy, for example radiotherapy, fistulae, diarrhoea, constipation, urinary tract infections, require additional vigilance with cleanliness and patients should be encouraged at every opportunity to perform this themselves (see Chapter 37, Sealed and Unsealed Radioactive Source Therapy).

Ideally the perineal hygiene should be attended to after the general bath or, at the very least, the water and wipes should be changed and clean ones utilized (Gooch, 1989; Gould, 1994) due to the large colonies of bacteria which tend to live in or around this area (Gould, 1994). Research has shown that soap and lotions administered improperly to the perineum/perianal area can cause irritation and infection. Many nurses will use soap or a similar chemical derivative in order to promote and ensure thorough cleaning, but frequently lack of knowledge can lead to further problems and discomfort for the patients (Lindell & Olsson, 1989). It was suggested that warm water alone be used to avoid irritating the mucous membranes which become sensitive during the ageing process. Care should be taken to maintain privacy and reduce embarrassment at all times, especially with regard to cultural influences.

Hair care

The way a person feels is often related to their appearance. Hair care can be complex – consideration should be given to the patient's personal preferences.

Washing of the hair can be difficult if a patient is bed bound but there are several ways to manage this. One example is by manoeuvring the patient to the top of the bed and hanging their head over the end (Wells & Trostle, 1984). If hair washing is not possible due to pain for example, then the use of an aerosol dry shampoo can be beneficial. Shampooing frequency depends on the patient's well-being and his/her hair condition.

Care of the beard and moustache are also important. Excess food can often become lodged here so regular grooming is essential for hygiene and comfort purposes. Beard trimmers can be used as appropriate.

Grooming the hair provides an ideal opportunity to observe for dandruff, psoriasis, flaky skin and head lice. Hair lice are extremely infectious so it is imperative to treat the hair with a medicated shampoo from the pharmacy as soon as possible. Careful washing of towels is necessary, and a separate towel should be used for each patient to avoid an outbreak of lice (Stichele *et al.*, 1995).

A patient's cultural and religious beliefs should always be taken into consideration when attending to hair. Some religions do not allow hair washing or brushing whilst others may require the hair to be covered by a turban. Similarly, in some countries facial hair is significant and should never be removed without the patient's/relatives' consent. Always establish any preferences before beginning care.

In the oncology setting chemotherapy is an established treatment and some cytotoxic drugs can cause alopecia (loss of hair). This is a particularly sensitive and traumatic event and skilled advice is required regarding adjustment to hair loss and the correct fitting of a wig (Tierney, 1987). A mild shampoo with a neutral pH is recommended for patients who are at risk of alopecia. Prevention of alopecia is discussed further in Chapter 36, Scalp Cooling.

Regular brushing and combing can avoid tangling and matting of the hair.

Care of the nails and feet

The feet and nails require special care in order to avoid pain and infection occurring. Nails should be trimmed correctly. Specialist advice from a chiropodist can be useful. Chronic diseases such as diabetes and the long term use of steroids can result in problems such as pressure ulcers, breakdown of the skin integrity and delays in the healing process. Special attention should be paid to cleaning the feet and in between the toes to avoid any fungal infection. Powders and creams are available that help with the treatment of infections and odour management.

Care of the ears and nose

Lack of attention to cleaning the ears and nose can lead to impairment of the senses. Usually these small organs require minimal care but observation for a build-up of wax in the ears and deposits in the nose is essential to maintain patency and efficacy.

Cotton buds and tap water are useful for gently cleaning the areas. Special care should be taken to avoid pushing too hard in the aural cavity with a risk of piercing the ear drum.

Patients undergoing enteral feeding and oxygen therapy should have regular nasal care to avoid excessive drying and excoriating of the delicate air passages. Gentle cleaning of the nasal mucosa with cotton buds and water is recommended and application of a thin coating of vaseline to prevent discomfort can be beneficial. Patients who have had piercing of the ears or nose will require cleansing of the holes to avoid the risk of infection. Body piercing is common practice in many countries now.

Eye care

Specific aspects of eye care, e.g. irrigation, are referred to in Chapter 20, Eye Care.

In general, the eye structure and delicate surface are protected by the tears that maintain the eye's moistness, but in a patient who is unconscious, drying of the eye may occur (Ross & Wilson, 1982). Gentle cleansing with low-linting gauze and 0.9% sodium chloride will be sufficient to prevent infection and will keep the eyes moist. The eye is an important organ of communication and consideration should always be given to a patient's sight aids, e.g. glasses, contact lenses. Assistance may be required to help clean these aids and advice regarding the most appropriate method should be sought, preferably from the patient.

Some patients may have an artificial eye and care should be taken to ensure this remains clean. Advice regarding the ideal method of removal and insertion should be sought.

Mouth care

Most aspects of mouth care, e.g. cleaning and infection control, are referred to in Chapter 26, Mouth Care.

Cleaning of equipment

Within an establishment the common use of cleaning equipment, e.g. washing bowls may lead to a high risk of infection. One bowl per patient should be allocated on admission and labelled accordingly to avoid cross-infection.

One study involving three wards in a general hospital showed the movement of three marked bowls, one in each ward. Regular observations were made regarding the drying and storage of these bowls and the results demonstrated clearly that drying and storage were haphazard and many bowls were contaminated (Greaves, 1985). The same study also looked at the misuse of face cloths. They were shown to be a source of infection as they were used for several patients and not washed sufficiently in between use. Recommendations from the survey were that either patients should be supplied with their own bowls or the bowls in general use should be thoroughly cleaned and dried and stacked pyramid fashion (Greaves, 1985; Gould, 1994).

Vigorous cleaning with a scouring powder is recommended for washing out the bowls and baths (Gould, 1994). If possible, each patient should have their own toiletries and towels which should be laundered regularly (Gould, 1994).

Summary

The patient is an individual who will depend on others to assist them in times of ill health. 'Whenever possible, patients should be enabled to perform their own hygiene, so that they can continue their usual practice' (Gooch, 1989). In this way patients will be able to maintain their own comfort and privacy for something that is a 'basic human right' (Young, 1991).

Care should be taken to observe the patient's cultural and religious beliefs and advice can be sought from the patient and relatives.

Attention should be paid to the cleaning of the equipment to avoid cross-infection. Personal hygiene is a simple procedure that can be performed for patients, but considerable thought should be given to individual preferences and patients' comfort.

It is clearly evident from the lack of research, that more work is required in this area to improve and raise standards of patient care.

References

Gooch, J. (1989) Skin hygiene. *Professional Nurse*, October, 13–17.

Gould, D. (1994) Helping the patient with personal hygiene. *Nursing Standard*, 8(34), 30–2.

Greaves, A. (1985) We'll just freshen you up, dear. *Journal of Infection Control Nursing, Nursing Times Supplement*, 6 March, 3–8.

Heath, B. M. H. (ed.) (1995) *Potter and Perry's Foundation in Nursing Theory and Practice*. Mosby–Wolfe Europe, London.

Henderson, V. (1966) *The Nature of Nursing*. Collier Macmillan, London.

Kershaw, B. & Salvage, J. (1992) *Models for Nursing*. John Wiley, London.

Lindell, M. & Olsson, H. (1989) Lack of care givers knowledge causes unnecessary suffering in elderly patients. *Journal of Advanced Nursing*, 14, 976–9.

Neuberger, J. (1987) *Caring for Dying People of Different Faiths*, 2nd edn. Mosby, London.

Orem, D. (1980) *Nursing – Concepts of Practice*, 2nd edn. McGraw Hill, New York.

Pearson, A. & Vaughan, B. (1988) *Nursing Models for Practice*. Heinemann, Oxford.

Roper, N. *et al.* (1981) *Learning to use the Process of Nursing*. Churchill Livingstone, Edinburgh.

Ross, J. & Wilson, K. (1982) *Foundations of Anatomy and Physiology*. Churchill Livingstone, Edinburgh.

Spiller, J. (1992) For whose sake – patient or nurse? *Professional Nurse*, April, 431–4.

Stitchele, V. *et al.* (1995) Systemic review of clinical efficacy of topical treatments for headlice. *British Medical Journal*, 311(7005), 604–8.

Tierney, A. J. (1987) Preventing chemotherapy induced alopeica in cancer patients: is scalp cooling worthwhile? *Journal of Advanced Nursing*, 12, 303–10.

Wagnild, G. & Manning, R. W. (1985) Convey respect during bathing procedures. *Journal of the Gerontology Nurse*, 11(12), 6.

Weller, B. & Wells, R. (1990) *Baillière's Nurses Dictionary*, 21st edn. Baillière Tindall, London.

Wells, R. & Trostle, K. (1984) Creative hairwashing techniques for immobilized patients. *Nursing*, 14(1), 47.

Wilson, M. (1986) Personal cleanliness. *Nursing*, 3(2), 80–2.

Wright, L. (1990) Bathing by towel. *Nursing Times*, 86(4), 36–9.

Young, L. (1991) The clean fight. *Nursing Standard*, 5(35), 54–5.

GUIDELINES: BED BATHING A PATIENT

PROCEDURE

Action	Rationale
1 Assess the patient's needs.	To plan care.

Guidelines: Bed bathing a patient (cont'd)

Action	Rationale
2 Plan care with the patient, noting his or her personal preferences.	To encourage participation and independence. To ensure patient comfort during procedure.
3 Collect all equipment by bedside: • clean bedlinen	To avoid leaving the patient during procedure.
• fleecy drawsheet or bath towel	To cover patient during procedure.
• laundry skip • towel(s) and flannel(s)	It may be necessary to provide disposable flannel if the patient does not use a separate flannel for face and body. They may however not wish this. To meet patient's preference.
• soap and toiletries as preferred by patient • clean night clothes • washbasin – reserved for patient – and warm water	To reduce risk of cross-infection (Greaves, 1985).
4 Clear area around bed; ensure that it is private and draught free.	To ensure space to carry out procedure and patient comfort.
5 Offer patient a urinal, bedpan or commode.	To reduce possibility of disruption to procedure and prevent any discomfort.
6 Cover patient with drawsheet or bath towel. Loosen top covers at foot of bed and fold back bed clothes.	To ensure bed clothes remain dry and patient remains warm.
7 Ask patient if they use soap on their face. Wash, rinse and dry face, neck and ears. Some patients may wish to do this themselves. Note: if additional care is required for the eyes and nose carry out on completion of bedbath. (Refer to section on care of eyes and nose.)	Many patients prefer plain water on their face. To promote cleanliness. To maintain independence. To ensure patient comfort and cleanliness.
8 Remove top half of night clothes and if an intravenous device is *in situ* or an extremity is injured remove night clothes on unaffected side first.	Leaving lower half of body clothed aids patient privacy and warmth. Removal of night clothes on unaffected side first is easier and more comfortable for the patient.
9 Wash, rinse and dry top half of body. Apply toiletries as required by patient. Replace night clothes. Change the water during procedure if cold and/or scummy.	To promote patient well-being and cleanliness. To ensure patient comfort and provide sufficient clean water to rinse off soap which might otherwise have a drying effect on the skin (Gooch, 1989).
10 Wash, rinse and dry lower half of body/ back. Replace night clothes. Change bottom sheet while patient is being turned, if they are to remain in bed.	To promote cleanliness. To reduce unnecessary activity for the patient and nurse.
11 Assist patient, if required, to brush teeth and/ or rinse mouth.	To freshen mouth and minimize plaque build up. (See Chapter 26, Mouth Care.)
12 Help patient to sit or lie in desired position.	To promote patient comfort. To reduce risk of pressure ulcers. (See Chapter 48, Wound Management.)

13 Comb patient's hair as desired.

To promote positive body image.

14 Remake bed.

To enhance patient comfort.

15 Remove equipment from bedside. Replace patient's possessions in their appropriate place. Place locker, bedside table and call bell within reach.

To clear working environment for patient and nurse.
To promote patient independence.

16 Wash hands.

To reduce risk of cross-infection.

Prior to each part of the procedure explain and obtain agreement from the patient. The procedure can allow time and opportunity for communication and interaction between the nurse and patient. (Adapted from *Foundation in Nursing Theory and Practice* by Potter & Perry, 1994. Mosby–Wolfe Europe Limited, London, UK.)

CHAPTER 35
Respiratory Therapy

Definition

Respiratory therapy is the administration of supplementary oxygen when tissue oxygenation is impaired. Oxygen is essential to allow aerobic metabolism to produce energy from the intake of food.

If tissue oxygenation becomes inadequate, anaerobic metabolism will lead to lactic acidosis and cell death (Oh, 1995).

Indications

There are many indications for respiratory therapy. The major ones are listed below:

(1) Acute respiratory failure – this can be subdivided into two groups, i.e. with or without carbon dioxide retention:
  (a) With carbon dioxide retention – the most common causes are chronic bronchitis, chest injuries, e.g. flail segment and rupture of the diaphragm, unconscious drug overdose, post-operative hypoxaemia and the neuromuscular diseases.
  (b) Without carbon dioxide retention – the most common causes are asthma, infective conditions, e.g. pneumonia and legionella, pulmonary oedema and pulmonary embolism (Oh, 1995).
(2) Acute myocardial infarction.
(3) Cardiac failure.
(4) Shock, particularly haemorrhagic, bacteraemic and cardiogenic.
(5) For a hypermetabolic state induced, for example, by major sepsis, trauma or burns.
(6) States where there is a reduced ability to transport oxygen, e.g. anaemia.
(7) Inability to utilize the oxygen carried, as in cyanide poisoning (Foss, 1990).
(8) During cardiorespiratory resuscitation.
(9) During anaesthesia for surgery.

REFERENCE MATERIAL

Physiology (see also Chapter 30, Observations)

Tissue oxygenation is reliant on the following factors:

(1) The oxygen cascade.
(2) Association and dissociation of haemoglobin and oxygen.
(3) Cardiac output (Oh, 1995).

An understanding of these factors and their interaction is essential in understanding the physiology of oxygen transport and transfer in the body.

The movement of oxygen from the alveoli in the lungs to the pulmonary blood is effected rapidly due to the pressure gradient that exists. The partial pressure of oxygen (PaO_2) in the alveoli is 13.7 kilopascals (kPa) as compared to 5.3 kPa in the pulmonary capillaries. This allows a swift exchange of oxygen through diffusion. Similarly oxygen is easily given up by the arterial blood to the tissues, again because of the steep pressure gradient. The partial pressure of arterial blood is 13.3 kPa and that of the tissues 2.7 kPa (Marieb, 1989). Table 35.1 and Fig. 35.1 show the various pressure gradients in the oxygen cascade.

Oxygen is carried in the blood in the following two

Table 35.1 Oxygen cascade. Pressure gradients for oxygen transfer from inspired gas to tissue cells.

	(kPa)
Inspired air	20.0
Alveolar	13.7
Arterial	13.3
Capillary	6.8
Tissue	2.7
Mitochondrial	0.13–1.3

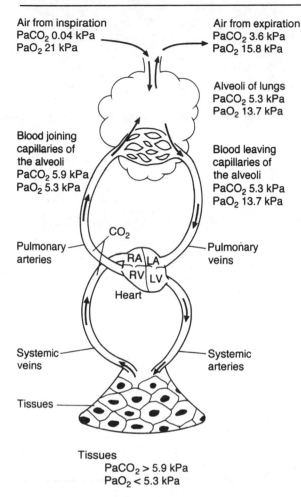

Air from inspiration
PaCO₂ 0.04 kPa
PaO₂ 21 kPa

Air from expiration
PaCO₂ 3.6 kPa
PaO₂ 15.8 kPa

Alveoli of lungs
PaCO₂ 5.3 kPa
PaO₂ 13.7 kPa

Blood joining
capillaries of
the alveoli
PaCO₂ 5.9 kPa
PaO₂ 5.3 kPa

Blood leaving
capillaries of
the alveoli
PaCO₂ 5.3 kPa
PaO₂ 13.7 kPa

CO₂

Pulmonary
arteries

RA LA
RV LV
Heart

Pulmonary
veins

Systemic
veins

Systemic
arteries

Tissues

Tissues
PaCO₂ > 5.9 kPa
PaO₂ < 5.3 kPa

Figure 35.1 Gas movement in the body is facilitated by partial pressure differences. The top of the figure illustrates the pressure gradients that facilitate oxygen and carbon dioxide exchange in the lungs. The bottom of the figure shows the pressure gradients that facilitate gas movements from the systemic capillaries to the tissues.

ways: dissolved in plasma; and bound to the haemoglobin within the red blood cells. Only about 1.5% of oxygen is carried in the plasma as oxygen is poorly soluble in water. Therefore, 98.5% of oxygen is transported around the body in a loose chemical alliance with haemoglobin (Marieb, 1989). Haemoglobin is made up of four polypeptide chains, each of which is bound to a heme group that contains iron. The iron groups bind to oxygen, and therefore each molecule of haemoglobin can combine with four molecules of oxygen. A haemoglobin molecule is said to be fully saturated with oxygen when all four heme groups are attached to oxygen. When less

than four are so attached, the haemoglobin is said to be partially saturated (Marieb, 1989).

The action of the four polypeptide molecules and their relationship to oxygen is interlinked so that when one molecule has taken up a molecule of oxygen, the others are facilitated to do the same. The same is also true for the opposite action when the heme molecules unload their oxygen molecules to the tissues (Marieb, 1989).

The timing of haemoglobin uptake and release of oxygen is affected by the following factors:

(1) The partial pressure of oxygen (PaO_2).
(2) Temperature.
(3) Blood pH.
(4) Partial pressure of carbon dioxide ($PaCO_2$) (Marieb, 1989).

The oxygen dissociation curve

This curve illustrates the factors affecting tissue oxygenation (Figs. 35.2, 35.3 and 35.4).

Haemoglobin and oxygenation

The extent of oxygen binding to haemoglobin depends on the PaO_2 of the blood, but the relationship is not precisely linear (see Fig. 35.2). The slope is steeply progressive between 1.5 kPa and 7 kPa and then plateaus out between 9 and 13.5 kPa. This is important for oxygen therapy because it illustrates that haemoglobin is almost completely saturated at 9 kPa and therefore further increases in the partial pressure of oxygen will cause only a slight rise in oxygen binding.

The most rapid uptake and delivery of oxygen to and from haemoglobin occurs during the steep portion of the curve (Marieb, 1989).

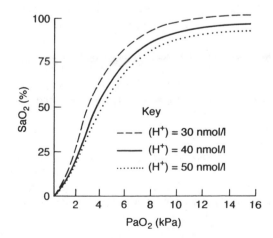

Key
– – – (H⁺) = 30 nmol/l
——— (H⁺) = 40 nmol/l
·········· (H⁺) = 50 nmol/l

SaO₂ (%)

PaO₂ (kPa)

Figure 35.2 The oxygen dissociation curve, illustrating the normal curve at 40 nmol/l.

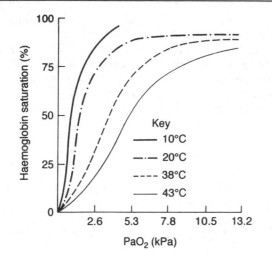

Figure 35.3 The oxygen dissociation curve and the effect of temperature changes. As the temperature rises the curve shifts to the right illustrating that oxygen unloading is accelerated as the temperature rises.

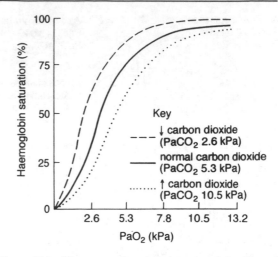

Figure 35.4 The oxygen dissociation curve and the effect of carbon dioxide changes. As the $PaCO_2$ rises the curve shifts to the right illustrating that oxygen unloading is accelerated as the $PaCO_2$ rises.

Haemoglobin, temperature and oxygen

As body temperature rises the affinity of haemoglobin for oxygen is reduced and less oxygen is bound while more oxygen is unloaded (Marieb, 1989) (Fig. 35.3).

Haemoglobin, pH and oxygen

As the pH of the blood declines (acidosis) the affinity of haemoglobin for oxygen decreases and more oxygen will be unloaded to the tissues. This is known as the Bohr effect. The same effect occurs when the partial pressure of carbon dioxide rises as this will also lead to a fall in blood pH and acidosis (Marieb, 1989) (Fig. 35.4).

Generally, a shift in the oxygen dissociation curve to the right will favour unloading of oxygen to the tissues, and a shift to the left will favour reduced tissue oxygenation. Factors that would influence a shift to the right are changes in temperature and pH. Factors that would influence a shift to the left are temperature and $PaCO_2$ changes (Oh, 1995).

Cardiac output

The final factor influencing tissue oxygenation is the cardiac output. When this is severely reduced, for example in shock states, there will be a severely reduced amount of oxygen available to the tissues (Edwards, 1988).

Oxygen consumption

At rest the normal oxygen consumption is approximately 200–250 millilitres per minute (ml/min). As the avail-able oxygen per minute in a normal man is about 700 ml, this means there is an oxygen reserve of 450–500 ml/min. Factors which increase the above consumption of oxygen include fever, sepsis, shivering, restlessness and increased metabolism (Oh, 1995). It is difficult to say at which absolute level oxygen therapy is necessary as each situation should be judged by the requirements for oxygen and the availability of oxygen. Therefore, all of the above information needs to be taken into account together with the measurement of the arterial blood gases.

Generally, additional oxygen will be required when the PaO_2 has fallen to 8 kPa or less (Oh, 1995). Oxygen saturation level at the tissues is also useful and can be measured using a pulse oximeter, which works by emitting narrow shafts of red and infra-red light through the tissue of a finger, toe or earlobe. Different amounts of light rays are absorbed by the arterial blood depending on its saturation with oxygen. The final oxygen saturation (SaO_2) is then calculated by computer (Ehrhardt & Graham, 1990).

Hazards of respiratory therapy

Carbon dioxide narcosis

Carbon dioxide is the chemical that most directly influences respiration by its direct effect on the efficiency of alveolar ventilation. The normal partial pressure of carbon dioxide in the blood is 4.0–5.5 kPa. When this level rises, the pH of the cerebrospinal fluid drops which in turn causes excitation of the central chemoreceptors, and hyperventilation occurs (Marieb, 1989).

In people who always retain carbon dioxide, and are therefore usually hypercapnic because of chronic pulmonary disease such as chronic bronchitis, the chemoreceptors are no longer sensitive to a raised level of carbon dioxide. In these cases the falling PaO_2 becomes the principle respiratory stimulus (the hypoxic drive) (Marieb, 1989). Therefore, if a high level of supplementary oxygen was delivered to such patients, severe respiratory depression would ensue and ultimately unconsciousness and death.

Oxygen toxicity

Pulmonary toxicity following prolonged higher percentages of oxygen therapy is recognized clinically, but there is still much to be learnt about the condition. The pattern is one of decreasing lung compliance as a result of a sequelae of haemorrhagic interstitial and intra-alveolar oedema, leading ultimately to fibrosis (Oh, 1995).

It is thought that where possible, long periods (that is 24 hours or more) of respiratory therapy above 50% should be avoided, although clinically it seems that there is much variance in the response of individual patients (Higgins, 1990).

Retrolental fibroplasia

This is a disease affecting premature babies that weigh under 1200 g (about 28 weeks' gestation) if they are exposed to high concentrations of oxygen. It appears that the oxygen stimulates immature blood vessels in the eye to vasoconstrict and obliterate, which results in neovascularization, accompanied by haemorrhage, fibrosis and then retinal detachment and blindness (Oh, 1995).

General considerations

(1) Oxygen is an odourless, tasteless, colourless, transparent gas that is slightly heavier than air.
(2) Oxygen supports combustion, therefore there is always a danger of fire when oxygen is being used. The following safety measures should be remembered:
  (a) Oil or grease around oxygen connections should be avoided.
  (b) Alcohol, ether and other inflammatory liquids should be used with caution in the vicinity of oxygen.
  (c) No electrical device must be used in or near an oxygen tent.
  (d) Oxygen cylinders should be kept secure in an upright position and away from heat.
  (e) There must be no smoking in the vicinity of oxygen.
  (f) A fire extinguisher should be readily available.

(g) Care should be taken with high concentrations of oxygen when using the defibrillator.

Equipment necessary to administer respiratory therapy

Any oxygen delivery system will include these basic components:

(1) Oxygen supply, either from a piped supply or a portable cylinder. All medical gas cylinders have to conform to a standardized colour coding: oxygen cylinders are black with a white shoulder and are labelled 'Oxygen' or 'O_2'.
(2) A reduction gauge – to reduce the pressure to that of atmospheric pressure.
(3) Flowmeter – a device which controls the flow of oxygen in litres per minute.
(4) Tubing – disposable tubing of varying diameter and length.
(5) Mechanism for delivery – a mask or nasal cannulae.
(6) Humidifier – to warm and moisten the oxygen before administration (Allan, 1988).

Methods of administration

Simple semi-rigid plastic masks (Fig. 35.5)

These are low-flow masks which entrain the air from the atmosphere and therefore are able to deliver a variable oxygen percentage (anything from 21 to 60%) (Allan, 1988). Large discrepancies between the delivered fractional inspired oxygen (FiO_2) and the actual amount received by the patient will occur with increased rate and depth of respiration (Oh, 1995).

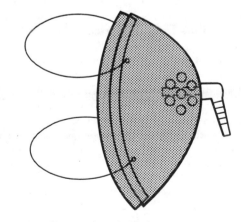

Figure 35.5 Semi-rigid plastic mask.

Nasal cannulae catheter (Fig. 35.6)

These provide an alternative to a mask but again there are great discrepancies between the delivered FiO_2 and the actual oxygen percentage received by the patient.

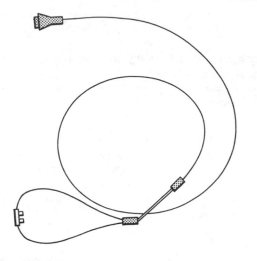

Figure 35.6 Nasal cannulae.

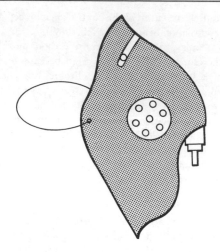

Figure 35.7 High-flow mask.

When used at low flow rates, for example 2 litres per minute, they are well tolerated and afford the patient more freedom than a mask. At high flow rates, above 8 litres per minute, they may cause discomfort and dryness of the nasal mucosa. Nasal cannulae cannot be attached satisfactorily to an external humidification device (Allan, 1988).

Fixed performance masks or high-flow masks (Venturi-type masks) (Fig. 35.7)
With these masks it is possible to achieve an unvarying mixture of gases and a known concentration of oxygen using the high air flow oxygen enrichment principle. These masks derive their name from the Venturi barrel in which a relatively low flow rate of oxygen is forced through a narrow jet. There are side holes in the barrel and this jet causes the air to be drawn in at a high rate. As the mixture of gas created is at a flow rate above that of inspiration, the mixture will be constant (Foss, 1990). There are many Venturi-type masks available but the larger-capacity masks are the most accurate and therefore the safest when a known concentration of oxygen is required or when efficient elimination of carbon dioxide is essential, for example, to provide respiratory therapy for the patient with chronic respiratory disease (Allan, 1988).

T-piece circuit
This is a simple, large-bore, non-rebreathing circuit which is attached directly to an endotracheal or tracheostomy tube. Humidified oxygen is delivered through one part of the T, and expired gases leave through the other part. This device may be used as part of the weaning process when a patient has been

ventilated previously by a mechanical ventilator (Oh, 1995).

CONTINUOUS POSITIVE AIRWAYS PRESSURE (CPAP)

Definition
CPAP therapy is the maintenance of a positive airway pressure greater than ambient pressure throughout inspiration and expiration. It can be delivered through a dedicated face mask to the spontaneously breathing patient, or through an endotracheal or tracheostomy tube (Oh, 1995).

Indications
(1) Acute respiratory failure. Can be used with spontaneously breathing patients who are able to protect their own airway. This includes situations where alveolar gas exchange is reduced (e.g. chest infection).
(2) As a method for weaning a patient from mechanical ventilation.
(3) After major surgery as a means of improving gaseous exchange.
(4) As a supportive measure in patients who are considered unsuitable for endotracheal intubation and mechanical ventilation.

REFERENCE MATERIAL
Use of the CPAP circuit dates back at least to 1912, when Bunnell used a primitive circuit during thoracic surgery. The first recorded use in intensive care was by Poulton

and Oxon in 1936. In the 1940s increased interest in CPAP was prompted by research into respiratory support in high altitude flying. Further developments occurred in the 1950s and 1960s, and in 1976 Greenbaum *et al.*, reported the use of CPAP with a face mask in adult respiratory distress syndrome (ARDS). In 1972 Williamson & Modell successfully used CPAP for selected spontaneously breathing patients with acute respiratory failure.

CPAP aids gaseous exchange by utilizing the following mechanisms:

(1) An increase in functional residual capacity (FRC).
(2) Reduction in intrapulmonary shunting.
(3) Potential reduction in pulmonary oedema.
(4) Symptomatic relief: the work of breathing is reduced.

Paediatric circuits

A child's compliance with oxygen masks or cannulae may be limited, requiring other devices to be used. Some examples of these are listed below:

(1) *Headbox or hood.* Oxygen can be delivered to infants and small children using a headbox or hood. The clear plastic box is fitted carefully over the child's head, encasing the head and neck. It is essential to monitor the oxygen concentration near the face to enable an accurate assessment of FiO_2 (Oh, 1995).
(2) *Oxygen tent/cot.* An oxygen tent can be used to supply oxygen therapy to larger children. The child is placed in a clear plastic tent which fits over the bed. The humidified oxygen supply is then directed into the tent. The advantages with the oxygen tent are that the child has freedom from any device over the face, and high degrees of humidity can be reached which may be especially useful in obstructive conditions e.g. croup (Allan, 1988) . The main disadvantage is the difficulty in maintaining a constant oxygen concentration (Oh, 1995).

Tracheostomy mask

These perform in a similar way to the simple semi-rigid plastic face mask, outlined above. The mask is placed over the tracheostomy tube or stoma, and the patient will receive less oxygen than is delivered as it will be diluted by room air (Oh, 1995).

Mechanical ventilation

This is indicated when there is reversible acute respiratory failure. The decision to use mechanical ventilation will be made after an assessment of respiratory mechanics, oxygenation and ventilation (Oh, 1995). There are a wide range of ventilators available and they all have slight differences of application but fall into two major groups:

(1) Positive pressure ventilators – these are the most widely used for the acute treatment of adults and children.
(2) Negative pressure ventilators – these are used much more rarely (usually for patients with chronic neurological problems such as poliomyelitis and some forms of muscular dystrophy) (Hinds, 1988). (For a detailed outline of respiratory therapy using mechanical ventilation, see Hinds, 1988; Oh, 1995.)

Hyperbaric respiratory therapy

This form of treatment is used mainly in the treatment of skin lesions and soft tissue injury and has also been used more recently for the patient with multiple sclerosis. The therapy is designed to administer 100% oxygen at a range of pressures greater than atmospheric pressure.

Hyperbaric therapy can be used topically or systemically depending on the patient's need, and the treatment is usually intermittent over a period of weeks or months (Oh, 1995).

Humidification

Humidity is the amount of water vapour present in a gaseous environment (Oh, 1995). For the purpose of clinical application, humidity is usually divided into absolute and relative humidity. Absolute humidity is a measurement of the total mass of water in a specified volume of gas at a known temperature. Relative humidity is the ratio (expressed as a percentage) of the mass of water in a given volume of gas (as above) with the mass of water required to saturate the same volume of gas at a given temperature (Oh, 1995).

Normally, the air travelling through the airways is warmed, moistened and filtered by the columnar mucus-secreting epithelial cells of the nasopharynx (Foss, 1990). The air entering the trachea will have a relative humidity of about 90% and a temperature between 32° and 36°C. The humidification and warming process then continues down the airways so that at the alveoli it is fully saturated at 37°C (Oh, 1995).

The humidification pathway is necessary to compensate for the normal loss of water from the respiratory tract (about 250 ml under resting conditions) (Oh, 1995). If the humidification apparatus is impaired due to disease such as upper respiratory tract infection or dehydration, alternative methods of humidification may need to be considered (Allan, 1988).

Respiratory therapy will compound these problems because the added gas will cause further dehydration of the mucous membranes and pulmonary secretions making it more difficult for the patient to expectorate (Foss, 1990). External humidification is essential when respiratory therapy is being delivered to a patient whose physiological humidification has been bypassed by an endotracheal or tracheostomy tube (Oh, 1995).

Methods of humidification

There are many devices that can be used to supply humidification, the best of these will fulfil the following requirements:

(1) The inspired gas must be delivered to the trachea at a room temperature of 32–36°C and should have a water content of 33–43 g/m³ (Oh, 1995).
(2) The set temperature should remain constant; humidification and temperature should not be affected by large ranges of flow.
(3) The device should have a safety and alarm system to guard against overheating, overhydration and electric shocks.
(4) It is important that the appliance should not increase resistance or affect the compliance to respiration.
(5) It is essential that whichever device is selected, wide-bore tubing (elephant tubing) must be used to allow efficient formation of water vapour.

Devices for humidification

(1) *Condensers*. These are also known as heat and moisture exchangers or 'Swedish nose'. They perform the function of the nasopharynx, retaining the heat and water from expired gas through condensation and returning them to the inspired gas. A new range of disposable condensers are now widely used to humidify oxygen delivered through an endotracheal or tracheostomy tube, but heated humidifiers may still be preferred for long-term use (Oh, 1995).
(2) *Cold water bubble humidifier*. This device delivers partially humidified oxygen that is about 50% relative humidity. Its use is not advised as it is so inefficient (Oh, 1995).
(3) *Water bath humidifiers*. With these devices, inspired gas is forced over or through a heated reservoir of water. To achieve an adequate humidity for the patient, the water bath must reach temperatures of 45–60°C. The gas will then cool as it moves down the breathing circuit to the patient, and a relative humidity of 100% will be reached. Hot water bath humidifiers are therefore very efficient and useful in the care of the immobile patient, particularly in an intensive therapy unit. However, they have four main disadvantages:

(a) Danger of overheating and causing damage to the trachea.
(b) Their efficiency can alter with changes in gas flow rate, surface area and the water temperature.
(c) Condensation and collection of water in the oxygen delivery tubes.
(d) The possibility of microcontamination of stagnant water (Tinker & Zapol, 1992).

(4) *Aerosol generators*. These devices are not governed by temperature, but provide micro-droplets of water suspended in the gas (Oh, 1995). The gas provided through aerosol devices can be very highly saturated with water, especially when ultrasonic nebulizers are used. There are three main types of aerosol humidifier:
(a) Gas-drive nebulizer.
(b) Mechanical (spinning disc) nebulizer.
(c) Ultrasonic nebulizer.

These devices are useful for the spontaneously breathing patient with chronic chest disease.

References and further reading

Allan, D. (1988) Making sense of oxygen delivery. *Nursing Times*, 83(18), 40–2.
Allison, R. C. (1991) Initial treatment of pulmonary oedema: a physiological approach. *American Journal of Medical Sciences*, 302(6), 385–91.
Edwards, D. (1988) Principles of oxygen transport. *Care of the Critically Ill*, 4(5), 13–16.
Ehrhardt, B. S. & Graham, M. (1990) Making sense of oxygen delivery. *Nursing* (US), March, 50–4.
Foss, M. A. (1990) Oxygen therapy. *Professional Nurse*, January, 180–90.
Greeg, R. W. *et al.* (1990) Continuous positive airway pressure by face mask in pneumocystis carinii pneumonia. *Critical Care Medicine*, 18(1), 21–4.
Greenbaum, D. M. *et al.* (1976) Continuous positive airways pressure without tracheal intubation in spontaneously breathing patients. *Chest*, 69, 615–20.
Higgins, J. (1990) Pulmonary oxygen toxicity. *Physiotherapy*, October, 76(10), 588–92.
Hinds, C. J. (1988) *Intensive Care. A Concise Textbook*. Baillière Tindall, London.
Marieb, E. N. (1989) *Human Anatomy and Physiology*. Benjamin Cummings Publishing, USA.
Oh, T. E. (1995) *Intensive Care Manual*. Butterworths, Sydney.
Tinker, J. & Zapol, W. (1992) *Care of the Critically Ill Patient*. Springer-Verlag, USA.
Williamson, D. C. & Modell, J. H. (1972) Intermittent continuous airways pressure by mask – its use in the treatment of atelectasis. *Archives of Surgery*, 177, 970–2.

CHAPTER 36

Scalp Cooling

Definition

Scalp cooling is a method of reducing scalp temperature and causing constriction of blood vessels, thus decreasing the amount of drug that can pass into the hair follicles and reducing cellular uptake of the drug.

Indications

The effectiveness of scalp cooling has been demonstrated satisfactorily only with doxorubicin and epirubicin (Dean *et al.*, 1979; Middleton *et al.*, 1982; Robinson, 1987). Patients receiving other cytotoxic drugs which may cause alopecia such as vindesine and vincristine, have undergone the procedure, although there are insufficient data to evaluate its effectiveness with these drugs. It is not performed routinely and the consultant's permission must be obtained as there is a risk of protecting scalp micrometastases, especially where there is the possibility of circulating cancer cells, e.g. in cases of leukaemia and lymphoma (Witman *et al.*, 1981). However, scalp cooling has been used successfully in relapsed lymphoma (Keller & Blausey, 1988; Pirohit *et al.*, 1992).

REFERENCE MATERIAL

Doxorubicin is one of the most active cytotoxic agents currently used in cancer chemotherapy. It belongs to the anthracycline antibiotic group of drugs and has a wide spectrum of activity (Benjamin *et al.*, 1974; Benjamin, 1975). Unfortunately, administration of doxorubicin is associated with alopecia in approximately 90% of cases, and this is often total. Hair loss is distressing for the patient and may lead to refusal to accept treatment (Dean *et al.*, 1979; Cline, 1984; Freedman, 1994).

Initial research into methods to prevent hair loss using a scalp tourniquet (Maxwell, 1980) or crushed ice (Dean *et al.*, 1979) was carried out in the USA. Promising results led to follow-up research at the Royal Marsden NHS Trust (Hunt *et al.*, 1982). The method, using a home-made cap (see Guidelines, below), differed on a number of points to previous work, and the results re-garding prevention of total hair loss were considerably better. The success rate in the research project was 85% and this has been maintained in everyday practice (David & Speechley, 1987).

Further work has been carried out to find a system that allows for more precise temperature control. The thermocirculator allows coolant to be pumped between two layers of a plastic cap at a constant temperature (Guy *et al.*, 1982). More recently a vortex refrigeration tube to provide cold air to the scalp has been produced (Symonds & McCormick, 1986; Adams *et al.*, 1992). The success of all these methods in preventing hair loss varies and the amount of hair loss experienced by the patient is dependent on a number of factors:

(1) Involvement of the liver with metastatic disease leads to elevated plasma levels of doxorubicin for a longer period. Extension of the cooling period does not seem to improve results (Satterwhite & Zimm, 1984).

(2) Inadequate cooling because of exceptionally thick hair may lead to partial loss. It has been demonstrated that maximum cooling occurs 20 minutes after the cap has been placed in position. The weight of the cap (as well as the temperature) is a factor, as this ensures that the contact is maintained over the complete scalp (Hunt *et al.*, 1982). Success does not appear to be dose dependent as was first thought (David & Speechley, 1987). It seems likely that when anthracyclines are used in combination with other drugs which cause alopecia (e.g. etoposide and cyclophosphamide) the success rate is not as high as with anthracyclines alone (Middleton *et al.*, 1985; Tierney, 1991).

Patients should be selected carefully for scalp cooling and should be well motivated to undertake the procedure. Patients must consent when they have been fully informed about the nature and length of the procedure, and know that they may discontinue the procedure at any time if they find it too traumatic, physically or psychologically (Tierney, 1987), or if they fail to retain hair.

Research shows that scalp cooling can be more distressing than originally thought (Tierney *et al.*, 1989), and work has now been carried out into how patients feel about the procedure and whether they find it worthwhile. In a small study 50% of patients found scalp cooling worthwhile and 70% would undergo the procedure again in order to prevent hair loss (Dougherty, 1996). Patients have reported adverse effects during and following treatment such as headaches, claustrophobia and 'ice phobias' (Tierney *et al.*, 1989).

It is important to ensure that if a patient refuses scalp cooling or fails to retain hair, adequate time is spent helping the patient to adapt to the hair loss physically, psychologically and socially. This can be achieved by ensuring that the patient sees the surgical appliance officer as soon as possible, in order to obtain a wig that can be matched to the style and colour of the patient's natural hair. Advice can be given on hair care and various ideas of hats, turbans and so on, and reinforced with a hair care information booklet.

References and further reading

Adams, L. *et al.* (1992) The prevention of hair loss from chemotherapy by the use of cold air scalp cooling. *European Journal of Cancer Care*, 15, 16–18.

Anderson, J. *et al.* (1981) Prevention of doxorubicin-induced alopecia by scalp cooling in patients with advanced breast cancer. *British Medical Journal*, 282, 423–4.

Baxley, K. O. *et al.* (1984) Alopecia: effect on cancer patients' body image. *Cancer Nursing*, December, 499–503.

Benjamin, R. S. (1975) A practical approach to Adriamycin toxicology. *Cancer Chemotherapy Reports*, 6, 319–27.

Benjamin, R. S. *et al.* (1974) Adriamycin chemotherapy – efficacy, safety and pharmacologic basis of an intermittent, single, high-dosage schedule. *Cancer*, 33, 19–27.

Cline, B. W. (1984) Prevention of chemotherapy-induced alopecia; a review of the literature. *Cancer Nursing*, June, 221–8.

David, J. A. & Speechley, V. (1987) Scalp cooling to prevent alopecia. *Nursing Times*, 83(32), 36–7.

Dean, J. C. *et al.* (1979) Prevention of doxorubicin-induced hair loss with scalp hypothermia. *New England Journal of Medicine*, 301, 1427–9.

Dougherty, L. (1996) Scalp cooling to prevent hair loss in chemotherapy. *Professional Nurse*, 11(8), 1–3.

Edelstyn, G. A. *et al.* (1977) Doxorubicin-induced hair loss and possible modification by scalp cooling. *Lancet*, 2, 253–4.

Freedman, T. G. (1994) Social and cultural dimensions of hair loss in women treated for breast cancer. *Cancer Nursing*, 17(4), 334–41.

Guy, R. *et al.* (1982) Scalp cooling by Thermocirculator. *Lancet*, 24 April, 937–8.

Hayward, J. L. (1977) Assessment of response to therapy in advanced breast cancer. *British Journal of Cancer*, 35, 292–8.

Hunt, J. *et al.* (1982) Scalp hypothermia to prevent Adriamycin-induced hair loss. *Cancer Nursing*, 5(1), 25–31.

Keller, J. F. & Blausey, L. A. (1988) Nursing issues and management in chemotherapy-induced alopecia. *Oncology Nursing Forum*, 15(5), 603–7.

Maxwell, M. B. (1980) Scalp tourniquets for chemotherapy-induced alopecia. *American Journal of Nursing*, 5, 900–2.

Middleton, J. *et al.* (1982) Prevention of doxorubicin-induced alopecia by scalp hypothermia: relation to degree of cooling. *British Medical Journal*, 284, 1674.

Middleton, J. *et al.* (1985) Failure of scalp hypothermia to prevent hair loss when cyclophosphamide is added to doxorubicin and vincristine. *Cancer Treatment Reports*, 69(4), 373–5.

Pirohit, O. P. *et al.* (1992) A six week chemotherapy regimen for relapsed lymphoma efficacy results and the influence of scalp cooling. *Annals of Oncology*, 3 (Supplement 5), 126.

Robinson, M. H. (1987) Effectiveness of scalp cooling in reducing alopecia caused by epirubicin treatment of advanced breast cancer. *Cancer Treatment Reports*, 71, 913–14.

Satterwhite, B. & Zimm, S. (1984) The use of scalp hypothermia in the prevention of doxorubicin-induced hair loss. *Cancer*, 54, 34–7.

Symonds, R. P. & McCormick, C. V. (1986) Adriamycin alopecia prevented by cold air scalp cooling. *American Journal of Clinical Oncology*, 9(5), 454–7.

Tierney, A. J. (1987) Preventing chemotherapy-induced alopecia in cancer patients: is scalp cooling worthwhile? *Journal of Advanced Nursing*, 12, 303–10.

Tierney, A. (1991) Chemotherapy-induced hair loss. *Nursing Standard*, 5(38), 29–31.

Tierney, A. J. *et al.* (1989) *A Study to Inform Nursing Support of Patients Coping with Chemotherapy for Breast Cancer*. Report prepared for the Scottish Home and Health Department.

Wagner, L. & Bye, M. G. (1979) Body image and patients experiencing alopecia as a result of cancer chemotherapy. *Cancer Nursing*, 2, 365–9.

Witman, G. *et al.* (1981) Misuse of scalp hypothermia. *Cancer Treatment Reports*, 65(5–6), 507–8.

GUIDELINES: SCALP COOLING

EQUIPMENT

1 A scalp cooling cap:
   (a) Commercial make.

(b) Home-made from eight hot/cold packs. These must be taped together and moulded around a wig stand. When bandaged in position, the cap is placed in a deep freeze (temperature approximately −18°C) for 24 hours.

(c) Rubber cap with tubing for thermocirculator machine.

2 Ear protection – gauze, cotton wool pads.

3 Bottle of hair conditioner.

4 Two crepe bandages (10 and 15cm wide).

5 Two towels.

6 Comfortable chair (recliner) or bed.

7 Extra pillows and blankets as required.

PROCEDURE

Action	Rationale
1 Before beginning, it is important to explain and discuss the procedure fully with the patient. The patient should understand that the scalp cooling can be discontinued at any time and that it will not jeopardize the chemotherapy.	To ensure that the patient understands the procedure and gives his/her valid consent.
2 If both machine and gel-pack method are available, the patient should be offered the choice, and told the advantages and disadvantages of each method.	To allow an informed choice to be made by the patient.
(a) Gel-pack method. *Advantages*: shorter procedure. *Disadvantages*: heavy and cold when initially placed on head.	
(b) Thermocirculator method. *Advantages*: cap placed on head first and then cooling allowed to occur gradually over 30 minutes. *Disadvantage*: longer procedure.	To prevent initial feeling of extreme cold when cap placed on head.
3 Check the cap has been in the deep freeze for 24 hours (gel-pack).	To ensure the cap is cold enough to be effective.
Ensure the machine is switched on and set at the correct temperature (machine).	To ensure coolant in pump can reach its correct temperature of −5°C.
4 Wet patient's hair thoroughly (gel-pack). Comb conditioner through the patient's hair (machine only).	To aid conduction of coldness and to aid with fitting of cap.
5 Place the ear protection in position.	To prevent cold injury.
6 Soak one crepe bandage in cold water and use it to bandage the patient's head tightly. The bandage should be applied evenly and should provide a thin layer over the scalp (gel-pack only).	To aid conduction of coldness. To compress the hair and prevent any air being trapped between the cap and scalp.
7 Place the cap on the patient's head making sure it fits closely and covers the whole hairline.	To ensure cooling over the head, including all the hair roots.
8 Add supplementary packs if necessary (gel-pack only).	To ensure adequate cooling of the scalp.
9 Bandage the cap in place.	To maintain even and close contact of the cap to the scalp and provide some insulation of the cold.

Guidelines: Scalp cooling (cont'd)

Action	Rationale
10 Switch the pump on (machine only).	To commence the flow of coolant around the cap and machine.
11 Add pillows, etc. as required.	To provide support for the patient's head and neck and to reduce the effect of the heaviness of the gel pack cap (approximately 2–3 kg).
12 Place a dry towel around the patient's shoulders.	To catch any water as the gel-pack cap defrosts.
13 Offer the patient the use of a blanket.	To prevent any chilling.
14 Leave the patient for at least 15 minutes before injection of the drug (gel-pack).	To obtain initial cooling of the scalp.
Leave the patient for at least 30 minutes (machine).	To allow for gradual cooling of the scalp.
15 Administer the drug by intravenous injection.	
16 Leave the patient for a further 45 minutes (both methods).	To maintain cooling until the plasma levels of drug have fallen (Hunt *et al.*, 1982).
17 When sufficient time has elapsed, remove the cap and bandages carefully.	To prevent damage to the scalp and hair.
18 Encourage the patient to rest, if desired.	To prevent faintness due to the weight being lifted off.
19 Towel the patient's hair dry (gel-pack). Rinse the conditioner from the patient's hair (machine). Allow the patient to style it.	To prevent damage to the hair. To ensure that the patient is comfortable and has a chance to rearrange hair before leaving hospital.
20 Ensure the patient is given a hair care information booklet in order to care for hair correctly between treatments.	To reinforce verbal information given during procedure.

NURSING CARE PLAN

Problem	Cause	Suggested action
Inadequate cooling: (a) Gel-pack cap (−20°C). (b) Machine cap (−5°C).	Poorly fitting cap. Incorrect temperature.	Follow the procedure carefully. Check the cap has been cooled to the correct temperature. Ensure the cap size is correct and that the hair roots are covered. If the patient has very thick hair, use the heaviest cap available.
Excess cooling.	Thin hair.	Use extra layers of bandages between the cap and scalp. If it

		is still painful then discontinue the procedure.
Complaints of headache.	Weight and coldness of cap.	Provide support and blankets as required.
Distressed patient.	Claustrophobia.	Support and reassure the patient. If necessary remove the cap.
	Ice phobia.	Be aware of this possible problem, encourage the patient to discuss feelings.
Hair loss.	Scalp cooling was not successful.	Offer the patient the opportunity to discontinue the scalp cooling. Make arrangements for the patient to see the appliance officer and obtain a wig. Discuss care of hair and scalp and give information booklet.

CHAPTER 37

Sealed and Unsealed Radioactive Source Therapy

Definition

Radioactive sources in clinical use can be broadly divided into two categories:

(1) Sealed sources
(2) Unsealed sources.

Sealed sources are usually powders or solids enclosed in a casing which is inserted into the patient. Generally there is little risk of spreading radioactive contamination from these sources, unless the casing is cracked during sterilization. Radioactive iridium-198 is a solid metal which may be made into alloy wires and used for direct insertion into tissues or cavities. Although not sealed in a metal casing the methods applied to the use of sealed sources are also applied to this substance. The principles of radiation protection: distance, time and shielding, which minimize personal exposure to radiation, must be applied when working with sealed sources to ensure all unnecessary exposure is avoided (Wootton, 1993).

Unsealed sources are radionuclides supplied in liquid or colloidal form, and are systemically administered orally or by injection. They are used in the treatment and diagnosis of malignant disease (Horwich, 1995; Souhami & Tobias, 1995). Unsealed sources carry an additional risk of environmental contamination, and additional protective measures are required to prevent contamination of persons and the environment (Wootton, 1993). For example, unsealed sources may concentrate in body fluids, in particular urine, which will then contain radioactivity, and when eliminated reduce the amount of radioactivity in the patient (Martin & Harbinson, 1979).

REFERENCE MATERIAL

Measures of radiation

Radiation kills by causing ionization within living cells. The activity of radioisotopes was at one time measured in millicuries (mc), but the standard unit is now the becquerel (Bq) (Wootton, 1993). A becquerel is the Système International (SI) unit of activity and is 1 disintegration per second.

$$k \left(kilo\right) = 1 \times 10^3$$

$$M \left(mega\right) = 1 \times 10^6 \text{ e.g. megabecquerel} \left(MBq\right)$$

$$G \left(giga\right) = 1 \times 10^9$$

The half-life of a radioactive substance is the time taken for half of the original number of radioactive atoms to decay and lose their radioactivity. The sensitive target appears to be deoxyribonucleic acid (DNA) in the nucleus of the cell. The ionizing radiation thus passes through the cells and tissues, and the dose of radiation received is measured in terms of energy absorbed. The unit of absorbed dose, the *rad* (radiation absorbed dose), has now been replaced by the gray, which equals 100 rads:

$$100 \text{ rads} = 100 \text{ centigray} \left(cGy\right) = 1 \text{ gray} \left(Gy\right)$$

For the purposes of radiation protection the dose to the whole body must be known. Whereas the absorbed dose is measured in gray, the dose to the whole body is in *sieverts*. For instance, for staff over 18 who are not pregnant, wearing a monitoring badge to monitor exposure to radiation, the maximum permissible dose is 50 millisieverts (0.05 sievert) per year (Department of Health and Social Security, 1985).

Ionizing radiation regulations

The use of ionizing radiation is governed by strict regulations. The principles of distance, shielding and time limitation must be observed to minimize radiation exposure in accordance with *The Ionising Radiations Regulations* (Department of Health and Social Security, 1985). An important principle for staff to observe is to keep all radiation exposure 'as low as reasonably achievable' (the ALARA principle).

The safety of patients exposed to ionizing radiation is regulated by the Ionising Radiations (Protection of Persons Undergoing Medical Examination or Treatment) (POPUMET) Regulations (1988). These regulations require that all staff who clinically or physically direct a medical exposure to ionizing radiation are adequately trained in the radiation protection of patients and staff. All staff should receive a 'core of knowledge' which conforms to the requirements of the POPUMET regulations.

SEALED RADIOACTIVE SOURCE THERAPY

Indications

Permanent or temporary insertions of small, sealed sources are used to deliver very high doses of radiation into tumours or tumour-bearing tissue while giving rapidly diminishing doses to adjacent structures. This will limit the damage caused to normal tissue. A specific dose of radiation will be received by the cancer. This is delivered continuously over a period of minutes, hours or days.

Radioactive isotopes used as sealed sources

Most radioactive isotopes used as sealed sources for brachytherapy emit both beta (β) and gamma (γ) radiation. Brachytherapy is where there is a very short distance between the radiation source and the tumour. It is either intracavitary, where radioisotope sources are placed in pre-existing body cavities, such as the uterine cavity or vagina, or interstitial, where radioisotope sources are inserted directly into the tissues in tubes or needles (Lambert & Blake, 1992).

The radiation useful in treating malignant disease includes X-rays, produced artificially by electron bombardment of a metal target, and gamma rays, a natural emission in the nuclear decay of radioisotopes. They are sometimes referred to as 'photon' radiation. Beta particles are also capable of ionization; these are distinguishable from electromagnetic radiation by their ability to carry an electrical charge (either positive or negative). Beta particles result when a neutron within the nucleus disintegrates to form a proton and an electron. The electron is ejected from the nucleus, producing beta radiation (Holmes, 1988).

Caesium-137

Caesium-137 is a radioisotope that can be used in the form of interstitial implants or in intracavitary applicators. It has a half-life of 30 years and has largely replaced radium as a source of brachytherapy.

Oral implants

Caesium-137 can be used in a needle-like implant that is inserted directly into the tissue surrounding the tumour. This is a fairly common treatment for early lesions of the cheek, lip and anterior two-thirds of the tongue. If bone involvement is suspected, e.g. in the mandible, alternative external treatment will be given.

The sources (Fig. 37.1) are inserted in theatre under a general anaesthetic. They are inserted individually in a predetermined pattern so that the implant covers the whole growth with a safety margin of at least 1 cm. Each needle is positioned by pushers so that its eye, through which silk is threaded, is just visible beneath the mucosal surface. Each silk is then stitched to the tongue with a single suture. When all the needles have been inserted, the silks are counted and gathered together. They are threaded through a piece of rubber to prevent friction and trauma to the mouth. The silks are strapped to the cheek to prevent any needle being swallowed should it work loose. Small beads are attached to the ends of the threads to facilitate counting the needles. X-rays are always taken to check the positions of the needles and to enable estimation of the dose distribution.

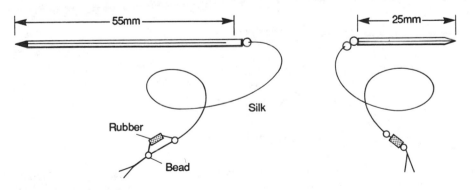

Figure 37.1   Caesium-137 needles.

Gynaecological applicators

Caesium-137 can be used in applicators. The commonest malignancies treated by the use of radioactive applicators are tumours of the female genital tract. Intracavitary applicators are used which deliver a high dose to the region of the cervix, the paracervical tissue, the upper part of the vagina and the uterine body.

Iridium-192

Iridium-192 is a radioisotope which can be used in the form of pins or wires as in interstitial therapy. Its half-life is 74.2 days. Iridium-192 is an ideal choice because of the low energy of its gamma emission, which simplifies radiation protection, and because in the form of a platinum-iridium alloy it can be drawn into thin flexible wires. The wires consist of an active platinum-iridium alloy core encased in a sheath of platinum $10\,\mu m$ thick, which screens out the beta radiation from the iridium-192.

Iridium-192 can now be made with a very high specific activity, that is, in a very radioactive form. High activity sources of iridium are used in high dose-rate remote afterloading systems, which reduce the amount of radiation to which radiotherapists and other staff are exposed.

Iridium-192 implants are used under the following circumstances:

(1) As a treatment for small primary lesions, especially tongue or breast lesions.
(2) As a 'boost' dose after external radiotherapy for larger primary tumours or where nodes are also involved.
(3) To treat recurrence.

Iridium-192 hair pin and single pin types of implants are usually used intraorally (Fig. 37.2). They are slotted into tissue using steel guides to obtain accurate alignment. Radiological examination is used to check the position of

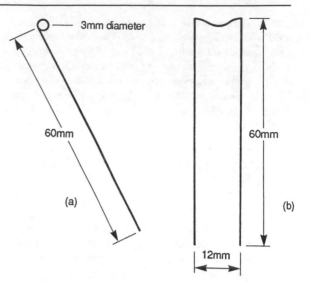

Figure 37.2 Iridium pins. (a) Iridium single pin. (b) Iridium-192 hair pin.

the guides before the iridium is inserted. The pins are held in place by sutures.

The staff of the physics department are normally responsible for calculating how long a radioactive implant is to stay in place. This is usually about six days, depending on the size of the tumour. Removal is carried out in theatre by the radiotherapist.

Iridium-192 wires are usually used for breast lesions or lesions of the vulva or perineum (Fig. 37.3). Polythene or metal cannulae are inserted under a general anaesthetic. In the case of breast lesions, both ends of each tube protrude through the skin. Correct alignment is established often with the aid of a perspex template which fits over the breast and holds the metal cannulae in the correct alignment. In the case of vulval or perineal insertions only one end of the tube protrudes. For these,

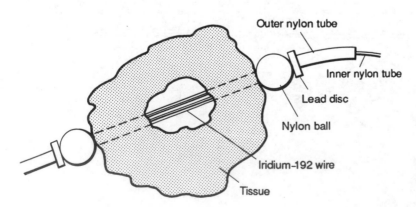

Figure 37.3 Iridium-192 wire in polythene cannula. Typical assembly in tissue.

alignment of the sources may be achieved by using a perspex template and vaginal obturator.

The iridium wire source is afterloaded, usually on the ward, and the wires are held in the cannulae with crimped lead washers. The tiny size of the high activity iridium-198 source in high dose rate machines may allow some interstitial brachytherapy to be given as a few treatments of several minutes each, in contrast to the single treatment of many hours duration which is necessary with low-activity iridium wire.

The radiotherapist is responsible for calculating how long a radioactive implant should stay in place. This is usually for 3–6 days, depending on the size of the tumour. Removal of the implant is usually carried out on the ward by the radiotherapist.

Iodine-125

Seeds of iodine-125 produce gamma rays that are less penetrating than those of gold-198. Therefore, these implants represent less of a hazard for staff and have replaced gold-198 in several centres. The half-life of iodine-125 is 60 days, much longer than that of gold-198. Some therapists believe that there is a radiobiological advantage to this longer half-life in treating slowly growing tumours such as carcinoma of the prostate.

Gold-198

Gold-198 was used as an interstitial source of radiation in the form of gold grains. It has largely been replaced by iodine-125 seeds. Its half-life is 2.76 days. Gamma and beta rays are emitted. The gamma rays are of relatively low energy and the beta rays are filtered out by platinum casing around the gold. Gold-198 grains are used primarily in the treatment of tumours of the lung, bladder neck, prostate and lymph nodes.

Gold-198 grains are 2.5 mm long and 0.5 mm in diameter, made of gold encased in platinum. Fourteen gold-198 grains are contained in an aluminium magazine which fits into the barrel of the implantation gun (Fig. 37.4). An injector needle is attached to the gun which is

inserted into the tissue that is to be irradiated. The patient requires a general anaesthetic for the insertion.

Gold grains have the following advantages over more classical methods of wires and pins in the irradiation of comparatively inaccessible tumours:

(1) Placing gold-198 grains is easier than placing needles or pins.
(2) Gold-198 grains do not need any fixing sutures.
(3) They are a permanent insertion, therefore the closure of any surgical wound can be immediate.

The disadvantage of this method is that higher numbers of gold-198 grains are required, which means that more precautions must be taken in order to achieve a regular geometrical arrangement to ensure satisfactory distribution of the dose. This can increase the length of time the doctors, nursing staff and other personnel present are exposed to irradiation.

Applicators

Small sealed sources inserted into the body may take the form of:

(1) *Intracavitary applicators*, i.e. sources that are placed in natural cavities and usually held in place by packing.
(2) *Interstitial implants*, i.e. sources that are inserted directly into the tumour-bearing tissue.

(*Note*: sources held in plastic surface applicators or moulds are applied directly to superficial cancers.)

Intracavitary applicators and interstitial implants can be used in three forms:

(1) The source is preloaded in the applicator before it is placed in the patient for a fixed length of time, e.g. caesium-137 needles and iridium-192 hair pins.
(2) Permanent insertion in the case of iodine-125 seeds or gold-198 grains which, once inserted, would be difficult to remove. In addition, as radioactive gold-198 grains have a half-life of less than 3 days this

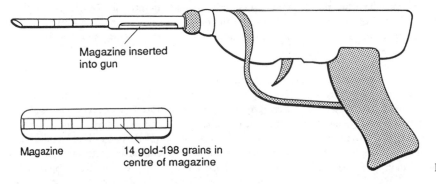

Magazine inserted into gun

Magazine

14 gold-198 grains in centre of magazine

Figure 37.4 Gold grain gun.

means that radiation protection restrictions will be relatively short.

(3) Afterloading systems – where the applicator is placed in position and the radioactive source is inserted when the position of the applicator and the condition of the patient are satisfactory. Insertion of the sealed source can be undertaken manually in the case of iridium-192 wires or by remote control, as in the case of the low dose rate Selectron machine and the Microselectron high dose rate machine.

Afterloading techniques have the advantage of allowing the source carrier to be accurately positioned (Cooper, 1993), and for the sources to be withdrawn to a radiation-proof safe during patient care, sparing staff from radiation exposure.

Historically, cervical cancer was one of the first tumours to be treated with radiotherapy, when radium was inserted into the endocervical canal and vagina to irradiate local disease. Techniques were developed in several centres, notably Paris, Stockholm and Manchester, which allowed consistency of treatment and, therefore, enabled the effectiveness and morbidity of treatment to be measured. A technique in common use today is the *Manchester* technique, in which an intrauterine tube and two vaginal ovoids are placed in the uterus and lateral vaginal fornices (Fig. 37.5e). The proportions of radioisotope (initially radium and latterly caesium) within the intrauterine tube and the vaginal ovoids were calculated to give a constant dose rate to a geometrical point A when using different lengths of intrauterine tube and different sizes of vaginal ovoids. This constancy of dose rate when using applicators of different sizes is an important aspect of the Manchester system.

Active sources. The radioisotope initially used for intracavitary brachytherapy was radium which, because of its gaseous daughter-product radon, is hazardous. Radium has, therefore, been replaced by caesium, but the hazards of handling active sources have largely led to the development of afterloading techniques minimizing source handling and staff exposure.

Afterloading brachytherapy. The basis of afterloading brachytherapy is that applicators are placed within the cervix and vaginal fornices, and that the radioisotope is only introduced into these when the applicators are correctly positioned, check radiographs have been taken and the patient is comfortable and in a protected environment. The sources may then be inserted either manually or by remote control. Manual methods are common and have the advantage of being cheap, but do not entirely protect staff as the sources have to be inserted by staff and cannot be removed for short periods while a patient's needs are attended to. Remote systems have the advantage of complete protection of staff, but have the

disadvantage of high cost and the need for interlocking mechanisms. These ensure that the correct source has been inserted into the correct applicator for the programmed length of time.

Remote afterloading systems allow the dose rate of brachytherapy to be increased. Classically, the dose rate with the Manchester system was approximately 50 cGy/hour to point A. With modern engineering methods, caesium pellets can be produced which will allow a dose rate of between 150 and 200 cGy/hour to point A. Many systems now use sources that allow a higher than standard dose rate to be delivered. This has the advantage of reducing treatment time, but does have radiobiological consequences necessitating a small reduction in dose (Brenner & Hall, 1991).

If the concept of increasing dose rate is taken further, high dose rate brachytherapy, delivering doses at rates in excess of 1 Gy/minute to point A, offers the possibility of very short treatment times. This allows complete geometrical stability of the applicator during the treatment and makes a higher patient throughput possible. However, there is considerably less time for repair of radiation damage to normal tissues in a high dose rate treatment and, therefore, such treatments have to be fractionated over several days, in contrast to the continuous treatment given by a low dose rate brachytherapy implant. Early clinical results show no difference between treatment at low dose rate and at high dose rate (Fu & Phillips, 1990), although mathematical modelling indicates that there is an increased risk of late tissue damage from fractionated high dose rate brachytherapy compared with a continuous low dose rate insertion.

Intracavitary applicators

The applicators are inserted under a general anaesthetic, and the position of the applicator is checked by X-ray before the patient returns to the ward. A urinary catheter is also inserted in theatre to reduce the risk of the sources becoming dislodged by the patient when micturating.

There are several different types of applicator available and choice is usually determined by the site of the tumour, the anatomy of the patient and the preference of the treatment centre. The most commonly used types of applicator are described below (see Fig. 37.5).

Manchester applicator

Manchester applicators are briefly described above. In their original form they were live sources enclosed in intrauterine tubes of varying lengths and vaginal applicators (ovoids) of varying sizes. The applicators were inserted under general anaesthetic and held in place by a gauze pack. More recently the applicators

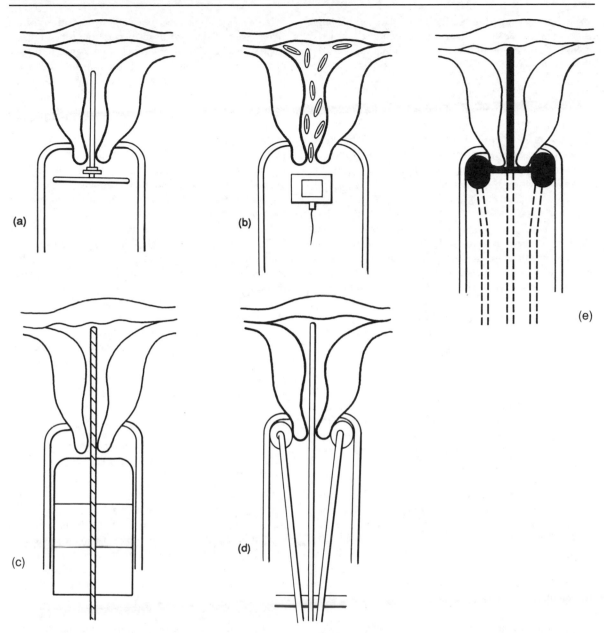

Figure 37.5 Gynaecological caesium applicators. The arrangement of brachytherapy sources in the uterus and vagina for the treatment of cervical carcinoma. The sources may be active or, more usually these days, afterloaded into the applicators along the catheters protruding from the vagina. (a) Modified Stockholm applicator. (b) Heyman's capsules and packet. (c) Dobbie applicator. (d) Fletcher applicator. (e) Manchester applicator.

have been modified for either manual or remote afterloading at either low or high dose rate, but the principle of the three applicator system remains. Removal of the applicators, or, if still used, the live sources is carried out on the ward and may require administration of Entonox for analgesia.

Stockholm applicator
This is used for carcinoma of the body of the uterus or cervix. Usually a uterine tube and two vaginal packets are inserted. Occasionally, if the vaginal vault is small, one packet is omitted or replaced by a vaginal tube. The radioactive material is held in place with a flavine-

soaked gauze pack. It is usually left in place for 22 hours. Tubes and packets have strings attached for removal and colour-coded beads indicate which should be removed first.

Modified Stockholm applicator
This is used for carcinoma of the body of the uterus and cervix. It consists of a uterine tube and a square box which connect together by a point and a hole. The vagina is then packed with gauze saturated with proflavine. They are usually left in place for 20 hours. The box should be removed first.

Fletcher applicator
This is used for carcinoma of the corpus or cervix, but the patient needs to have a fairly capacious vaginal vault. Hollow applicators, a uterine tube and two vaginal ovoids are inserted in theatre and loaded with the radioactive sources later, on the ward, by the radiotherapist. The apparatus is held in place with a flavine pack. Long ends project through the vulva so that afterloading can be done. These insertions are usually left in place for 60–72 hours. No strings are needed as the apparatus itself projects from the vulva.

Heyman's capsules
These are used for carcinoma of the corpus where there is enlargement of the uterus and expanded uterine cavity. They consist of small metal capsules, each of which contains a small, radioactive source. As many capsules as possible are placed into the uterus. Usually two vaginal packets are used as well. They are held in place by a flavine gauze pack and are left in for about 12–18 hours. Each capsule has a flexible wire attached, strapped to the thigh, for removal, and a numbered tag to indicate the order of removal.

Heyman's capsules are rarely used now as imrovements in anaesthetics allow the great majority of patients with endometrial cancer to undergo hysterectomy.

Dobbie applicator
This is used to irradiate the whole vagina. A perspex cylindrical applicator, with radioactive sources in the centre, is inserted into the vagina and sutured in place to the vulva. It may be used with low or high dose rate sources. Strings are attached to the applicator for removal.

Manual afterloading systems
Manual afterloading systems are largely being replaced by remote systems, but they are still used in a few centres and are widely used in developing countries.

The plastic applicator tubes follow the pattern of the Manchester system with an intrauterine tube and two vaginal ovoids. The plastic tubes are designed to be disposed of after a single use. Insertion of the tubes takes place under general anaesthetic, after which confirmatory X-rays are taken with dummy sources in place. As with the classical Manchester system there are varying lengths of intrauterine tube and sizes of ovoids.

If the X-rays are satisfactory and the dosimetry has been calculated the radioactive caesium sources are introduced on their carrying rods using long-handled forceps. Once in place inside the plastic tube a silver metal cap is screwed over the end of the plastic tube to hold the sources securely.

Manual afterloading does not permit, for reasons of staff safety, the use of high activity sources and treatment may last many hours or even several days. When treatment is complete the caps are removed from the tubes and the sources are withdrawn and placed immediately in a lead storage vessel. The plastic applicator tubes are then removed.

It is particularly important to observe for displacement or extrusion of the applicator tubes over the long treatment times. It is customary to mark the thigh level with the end of the applicator tubes and to compare this alignment at regular intervals as the treatment progresses. In addition, the silver metal caps should be monitored regularly for any loosening or displacement.

REMOTE AFTERLOADING

Definition
Remote controlled afterloading machines transfer active sources from a radiation-proof safe to the patient only when it is safe to do so. The transfer may be pneumatic or cable-driven. The low dose-rate Selectron machine operates pneumatically, whereas the high dose rate Microselectron is cable driven (Wilkinson et al., 1983).

Indication
Remote-controlled afterloading machines are gradually replacing conventional intracavitary radium and caesium applicators as well as other manual and mechanical afterloading techniques.

The low dose-rate Selectron has been used predominantly for the treatment of gynaecological cancers, but may also be useful in the treatment of a number of other tumours such as cancer of the oesophagus and colon. Whilst the high dose rate Microselectron is also regularly used in the treatment of gynaecological cancers, in some cases it may also be useful in the treatment of bronchial carcinoma (Bomford et al., 1993).

REFERENCE MATERIAL

The low dose rate Selectron

The Selectron unit comprises a lead-shielded safe containing caesium-137 sources in the form of small spherical pellets, a microprocessor, keyboard, display unit and printer (Fig. 37.6). Leading from the Selectron unit are either three or six flexible plastic transfer tubes corresponding to numbered treatment channels. Each tube ends in a fragile plastic catheter which is inserted into the appropriately numbered applicator and secured by a coupling device. The unit has a supply of compressed air and it is air pressure that the system uses to transfer the sources from the safe within the unit to the applicators along the connecting tubes. Operation of the unit is initiated from a remote-control unit situated outside the protected treatment area. Together these components form the basis of the remote-controlled afterloading system (Blake, 1991).

The Selectron provides an accurate and safe method of radiotherapy treatment for cancers of the cervix, uterus and upper part of the vagina.

The advantages of the Selectron system are threefold:

(1) Remote afterloading eliminates contact with radioactive material and protects personnel.
(2) It allows highly accurate dosimetry.
(3) The activity of the caesium-137 sources is such (up to 40 millicurie (mc)) that treatment times for patients are considerably shorter than for conventional techniques.

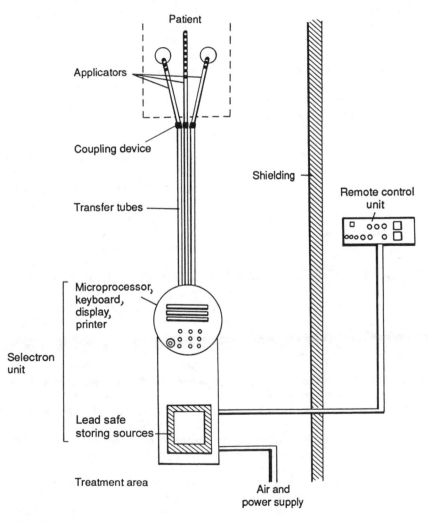

Figure 37.6 Selectron unit.

While the Selectron has been used predominantly for the treatment of gynaecological cancers, features of its design render it potentially useful for treating a number of other tumours such as cancers of the oesophagus or colon.

Patients have hollow, lightweight stainless steel applicators positioned in the operating theatre under a general anaesthetic. These are usually modified Manchester or Fletcher type applicators consisting of a uterine tube and two vaginal ovoids held in place with a proflavine-soaked vaginal packing. However, several other applicators are available. Accurate positioning of the applicators is confirmed by taking X-rays with dummy sources *in situ* and the optimum source configuration is selected, taking account of individual anatomical variations.

The Selectron is programmed by the physicist. For each treatment channel being used, active source pellets are interspersed with inactive stainless steel space pellets to achieve the desired dose distribution. The treatment time required to reach the prescribed dose is also entered. With a six-channel Selectron unit it is possible to treat two patients with three applicators each simultaneously. The radiotherapist is responsible for connecting the transfer tubes to the applicators. The transfer tubes are led over a bed bracket which supports the weight of the tubes and prevents traction being applied to the applicators in the patient. If the wrong catheter is connected to the applicator, the system will fail to operate.

Operating the Selectron

Treatment is commenced by activation of the remote control unit when all staff have left the treatment area. While treatment is in progress it can be interrupted and restarted from the remote control unit by pressing the stop and start buttons. The display panel indicates which channels are being used for treatment and which are unused with red and green lights respectively. The time of the longest treatment is displayed in decimal hours and a telephone intercom system allows for communication with the patient without the need to interrupt treatment.

Interrupting the treatment by pressing the green stop button results in the sources being withdrawn into the Selectron unit and stops the timer. This allows nursing staff to enter the treatment area in safety and give routine or specific care to the patient. Pressing the red start button transfers the sources back into the applicators and restarts the timer. The red lights demonstrate that the channels are operating again satisfactorily.

The system has built-in safety features. In the event of a failure in the system, treatment stops automatically. An audible and visual alarm at the remote control unit alerts staff to a problem and indicates whether this is a fault related to the air or power supply, the pellets or the timer. There is an optional nurse station display unit with a similar alarm indicator which also emits an audible signal when treatment has been interrupted. This helps to prevent treatment being inadvertently left interrupted for long periods.

A record of any break in treatment is shown on the print-out from the unit itself, together with any programming or system fault. These appear as an error code and can be identified by reference to the Selectron users' manual.

At the end of the treatment time, all sources will be withdrawn automatically from the applicators back into the Selectron unit. When two patients are being treated simultaneously termination of the treatment of one patient may be some time before that of the other. This means the timer will register the longer treatment time but the indicator lights for the channels used for the first patient will have changed from red to green.

Additional safety features include a door switch facility to retract sources immediately if the door to the treatment area is opened when treatment is in progress, and/or Geiger dose meters visible when entering the treatment area and approaching the patient, which indicate when there are radioactive sources either in the patient or in the connecting tubes.

The high dose rate (HDR) Microselectron

The operating principles of the HDR Microselectron are similar to those of the low dose rate Selectron. Low dose rate Selectron applicators are afterloaded with active sources interspersed with inactive spacers to produce the correct isodose pattern. HDR Microselectron machines, on the other hand, achieve the desired isodose pattern with a single cobalt-60 or iridium-192 source which moves within the applicators and stops at pre-set positions for predetermined dwell times.

The HDR Microselectron delivers radiation at approximately 100 times the rate of the LDR Selectron and treatment times are therefore much shorter. It has the added advantage of applicators with a smaller diameter which can be put in place under local anaesthetic in the outpatients' department (Blake, 1989).

Once in position, HDR Microselectron intracavitary applicators are fixed to the treatment couch by means of an adjustable clamp (Patel *et al.*, 1994). Movement of the applicators is therefore minimal and dosimetry calculations accurately represent actual treatment (Crook & Esche, 1993). In addition, more constant and reproducible geometry of source positioning is possible (Perez *et al.*, 1992).

Treatment protocols generally consist of two treatments but can involve as many as five. Following explanation and support for the patient the procedure, which lasts between 20 and 30 minutes, is carried out under local anaesthetic (Blake, 1989). For the first treatment a urinary catheter is passed and the balloon inflated with dilute contrast medium. Check radiographs are taken once the applicator tubes are in place to collect information which is fed into the Selectron planning computer and used to calculate the treatment time.

The HDR Microselectron follows the same principles for programming and treatment as the LDR Selectron. When treatment is complete the applicators and catheter are removed and the patient is free to go home. A study by Blake (1989) found that patients undergoing treatment with the HDR Microselectron for gynaecological cancer have found the experience acceptable, and responded positively to being treated as outpatients.

Adequate preparation of the patient is essential. Brown (1990) suggests that time spent preparing the patient increases tolerance of the implant procedure, and that badly prepared patients may be more anxious and less able to follow instructions. An assessment of patients' physical and emotional needs must be made prior to each treatment to identify if any aspect of the treatment is problematic.

The advantages of the HDR Microselectron are threefold:

(1) The shorter treatment time reduces variations in the patient's position and allows more accurate dosimetry (Perez et al., 1992).
(2) Treatment lasts only minutes, minimizing the need for immobilization and reducing discomfort and the risk of complications associated with bed-rest.
(3) Treatment can be offered on an outpatient basis with a consequent reduction in cost (Blake, 1989).

Complications of intracavitary radiotherapy for gynaecological cancers

Radiation-induced early complications of intracavitary treatment are generally mild. They include proctitis and cystitis. Severe reactions are rare, but may include severe or prolonged proctitis in patients with pre-existing bowel disease, and urgency and freqency of micturition, nocturia and dysuria. Late complications may include bowel and bladder strictures, ulceration, and occasionally, fistula formation (Sutton, 1986). Perez et al. (1992), following a review of the research literature, found that major rectal complications were reported in 1.4% to 10% of cases, whereas minor or moderate complications were found in 0.7% to 24% of cases. Bladder complications were reported in 0.3% to 4% of cases.

Preparation of patient

Information about radiation therapy should be given to patients and carers when therapy is first discussed to allay fears and misconceptions about radiotherapy. Verbal information should be reinforced with written material to prepare the patient, reduce anxiety and promote coping. A contact name and telephone number are useful for patients who wish to obtain further information at a later date.

Information for gynaecological patients receiving radiotherapy can be divided into three categories: disease and treatment, short- and long-term side-effects and sexuality.

It should be explained that patients will require an indwelling urinary catheter and that they will be connected to the Selectron unit with flexible plastic tubes. Movement in bed will be restricted. Patients should be prepared for the noises made by the Selectron system, especially when sources are being transferred in and out of the applicators. Some patients find the prospect of treatment alarming and may prefer to receive regular sedation for the duration of the treatment. It is reassuring for patients to know that they will be monitored closely by nursing staff using a closed-circuit television system. A personal telephone line and a nurse call system must also be provided to enable patients to communicate with staff.

Vaginal care following intracavitary treatment

Because the vaginal canal is included in the radiation field, vaginal stenosis, fibrosis, loss of elasticity and lubrication, and a decrease in sensation may develop after treatment if prophylactic measures are not taken (Jenkins, 1986).

To help prevent changes due to radiation, women who are sexually active should continue to have regular intercourse after any discomfort caused by an acute radiation reaction has resolved. Alternatively, a dilator can be used to keep the vagina open and stretched. Water-soluble lubricants may alleviate the dry mucosa, and hormone therapy, if appropriate, may be given orally or vaginally to increase natural lubrication (Lambert & Blake, 1992).

Women should begin using a dilator two weeks after treatment has finished. Initially the dilator should be inserted into the vagina daily for 5–10 minutes (removing and reinserting three or four times). A water-soluble lubricant should be used to ensure ease of insertion (Dolan, 1987; Martin & Braly, 1991). Following advice from a doctor or nurse specialist, frequency of dilatation can be reduced to between three times and once per week. However, dilatation should continue for life if the patient wishes to maintain vaginal patency (Dolan, 1987). Dilatation should maintain vaginal patency and allow follow-up vaginal examination and smears to be performed without undue discomfort. It should also help comfortable resumption of intercourse.

Some clinical oncologists additionally recommend douching during radiotherapy and following brachytherapy, continuing for up to 8 weeks, to avoid infections and the formation of adhesions. Douching should not be carried out, however, if there is a risk of haemorrhage from persistent tumour (Lambert & Blake, 1992).

Patients are encouraged to douche once per day using a disposable douche and tap water. Douching should continue until symptoms have resolved and advice has been given by a doctor or nurse specialist.

Follow-up care

Possible acute side-effects of intracavitary radiotherapy include a sensation of abdominal fullness, cramping, lower back pain and an urge to urinate. An appropriate analgesic should be prescribed. Prior to the insertion of the applicators and during treatment anti-embolic stockings should be worn to reduce the risk of deep vein thrombosis and pulmonary emboli.

Potential long-term side-effects include fibrosis (scarring) of vaginal tissues leading to narrowing and shortening of the vagina. In addition, permanent loss of vaginal lubrication and reduced elasticity of the vaginal wall may also occur. This can cause dyspareunia (painful intercourse) in 25–65% of patients. Oestrogen therapy may help to relieve these symptoms in up to 50% of women.

Gynaecological patients of all ages should be given information about the sexual changes which might occur as a result of their disease and/or treatment. They should be reassured that many women regain their capacity for sexual activity and enjoyment. Bruner et al. (1993) reported an overall decrease of 22% in coital frequency following treatment with intracavitary implants: 15% for patients with endometrial cancer and 32% for patients with cervical cancer. An overall decrease of 37% in sexual satisfaction following treatment with intracavitary implants was also reported: 30% for patients with endometrial cancer and 48% for patients with cervical cancer.

Anxiety and depression can create barriers to sexual activity and some patients may need to be referred for specialized psychological support. Women may experience a decrease in self-esteem together with deep concern about a loss of femininity when undergoing apparently simple gynaecological examinations. They may consequently experience some form of sexual dysfunction.

Younger women are more likely to attribute personal and marital stress to sexual problems. Patients prefer discussions about sexual function to be initiated by clinical staff, often nurses in particular. Intensive intervention in the post-treatment period may help women to cope more easily with changes in their bodies and sexual issues, whether these are due to disease, treatment, or the cancer diagnosis itself.

Discharge of the patient

Patients are usually discharged on the day of completion of brachytherapy. They must void urine normally following removal of the urinary catheter. Patients are sometimes unsteady on their feet after prolonged bed rest and may require assistance. They should be informed that normal bowel actions may not return for a day or so; advice on managing diarrhoea or constipation should be given. Light spotting or discharge from the vagina is normal. If patients experience pain or any more marked bleeding hospital staff should be contacted immediately. Symptoms of urinary tract infection such as dysuria and/or elevated temperature should also be reported.

References and further reading

Anderson, B. L. (1994) Yes, there are sexual problems: now, what can we do about them? *Gynecologic Oncology*, 52(1), 10–13.

Baker, J. (1979) Implants and applications. In: Scan-technology in nursing – radiotherapy, (ed. R. Tiffany), *Nursing Times*, 148, Supplement, part 10, 37–40.

Blake, P. R. (1989) Intracavitary therapy and the use of the Microselectron-HDR at the Royal Marsden Hospital, London. *Activity. The Selectron Users' Newsletter*, 2, 4–7.

Blake, P. R. (1991) Radiotherapy and chemotherapy in the treatment of gynaecologic cancer. In: *Textbook of Gynaecology*, (ed. R. Varma). Edward Arnold, London.

Bomford, C. K. et al. (1993) *Textbook of Radiotherapy*. Churchill Livingstone, Edinburgh.

Brenner, D. J. & Hall, E. J. (1991) Fractionated high dose rate versus low dose rate regimens for intracavitary brachytherapy of the cervix. *British Journal of Radiology*, 64, 133–41.

Brown, D. (1990) The role of the nurse in brachytherapy. *Activity*, 4(3), 53–5.

Bruner, D. W. et al. (1993) Vaginal stenosis and sexual function following intracavitary radiation for the treatment of cervical and endometrial carcinoma. *International Journal of Radiation Oncology, Biology, and Physics*, 27, 825–30.

Cooper, J. S. (1993) Carcinomas of the oral cavity and oropharynx. In: *Moss' Radiation Oncology. Rationale, Techniques, Results*, (eds. D. Cox & J. D. Cox), 7th edn. Mosby, St Louis.

Crook, J. & Esche, B. A. (1993) The uterine cervix. In: *Moss' Radiation Oncology. Rationale, Techniques, Results*, (eds D. Cox & J. D. Cox), 7th edn., pp. 617–82. Mosby, St Louis.

Dean, E. M. et al. (1988) Gynaecological treatments using the Selectron remote afterloading system. *British Journal of Radiology*, 61(731), 1053–7.

Department of Health and Social Security (1985) *The Ionising Radiations Regulations Schedule 1*. HMSO, London.

Department of Health and Social Security (1988) *Ionising Radiation Regulations (Protection of Persons Undergoing Medical Examination or Treatment)*. HMSO, London.

Dolan, M. E. (1987) Sexuality in gynaecological patients undergoing radiation therapy treatments. In: *Radiation Therapy of Gynaecological Cancers*, (eds D. Nori & B. S. Helias), pp. 399–407. Alan Liss, New York.

Dudjak, L. (1988) Radiation therapy nursing care record: a tool for documentation. *Oncology Nursing Forum*, 15(6), 763–77.

Dunne-Daly, C. F. (1994) Education and nursing care of brachytherapy patients. *Cancer Nursing*, 17(5), 434–45.

Eardley, A. (1992) Standards of care for the patient having radiotherapy: can they be achieved? *Journal of Cancer Care*, 1, 151–5.

Frith, B. (1991) Giving information to radiotherapy patients. *Nursing Standard*, 5(34), 33–5.

Fu, K. & Phillips, T. (1990) High dose rate versus low dose rate intracavitary brachytherapy for carcinoma of the cervix. *International Journal of Radiation Oncology, Biology, Physics*, 19, 791–6.

Gibbs, J. (1991) Radiation hazards. *Nursing Times*, 87(27), 46–7.

Hassey, K. M. (1987) Principles of radiation safety and protection. *Seminars in Oncology Nursing*, 3(1), 23–9.

Hodt, H. J. *et al.* (1952) A gun for interstitial implantation of radioactive gold grains. *British Journal of Radiology*, 25, 419–21.

Holmes, S. (1988) *Radiotherapy. The Lisa Sainsbury Foundation Series*. Austen Cornish, London.

Horwich, A. (1995) *Oncology: A Multidisciplinary Textbook*. Chapman & Hall Medical, London.

Hussey, K. (1985) Demystifying the care of patients with radioactive implants. *American Journal of Nursing*, 85, 789–92.

Jenkins, B. (1986) Sexual healing after pelvic irradiation. *American Journal of Nursing*, 86(8), 920–22.

Jenkins, B. (1988) Patients' reports of sexual changes after treatment for gynaecological cancer. *Oncology Nursing Forum*, 15(3), 349–54.

Klevenhagen, S. C. (1986) The role of the physicist in radiotherapy. In: *Radiotherapy in Clinical Practice*, (ed. H. E. Hope-Stone), pp. 411–32. Butterworths, London.

Lamb, M. A. (1990) Psychosexual issues: the women with gynaecological cancer. *Seminars in Oncology Nursing*, 6(3), 237–43.

Lambert, J. E. & Blake, P. R. (1992) *A Guide to Gynaecology Oncology*. Oxford University Press, London.

Martin, L. F. & Braly, P. S. (1991) Gynaecological cancers. In: *Cancer Nursing*, (eds S. B. Baird *et al.*), pp. 502–35. W. B. Saunders, Philadelphia.

Martin, A. & Harbinson, S. (1979) *An Introduction to Radiation Protection*, 2nd edn. Chapman & Hall, London.

Nucletron Engineering (1981) *Selectron Users' Manual*, Nucletron Engineering, Chester.

Paine, C. H. (1972) Modern afterloading methods for interstitial radiotherapy. *Clinical Radiology*, 23, 263–72.

Patel, F. D. *et al.* (1994) Low dose vs high dose-rate brachytherapy in the treatment of carcinoma of the uterine cervix: a clinical trial. *International Journal of Radiation Oncology, Biology and Physics*, 28, 335–41.

Perez, C. A. *et al.* (1992) Clinical applications of brachytherapy. In: *Principles and Practice of Radiation Oncology*, (eds C. A. Perez & L. W. Brady). J. B. Lippincott, Philadelphia.

Pierquin, B. *et al.* (1978) The Paris system in interstitial radiation therapy. *Acta Radiologica: Oncology, Radiation, Physics, Biology*, 17(1), 33–48.

Royal College of Nursing (1991) *Standards of Care for Cancer Nursing*. Royal College of Nursing Cancer Nursing Society, London.

Royal Marsden NHS Trust (1994) *Local Rules for the Protection of Ward and Theatre Staff against Ionising Radiation arising from Patients administered with Radioactive Material*. Royal Marsden NHS Trust, London.

Rushton, M. (1991) Nursing patients with gynaecological malignancies. In: *Oncology for Nurses and Health Care Professionals*, (eds R. Tiffany & D. Borley), 2nd edn., pp. 340–65, Harper & Row, Beaconsfield.

Shell, J. & Carter, J. (1987) The gynaecological implant patient. *Seminars in Oncology Nursing*, 3(1), 54–66.

Shepherd, J. H. & Monaghan, J. M. (1990) *Clinical Gynaecological Oncology*, 2nd edn. Blackwell Scientific Publications, Oxford.

Souhami, R. & Tobias, J. (1995) *Cancer and its Management*. Blackwell Science, Oxford.

Sutton, M. L. (1986) Gynaecological radiotherapy. In: *Radiotherapy in Clinical Practice*, (ed. H. F. Hope-Stone), pp. 203–37. Butterworths, London.

Thranov, I. & Klee, M. (1994) Sexuality among gynecologic cancer patients: a cross-sectional study. *Gynecologic Oncology*, 52(1), 14–19.

Tiffany, R. (1979) *Cancer Nursing – Radiotherapy*. Faber & Faber, London.

Welby-Allen, M. (1982) Selectron treatment in gynaecology. *Nursing Times*, 78(46), 1948–50.

Whale, Z. (1991) A threat to femininity? Minimising side-effects in pelvic irradiation. *Professional Nurse*, 6(6), 309–11.

Wilkinson, J. M. *et al.* (1983) The use of Selectron afterloading equipment to simulate and extend the Manchester system for intracavitary therapy of the cervix uteri. *British Journal of Radiotherapy*, 56, 409–14.

Wootton, R. (1993) *Radiation Protection of Patients*. Cambridge University Press, London.

GUIDELINES: CARE OF PATIENTS WITH INSERTIONS OF SEALED RADIOACTIVE SOURCES

Action

1 When transferring patients from theatre to ward, the nurse and porter should remain at

Rationale

To minimize the risk of exposure to radiation.

Guidelines: Care of patients with insertions of sealed radioactive sources (cont'd)

Action	Rationale
the head and foot of the bed and at least 120 cm from the centre of the bed in the event of any delay in the transfer. If the source is intra-oral, the nurse should stand at the foot of the bed.	
2 A yellow radiation hazard board should accompany the patient back from theatre. This must remain at the bottom of the bed or outside the cubicle until the source is removed.	To warn everybody that the patient has a radioactive source.
3 Nursing staff must calculate the time allowed with the patient in any 24-hour period. This time should be written on the yellow hazard notice on the bed or cubicle door.	To minimize exposure to radiation.
4 A Geiger counter should be available on the ward.	To monitor radioactivity if a dislodged source is suspected, e.g. in the bed linen.
5 One nurse should be delegated responsibility for the nursing care of the patient. The time spent with the patient should be shared between all of the staff on duty, and time spent in nursing procedures must be kept to a minimum.	To minimize the risk of overexposure to radiation.
6 Every nurse must wear a radiation badge above the level of the lead shield.	To record the extent of exposure to radiation.
7 All bed linen and waste materials removed from the patient area should be monitored before being removed from the ward.	To prevent loss of an accidentally dislodged source.
8 If a source becomes dislodged, use the long-handled forceps to put the source into a lead pot. Care should be taken not to damage the source. It must never be handled directly with the fingers.	To minimize the dose of radiation received.
9 Visitors must remain at least 120 cm away from the patient. The visit should not last longer than the time shown on the warning notice. No children or pregnant women are allowed to visit.	To minimize the risk of overexposure to radiation.

GUIDELINES: CARE OF PATIENTS WITH INTRA-ORAL SOURCES

PREPARATION OF THE PATIENT

Dental assessment of the patient is usually carried out before oral brachytherapy so that caries, mouth infections and dental extractions may be dealt with in case of the oral blood supply being impaired by the treatment. The patient is usually admitted 24 hours before the implant, during which time the nature of the procedure and the implications of having a radioactive source should be explained to the patient. Ideally, the patient should be nursed in a cubicle or in a bed away from other patients to reduce the amount of radiation exposure to other people.

Action	Rationale
1 Encourage frequent mouth care. The patient should void the solution into a bowl and not into a handbasin.	To reduce the risk of infection. To prevent the loss of a dislodged source.
2 Provide a soft, puréed or liquid diet.	To reduce the risk of the patient biting into the source or tongue. Eating is often difficult when implants are present.
3 Avoid spicy and/or hot foods. Discourage the patient from smoking and/or drinking alcohol.	To prevent exacerbation of local reaction or soreness.
4 Encourage ingestion of carbonated drinks.	To alleviate dryness.
5 Provide crushed ice for the patient to suck and/or soluble aspirin as a mouthwash.	To minimize oral pain and discomfort.
6 Give steroids as prescribed.	To prevent and/or minimize swelling.
7 Provide writing equipment for the patient.	To reduce the need for oral communication. This is liable to increase soreness and alter the distribution of the sources.
8 Provide paper tissues and a bowl for saliva.	The patient may have difficulty in swallowing due to soreness and oedema.
9 The sources should be checked at regular intervals, e.g. at the beginning of a span of duty.	To make sure that the sources have not become dislodged.
10 The patient must be confined to the cubicle or the space around the bed. Washing is carried out in the bed area, but the general toilet facilities should be used, provided that the patient remains at a distance from other people.	To minimize the risk of radiation exposure to other people on the ward.

DISCHARGE OF THE PATIENT

The patient is usually discharged the day after the removal of the implant. The patient should be warned about the brisk local reaction which may be experienced due to rapid cell breakdown induced by the radiation. In order to minimize the risk of infection or soreness, the patient should be taught how to care for the treated area, e.g. frequent oral toilet.

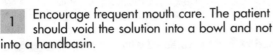

GUIDELINES: CARE OF PATIENTS WITH GYNAECOLOGICAL SOURCES

PREPARATION OF THE PATIENT

The patient is usually admitted 12–48 hours before the procedure so that any pre-anaesthetic investigations may be performed. An enema or suppositories are usually given to reduce the chance of the patient having

Guidelines: Care of patients with gynaecological sources (cont'd)

a bowel action while the sources are in place, which could dislodge the sources. Some patients, however, have diarrhoea on admission due to previous radiotherapy and will need regular medication, such as codeine phosphate, both before and during the application of the sources. A full explanation should be given to the patient along with information about the implications of having a radioactive source inside her and informed consent obtained. The patient should be bathed before any premedication is administered.

Action	Rationale
1 The patient must remain in bed in a recumbent or semi-recumbent position while the applicators or implants are in place.	To prevent the applicators becoming dislodged or changing their position in relation to the internal organs.
2 Rolling from side to side is permitted and should be encouraged if the patient is at risk of developing a pressure sore.	To promote comfort and to relieve prolonged pressure on any one area.
3 On return from theatre, the sanitary towel should be checked for discharge. Disposable pants may be worn. Check that the catheter is correctly positioned to allow drainage.	To secure the position of the sanitary towel. To ensure that urine is draining freely.
4 Observe for any blood or other discharge from the vagina. Check the temperature and pulse every 2 hours.	To monitor haemorrhage, shock and other post-operative complications.
5 Administer prescribed analgesics, antiemetics and antidiarrhoeal agents.	For the patient's comfort.
6 Encourage fluid intake as soon as the patient is allowed to drink. If the source is to be in for longer than 24 hours:	
(a) Encourage a fluid intake of 50–100% a day over and above the patient's normal intake.	To ensure adequate hydration. To reduce the risk of urinary tract infection.
(b) A low-residue diet may be taken.	To prevent the stimulation of a bowel action.

GUIDELINES: REMOVAL OF GYNAECOLOGICAL CAESIUM

The removal of applicators is usually performed by suitably qualified and competent nursing staff.

EQUIPMENT

1 Sterile gynaecological pack containing large receiver, green towel, paper towel, long dissecting forceps, sanitary towel, cotton wool balls.
2 Equipment for the administration of Entonox.
3 Solutions of choice for swabbing, e.g. 0.9% sodium chloride.
4 Gloves.
5 Sterile scissors or stitch cutter.
6 Clean draw sheet.
7 Geiger counter.

PROCEDURE

Action	Rationale
1 Explain and discuss the procedure with the patient.	To ensure that the patient understands the procedure and gives her valid consent.
2 Check the date and time for removal on the form that was received from the physics department when sources were inserted.	The accurate timing of the removal is essential for the administration of the correct therapeutic dose of radiation.
3 Check that any pre-removal drugs (e.g. sedatives, analgesics) have been administered.	
4 Check, with another nurse, the exact time of removal and the number of applicators.	To reduce the risk of error.
5 Ensure that:	
(a) The lead shield is suitably positioned beside the patient.	To shield the nurse from exposure to radiation.
(b) The lead pot is also suitably positioned with the lid removed.	So that sources can be placed in the pot immediately after removal.
6 Begin the administration of Entonox at least 2 minutes before commencing the procedure.	To allow time for the effects of the gas to be felt. (For further information on Entonox administration, see Chapter 17.)
7 Prepare a trolley, put on gloves and open the pack before going to the bedside.	This is a clinically clean, not an aseptic procedure. To reduce the time spent in close proximity to the source.
8 Working from behind the lead shield, assist the patient into the dorsal position with knees apart. Remove the sanitary towel.	To obtain access to the sources.
9 Remove any sutures, if present. Remove the vaginal packing.	
10 Remove the caesium sources in reverse order of insertion. Contact the clinical oncologist immediately if difficulty is encountered in removing a source.	
Place the removed sources in a lead pot immediately and cover with the lid.	To contain radioactivity.
11 Remove the lead pot to a designated area, e.g. an isotope sluice or safe. Ensure that the lid of the pot or the sluice door is locked.	To remove the radioactive source from the ward area. To prevent unauthorized access to the source.
12 Monitor the patient's level of radioactivity.	To ensure that no sources remain inside the patient.
13 Remove the urinary catheter.	
14 Swab the vulva and perineal area with a solution such as 0.9% sodium chloride.	To promote patient hygiene and comfort.
Ensure that the patient has a clean sanitary towel in position and is made comfortable.	

Guidelines: Removal of gynaecological caesium (cont'd)

Action	Rationale
15 Monitor the bed linen, paper bags, vaginal packing and other waste material. (Two nurses should monitor the patient independently.)	To ensure that no source has been lost or remains inside the patient.
16 The patient should remain in bed until the physics department staff are satisfied that all sources are accounted for.	To ensure that all sources have been accounted for before the patient moves around.
17 Remove the radiation warning notice.	

NURSING CARE PLAN

Problem	Cause	Suggested action
Patient has a bowel action.		Inform the radiotherapist.
Patient removes caesium source herself:	Confusion, e.g. post-anaesthetic.	Using long-handled forceps place the source in the lead container or safe. Inform the radiotherapist and the physics department.
Pyrexia.	Pelvic cellulitis or abscess. Reaction to the proflavine pack. Urinary infection. Physiological reaction to the breakdown of the tumour. Chest infection. Peritonitis due to perforation of the uterus.	If the patient's temperature remains over 37.5°C for two consecutive readings, inform the radiotherapist. The caesium may have to be removed if the pyrexia persists.

GUIDELINES: CARE OF PATIENTS UNDERGOING SELECTRON TREATMENT

Action	Rationale
1 Nurse the patient on a pressure-relieving mattress or with a foam wedge under her buttocks.	To promote comfort and to relieve backache since rolling is not permitted.
2 Ensure the plastic transfer tubes are supported securely in the bed bracket, leaving slight slack.	To enable the patient to change position slightly without putting traction on the applicators.
3 Limit the frequency and duration of interruption to treatment. Visitors are discouraged unless the patient is markedly distressed.	To prevent unnecessary prolongation of treatment time.

4   Unless otherwise indicated by the patient's physical or psychological mental condition, check 2-hourly:

(a) Temperature, pulse and vaginal loss.

To monitor for haemorrhage, shock or other postoperative complications.

(b) Contents of catheter drainage bag.

To ensure urine is draining freely.

(c) Assist patient to adjust her position.

To promote comfort and relieve prolonged pressure on any one area.

5   Administer prescribed analgesics, antiemetics antidiarrhoeal and sedative agents as appropriate and evaluate effect.

To promote the patient's comfort and well-being.

6   Encourage fluid intake as soon as the patient is able to drink.

To ensure adequate hydration and reduce the risk of urinary tract infection.

7   If the patient wishes to eat, a light, low-residue diet may be taken.

To prevent stimulation of a bowel action.

GUIDELINES: REMOVAL OF SELECTRON APPLICATORS

If two patients are being treated simultaneously, removal of the applicators may be delayed until both patients have finished treatment, depending on the individual treatment times.

EQUIPMENT

As for removal of other gynaecological applicators see Guidelines: Removal of gynaecological caesium, above, (items 1–7) plus:

8 Rubber caps for the applicators.

PROCEDURE

Action	Rationale
1 Check treatment has been terminated by: (a) Ensuring the appropriate channel lights are green. If the other patient's treatment is continuing, interrupt treatment. (b) Ensure time display on the Selectron unit reads zero for the appropriate channels. (c) Ensure the print-out indicates treatment has stopped for those channels.	The applicators should be removed only on completion of treatment.
2 Record the finish time on the patient's dosimetry sheet.	This is kept as a record in the patient's notes.
3 Check that the closed-circuit television camera is not focused on the patient.	To ensure privacy.
4 Explain and discuss the procedure with the patient.	To ensure that the patient understands the procedure and gives his/her valid consent.
5 Ensure any pre-removal drugs have been administered.	To allow analgesic or sedative to be felt.

Guidelines: Removal of Selectron applicators (cont'd)

Action	Rationale
6 Assist the patient into a comfortable position with her knees apart.	To allow access to the applicators.
7 Uncouple the plastic transfer tubes by rotating the black coupling anticlockwise in the direction of the arrow and very carefully store the tubes on the plastic supporting mantle attached to the Selectron unit.	To prevent the plastic catheter becoming damaged or kinked.
8 Place rubber caps on the ends of the applicators.	To ensure no fluid or debris is allowed to enter the applicator tubes.
9 Commence administration of Entonox (see Chapter 17) at least 2 minutes before removal of the applicators.	To allow the effect of the gas to be felt.
10 Prepare the equipment and put on gloves.	The procedure is clinically clean and not aseptic.
11 Remove the vulval dressing pads, any sutures and vaginal packing.	These must be removed before the applicators can be eased out.
12 Dismantle the applicators by loosening the screws holding them together.	To promote ease of removal.
Remove the uterine tube first, ensuring it is taken out complete with its small white flange, followed by the ovoids.	To prevent the flange being left in the patient's vagina.
13 Remove the catheter, swab the vulval area and ensure the patient has a clean sanitary pad and a fresh draw sheet.	To promote cleanliness and patient comfort.
14 The patient can then be assisted into a comfortable position and is permitted up to have a bath.	The patient is reassured that the procedure has been completed, that she is no longer radioactive and can resume normal activities.

Applicators are retained carefully for cleaning in accordance with local policies. Remaining treatment can then be given to the second patient.

NURSING CARE PLAN

See also 'Nursing care plan' for conventional gynaecological sources, above.

Problem	Cause	Suggested action
Patient removes the applicators herself.	Confusion, e.g. post-anaesthetic.	Interrupt treatment. Deposit applicators and attached tubing in the lead pot. Inform radiotherapist and physicist. Restart treatment if two patients are being treated.

Applicator is partially dislodged.	Patient may have moved too much or too vigorously.	Interrupt treatment. Inform physicist and radiotherapist. The applicator may have to be removed as above.
Alarm sounding at nurse station.	Treatment has been interrupted and inadvertently left off.	Check patient is unattended and recommence treatment.
Sources are not transferred to the applicators.	Incorrect coupling or loose connection.	Check print-out to identify which channel is at fault. Tighten appropriate coupling device.
Alarm activated at remote control unit.	Failure in the system.	Check the error code on the print-out with the Selectron users' manual. Rectify as indicated in the manual or seek technical assistance from the physics department.
Pellets stuck in the applicator or transfer tubing.	A damaged or kinked catheter.	Inform the physics department. Withdraw the plastic catheter using long-handled forceps and deposit in the protected container until technical assistance can be provided. Reassure the patient.

GUIDELINES: CARING FOR THE PATIENT WITH RADIOACTIVE SEEDS OR GRAINS (E.G. IODINE-125 OR GOLD-198)

PREPARATION OF THE PATIENT

The patient is usually admitted at least one day before treatment: Patients should be nursed ideally in a single room but, more importantly, in a bed away from the main thoroughfare.

Grains or seeds are implanted permanently into the tissue and therefore the patient must agree to stay in hospital until the physics staff state that the radioactivity is at a legally permissible level for discharge.

Breast and lymph node implantation

Action

1 The dressing to be left securely in position unless special instructions are given by the radiotherapist.

2 If dressing becomes dislodged leave it at the bedside, preferably in a lead pot and inform the physics staff.

3 If there is any possibility that the sources have become detached inform physics department staff immediately and do not remove anything from the room.

Rationale

Sources may became detached, dressings will prevent them from becoming lost.

If sources have became detached and are in the dressings physics staff will take the necessary action.

It is important that the source is not lost as this could result in contamination of the environment. The patient's total dose will be altered and the medical staff will need to be informed.

Guidelines: Caring for the patient with radioactive seeds or grains (cont'd)

Lung implantation

Action	Rationale
1 Check all sputum and drainage from the chest with the Geiger counter. If no radioactivity is found the sputum and drainage may be disposed of in the usual way unless special instructions are given by the physics department or radiotherapy staff.	To check for radioactivity in case any sources are coughed up or expelled in the drainage.
2 If radioactivity is detected, inform physics department staff immediately. Save the sputum or drainage for them to deal with.	To prevent contamination of the hospital environment.

Bladder and prostate implantation

Action	Rationale
1 Check all urine with the Geiger counter. If no radioactivity is found the urine may be disposed of in the usual way.	To check for radioactivity in case any sources are expelled in the urine.
2 If radioactivity is detected inform physics staff immediately and save urine for them to deal with.	To prevent contamination of the hospital environment.
3 Leave suspect urine in a safe place at the bedside, e.g. under the bed.	To prevent accidental disposal.

GUIDELINES: CARE OF PATIENTS WITH BREAST SOURCES

PREPARATION OF THE PATIENT

The patient will usually be admitted for local excision of the breast tumour and an axillary clearance. Drains are inserted and these are usually removed before the iridium wire sources are loaded 24–48 hours after surgery. When the sources are loaded, the patient should be nursed in a bed away from other patients.

Action	Rationale
1 Any dressing is left undisturbed for the duration of treatment.	To minimize the time spent in proximity to the patient.
2 The patient is confined to the cubicle or the space around the bed. Washing is carried out at the bed area. If general toilet facilities have to be used the patient must remain at a distance from other people.	To minimize the risk of radiation to other people on the ward.
3 Administer prescribed analgesia as required throughout the treatment period and before removal.	For the patient's comfort.

DISCHARGE OF THE PATIENT

The patient should normally be discharged the day after the removal of the implant. The patient should be warned about the brisk local reaction which she may experience due to the rapid cell breakdown induced by the radiation. In order to minimize the risk of infection or soreness, the patient should be taught how to care far the treated area.

UNSEALED RADIOACTIVE SOURCE THERAPY

REFERENCE MATERIAL

Unsealed sources are used to concentrate a radioisotope in a particular part of the body. Four unsealed sources will be discussed here:

(1) Rhenium-186 hydroxyethylidene diphosphonate (Re186 HEDP), used in the treatment of bone metastases.
(2) Iodine-131, used in the treatment of thyroid disorders.
(3) Meta-iodobenzylguanidine (MIBG), used in the treatment of neuroblastoma.
(4) Monoclonal antibodies labelled with iodine-131, used in the treatment of recurrent cystic glioblastoma.

Rhenium-186 hydroxyethylidene diphosphonate (Re186 HEDP)

Definition

Rhenium-186 forms a stable diphosphonate chelate with hydroxyethylidene diphosphonate (HEDP) forming rhenium-186 hydroxyethylidene diphosphonate (Re186 HEDP) (Lewington, 1993). The linking of the radionuclide rhenium-186 to a suitable chemical compound produces a radiopharmaceutical which is localized in metastatic foci in bone (Donald et al., 1989). Rhenium-186 HEDP is a beta–emitting radionuclide with a maximum beta energy of 1.07 MeV (megaelectron volts). It has a gamma ray emission of 137 keV (Maxon et al., 1988).

The beta particles travel only short distances and, therefore, their energy deposition is localized in metastatic foci in bone, delivering a therapeutic radiation dose directly to the metastases whilst delivering a much lower dose to normal bone marrow. Because Re186 HEDP also emits gamma rays, which can be located by diagnostic imaging techniques, it is possible to verify its location in areas of metastatic disease, and to measure the dose of radiation delivered to the tumour and bone marrow (Maxon et al., 1992).

Use

Bone metastases are the commonest cause of cancer pain, and can lead to immobility, pathological fractures, bone marrow failure, neurological symptoms and hypercalcaemia (Lewington, 1993). Approximately 80% of patients with prostate cancer develop bone metastases (Maxon et al., 1991) in spite of surgery, hormone therapy, external beam radiotherapy and chemotherapy (Maxon et al., 1988). In 1991 prostate cancer was the second most common cause of death from malignant disease in men (Dearnaley, 1994). Studies using Re186 HEDP as targeted radiotherapy have shown that it can provide prompt and significant relief of pain in approximately 80% of patients (Maxon et al., 1990). It has advantages over conventional external beam radiotherapy because it is tumour specific with relative sparing of surrounding healthy tissue (Lewington, 1993). Whilst thrombocytopenia is a dose-limiting toxicity, leucopenia is less severe (Klerk et al., 1994). A mild transient increase in pain may occur within a few days of administering Re186 HEDP (Maxon et al., 1992).

Rhenium-186 HEDP is administered by intravenous injection. Because Re186 HEDP is excreted in the urine, urinary catheterization is carried out prior to treatment to ensure that the bladder remains empty and the radiation dose to the bladder is minimized. Therefore caution must be exercised when emptying the catheter bag (see 'Preparation of the therapy room', below). Because the half-life of Re186 HEDP is only 90 hours (Maxon et al., 1988), patients may only need to be segregated after it has been administered for between 24 and 48 hours (Maxon et al., 1988).

Iodine-131

Definition

Radioactive iodine-131 is a beta-gamma emitter with a half-life of 8 days, and is used mainly in the form of iodide solution. The beta radiation gives a high, local dose in iodine concentrating tissue. The gamma component is useful for external measurement and scanning (Pointon, 1991).

Use

Thyroid tissue selectively concentrates iodide, which enables iodine-131 to be used in the diagnosis and treatment of thyroid disorders:

(1) Thyrotoxicosis. Treatment doses between 75 and 400 megabecquerels (MBq) activity of iodine-131 can be usually given, often on an outpatient basis.
(2) Well differentiated thyroid cancers (papillary and follicular) and metastases that function similarly to the thyroid tissue. Treatment is usually on an inpatient basis because of the higher activities involved.

Iodine-131 is normally administered as a solution taken orally by the patient, or it may be given in the form of capsules. It can also be administered intravenously.

Treatment programme for carcinoma of the thyroid

(1) *Surgical removal of the thyroid.* Normal thyroid tissue concentrates iodine more efficiently than malignant tissue, and some malignant tissues concentrate iodine-131 only after removal of normal tissue (Pointon, 1991). It is recommended, therefore, that a surgical near-total thyroidectomy is performed before administration of iodine-131.
(2) *Iodine-131 treatment.* Following thyroidectomy an ablation dose of, typically, 3 GBq of iodine-131 is administered to ablate the remnants of thyroid tissue. Further treatments of 5.5 GBq may be necessary to destroy deposits in local lymph nodes and distant metastases.

Preparation of the patient before admission

(1) *Twenty-one days before admission*: patients taking tetraiodothyronine (T_4) (thyroxine) must stop taking this medication.
(2) *Ten days before admission*: patients taking triiodothyronine (T_3) must stop taking this medication.
(3) *Three days before admission*: occasionally, to enhance the uptake of iodine-131, three daily injections of thyroid-stimulating hormone are administered.

Meta-iodobenzylguanidine (MIBG)

Definition
Meta-iodobenzylguanidine is a synthetic physiological guanethidine analogue which is structurally similar to both the neurotransmitter hormone norepinephrine and the ganglionic blocking drug guanethidine. MIBG will localize in a wide variety of neuroendocrine tumours including neuroblastomas and phaeochromocytomas (Barry *et al.*, 1990) yet in relatively few normal cells (Kemshead *et al.*, 1990).

MIBG can be linked to iodine-131 (a radionuclide) to produce the radiopharmaceutical 131-I MIBG. A radiopharmaceutical is a radionuclide linked to a suitable chemical compound whose biochemical properties allow the radionuclide to be localized in the desired tissue (Donald *et al.*, 1989).

Use
131-I MIBG can be used as a safe, effective, non-invasive method of localizing both primary and meta-static neuroendocrine tumours (Barry *et al.*, 1990). Therapeutic doses of 131-I MIBG can be given to patients in whom standard surgical and chemotherapeutic treatments have failed to control primary tumours, or can be used as an adjuvant to these treatments to prevent recurrence of the tumour (Fielding *et al.*, 1991).

Prior to therapy patients undergo scanning investigations using a tracer dose of 131-I MIBG which allows calculation of the treatment dose. Therapeutic doses of 131-I MIBG are custom-synthesized for each patient and kept frozen from the time of synthesis until the dose is administered to reduce the risk of autoradiolysis. The solution is thawed, diluted and infused intravenously over 30–60 minutes using a shielded syringe pump. During infusion pulse, blood pressure and electrocardiogram are monitored (Barry *et al.*, 1990).

Side-effects include anorexia and mild nausea and vomiting, which can be controlled with anti-emetics and an adequate intake of fluids. The major toxicities are to bone marrow, with a higher incidence of significant thrombocytopenia than neutropenia (Hoefnagel *et al.*, 1987), and to the bladder (Fielding *et al.*, 1991).

Principles of protection policies
Iodine-131 is excreted rapidly in patients who have had a thyroidectomy via all body fluids, especially the urine. In those patients who have not undergone thyroidectomy, excretion is rapid initially, slowing as the iodine-131 is bound by the thyroid tissue. Consequently, great care must be taken with all body fluids, especially during the first few days.

Preparation of the patient
To prevent the uptake of any free iodine-131, the uptake of radioactive iodine by the thyroid gland is blocked by giving patients excess oral iodine 3 days before and 3 weeks after administration of MIBG.

As MIBG stimulates noradrenaline, drugs which act as antagonists (e.g. phenothiazines) are contraindicated during treatment (Shulkin & Shapiro, 1990).

Monoclonal antibodies labelled with iodine-131 for recurrent cystic glioblastoma

Definition
Monoclonal antibodies specific to glioma antigens can be radiolabelled with iodine-131 and administered as

therapy for patients with cystic gliomas. The tumour is targeted by the monoclonal antibodies which deliver the radiation dose to the tumour. Because the antibodies are specific to glioma tissue, the exposure of normal tissues is limited (Lashford *et al.*, 1988).

An antibody is a protein which is produced as a result of the introduction of an antigen. It has the ability to combine with the antigen that stimulated its production. Monoclonal antibodies are identical copies of a single antibody (Stites & Terr, 1991). It is possible to produce monoclonal antibodies that are specific to tumour cells, which can be labelled with a radioisotope. When administered to the patient, the labelled monoclonal antibody seeks, attaches itself to, and then as the radioisotope decays, emitting radiation, it destroys malignant cells which carry the appropriate specific antigen (Epenetos, 1993).

Use
High-grade malignant gliomas are at present not curable with conventional treatment (surgery, radiotherapy and chemotherapy) (Brada, 1989). Small studies of monoclonal antibodies labelled with iodine-131 administered intrathecally have shown that some patients have a significant and lasting therapeutic response without significant immediate or lasting toxicity (Lashford *et al.*, 1988).

The procedure consists of surgically inserting a catheter into the tumour, and then administering a diagnostic dose of monoclonal antibody labelled iodine-124. Following positron emission tomography (PET), a technique for imaging the distribution of radiolabelled pharmaceuticals (Horwich, 1995) it is possible to calculate the therapeutic dose of antibody labelled with iodine-131. The therapeutic dose is administered slowly into the catheter by the patient's physician.

Following administration, it is important to carry out careful neurological observations to identify complications related to placement of the catheter, allergic reactions to the monoclonal antibody labelled with iodine-131 or possible toxicities associated with instillation of intracystic therapies.

The principles of protection policies must be followed. Education and support for patients and carers is particularly important because of the nature of this rarely used therapy.

Principles of radiation protection
The following radiation protection policies and nursing guidelines are written to conform with the *Ionizing Radiations Regulations, 1985* and *1988* and associated guidance notes. They are applicable where dedicated single-bed treatment rooms with en suite toilet and bathing facilities are available.

Further precautions may be necessary when these conditions are not met. The advice of the radiation protection advisor must always be sought.

When patients are treated with radioactive sources it may be necessary to limit the time staff and others spend in close proximity to the patient. A controlled area notice with a radiation trefoil and a *no unauthorized entry* sign is displayed to restrict access to the patient. Entry to this controlled area is governed by a written work protocol supported by local rules which are compiled and employed to ensure that all persons entering a controlled area adopt safe working procedures. Radiation protection supervisors are appointed to each controlled area to ensure local rules are followed (Department of Health and Social Security, 1985).

Nurses must follow the procedures set out for the period when controlled area restrictions apply. This, and careful planning of work, will ensure that exposure to radiation is minimized in a way that is compatible with good nursing care. Patients are cared for in a shielded room using the radiation protection principles of distance, shielding and time minimization, as for iodine-131 therapy (see below).

Controlled area
The entrance to the controlled area must be marked with a warning sign. Information is displayed to indicate the following:

(1) The radioactive material and activity administered.
(2) The nursing time allowed per day:
    (a) Essential nursing procedures only should be carried out and unnecessary time must not be spent in close proximity to the patient while the sign is displayed.
    (b) The time given is such that a nurse remaining at a distance of approximately 60 cm from the patient for the time indicated each day would, after 5 consecutive days, receive the maximum permissible dose for the working week.

Appropriate barriers, i.e. lead shields, should be placed at the entrance to:

(1) Prevent inadvertent entry by unauthorized personnel.
(2) Reduce radiation exposure to visitors and staff.

Patients treated with unsealed radioactive sources should be confined to their rooms, except for special medical or nursing procedures, when they must be accompanied by suitably trained staff.

Film badges
Film badges should be worn at all times when on duty.

Contamination control

With unsealed sources, it is important to guard against contamination both of personnel and the hospital environment by the correct use of protective gloves, gowns and overshoes. The patient's body fluids are highly radioactive, especially in the days immediately after iodine-131 has been administered. The application of cosmetics, eating, drinking or smoking while there is any possibility that the hands are contaminated is prohibited.

In the event of any incident involving radioactive material, the physics department must be advised immediately, even if the incident occurs outside normal working hours.

Preparation of the therapy room

Equipment

Equipment should be kept to a minimum. It must be checked to ensure that it is in working order, as maintenance staff will only be allowed into the room in exceptional circumstances.

Bed linen and disposable items (gloves, aprons, overshoes, cutlery and crockery) should be kept in a utility room or ante-room along with the patient's treatment chart and a radiation monitor.

Personal items

Nurses should be sensitive to the psychological implications for patients of being labelled 'radioactive' and confined in isolation. Although patients may want to bring some personal belongings with them, they should be advised to keep these to a minimum, as items may become contaminated and need to be stored until radioactivity has decayed.

Protective floor covering

Plastic-backed absorbent paper, kept in place by adhesive tape, is used to retain accidental urine spills or splashes on the floor immediately surrounding the toilet. Each patient is assessed to decide if further floor covering is necessary, e.g. catheterized patients will require floor covering below a catheter bag.

Cleaning the treatment room

During occupancy of the treatment room by the patient, cleaning of the room is kept to a minimum and should be supervised by the physics staff. After the patient is discharged, monitoring and any necessary decontamination of the room will be arranged by the physics department, which will inform the relevant personnel when this has been completed. Only then may the room be entered and thoroughly cleaned.

Preparation of the patient

Consent

Patients are required to sign a consent form agreeing to treatment, following a full explanation from the treating clinician. This is to comply with medical, ethical and legal requirements and local hospital policy. Consent is usually obtained in the outpatient clinic before ordering the radioactive material.

On admission

Before the administration of unsealed sources, any symptoms of diarrhoea or constipation must be remedied. Diarrhoea could result in contamination of the treatment area. Constipation not only inhibits the elimination of radioactivity but could also obscure radiological investigations, e.g. scanning.

Patients and relatives should be educated about the principles of radiation protection and the procedures with which the patient has to comply while in isolation. It is important to identify potential anxieties before administration while the nurse is able to reassure the patient and is unconstrained by time limits.

The patient must also agree to stay in hospital until the physics department advises that the level of radioactivity permits discharge.

Discharge of the patient

A patient should not be discharged from hospital until the activity retained has fallen below recommended levels. This level will depend on several factors, including:

(1) Mode of transport on leaving hospital.
(2) Journey time involved.
(3) Personal circumstances, i.e. young children or pregnant women at home.

Patients will be assessed individually for radiation clearance by the physics department before discharge. The treating physician will then be advised of the results of the assessment. Advice will be given to patients on issues such as return to work and visits to public places. Patients who are discharged with more than 150 MBq of radioactivity retained will be given appropriate information in the form of an instruction card carrying details of precautions to be taken. This card must be signed by the treating clinician.

It must be emphasized that this card is to be carried and the instructions followed until the latest date shown so that, for instance, staff would be alerted should the patient be readmitted to hospital. Additional verbal instructions may be necessary.

Regulations

Ionizing Radiations Regulations (1985). HMSO, London.
Ionizing Radiations (Protection of Persons Undergoing Medical Examination or Treatment) Regulations (1988). HMSO, London.

References and further reading

Barry, L. *et al*. (1990) Radioiodinated metaiodobenzylguanidine (MIBG) in the management of neuroblastomas. In: *Neuroblastoma Tumor Biology and Therapy*, (ed. C. Poshedly). CRC Press, Boston.

Brada, M. (1989) Back to the future: radiotherapy in high grade gliomas. *British Journal of Cancer*, 60, 14.

Dearnaley, D. P. (1994) Cancer of the prostate. *British Medical Journal*, 308, 780–84.

Department of Health and Social Security (1985) *Ionizing Radiation Regulations*. HMSO, London.

Donald, R. B. *et al*. (1989) *Nuclear Medicine Technology and Techniques*. C. V. Mosby, Baltimore.

Epenetos, A. A. (1993) *Monoclonal Antibodies: Two Applications in Clinical Oncology*. Chapman & Hall Medical, London.

Fielding, S. L. *et al*. (1991) Dosimetry of 131 I MIBG for treatment of resistant neuroblastoma: results of a UK study. *European Journal of Nuclear Medicine*, 18, 308–16.

Hoefnagel, C. A. *et al*. (1987) Radionuclide diagnosis and therapy of neural crest tumors using 131 I MIBG. *Journal of Nuclear Medicine*, 28, 308–14.

Horwich, A. (ed.) (1995) *Oncology: A Multidisciplinary Textbook*. Chapman & Hall Medical, London.

International Commission on Radiological Protection Publication 57: Radiological Protection of the Worker in Medicine and Dentistry (1990). Pergamon Press, Oxford.

Kemshead, J. T. *et al*. (1990) Neuroblastoma: perspectives for future research. In: *Neuroblastoma Tumor Biology and Therapy*, (ed. C. Pochedly). CRC Press, Boston.

Klerk, J. M. H. *et al*. (1994) Dose escalation study of rhenium-186 hydroxyethylidene diphosphonate in patients with metastatic prostate cancer. *European Journal of Nuclear Medicine*, 21(10), 1114–20.

Lashford, L. S. *et al*. (1988) A pilot study of iodine-131 monoclonal antibodies in the therapy of leptomeningeal tumours. *Cancer*, 61, 857–68.

Lewington, V. J. (1993) Targeted radionuclide therapy for bone metastases. *European Journal of Nuclear Medicine*, 20, 66–74.

Martin, A. & Harbinson, S. (1979) *An Introduction to Radiation Protection*. Chapman & Hall Medical, London.

Mayes, J. *et al*. (1989) *Neuroblastoma: MIBG in its Diagnosis and Management*. Springer Verlag, London.

Maxon, H. R. *et al*. (1988) Re-186 HEDP for treatment of multiple metastatic foci in bone: human biodistribution and dosimetric studies. *Radiology*, 166, 505–7.

Maxon, H. R. *et al*. (1990) Re-186 treatment of painful osseous metastases: initial clinical experience in 20 patients with hormone resistant prostate cancer. *Radiology*, 176, 155–9.

Maxon, H. R. *et al*. (1991) Rhenium-186 HEDP for treatment of painful osseous metastases: results of a double-blind crossover comparison with placebo. *Journal of Nuclear Medicine*, 32, 1877–81.

Maxon, H. R. *et al*. (1992) Rheninm – 186 hydroxyethylidene diphosphonate for the treatment of painful osseous metastases. *Seminars in Nuclear Medicine*, 22(1), 33–40.

Mould, R. F. (1985) *Radiation Protection in Hospitals*. Adam Hilger, Bristol and Boston.

National Council for Radiation Protection (NCRP) Report 105 (1989) *Radiation Protection for Medical and Allied Health Personnel*. NCRP.

National Radiological Protection Board (NRPB) (1988) *Guidance Notes For the Protection of Persons Against Ionizing Radiations Arising from Medical Use*. HMSO, London.

Pointon, R. C. S. (1991) *The Radiotherapy of Malignant Disease*. Springer Verlag, London.

Shulkin, B. L. & Shapiro, B. (1990) Radioiodinated MIBG in the management of neuroblastoma. In: *Neuroblastoma Tumor Biology and Therapy*, (ed. C. Pochedly). CRC Press, Boston.

Sisson, J. C. *et al*. (1984) Radiopharmaceutical treatment of malignant phaeochromocytoma. *Journal of Nuclear Medicine*, 24, 197–206.

Souhami, R. & Tobias, J. (1995) *Cancer and its Management*. Blackwell Science, Oxford.

Stites, D. P. & Terr, A. I. (1991) *The Basis of Human Immunology*. Prentice-Hall International, London.

Tiffany, R. (ed.) (1987) *Cancer Nursing: Radiotherapy*. Faber and Faber, London.

Tiffany, R. (ed.) (1988) *Oncology for Nurses and Health Care Professionals*, Vols 1 and 2. George Allen & Unwin, London.

Walter, J. (1977) *Cancer and Radiotherapy*. Churchill Livingstone, Edinburgh.

Wootton, R. (1993) *Radiation Protection of Patients*. Cambridge University Press, Cambridge.

GUIDELINES: NURSING THE PATIENT BEFORE THE ADMINISTRATION OF IODINE-131

	Action	Rationale
1	Explain and discuss the procedure with the patient.	To ensure that the patient understands the procedure and gives his/her valid consent.
2	The patient is to be fasted for two hours before and after administration of an	To reduce the risk of nausea and/or vomiting.

Guidelines: Nursing the patient before the administration of iodine-131 (cont'd)

Action	Rationale
iodine-131 dose. Offer a light diet for the remainder of the day.	
3 Administer a prophylactic antiemetic 30 minutes before scheduled administration of the dose.	To prevent nausea and vomiting.
4 Check that the preparation of the room and the patient is complete. Ensure that any surplus items have been removed.	To prevent contamination of extraneous equipment.
5 Apply a wristband showing the radiation warning symbol to the patient's wrist.	To identify the patient as radioactive.
6 Place the radiation warning sign at the entrance to the therapy room.	To identify the room as a controlled area.

GUIDELINES: NURSING THE PATIENT RECEIVING IODINE-131 THYROID TREATMENT

Action	Rationale
1 Explain and discuss the procedure with the patient.	To ensure that the patient understands the procedure and gives his/her valid consent.
2 Assist the patient to remove dentures/bridges.	To prevent radioactive material being trapped behind dental plates.
3 The patient swallows the capsule or drinks the iodine-131 through a straw, physically directed by an authorized physicist in the presence of the clinician directing treatment.	Drinking through a straw reduces the amount of radioactive material left around the mouth. To meet current regulations.
4 Offer the patient a drink of water to rinse out the mouth. (This must be swallowed.) Assist the patient to replace dentures.	To remove any iodine-131 from inside the mouth.

GUIDELINES: NURSING THE PATIENT RECEIVING IODINE-131 MIBG TREATMENT

Action	Rationale
1 Explain and discuss the procedure with the patient.	To ensure that the patient understands the procedure and gives his/her valid consent.
2 Apply a vital signs monitor with a variable time setting mode to the patient that will be visible to staff from outside the room.	Following the administration of MIBG, a transient rise in blood pressure and pulse may occur.

3	Check that the patient has been cannulated, and commence prescribed intravenous fluids three hours before iodine-131 MIBG administration.	Iodine-131 MIBG is administered intravenously through a three-way tap attached to the giving set.
4	Set up iodine-131 MIBG infusion and give over 30–60 minutes.	To minimize transient rise in blood pressure and pulse.
5	Monitor blood pressure and pulse: (a) Every 5 minutes during infusion; (b) Every 10 minutes for the first 45 minutes post-infusion; (c) Hourly for 4 hours; (d) Four-hourly; or more frequently if required.	To detect and monitor any change.
6	Continue intravenous hydration for 24 hours post-infusion and simultaneously encourage oral fluids.	To increase the urinary output and elimination of radioactivity from the bladder.

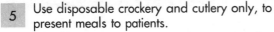

GUIDELINES: NURSING THE PATIENT AFTER ADMINISTRATION OF UNSEALED SOURCES

Entering the room

Action	Rationale
1 Put on disposable gloves.	To prevent contamination of the hands.
2 Put on disposable overshoes.	To prevent spread of contamination outside the treatment area.
3 Put on a suitable protective gown: (a) Long-sleeve cotton gown, e.g. for lifting patient. (b) Disposable water-repellent gown, e.g. for dealing with vomit or incontinence.	To protect against low levels of contamination, e.g. from the patient's skin. To protect against high levels of contamination.
4 Plan work before entering the controlled area and then work quickly and efficiently, keeping within the time allowance stated.	To minimize radiation exposure, as consistent with good nursing core.
5 Use disposable crockery and cutlery only, to present meals to patients.	China crockery and cutlery may become contaminated.

Maintaining patient comfort and hygiene

Action	Rationale
1 Encourage the patient to bathe/shower frequently, at least once a day.	To reduce any radioactive perspiration on the skin.
2 Encourage the patient to wash the hands thoroughly after each possible contact with bodily fluids, e.g. cleaning teeth, going to the toilet, etc.	To remove radioactivity from the hands.

Guidelines: Nursing the patient after administration of unsealed sources (cont'd)

Action	Rationale
3 The patient should regularly remove any dentures and clean under running water.	To remove radioactive saliva from around dentures.
4 The patient should regularly remove any contact lenses and rinse in their usual cleaning fluid.	To remove any radioactive tears from lenses
5 Encourage a good fluid intake of between 2 and 3 litres per day.	To increase the urinary output and elimination of radioactivity from the bladder.
6 Ensure that the patient has own personal toilet facilities and flushes the toilet twice after use.	To reduce contamination of others and of the environment. Urine of patients treated with iodine-131 is initially highly radioactive.
7 Bedbound patients should be catheterized before the dose is given. Empty the catheter bag every 4–6 hours, or more frequently if necessary.	Catheterization reduces the nursing time spent with the patient and the likelihood of contamination. Frequent emptying of the bag reduces the radiation level in the room.
8 If the patient requires a bedpan or urinal, this item must be kept solely for this patient's use. The bedpan or urinal must be handled carefully with gloved hands and the contents disposed of in the toilet, which is flushed twice. The bedpan or urinal may be washed in the bedpan washer. It should be sealed in a plastic bag for the journey to and from the sluice.	To reduce contamination of the environment and of other patients and staff.
9 If leakage occurs from injection sites, wound sites etc., the nurse should contact the medical staff and the physics department immediately. Any contact with the dressing should be done with long-handled forceps.	It must be remembered that all body fluids are potentially radioactive.
10 Gloves and a protective gown must be worn whenever handling soiled bed linen.	To prevent contamination.
11 All soiled linen must be deposited in a special container provided for this purpose.	Soiled linen must be monitored for contamination before going to the laundry.

Visitors

Action	Rationale
 **1** Visiting time is limited as advised by the physicist during the first day following administration of an unsealed source.	The patient is highly radioactive during this period.
2 On subsequent days visiting is unlimited providing visitors remain outside the room behind the lead screen.	To minimize the exposure of visitors to radiation.
3 Physical contact with the patient or bed linen is not allowed as protective clothing is not available to visitors.	To prevent contamination of visitors.

	Action	Rationale
4	Children under 16 years of age and pregnant women should be discouraged from visiting.	Radiation exposure of children and the unborn must be kept as low as practicable.

On leaving the room

	Action	Rationale
1	Remove overshoes, taking care not to touch the shoes worn underneath.	These are removed first while gloves are still being worn to prevent the spread of contamination to hands or the floor outside the room.
2	Remove the plastic apron, by holding the front of apron and breaking the neck and waist ties.	
3	Remove gloves by peeling them off the hands, taking care not to touch the outside surfaces with bare hands, and discard them in the clinical waste bag provided.	To prevent transfer of contamination from the gloves' outer surfaces to the hands.
4	Wash hands thoroughly using soap and water.	To remove any contamination.
5	Use the radiation monitor each time when leaving the room and monitor for contamination of the hands, feet and clothing. If contamination has occurred, inform the physics department immediately and follow the decontamination procedure.	To ensure that the nurse is not contaminated.
6	If contamination is suspected whole body monitoring will be undertaken.	To check for thyroid and lung uptake.

GUIDELINES: EMERGENCY PROCEDURES

In an emergency, the safety and medical care of the patient must take precedence over any potential radiation hazards to staff. Written radiation safety instructions must be available in all radiation areas where an emergency may arise. These instructions must contain a detailed description of how to manage a patient in the event of a medical emergency and the action required in other emergency situations such as fire. The course of action in an emergency procedure depends on local circumstances and the nature of the emergency.

An incident occurring within the first 24 hours of iodine-131 being administered is obviously a greater hazard than a similar incident on the day of discharge.

Incontinence and/or vomiting

	Action	Rationale
1	Inform the physics department immediately.	So that the physics department can advise on radiation protection as soon as possible.
2	If physics department staff are not immediately available, use a radiation monitor to assess the extent of the spillage.	To define extent of contamination and determine what further measures need to be taken.

Guidelines: Emergency procedures (cont'd)

Action	Rationale
3 Put some absorbent material on top of all the radioactive wet area.	To absorb contamination.
4 Leave the area until physics department staff arrive. Polythene sheets may be placed over all of the contaminated area.	To prevent spread of contamination.

Contamination of bare hands

Action	Rationale
1 Wash hands in warm soapy water, paying special attention to the areas around the fingernails, between the fingers and on the outer edges of the hands. Continue washing until contamination is below the permissible limits indicated by local monitoring protocols.	To remove radioactive material from any areas where it might be trapped.
2 If a wound is produced in a contamination accident, wash thoroughly under running water, opening the edges of the cut. This should be continued until physics department staff can demonstrate that no residual radioactivity remains in the wound.	To stimulate bleeding and permit thorough flushing of the cut.

Death

Action	Rationale
1 Inform the physics department immediately.	So that the physics department staff can begin making the necessary arrangements for removal of the body to the mortuary.
2 Two nurses wearing gloves, plastic aprons, gowns and overshoes should perform last offices. All orifices must be packed carefully. Any vomit, blood, faeces or urine must be cleaned from the body.	To avoid contamination with body fluids. Minimal handling of the body reduces the risk of contamination.
3 The body should be totally enclosed in a plastic cadaver bag.	To avoid contamination of the porters and the mortuary staff.
4 Transfer of the body should be arranged with the physics department.	The physics department will supervise the transfer of the body.

Cardiac arrest

Action	Rationale
1 The switchboard must be told to inform the physics department as soon as possible after alerting the emergency resuscitation team.	So that the physics department can advise on radiation protection as soon as possible.

2	Do not use mouth-to-mouth resuscitation. All areas must be supplied with an Ambu bag for this purpose.	Mouth-to-mouth contact could result in contamination of the resuscitator.
3	Overshoes, gloves and gowns must be put on as soon as it is practicably possible.	To minimize personal contamination.
4	All emergency equipment must be monitored and decontaminated as necessary before being returned to general use.	To prevent contaminated equipment leaving the controlled area.

Fire

Action   **Rationale**

1	Every effort should be made to contact the physics department without compromising the patient's safety.	To help in the evacuation of the patients treated with iodine-131
2	Following evacuation, patients treated with iodine-131 should be kept at a distance from other patients and staff.	To minimize exposure of others to radiation.

CHAPTER 38
Specimen Collection

Definition
Specimen collection is the collection of a required amount of tissue or fluid for laboratory examination.

Indications
Specimen collection is required when microbiological, biochemical or other laboratory investigations are indicated. Nursing staff should be able to identify the need for microbiological investigations and, if appropriate, initiate the taking of specimens. Specimen collection is often a first crucial step in investigations that define the nature of the disease and determine diagnosis and the mode of treatment.

REFERENCE MATERIAL

General principles
Successful laboratory diagnosis depends on the collection of specimens at the appropriate time, using the correct technique and equipment and transporting them to the designated laboratory safely without delay. For this to be achieved, good liaison is essential between medical, nursing, portering and laboratory staff. The nurse's role is:

(1) To identify the need for and importance of micro-biological investigation.
(2) To initiate, if appropriate, the taking of a swab or specimen, e.g. during wound dressing it is usually the nurse who identifies signs of infection.
(3) To know the appropriate investigation to be taken so as to avoid indiscriminate specimen collection which wastes time and money.
(4) To collect the desired material in the correct container.
(5) To arrange prompt delivery to the laboratory.

Collection of specimens
The greater the quantity of material sent for laboratory examination, the greater the chance of isolating a causa-tive organism. Anaerobic and other fastidious micro-organisms particularly are more likely to survive. It is, therefore, preferable to send a few millimeters of pus aspirated with a sterile syringe than to send a swab. Specimens are readily contaminated by poor technique. Cultures taken from such specimens often result in confusing or misleading results.

Aseptic technique must be used when collecting specimens to avoid inadvertent contamination of the site of sample or the specimen (Macleod, 1992). Specimens must be collected in sterile containers with close-fitting lids and swabs must never be removed from their sterile containers until everything is ready for taking the sample.

Ideally, samples should be collected before beginning any treatment, e.g. antibiotics or antiseptics. If the patient is receiving such treatment at the same time the specimen is collected, the laboratory staff must be informed. Both antibiotics and antiseptics may destroy organisms that are, in fact, active in the patient and will affect the outcome of the laboratory test. Specimens should also be obtained using safe technique and practices (Hart, 1991). For example, gloves should always be worn when handling all body fluids.

Documentation
Requests for microbiological investigations must include the following information:

(1) Patient's name, ward and/or department.
(2) Hospital number.
(3) Date collected.
(4) Time collected.
(5) Diagnosis.
(6) Relevant signs and symptoms.
(7) Relevant history, e.g. recent foreign travel.
(8) Any antimicrobial drug being taken by the patient.
(9) Type of specimen.
(10) Consultant's name.
(11) Name of the doctor who ordered the investigation,

as it may be necessary to telephone the result before the typed report is dispatched.

Without full information, it is impossible to examine a specimen adequately or to report it accurately.

Transportation of specimens

Guidelines are now available on the labelling, transport and reception of specimens (Health Services Advisory Committee, 1986). The sooner a specimen arrives in the laboratory, the greater is the chance of organisms present surviving and being identified. Delays will cause changes that may radically alter the result. The laboratory count of bacteria in a delayed specimen could be significantly different to that of the specimen when it was collected. Urine for example is normally sterile, whilst the urethra is not sterile and even a carefully taken urine specimen may contain a few microbes which will flourish and provide misleading results (Stokes & Ridgeway, 1980).

If specimens cannot be sent to a laboratory immediately, they should be stored as follows:

(1) Blood culture samples in a 37°C incubator.
(2) All other specimens in a specimen refrigerator at a temperature of 4°C.

In diagnostic pathology it is likely that at any given time there will be a number of specimens that present a risk of infection. Every health authority, therefore, must ensure that medical, nursing, phlebotomy, laboratory, portering and any other staff involved in handling specimens are trained to do so. Specimen containers must be sufficiently robust and must not leak when used. They must also be closed securely and any accidental spillage cleaned immediately. Ideally, all specimens should be placed in a double self-sealing bag with one compartment containing the request form and the other the specimen. Specimens should be transported to the laboratory in washable baskets or trays.

It is the responsibility of the person who requests and takes specimens that are known to be infectious to ensure that both the form and the container are labelled with biohazard labels.

Types of investigation

Bacterial

A wide range of methods is available for obtaining cultures and identifying organisms from a specimen or swab. To employ all these tests would be time consuming and costly. Testing, therefore, tends to be selective. It is at this stage that the laboratory request form plays a particularly important part. A faecal specimen, for example, from a patient with diarrhoea who also has a recent history of foreign travel, would be investigated for organisms not normally looked for in faecal specimens from patients without such a history.

The majority of specimens undergo microscopic investigation. This is valuable as an early indication of the causative organisms in an infection. The specimen is often cultured for 24–48 hours longer in the case of blood cultures. Prolonged incubation (up to 21 days) may be required for growth of some organisms, e.g. *Brucella* species (Mims *et al.*, 1993). This is followed by antibiotic sensitivity testing on any pathogenic organisms that are isolated. This involves the application of paper discs impregnated with antibiotics onto the agar plates. After overnight incubation during which time the growth of bacteria may be inhibited by the antibiotic disc, the zones of inhibition can be observed for the degree of sensitivity of the organism (Mims *et al.*, 1993).

Viral

Three types of technique are available for the diagnosis of viral infections:

(1) Electron microscopy.
(2) Culture.
(3) Serology.

For culture specimens the use of viral transport media and speed of delivery to the laboratory are important as viruses do not survive well outside the body. With good liaison, the nursing personnel should obtain the specimen when the laboratory staff have the transport ready to take it to the virus laboratories. If delays occur, the specimen should be refrigerated at a temperature of 4°C.

The time at which specimens are collected for viral investigations is important. Many viral illnesses have a prodromal phase during which the multiplication and shedding of the virus are at a peak and the patient is most infectious (Mims & White, 1984).

Serological

Serological testing for the presence of antigens and antibodies is used when it is not possible to isolate the organism from the patient's tissue easily. By demonstrating serum antibodies to suspected organisms it is inferred that the patient is, or has been, infected with the organism. A single test is inadequate as if the titres (the concentration of the substance being measured) are raised it is impossible to determine whether this is due to past or present infection. Two tests need to be carried out, both of which involve the collection of 10 ml of blood once at the beginning of the illness and again 10–14 days later. If a rising titre level is demonstrated it suggests the patient's infection is current (Mims *et al.*, 1993).

Mycosis

Although many pathogenic fungi will grow on ordinary bacteriological culture media, they grow better and with less risk of bacterial overgrowth on special mycological media. The presence of fungi in clinical specimens is difficult to interpret as *Candida albicans*, for example, is commonly present in the upper respiratory, alimentary and female genital tract and on the skin of healthy people (Meunier, 1988).

Mycobacteriological

For further information, please refer to the procedure on tuberculosis (Chapter 5).

Protozoa

Most protozoa do not cause disease but those that do, e.g. malaria, make a formidable contribution to human illness (Akinola, 1984). Laboratory investigations depend on direct microscopy which necessitates specimens being delivered to the laboratory as quickly as possible, whilst the protozoa are mobile and therefore visible.

Blood

When blood specimens are obtained from existing intravenous lines it is essential that the line is flushed thoroughly before use and that the first sample is discarded to prevent erroneous results (Johnston & Messina, 1991). For further information on the collection of blood see the procedure for venepuncture (Chapter 46).

Quantitative analysis of drugs in blood

Therapeutic drug monitoring by blood analysis can provide valuable information to guide clinicians in achieving optimal treatment with selected therapeutic agents.

With drugs that possess a narrow therapeutic range in serum, as with the aminoglycoside antibiotics (Barza *et al.*, 1978), if the serum levels are too low the patient is jeopardized by the probable lack of efficacy. However, if the serum concentration is excessive, the patient may suffer serious toxicity. In the case of gentamicin, exposure to high serum levels for a prolonged period may cause renal impairment or ototoxicity (Cipolle *et al.*, 1981). However, when the serum levels are within the normal range, the incidence of dose-related side-effects is minimal in most patients (Koch-Weser, 1972).

In order to correctly individualize drug dosage, and then to monitor the drug effectively, the doctor needs to be familiar with the metabolic processes and relationships between a drug dose and drug concentration in biological fluids (Greenblatt *et al.*, 1975). This is affected by many factors, such as route of administration (Riegelman, 1973) and age (Rane, 1976). Disease proc-

esses, for example liver (Blaschke, 1977) and renal disease (Peters *et al.*, 1978), will also affect metabolism and excretion of the drug.

Drug monitoring is time consuming and costly. However, it is important to evaluate the cost of the test in the light of the information it yields both to ensure that therapeutic concentrations of the drug are achieved and to prevent toxicity (Mims *et al.*, 1993).

Analysis involves laboratory testing of blood serum. Although this knowledge can be gained from random sampling, most benefit will be obtained by the correct timing of sample collection. This will provide a direct relationship to drug administration, and therefore give the correct interpretation of the serum concentration results.

Ideally, a trough sample just before the next scheduled dose, plus a peak level at a set time following the administration of the drug, will provide the most useful information (Mims *et al.*, 1993)

In the procedure guidelines below two examples of drug analysis have been discussed; the laboratory will supply specific times for blood sampling for other drugs.

References and further reading

Akinola, J. (1984) Malaria. *Nursing Times*, 80(38), 40–3.

Ayton, M. (1982) Microbiological investigations. *Nursing*, 2(8), 26–9, 232.

Barza, M. *et al.* (1978) Why monitor serum levels of gentamicin? *Clinical Pharmacokinetics*, 3, 202–15.

Barton, S. & Jenkins, D. (1989) An exploration for the problems of the false negative cervical smear. *British Journal of Obstetrics and Gynaecology*, 96, 492–9.

Blaschke, T. F. (1977) Protein binding and kinetics of drugs in liver disease. *Clinical Pharmacokinetics*, 2, 32–44.

Cipolle, R. J. *et al.* (1981) Therapeutic use and serum concentration monitoring. In: *Individualizing Drug Therapy: Practical Applications of Drug Monitoring*, (eds W. J. Taylor & A. L. Finn). Gross, Townsend & Frank, New York.

Greenblatt, D. J. *et al.* (1975) Clinical pharmacokinetics. *New England Journal of Medicine*, 293, 964–70.

Hargiss, C. O. & Larson, E. (1981) How to collect specimens and evaluate results. *American Journal of Nursing*, 81, 2166–74.

Hart, S. (1991) Blood and body fluid precautions. *Nursing Standard*, 5, 25–7.

Health Services Advisory Committee (1986) *Safety in Health Services Laboratories: The Labelling, Transport and Reception of Specimens*. HMSO, London.

Johnston, J. B. & Messina, M. (1991) Erroneous laboratory values obtained from central catheters. *Journal of Intravenous Nursing*, 14(1), 13–15.

Koch-Weser, R. J. (1972) Serum drug concentration as therapeutic guides. *New England Journal of Medicine*, 287, 227–31.

Macleod, J. A. (1992) Collecting specimens for the laboratory tests. *Nursing Standard*, 6(20), 36–7.

Meunier, F. (1988) Fungal infection in the compromised host.

In: *Clinical Approach to Infection in the Compromised Host*, (eds R. H. Rubin & L. S. Young), pp. 193–212. Plenum, New York.

Mims, C. A. & White, D. O. (1984) *Viral Pathogenesis and Immunology*. Blackwell Science, Oxford.

Mims, C. A. *et al.* (1993) *Medical Microbiology*. C. V. Mosby, St Louis.

Parker, M. J. (1982) *Microbiology for Nurses*, 6th edn. Baillière Tindall, London.

Peters, U. *et al.* (1978) Digoxin metabolism in patients. *Archives of Internal Medicine*, 138, 1074–6.

Rane, A. *et al.* (1976) Clinical pharmacokinetics in infants and children. *Clinical Pharmacokinetics*, 1, 2–24.

Riegelman, S. (1973) Effects of route of administration on drug disposition. *Journal of Pharmacokinetics and Biopharmaceutics* 1, 419–34.

Singer, A. *et al.* (1994) *Lower Genital Tract Pre-cancer*. Blackwell Science, Oxford.

Smith, A. L. (1985) *Principles of Microbiology*, 10th edn. C. V. Mosby, St Louis.

Stokes, E. J. & Ridgeway, G. L. (1980) *Clinical Bacteriology*, 5th edn. Edward Arnold, London.

Wilson, M. E. & Mizer, H. E. (1969) *Microbiology in Nursing Practice*. Macmillan, London.

GUIDELINES: SPECIMEN COLLECTION

PROCEDURE

Action	Rationale
1 Explain and discuss the procedure with the patient and ensure privacy while the procedure is being carried out.	To ensure that the patient understands the procedure and gives his/her valid consent.
2 Wash hands using bactericidal soap and water or bactericidal alcohol hand rub.	Hand washing greatly reduces the risk of infection transfer.
3 Place specimens and swabs in the appropriate, correctly labelled containers.	To ensure that only organisms for investigation are preserved.
4 Dispatch specimens promptly to the laboratory with the completed request form.	To ensure the best possible conditions for any laboratory examinations.

Eye swab

Action	Rationale
1 Using either a plastic loop or a cotton wool-covered wooden stick, hold the swab parallel to the cornea and gently rub the conjunctiva in the lower eyelid.	To ensure that a swab of the correct site is taken. To avoid contamination by touching the eyelid.
2 If possible, smear the conjunctival swab on an agar plate at the bedside.	Eye swabs are often unsatisfactory because of the action of tears, which contain the enzyme lysozyme which acts as an antiseptic. Conjunctival scrapings are preferable. This procedure is usually performed by medical staff.

Nose swab

Action	Rationale
1 Moisten the swab beforehand with sterile water.	To prevent discomfort to the patient. The healthy nose is virtually dry and a dry swab may cause discomfort.

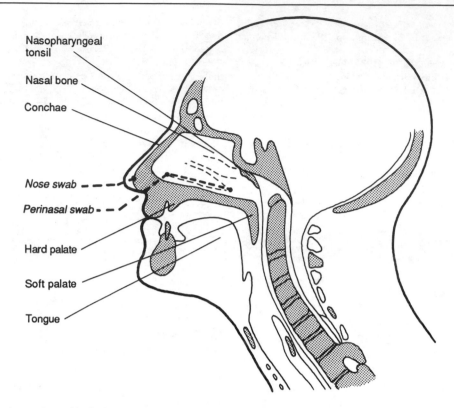

Nasopharyngeal
tonsil

Nasal bone

Conchae

Nose swab

Perinasal swab

Hard palate

Soft palate

Tongue

Figure 38.1   Area to be swabbed when sampling the nose.

Guidelines: Specimen collection (cont'd)

Action

 2 Move the swab from the anterior nares and direct it upwards into the tip of the nose (Fig. 38.1).

3 Gently rotate the swab.

Rationale

To swab the correct site and to obtain the required sample.

Perinasal swab (for whooping cough)

Action

1 Using a special soft-wire mounted swab, pass it along the floor of the nasal cavity to the posterior wall of the nasopharynx (Fig. 38.1).

2 Rotate the swab gently.

Rationale

To minimize trauma to nasal tissue. To obtain a swab from the correct site.

Sputum

Action

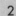 **1** Use a specimen container that is free from organisms of respiratory origin. This need not, therefore, be a sterile container.

Rationale

Sputum is never free from organisms since material originating in the bronchi and alveoli has to pass through the pharynx and mouth, areas that have a normal commensal population of bacteria.

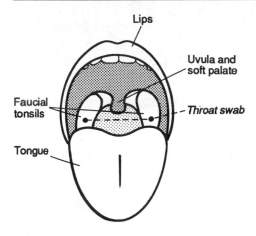

Figure 38.2 Area to be swabbed when sampling the throat.

Action	Rationale
2 Care should be taken to ensure that the material sent for investigations is sputum, not saliva.	To obtain the required sample.
3 Encourage patients who have difficulty producing sputum to cough deeply first thing in the morning. Alternatively, a physiotherapist should be called to assist.	To facilitate expectoration.
4 Send any sputum specimen to the laboratory immediately.	The bacterial population alters rapidly and rapid dispatch should ensure accurate results.

Throat swab

Action	Rationale
1 Ask the patient to sit in such a position that he/she is facing a strong light source. Depress the patient's tongue with a spatula.	To ensure maximum visibility of the area to be swabbed. The procedure is one that is likely to cause the patient to gag and the tongue will move to the roof of the mouth, contaminating the specimen.
2 Quickly, but gently, rub the swab over the prescribed area, usually the tonsillar fossa or any area with a lesion or visible exudate (Fig. 38.2).	To obtain the required sample.
3 Avoid touching any other area of the mouth or tongue with the swab.	To prevent contamination by other organisms.

Ear swab

Action	Rationale
1 No antibiotics or other chemotherapeutic agents should have been used in the aural region three hours before taking the swab.	To prevent collection of traces of such therapeutic agents.
2 Place the swab into the outer ear as shown in Fig. 38.3. Rotate the swab gently.	To avoid trauma to the ear. To collect any secretions.

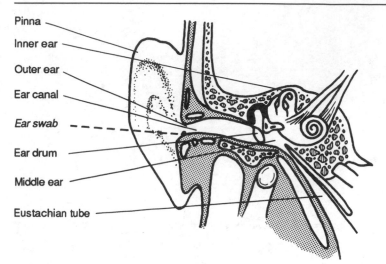

Pinna

Inner ear

Outer ear

Ear canal

Ear swab

Ear drum

Middle ear

Eustachian tube

Figure 38.3 Area to be swabbed when sampling the outer ear.

Guidelines: Specimen collection (cont'd)

Wound swab

Action

Action	Rationale
1 Take any swabs required before dressing procedure begins.	To prevent collection of any therapeutic agents that may be employed in the dressing procedure.
2 Rotate the swab gently.	To collect samples. It is preferable to send samples of purulent discharge instead of swabs.

Note: The use of disposable gloves is recommended in the following procedures in order to prevent cross-infection.

Vaginal swab

Action	Rationale
1 Introduce a speculum into the vagina to separate the vaginal walls. Take the swab as high as possible in the vaginal vault.	To ensure maximum visibility of the area to be swabbed. To ensure that the swab is taken from the best site. If infection by *Trichomonas* species is suspected, a charcoal-impregnated swab is recommended as this organism survives longer in this medium.

Penile swab

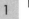

Action	Rationale
1 Retract prepuce.	To obtain maximum visibility of area to be swabbed.
2 Rotate swab gently in the urethral meatus.	To collect any secretions.

Rectal swab

Action	Rationale
1 Pass the swab, with care, through the anus into the rectum.	To avoid trauma. To ensure a rectal and not an anal sample is obtained.

| 2 | Rotate gently. | To avoid trauma. |

| 3 | In patients suspected of suffering from threadworms, take the swab from the perianal region. | Threadworms lay their ova on the perianal skin. |

Faeces

Action		Rationale
1	Ask the patient to defaecate into a clinically clean bedpan.	To avoid unnecessary contamination from other organisms.
2	Scoop enough material to fill a third of the specimen container using a spatula or a spoon, often incorporated in the specimen container.	To obtain a usable amount of specimen. To prevent contamination.
3	Examine the specimen for such features as colour, consistency and odour, and record your observations.	To monitor any fluctuations and trends.
4	Segments of tapeworm are seen easily in faeces and any such segments should be sent to the laboratory for identification.	Unless the head is dislodged, the tapeworm will continue to grow. Laboratory confirmation of the presence of the head is essential.
5	Patients suspected of suffering from amoebic dysentery should have any stool specimens dispatched to the laboratory immediately.	The parasite causing amoebic dysentery exists in a free-living nonmotile cyst. *Both* are characteristic in their fresh state but are difficult to identify when dead.

Urine

Action		Rationale
1	Specimens of urine should be collected as soon as possible after the patient wakens in the morning and at the same time each morning if more than one specimen is required.	The bladder will be full as urine has accumulated overnight. If specimens are taken at other times, the urine may be diluted. All specimens will be comparable if taken at the same time each morning.
2	Dispatch all specimens to the laboratory as soon after collection as possible.	Urine specimens should be examined within 2 hours of collection or 24 hours if kept refrigerated at a temperature of 4°C. At room temperature overgrowth will occur and lead to misinterpretation.

Midstream specimen of urine: male

Action		Rationale
1	Retract the prepuce and clean the skin surrounding the urethral meatus with soap and water, saline or a solution that does not contain a disinfectant.	To prevent other organisms contaminating the specimen. Disinfectants may irritate or be painful to the urethral mucous membrane.
2	Ask the patient to direct the first and last part of his stream into a urinal or toilet but to collect the middle part of his stream into a sterile container.	To avoid contamination of the specimen with organisms normally present on the skin.

Guidelines: Specimen collection (cont'd)

Midstream specimen of urine: female

Action	Rationale
1 Clean the urethral meatus with soap and water, saline or a solution that does not contain a disinfectant.	To prevent other organisms contaminating the specimen. Disinfectants may irritate or be painful to the urethral mucous membrane.
2 (a) Use a separate wool swab for each swab. (b) Swab from the front to the back.	To prevent cross-infection. To prevent perianal contamination.
3 Ask the patient to micturate into a bedpan or toilet. Place a sterile receiver or a wide-mouthed container under the stream and remove before the stream ceases.	To avoid contamination of the specimen with organisms normally present on the skin.
4 Transfer the specimen into a sterile container.	

Specimen of urine from an ileal conduit

For further information see the relevant section in the procedure on stoma care (Chapter 39).

Catheter specimen of urine

For further information see the relevant section in the procedure on urinary catheterization (Chapter 45).

24-hour urine collection

Action	Rationale
1 Request the patient to void the bladder at the time appointed to begin this procedure. Discard this specimen.	To ensure the urine collected is that produced in the 24 hours stated.
2 All urine passed in the next 24 hours is collected in a large specimen bottle. The final specimen is collected at exactly the same time the bladder was voided 24 hours earlier.	Body chemistry alters constantly. A 24-hour collection will accommodate all the variables within a representative period.
3 Care must be taken to ensure the patient understands the procedure in order to eliminate the risk of an incomplete collection.	A 24-hour collection will not be obtained if one sample is lost and the results will be invalid.

Semen

Action	Rationale
1 Sexual intercourse should not have taken place for 3–4 days before the specimen is collected.	To ensure the sperm count will be at maximum levels. It takes between 3 and 4 days for the sperm count to return to normal after ejaculation.
2 A fresh masturbated specimen must be collected in a sterile container and delivered	Sperm will die if there is a delay in testing. Specimens must not be collected in a condom as

to the laboratory within 2 hours of the collection of the specimen.

sperm die when in contact with materials such as rubber.

Cervical scrape

Action

1 The ideal time for smear testing is mid-cycle.

2 The menses should be avoided.

3 The smear must be taken before a vaginal examination is carried out.

4 Label the ground glass end of the slide with the patient's name.

5 Expose the cervix by using a dry speculum or one moistened with warm tap water.

6 Using the bi-lobed end of the cervical spatula, scrape firmly but gently around the squamocolumnar junction of the cervix. If the os is splayed open or scarred, a wider sweep with the broad end of the spatula may be necessary.

7 Smear both sides of the spatula evenly on the slide with one stroke from each side of the spatula.

8 Fix immediately.

9 Allow the fixing agents to dry.

10 Place the slides in a transport container.

11 Small endocervical lesions, which could be missed by the use of a spatula, may be sampled using an endocervical plastic brush (Singer *et al.*, 1994).

12 Identify and insert and gently rotate the brush in the cervical canal.

13 Withdraw the brush and gently smear the brush evenly on on the slide (treat slide as above, see 8, 9 and 10).

14 Send, with a completed cervical cytology request form, to the appropriate laboratory.

Rationale

To allow for accuracy of results as the cervix is usually free of contamination from menstrual flow at this time.

This is less uncomfortable for the patient.

To ensure normal tissue samples are obtained.

To ensure patient identification.

To ensure maximum visibility. Greasy lubricants inhibit specimen collection.

To obtain a usable amount of specimen.

To ensure complete specimens.

To preserve the specimen and ensure accurate results.

Dry specimens are less likely to be damaged.

To safeguard delicate glass slides.

This brush with its narrow tip can be inserted into the cervical canal improving the quality of smear taken from the endocervix (Barton & Jenkins, 1989).

To obtain a usable amount of specimen.

To ensure a complete specimen.

GUIDELINES: ANALYSIS OF DRUG LEVELS IN BLOOD

PROCEDURE

Gentamicin levels

Action

1 Following venepuncture guidelines (Chapter 46), withdraw 10 ml blood to obtain specimen for clotted sample to provide trough level serum using a new needle or winged infusion device. Blood specimen container to be clearly labelled 'pre-gentamicin administration blood'.

2 Administer intravenous gentamicin as patient's prescription states (following procedure for administration of drugs by direct injection, bolus, or push; see Guidelines, Chapter 23) via patient's established cannula.

3 One hour after administration of gentamicin withdraw 10 ml blood to obtain specimen for clotted sample to provide peak level serum either using the needle from which the pre-gentamicin administration blood was withdrawn or a new device. Blood specimen container to be clearly labelled 'post-gentamicin administration blood'.

4 Rarely but occasionally when only poor and limited venous access is available, the blood specimens may have to be obtained from the patient's existing device.
The device must be flushed thoroughly before taking the blood sample.
The blood specimen container and request form must be labelled to indicate this deviation from the usual procedure.

Rationale

To obtain a blood sample safely via an intravenous device that is not contaminated by previous administration of gentamicin residue, which could provide an inaccurate result.

To continue with patient's prescribed drug regime.

Time gap allows for even distribution of gentamicin thorough the blood and for peak blood levels to be achieved.

The possibility of these specimens being contaminated with residue drug is high.

Contamination can be reduced by thorough flushing of the line.
The clinician interpreting the result will be aware of the method of obtaining the blood specimen.

Vancomycin levels

Action

1 Following venepuncture guidelines (Chapter 46), withdraw 10 ml blood to obtain specimen for clotted sample to provide trough level serum using a new needle or winged infusion device. Blood specimen container must be clearly labelled 'pre-vancomyin administration blood'.

2 Administer vancomycin intravenously as patient's prescription states (following administration of drugs by continuous infusion; see procedure for Guidelines, Chapter 23) via patient's established cannula.

Rationale

To obtain a blood sample safely via an intravenous device that is not contaminated by previous administration of vancomycin, which could provide an inaccurate result.

To continue with patient's prescribed drug regime.

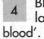 One hour after completion of administration of vancomycin, withdraw 10ml blood to obtain specimen for clotted sample to provide peak level serum.

Time span allows for even distribution of vancomycin throughout the blood and for peak blood levels to be achieved.

4 Blood specimen container to be clearly labelled 'post-vancomycin administration blood'.

CHAPTER 39

Stoma Care

Definition

'Stoma' is a word of Greek origin meaning 'mouth' or 'opening' (Black, 1994a). A bowel or urinary stoma is usually created on the abdominal wall as a diversionary procedure because the urinary or colonic tract beyond the position of the stoma is no longer viable.

Indications

Stoma care is required for the following purposes:

(1) To collect urine or faeces in an appropriate appliance.
(2) To achieve and maintain patient comfort and security.
(3) To maintain good skin and stoma hygiene.

REFERENCE MATERIAL

Types of stoma

Colostomy

In a colostomy the stoma may be formed from any section of the large bowel, e.g. 'end' or 'terminal' sigmoid colostomy (usually permanent, Fig. 39.1). A temporary (usually transverse) colostomy may be raised to divert the faecal output, thus allowing healing of an anastamosis further along the colon. With a defunctioning loop colostomy, a rod or bridge may be used to maintain a hold on the abdominal surface. Such a rod or bridge is removed 7–10 days after insertion (Fig. 39.2). The term 'defunctioning' is used to indicate that the bowel distal to the stoma is being rested (Borwell, 1994).

Ileostomy

In an ileostomy the ileum is brought out onto the abdominal wall (Fig. 39.2), as when, for example, the large colon is affected by inflammatory disease. Many patients with ulcerative colitis are offered a Park's pouch and therefore do not have to have a permanent stoma. For this operation a colectomy is performed and the terminal ileum is made into a reservoir (pouch) and brought down and attached to the anus. A temporary ileostomy allows the pouch to heal (Nemer & Rolstad, 1985).

Ileal loop, ileal conduit or urostomy

The performance of such operations (when the bladder is removed or diseased), requires the ureters to be transplanted from the bladder into a length, approximately 15 cm, of ileum which has been isolated, along with its mesentery, from the remainder of the small bowel. One end of the ileum, with the resected ureters, remains inside the abdomen, while the other is brought out on to the abdominal wall and everted to form a slightly protruding stoma (Fig. 39.3).

Other types of urinary diversion

Other types of urinary diversion include ureterostomy, a procedure that brings the ureters out onto the abdominal wall together (one stoma) or separately (two stomas). It may be possible for some patients with bladder disease to have a continent pouch or 'new' bladder formed internally. One example of this is the Mitrofanoff technique

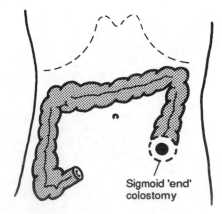

Figure 39.1 Sigmoid 'end' colostomy.

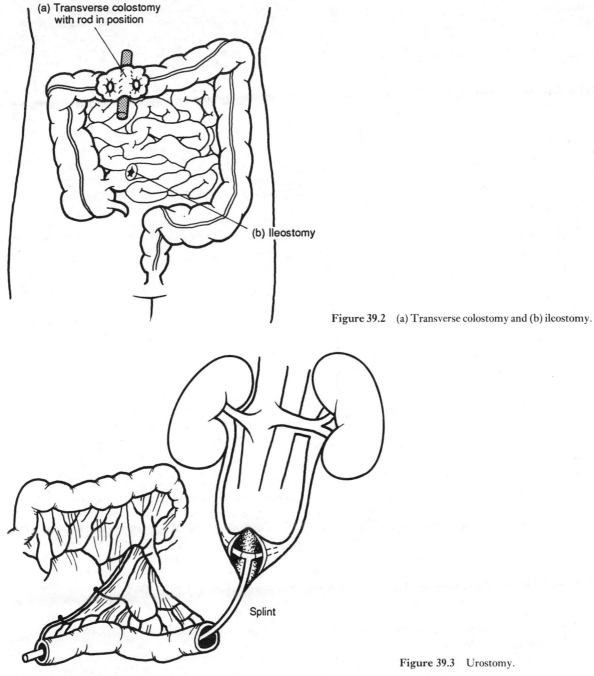

Figure 39.2   (a) Transverse colostomy and (b) ileostomy.

(a) Transverse colostomy
with rod in position

(b) Ileostomy

Splint

Figure 39.3   Urostomy.

(Horn, 1991; Gelister & Woodhouse, 1991). For further information on these continent urinary diversions, see Chapter 12.

Indications for bowel stoma

(1) Cancer of the bowel.
(2) Cancer of the pelvis.
(3) Trauma.
(4) Neurological damage.
(5) Congenital disorders.
(6) Ulcerative colitis.
(7) Crohn's disease.
(8) Diverticular disease.
(9) Familial polyposis coli.

(10) Intractable incontinence.

(11) Radiation enteritis.

Indications for urinary stoma

(1) Cancer of the bladder.

(2) Cancer of the pelvis.

(3) Trauma.

(4) Congential disorders.

(5) Neurological damage.

(6) Intractable incontinence.

(Black, 1994a.)

Pre-operative preparation for stoma surgery

Physical preparation of the patient will vary according to the type of operation and the policies of individual surgeons and hospitals. This will involve the usual preparation for anaesthesia (Chapter 32, Peri-operative Care), preparation of the area of the body involved and of the bowel. Other specific procedures may also be included.

Psychological preparation of the individual facing stoma surgery should begin as soon as surgery has been considered, preferably by utilizing the skills of a trained stoma care nurse. Boore (1978), Hayward (1978) and Janis & Rodin (1982) have illustrated the importance of pre-operative information and explanation in reducing postoperative physical and psychological stress. Information giving and discussion with patients about their stoma and lifestyle starts pre-operatively and continues throughout the patient's stoma experience. The aims of these interactions are as follows:

(1) To help the individual with a stoma to return to their previous place in society whenever possible.

(2) To help in the process of adapting to a changed body image (Price, 1990; Salter, 1988a).

(3) To reduce anxiety. The patient's perception of life with a stoma may have a positive or detrimental influence on rehabilitation. There may be myths and wrong information to dispel, and the patient's awareness of the experiences of another ostomist to discuss (Bryant, 1993; Salter, 1992).

(4) To explain that the presence of a stoma need not adversely affect any previous quality of life such as hobbies, work, social life or any other interests, although the underlying disease might (Salter, 1992; Joels, 1989).

(5) To prepare the patient for the appearance and likely behaviour pattern of the stoma (Black, 1985a).

(6) To reassure patients that they will be able to manage an appliance whatever the environment (Salter, 1995).

(7) To assure patients that they will be supported fully while in hospital and will not be discharged until they are confident about the stoma's care and that continuing support will be available in the community (Salter, 1995).

Such pre-operative education has been shown to increase cooperation and trust and reduce anxiety, the length of time the patient remains in hospital and the amount of postoperative analgesia required (Wade, 1989). It should be borne in mind that any information given should be relevant to the patient's needs. Family and/or close friends may also be involved, when appropriate, on agreement with the patient (Salter, 1992).

Diet

All patients should be encouraged to eat a wide variety of foods.

Colostomy

Certain foods, e.g. large portions of fruit and vegetables (onions, sprouts, cabbage, etc.) may cause diarrhoea or excess flatus (Little, 1989). It is suggested that rather than eliminate these items from the diet, the foods identified should be tried again in smaller portions. No food item affects everyone in the same way and it is best for the individual to experiment. It might be preferable to reduce the portion and prepare for the consequences. Beer and fizzy drinks may cause excess flatus. Beer and other forms of alcohol will affect the ostomist as they do everyone else (Little, 1989).

Ileostomy

Certain foods will cause excess flatus. Pulses, dried fruit, peanuts and coconut are digested slowly and so they will need to be masticated well before swallowing.

If these foods are taken in excess and not masticated well they could swell in the gut and cause a 'bolus' obstruction. Some foods, e.g. tomato skins or pips, may pass into the appliance unaltered due to a more rapid transit time (Black, 1985b). Care should also be taken by patients using oral contraception as absorption may be impaired (Black, 1994b).

Urostomy

There are no dietary restrictions. It must be stressed, however, that an adequate fluid intake must be maintained to minimize the risk of urinary infection. Approximately 1.5 litres (or 12 cups per day) is the recommended minimum (Black, 1989). The slow return of both a normal appetite and bowel function is a common feature following this operation (due to bowel handling in surgery) and it gives cause for much anxiety. The patient should be warned of this and advised to take small, light meals supplemented by nutritious drinks.

Normal appetite may not return for 2 or 3 months after the operation.

Fear of malodour

This is a common fear for patients with bowel stomas, often based on hearsay or experience with other ostomists in hospital or the community. Appliances are odour free when fitted correctly. Flatus may be released via charcoal filters and deodorizers are available. The individual must be reassured, however, that any problems that occur post-operatively will be investigated, with a good possibility of them being solved by such means as the use of alternative appliances.

Sex and the ostomist

The possibility of sexual impairment for both men and women after stoma surgery depends on the nature of the operation, the ensuing damage to the nerves and tissues involved. The psychological impact of the surgery and its effect on the individual's body image must also be taken into consideration. Surgery that results in physical sexual disability will have psychological repercussions, while some sexual difficulties may be of psychological origin (Model, 1990). Impairment may be permanent or temporary. In the latter case, resolution of the difficulty may take anything up to two years. Pre- and post-operative counselling should be offered for both patient and partner. In cases of male impotence, surgical intervention, such as insertion of penile implants, may be appropriate if impairment becomes permanent. Vacuum devices and intercavernosal self-injections of alprostadil, a prostoglandin E_1, (Caverject) may also be used to induce an erection (Padma-Nathan, 1993; *ABPI Data Sheets Compendium 1995–96*).

Female patients may experience dyspareunia; this may be due to narrowing or shortening of the vagina or a reduction in the volume of vaginal secretions (Schover, 1986). The use of a lubricant, adopting different positions during lovemaking or encouraging greater relaxation by extending foreplay may help resolve painful intercourse (Topping, 1990).

Useful references on the psychological and sexual aspects of care may be found in Wells (1990), Van De Wiel *et al.* (1991) and Anders (1993).

Personnel who may be expected to provide information

(1) Medical staff.
(2) Stoma care nurse.
(3) Nursing staff on ward.
(4) Primary health care team.
(5) Another suitable ostomist. 'Visitors' are trained by the voluntary associations and, ideally, should be of similar age, sex and background to the patient to enable the patient to discuss problems of adapting to life with a stoma.

Useful aids

(1) Information booklets.
(2) Samples of the various appliances.
(3) Diagrams.
(4) Audio tapes.
(5) Video tapes.

These aids are valuable to reinforce and clarify the verbal information.

Pre-operative assessment

It is important to determine whether a patient will be able to manage a stoma by assessing the following:

(1) Eyesight.
(2) Manual dexterity.
(3) The presence of other debilitating diseases, e.g. Parkinson's disease or arthritis.
(4) Mental state.
(5) Loss of an upper limb.
(6) Skin conditions.
(7) Abnormal contours, e.g. the changes that occur with spina bifida.

Siting of the stoma is one of the most important preoperative tasks to be carried out by the doctor, stoma care nurse or experienced ward nurse (Figs 39.4 and 39.5). This minimizes future difficulties such as interference by the stoma with clothes, or skin problems caused by leakage of the appliance due to a badly sited stoma (e.g. on the waistline or in a body crease). When siting the stoma, consideration should be given to the following:

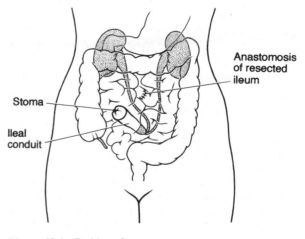

Figure 39.4 Position of stoma.

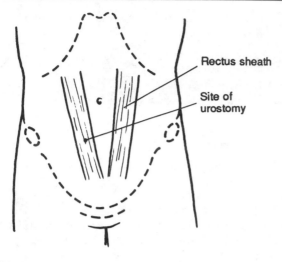

Figure 39.5   Site of urostomy.

(1) A flat area of the skin to facilitate safe adhesion of the appliance.
(2) Avoidance of bony prominences such as hips and ribs which may interfere with the adhesion of the appliance, or pendulous breasts which may obscure the stoma from the patient's view, making self-care impossible.
(3) Avoidance of skin creases, especially in the region of the groin or the umbilicus, to avoid urine or faecal matter tracking along the skin creases.
(4) Avoidance of scars, which may cause skin creases which may lead to leakages.
(5) Avoidance of wasitline or belt areas, as patient's clothing may put pressure on the stoma which may lead to leaks or trauma.
(6) Maintenance of the stoma within the rectus sheath, as this reduces the risk of herniation later (Black, 1989; Ortiz *et al.* 1993; Kelly, 1995). The muscle may be identified by asking the patient to lie flat then to raise the head. The muscle may also be palpated and easily felt when the patient coughs.
(7) Ideally, the patient should be able to see the stoma site.

The patient must be observed while lying, sitting in a comfortable chair, with the abdominal muscles relaxed, and standing. Consideration must be given to any bending or lifting involved with the patient's work and any other activities in which the patient partakes. Account must also be taken of any weight gain or loss in the post-operative period, as this may change the contours of the abdomen and hence the position of the stoma.

Post-operative period

Control of stoma action

Ileal loop
Urine will dribble from the stoma every 20–30 seconds. The output may be slightly less after periods of reduced fluid intake, e.g. at night. An appliance has to be worn at all times.

Ileostomy
Once the stoma starts to act a few days after surgery, the fluid output, normally 500–850 ml every 24 hours, takes on a porridge consistency once a normal intake of food is established (Foulkes, 1981). The effluent contains enzymes that will excoriate the skin if contact is allowed. While the effluent cannot be controlled, the ostomist may find that the stoma is more active after main meals.

Colostomym
Due to its position, only a small amount of water will be reabsorbed from the faecal matter which is passed via a transverse colostomy, therefore the effluent will be unformed. Patients with a sigmoid colostomy may find that wholemeal foods assist in producing a formed stool once or twice daily.

Medications that reduce peristaltic action, e.g. codeine phosphate, may also be used to control diarrhoea. The only means of controlling a sigmoid colostomy, however, is by regular irrigation or by use of a Conseal plug system. This method must be taught under supervision to suitable ostomates.

Irrigation
Irrigation is a method of controlling the output of a colostomy by means of washing out the stoma with warm tap water (with the use of a coned irrigation set), every 24–48 hours.

The advantage of successful colostomy irrigation is that there is no stool leakage between irrigations (De-Hong, 1991).

Post-operative stages

Stage I
In theatre an appropriately sized skin-protective wafer should be applied around the stoma, followed by a drainable, transparent appliance, which should be left on for approximately 5 days. For the first 48 hours post-operatively, observe stoma colour (pink and healthy appearance indicates a good blood supply), size and stoma output (bearing in mind that it may take a few days for a bowel stoma to act). The drainable appliance should

always be emptied frequently, gas should be allowed to escape and the appliance should not be allowed to get more than half full with effluent. If the appliance becomes too full leaks may occur and the weight from the effluent or the pressure from gas may cause the appliance to fall off.

Immediately post-operatively patients would not be expected to perform their own stoma care but would be encouraged to observe the nurse caring for them and may discuss it with the nurse. Viewing the stoma may be difficult for the patient, who may be very aware of other people's reaction to it (Price, 1993).

Stage II

As the patient's condition improves, a demonstration change of the appliance will be given with full explanation of the principles of stoma care. This will be followed by further opportunities to discuss any problems or raise new queries. Provided the patient agrees, it is useful to involve the patient's partner or close friends or relatives at this stage. Their acceptance of the stoma may encourage the patient and help to restore the patient's self-esteem (Salter, 1995). In the following days patients will be encouraged to participate in and gradually assume responsibility for their own stoma care. They may now be ready to discuss appliances and choose the one that they wish to use at home. Preparation for discharge will be discussed.

Stage III

Ideally, the patient should now be independent, eating a normal diet, be ready for discharge and should be confident in stoma care.

If the family or close friends are closely involved during all stages and are supportive, patients are better able to adapt to the threat of mutilating surgery and altered pattern of elimination (Price, 1993). The family or close friends are also likely to require support and information so that they are in a position to help the ostomate. Acceptance of the stoma is a gradual process and, on discharge from hospital, patients may only be beginning to adapt to life with a stoma.

Specific discharge plans

Follow-up support

The patient is discharged with adequate supplies until a prescription is obtained from the general practitioner. Written reminders are provided of how to care for the stoma, how to obtain supplies of appliances, and any other information that may be required. The patient should have details of non-medical stoma clinics, details about the relevant agencies and information about vol-

untary associations. Arrangements should also have been made for a home visit from the stoma care nurse and/or the community nurse.

Obtaining supplies

All National Health Service patients with a permanent stoma are entitled to free prescriptions for their stoma care products, and should complete the relevant forms for exemption from payment. Appliances can then be obtained from the local chemist, a free home delivery service or directly from the appropriate manufacturers.

Stoma appliances and accessories

Many of the appliances now available are very similar in style, colour and efficiency and often there is very little to choose between them when the time comes for the ostomate to decide what to wear.

The aim of good stoma care is to return patients to their place in society (Black, 1994c). One of the ways in which this can be facilitated is to provide them with a safe, reliable appliance. This means that there must be no fear of leakage or odour and the appliance should be comfortable, unobtrusive and easy to handle. The ostomist should also be allowed a choice of bag from a selection of appropriate appliances. It is also necessary to ensure that there are no problems with the stoma or peristomal skin.

Appliances

Choosing the right size of appliance

Bags are labelled according to the size of the opening that fits around the stoma. To keep the skin unblemished, it must be protected from the stoma output. The size chosen, therefore, should be one that fits snugly around the stoma to within 0.5 cm of the stoma edge. This narrow edge of skin is left exposed to prevent any of the adhesives, some of which are more rigid than others, rubbing against the stoma. The appliances usually come with measuring guides to allow for correct choice of size. During the first weeks the oedematous stoma will reduce in size and the bags or flange of the two-piece type appliances will have to be changed accordingly.

Types of appliance

Although some people whose stomas were created several years ago are wearing non-disposable rubber bags, most appliances used today are made of a specially designed laminate composed of three types of plastic. This should ensure that the appliances are:

(1) Leak proof.
(2) Odour proof.
(3) Unobtrusive.

(4) Noiseless.

(5) Disposable.

The appliances differ slightly according to the stoma for which they are meant. All types, however, fall within one of two broad categories:

(1) One-piece. This comprises a bag with an adhesive wafer that fits around the stoma. When the bag is renewed, the adhesive is removed from the skin. Its advantage is that it is easy to handle, e.g. by an ostomate suffering from arthritis.

(2) Two-piece. This comprises a flange for the skin that fits around the stoma and a bag that clips on to the flange. It can be used with sore and sensitive skin as when bags are removed from the flange, the skin is left undisturbed. However, the patient must have the dexterity to clip the bag securely onto the flange.

Drainable bags

(1) Bowel stoma bags (Fig. 39.6a).
Suitable for: ileostomy, transverse colostomy.
Stoma output: fluid to semiformed (volume is too great for closed bags).
Use: emptied frequently, taking care to rinse outlet afterwards; may be left on for up to three days.
Additional features: flatus filters are absent in some as the fluid would obstruct the charcoal, rendering it useless, or will leak through the small opening; the outlet may have a separate clip or fixed 'roll-up' closure.
Colour: clear, white, pink/beige.

(2) Urinary stoma bags (Fig. 39.6b).
Suitable for: urostomy.
Stoma output: urine.
Use: emptied frequently via a fixed tap; may be left on for up to 3 days.
Additional features: may be used with large collecting bag and tubing for night drainage.
Colour: clear or semi-opaque.

(3) Closed bags (Fig. 39.6c).
Suitable for: sigmoid colostomy.

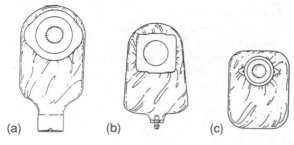

Figure 39.6 Stoma equipment.

Stoma output: a formed stool.
Use: changed once or twice a day.
Additional features: some have incorporated flatus filters that allow the release of flatus through charcoal patches that absorb the odour.
Colour: clear, white or pink/beige.

Some may be fitted with protective adhesive especially for sensitive skin and many now have a cotton-weave backing to reduce and absorb perspiration and to prevent the plastic from sticking to the skin.

Accessories

The specific products in this section have been mentioned as examples of what aids are available and reference to them is not necessarily intended as a recommendation.

Solutions for skin and stoma cleaning

Mild soap and water, or water only, are sufficient. Detergents, disinfectants and antiseptics cause dryness and irritation and should not be used. The stoma is not a wound or a lesion and should be regarded as a resited urethra or anus.

Skin barriers

(1) Creams.
Unless made specifically for use on peristomal skin, these should not be used, as the residual surface film of grease prevents adherence of the appliance. Creams usually have a smoothing and moisturizing effect.
Use: for sensitive skin, as a protective measure.
Method: use sparingly; massage gently into the skin until completely absorbed; excess grease may be wiped off with a soft tissue.
Example: Chiron barrier cream (aluminium chlorohydrate 2% in an emulsified base) (Martindale, 1993).
Precaution: not to be used on broken or sore skin.

(2) Skin gels/sealants.
Use: act as a film on the skin, first to prevent irritation and, second, to give protection as it is removed with the adhesive of the bag, thus preventing removal of the stratum corneum of the skin.
Method: use sparingly; pat onto the skin gently; dries quickly.
Examples: Skin Gel, Skin Prep.
Precaution: should not be used on broken skin as they contain alcohol and cause stinging (Martindale, 1993).

(3) Protective wafers.
Use: these are hypoallergenic and are designed to cover and protect skin, and allow healing if the skin

is sore or broken. May be useful in cases of skin reaction or allergy to the adhesive or an appliance.
Method: the wafers may be cut with the aid of a template (pattern) to the required shape and fitted on to the skin. The appliances are then attached to the wafer. The rim of the wafer should not press against the stoma but should fit to 0.5 cm around it.
Examples: Stomahesive or Comfeel type of wafers. (Stomahesive is composed of gelatin, pectin, sodium carboxymethycellulose, and polyisobutylene (Martindale, 1993); it adheres painlessly to normal, erythematous, moist or broken skin; it is available in three sizes.)
Precautions: allergy may occur, but rarely.

(4) Protective rings.
Use: protective rings are used to provide skin protection around the stoma; they will protect a smaller area than the wafers mentioned above. They are also useful to fill in 'dips' or 'gulleys' in the skin.
Method: like the wafers, they have an adhesive side and may be applied directly to the skin. They form an integral part of some of the appliances.
Example: Salts Cohesive seals.
Precautions: as for protective wafers above.

(5) Pastes.
Use: useful to fill in crevices and 'gulleys' in the skin to provide a smooth surface for an appliance.
Method: *Stomahesive* – either leave for 60 seconds after applying to the skin, when the surface will be dry, making the paste easier to mould into the skin contour, or apply with a spatula, or wet the finger first to prevent the paste sticking and mould the paste immediately. Will sting on raw areas as it contains alcohol. Apply a little Orahesive powder to these areas first. *Orabase* – similar to Stomahesive in composition but with the addition of liquid paraffin. For protection of raw areas. Does not contain alcohol so will not cause local irritation.
Examples: Stomahesive paste, soft paste and Orabase paste.

(6) Powders.
Use: for protection of sore or raw areas without impeding adhesion of the appliance.
Method: sprinkle on affected areas.
Example: Orahesive powder.

Adhesive preparations
Lotions.
Use: only required when appliance does not adhere well to the skin, e.g. because of leakage, uneven site, or if abdominal fistulae present.
Method: pat gently onto skin. The individual products differ considerably in their method of application and it is recommended that the user consults the manufacturer's instructions.
Example: Saltair solution.

Convex devices
Use: these devices are designed to be used with retracted stomas. The convex shape allows a greater seal round the stoma by filling in any crevices caused by retraction, scars or skin creases.
Method: convexity may be achieved by fitting specially designed plastic inserts into the baseplate of a two piece appliance or by using appliances with built in convexity.
Examples: convex inserts, Impression range of appliances.

Deodorants

(1) Aerosols.
Use: absorb odour.
Method: one or two puffs into the air before emptying or removal of appliance.
Examples: Atmacol, Oziom, Limone.
(2) Drops and powders.
Use: for deodorizing bag contents.
Method: squeeze tube two or three times and then shake appliance to fully disperse the powder.
Examples: Ostobon deodorant powder.
(3) Flatus filters (charcoal filled) usually incorporated into the bag.
Use: to allow gradual release of flatus from the bag while allowing absorption of odour by the charcoal. The charcoal may only be effective for between 6 and 12 hours, depending on brand of filter.
Precaution: use of flatus filters is not advised when the stoma effluent is very fluid as the charcoal may become moist and the air outlet blocked.

Useful addresses

(1) Association for Spina Bifida and Hydrocephalus (ASBAH), 42, Park Road, Peterborough PE1 2UQ (Tel: 01733 555988).
(2) British Colostomy Association, 13–15 Station Road, Reading, Berkshire RG1 1LG (Tel: 01734 391537).
(3) IA (Ileostomy and Internal Pouch Support Group), PO Box 23, Mansfield, Nottingham NG18 47T (Tel: 01623 28099).
(4) Urostomy Association, 'Buckland', Beaumont Park, Danbury, Essex CM3 4DE (Tel: 0124 522 4294).

References and further reading

Anders, K. (1993) Open communication can restore self-esteem: sexuality issues related to cystectomy for stoma formation. *Professional Nurse*, 8(10), 638–43.
APBI Data Sheets Compendium 1995–96, (compiler G. Walker). Datapharm Publications.

Bell, N. (1989) Sexuality: promoting fulfilment. *Nursing Times*, 85(6), 35–7.

Black, P. K. (1985a) Selecting a site. *Nursing Mirror*, 16(9), 22–4.

Black, P. K. (1985b) Drugs and diet. *Nursing Mirror*, 161, 26–8.

Black, P. K. (1989) Complications associated with a stoma. *Surgical Nurse*, 2(6), Supplement, i–v.

Black, P. K. (1994a) Stoma care: a practical approach. *Nursing Standard*, 8(34), *RCN Nursing Update*, Learning Unit 045.

Black, P. K. (1994b) Hidden problems of stoma care. *British Journal of Nursing*, 3(14), 707–11.

Black, P. K. (1994c) Choosing the correct stoma appliance. *British Journal of Nursing*, 3(11), 545–6, 548, 550.

Boore, J. R. P. (1978) *A Prescription for Recovery: the Effect of Preoperative Preparation of Surgical Patients on Postoperative Stress, Recovery and Infection*. Royal College of Nursing, London.

Borwell, B. (1994) Colostomies and their management. *Nursing Standard*, 8(45), CE article 332.

Breckman, B. (1981) *Stoma Care*. Beaconsfield Publishers, Beaconsfield.

Brindley, G. (1986) Pilot experiments on the actions of drugs injected into the human corpus cavernosum penis. *British Journal of Pharmacology*, 87, 495–500.

Broadwell, D. C. (1987) Peristomal skin integrity. *Nursing Clinics of North America*, 22(2), 321–32.

Broadwell, D. C. & Jackson, B. S. (1982) *Principles of Ostomy Care*. C. V. Mosby, St Louis.

Brooke, B. N. *et al.* (1982) *Stomas*. W. B. Saunders, London.

Bryant, R. A. (1993) Ostomy patient management: care that engenders adaptation. *Cancer Investigation*, 11(5), 565–77.

Coloplast (undated) *Back on Your Feet Again*, Coloplast.

Davies, K. (1990) Impotence after surgery. *Nursing*, 4(18), 13–26.

De-Hong, Y. (1991) An assessment of colostomy irrigation. *Ostomy International*, 11(2), *Nursing* (1st series), 17, 727–9.

Dyer, S. (1988) Stoma care: choosing the right appliance. *Professional Nurse*, 3(8), 278–80, 282–3.

Elcoat, C. (1986) *Stoma Care Nursing*. Baillière Tindall, London.

Etnyre, W. (1990) Meeting the needs of gay and lesbian ostomates. *Proceeding of 8th Biennial Congress World Council of Enterostomal Therapists*.

Faller, N. & Lawrence, K. (1992) A pictorial workshop: 'Tips on clips: hints on tail closures', 'Ideas sobre pinzas'. *World Council of Enterostomal Therapists Journal*, 12(4), 26–7.

Foulkes, B. (1981) Specific aspects of ileostomy care. In: *Stoma Care*, (ed. B. Breckman). Beaconsfield Publishers, Beaconsfield.

Gelister, J. F. & Woodhouse, C. R. (1991) Role of continent suprapubic diversion in pelvic cancer. *British Journal of Urology*, 68, 376–9.

Hayward, J. (1978) *Information – A Prescription Against Pain*. Royal College of Nursing, London.

Horn, S. (1991) Nursing patients with a continent urinary diversion. *Nursing Standard*, 4(21), 24–6.

Janis, I. L. & Rodin, J. (1982) Attribution centred and decision making: social psychology and health care. In: *Health Psychology*, (eds G. C. Stone *et al.*). Jossey-Bass, London.

Joels, J. (1989) Psychological implications of having a stoma. *Surgical Nurse*, 2(6), Supplement, x–xii.

Kelly, L. (1995) Patients becoming people. *Journal of Community Nursing*, August, 12–16.

Klopp, A. (1990) Body image and self-concept among individuals with stomas. *Journal of Enterostomal Therapy*, 17(3), 98–105.

Krasner, D. (1993) Six steps to successful stoma care. *Registered Nurse*, July.

Little, G. R. (1989) The dietary implications of having a stoma. *Surgical Nurse*, 2(6), Supplement, vi–ix.

MacDonald, K. & Joels, J. (1990) Stoma care: which appliance to choose? *Surgical Nurse*, 3(1), i–vi.

MacDonald, L. (1982) Problems of the colostomy population. *Stoma Care News*, 1, p. 45, in *Nursing Mirror* (1983) Clinical Forum 8: Stoma Care, *Nursing Mirror*, 157(11), Supplement.

Martindale (1993) *The Extra Pharmacopoeia*, (ed. J. E. F. Reynolds), 13th edn. The Pharmaceutical Press, London.

Model, G. (1990) A new image to accept: psychological aspects of stoma care. *Professional Nurse*, 5(6), 310–16.

Nemer, E. & Rolstad, B. (1985) The role of the ileo–anal reservoir in patients with ulcerative colitis and familial polyposis. *Journal of Enterostomal Therapy*, 12(3), 74–83.

Ortiz, H. *et al.* (1993) Does the frequency of colostomy hernia depend on the colostomy location in the abdominal wall? *World Council of Enterostomal Therapists Journal*, 13(2), 13–14.

Padma-Nathan, H. (1993) Intracavernosal pharmacotherapy. *Current Opinions in Urology*, 3, 492–5.

Price, B. (1990) *Body Image Nursing: Concepts and Care*. Prentice Hall, New York.

Price, B. (1993) Profiling the high risk altered body image patient. *Senior Nurse*, 13(4), 17–21.

Price, B. (1994) Understanding the experience of an altered body image. *Eurostoma*, 5, 10–11.

Salter, M. (1986) Self-image and sexuality. *Primary Health Care*, 4(3), 8–9.

Salter, M. (1988a) *Body Image – The Nurse's Role*. Scutari Press, London.

Salter, M. (1988b) Preoperative education and counselling. *Practice Nurse*, October, 226–8, 230.

Salter, M. (1992) Body image: The person with a stoma, Part 1. *Wound Management*, 2(2), 8–9.

Salter, M. (1995) Guest editorial: some observations on body image. *World Council of Enterostomal Therapists*, 15(3), 4–7.

Schover, L. R. (1986) Sexual rehabilitation of the ostomy patient. In: *Ostomy Care and the Cancer Patient*, (eds D. B. Smith & D. E. Johnson). Grune & Stratton, Orlando.

Tomaselli, N. & Morin, K. (1991) Body image in patients with stomas: a critical review of the literature. *Journal of Enterostomal Therapy*, 18(3), 95–9.

Topping, A. (1990) Sexual activity and the stoma patient. *Nursing Standard*, 4(41), 24–6.

Van De Wiel, H. B. M. *et al.* (1991) Sexual functioning after ostomy surgery. *Sexual and Marital Therapy*, 6(2),

196–209.
Wade, B. (1989) Nursing care of the stoma patient. *Surgical Nurse*, 2(5), Supplement, ix–xii.
Wade, B. (1990) Patients' fears after stoma surgery. *Nursing*

Standard, 55(3).
Wells, R. (1990) Sexuality: an unknown word for patients with a stoma? *Second International Symposium on Supportive Care in Cancer Patients*, St Gallen (unpublished paper).

GUIDELINES: STOMA CARE

These procedural guidelines contain the basic information needed for changing a stoma appliance. Modifications may be made according to the following factors:

1 The place of change, i.e. bathroom, bedside, availability of sink, etc.
2 The person changing the appliance, i.e. nurse or patient.
3 Type of appliance used, e.g. one- or two-piece, closed or drainable.
4 Any accessories used, e.g. flatus filters, hypoallergenic tape, barrier creams, etc.

EQUIPMENT

1 Clean tray holding:
  (a) Tissues.
  (b) New appliances.
  (c) Disposal bags for used appliances and tissues.
  (d) Relevant accessories, e.g. flatus filters, tape, etc.
2 Bowl of warm water.
3 Soap.
4 Jug for contents of appliance.
5 Gloves. (It is now common practice and, in many cases, hospital policy, to wear gloves when dealing with blood and body fluids due to the risk of infections. Thus they should be worn for cleaning stomas. It is recognized that it could be difficult to attach an appliance with gloves *in situ* (due to the adhesive), but once the stoma has been cleaned of excreta and blood, the gloves may be removed to apply the bag.) This practice should be explained to the patient so that they do not feel it is just because they have a stoma that gloves are worn.

PROCEDURE

Action	Rationale
1 Explain and discuss the procedure with the patient.	To ensure that the patient understands the procedure and gives his/her valid consent.
2 Explain the procedure.	To familiarize the patient with the procedure.
3 Ensure that the patient is in a suitable and comfortable position where the patient will be able to watch the procedure; if well enough a mirror may be used to aid visualization.	To allow good access to the stoma for cleaning and for secure application of the stoma bag. The patient will become familiar with the stoma and will also learn much about the care of the stoma by observation of the nurse (Bryant, 1993).
4 Use a small protective pad to protect the patient's clothing from drips if the effluent is fluid and apply gloves for nurse's protection.	Avoids the necessity for renewing clothing or bedclothes and demoralization of the patient as a result of soiling.

Guidelines: Stoma care (cont'd)

Action	Rationale
5 If the bag is of the drainable type, empty the contents into a jug before removing the bag.	For ease of handling the appliance and prevention of spillage.
6 Remove the appliance. Peel the adhesive off the skin with one hand while exerting gentle pressure on the skin with the other.	To reduce trauma to the skin. Erythema as a result of removing the appliance is normal and quickly settles (Broadwell, 1987).
7 Remove excess faeces or mucus from the stoma with a damp tissue.	So that the stoma and surrounding skin are clearly visible.
8 Examine the skin and stoma for soreness, ulceration or other unusual phenomena. If the skin is unblemished and the stoma is a healthy red colour, proceed.	For the prevention of complications or the treatment of existing problems (see Nursing care plan).
9 Wash the skin and stoma gently until they are clean.	To promote cleanliness and prevent skin excoriation.
10 Dry the skin and stoma gently but thoroughly.	The appliance will attach more securely to dry skin.
11 Apply a clean appliance.	
12 Dispose of soiled tissues and the used bag. Rinse the bag through in the sluice with water, wrap it in a disposable bag and place it in an appropriate plastic bin. At home the bag should be emptied into the toilet; a closed bag may be cut at the lower end, then rinsed using a jug or by holding it under the flushing water. Wrap the bag in newspaper, tie it in a plastic bag and dispose of it in a rubbish bag.	Faecal material in waste bags is a potential source of infection. Excreta should be disposed of down the sluice.
13 Wash hands thoroughly using bactericidal soap and water or bactericidal alcohol hand rub.	To prevent spread of infection by contaminated hands.

GUIDELINES: COLLECTION OF A SPECIMEN OF URINE FROM AN ILEAL CONDUIT OR UROSTOMY

EQUIPMENT

1 Sterile dressing pack.
2 Soft catheter – Nelaton type, not larger than 12 or 14 Fr.
3 Disposable plastic apron.
4 Universal specimen container.
5 Skin-cleansing solution.
6 Bactericidal alcohol hand rub.
7 Clean stoma appliance.

PROCEDURE

Action	Rationale
1 Explain and discuss the procedure with the patient.	To ensure that the patient understands the procedure and gives his/her valid consent.
2 Ensure that the patient is in a comfortable position, e.g. sitting up, supported by pillows, and that the stoma is easily accessible.	For patient comfort and to allow access to stoma.
3 Screen the bed, then wash hands using bactericidal soap and water or bactericidal alcohol hand rub. Then dry them.	For the patient's privacy and to reduce the risk of cross-infection. Curtains are drawn at this stage so that dust and airborne organisms disturbed by the curtains do not settle on the sterile trolley.
4 Prepare the trolley and take it to the patient's bedside.	To ensure equipment is easily available.
5 Put on a disposable plastic apron.	To reduce risk of cross-infection.
6 Remove the sterile dressing pack, catheter and receiver from their outer wrappings. Place them on the top shelf of the trolley.	To prepare equipment.
7 Remove the appliance from the stoma and cover the stoma with a clean topical swab.	To absorb spillage from the stoma.
8 Clean hands with a bactericidal alcohol hand rub, and put on clean disposable gloves before opening the sterile field on the trolley.	To reduce the risk of introducing infection into the stoma during the procedure.
9 Remove the non-linting gauze with forceps, check and discard it. Arrange a towel to absorb spillage from the stoma.	To keep the areas as clean as possible and to protect the patient and the bedclothes from spilled urine.
10 Clean around the stoma with water or saline, from the centre outwards.	Good cleansing of the area reduces the risk of introduction of surface pathogens into the ileal loop.
11 Apply gentle skin traction to allow stomal opening to be more visible. Insert the catheter tip gently to a depth of 2.5–5 cm only and wait for urine to drain through. Collect the sample in the specimen container. The recommended volume is 3–5 ml.	To avoid catheter coming into contact with external surfaces of stoma. Gentle handling reduces the risk of ileal perforation and is more comfortable for the patient. To ensure adequate sample of urine for bacteriological assessment.
12 Remove the catheter and seal in the specimen container. Remove gloves and attend to stoma care and apply a pouch as usual. Make the patient comfortable.	To prevent spillage of sample. To ensure patient comfort.
13 Dispose of equipment.	
14 Wash hands with bactericidal soap and water and dry.	To reduce risk of cross-infection.
15 Check that the specimen is labelled correctly and dispatch it to the laboratory with the appropriate forms.	

NURSING CARE PLAN

Problem	Cause	Suggested action
Leakage of urine or faeces.	Ill-fitting appliance.	Remeasure stoma and ensure a snug fitting appliance. Prepare template for future use.
	Skin creases or 'gulleys' preventing correct application of adhesive.	Build up indented areas and fill in gulleys to create a smooth surface e.g. using paste.
	Infrequent emptying of drainable bag leading to stress on adhesion.	Drainable bags should be emptied frequently, e.g. 2- to 3-hourly if necessary.
Sore skin.	Leakage.	As above.
	Skin reaction to adhesive.	Change the make of appliance or apply a protective square between skin and adhesive. Anti-inflammatory agents may be required for very severe reactions.
	Poor hygiene.	Improve the technique of nurses or patient.
Odour.	Ill-fitting appliance; lack of seal between skin and adhesive.	Fit the appliance with care. Consider a change of the type of appliance.
	Poor hygiene.	Improve the technique of nurses or patient.
	Poor technique, e.g. when emptying drainable bag.	Empty the bag, then rinse the end with water to ensure that it is clean before closing.

Urostomy specimen

Problem	Cause	Suggested action
Stoma specimen of urine contaminated.	Contaminants introduced during specimen collection.	Take a repeat specimen, observing aseptic procedure and cleaning the stoma well.
Ileum perforated during specimen collection.	Catheter too hard or inserted too roughly.	Report to a doctor immediately.
Difficulty passing catheter into conduit.	Small degree of retraction of ileum.	Apply gentle pressure to the area around the stoma to make it protrude.
	Unpredictable direction of ileum.	Gently insert your little (gloved) finger into the stoma to determine the direction of the conduit. Insert the catheter tip along this line.

CHAPTER 40
Syringe Drivers

Definition
A syringe driver is a portable battery-operated infusion pump weighing approximately 175 g (including the battery) and measuring 165 mm by 53 mm by 23 mm.

Indications
The syringe driver is used to deliver drugs at a predetermined rate via the appropriate parenteral route. Typical applications include its use in pain control, cytotoxic chemotherapy, coronary care and neonatal care. It may also be used for the administration of heparin and insulin, and treatment of thalassaemia. This chapter focuses on the clinical application of the syringe driver in the administration of subcutaneous drugs.

REFERENCE MATERIAL
The syringe driver was developed in 1979 by Dr Martin Wright for use in treating thalassaemia with infusions of desferrioxamine (Wright & Callam, 1979).

The use of a portable battery operated syringe driver for subcutaneous medications is now a well established technique in palliative care and is used to administer analgesics and anti-emetics, anxiolytic sedatives and dexamethasone (Coyle et al., 1986; Dover, 1987; Oliver, 1988; Bottomley & Hanks, 1990 as cited in Doyle et al., 1993) and more recently ketorolac (Blackwell et al., 1993) and octreotide (Mercadante, 1992).

The Graseby Medical MS16A and Graseby MS26 syringe drivers are typical examples of the drivers in use; however, other types are available and nurses should follow the manufacturer's instruction manual for details of their use. The Graseby Medical MS16A syringe driver allows drug administration on an hourly rate (Fig. 40.1). This pump is now clearly marked with pink highlighted '1 HR' in the bottom right-hand corner of the driver. The MS26 delivers drugs on a 24-hourly rate. It is important that users are aware that the MS16A syringe driver is calibrated in mm per hour, and the MS26 is calibrated in mm per day. The MS26 model is now marked with '24 HR' in the bottom right-hand corner to avoid error. The MS series of syringe drivers may be used with most sizes and makes of plastic syringes, although it is preferable to use those with Luer lock facility to avoid leakage or accidental disconnection.

Indications for use
The syringe driver should be used for patients who are unable to tolerate oral medication for whatever reason – nausea and vomiting, dysphagia, intestinal obstruction, local disease or sometimes in intractable pain unrelieved by oral medications and where rapid dose titration is required.

Advantages in the use of the syringe driver

(1) Avoids the necessity of intermittent injections.
(2) Mixtures of drugs may be administered (see Drug stability and compatibility, below).
(3) Infusion timing is accurate, which is particularly advantageous in the community.
(4) The device is lightweight and compact allowing mobility and independence.
(5) Rate can be increased (see Additional notes at end of chapter).
(6) Simple calculations of dosage are required over a 12- or 24-hour period.

Disadvantages in the use of the syringe driver

(1) Patient may become psychologically dependent on the device.
(2) Inflammation or infection may occur at the site of the cannula insertion.
(3) Rate calculation can be confusing for the novice because there are two different types of pumps, particularly if the patient's dose requirements alter (see Additional notes, below).
(4) The alarm system of some syringe drivers, e.g. the

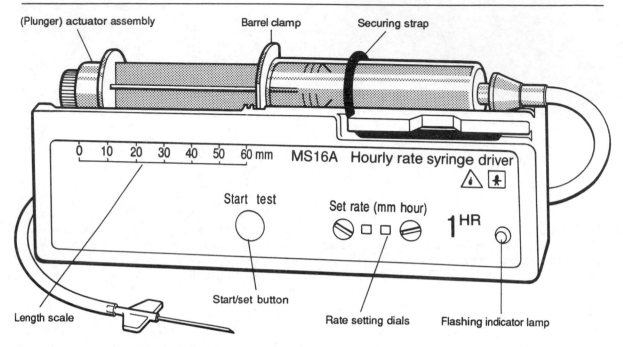

Figure 40.1   Graseby Medical MS16A hourly rate syringe driver.

Graseby, operates only if the plunger is obstructed. It does not alert the nurse if the flow is too rapid or if the skin site has perished.

Skin site selection for subcutaneous infusion

The best sites to use for continuous infusion of drugs are the lateral aspects of the upper arms and thighs, the abdomen, the anterior chest below the clavicle and, occasionally, the back (Nicholson, 1986). Areas which should not be used for cannula placement are:

(1) Lymphoedematous limbs. The rate of absorption from a skin site would be adversely affected. A cannula breaches skin integrity thus increasing the risk of infection in a limb which is already susceptible.
(2) Sites over bony prominences: the amount of subcutaneous tissue will be diminished, impairing the rate of drug absorption.
(3) Previously irradiated skin area. Radiotherapy can cause sclerosis of small blood vessels, thus reducing skin perfusion (Tiffany, 1988).
(4) Sites near a joint: excessive movement may cause cannula displacement and patient discomfort.

Care of the skin site

The infusion site should be renewed when there is evidence of inflammation (erythema or reddening) or poor absorption (a hard subcutaneous swelling). The time taken for this to occur can vary from hours to over three weeks, dependent on the patient, and the drug(s) being infused (Regnard & Newbury, 1983; Coyle et al., 1986; Nicholson, 1986; Brenneis et al., 1987; Bruera et al., 1987). There would appear to be a relationship between the concentration of drug(s) being infused, and the duration of a skin site (Nicholson, 1986). In one study, the average frequency of needle resiting was 5.1 days for patients receiving 7.5–30 mg of diamorphine per 24 hours, but only 2.4 days for those receiving 1000–2000 mg per 24 hours (Nicholson, 1986).

Another study noted no statistically significant relationship between duration of skin site and sex and age of patients, type or dose of narcotic, rate of infusion, or triceps skinfold measurement (Brenneis et al., 1987). Clearly, further research into the factors influencing skin site survival is required.

If skin sites break down rapidly, suggestions include:

(1) Further dilute the drug infused.
(2) Change the infusion device.
(3) Use a different site cleanser.
(4) Change the site dressing.

Drug stability and compatibility

In the context of single drug infusions, instability is not a clinically significant problem. The drug simply has to be:

(1) Available in injectable form.

(2) Suitable for subcutaneous administration.

(3) Stable in solution for the duration of the infusion (usually 12–48 hours).

For example, diamorphine hydrochloride is stable, in solution, for up to two weeks (Jones & Hanks, 1986).

Problems of drug instability and incompatibility arise when higher drug concentrations and combinations of two or more drugs are used. In addition, exposure of drug solutions to direct light and increased storage temperatures (up to 32°C) may exacerbate the problem.

Where drug combinations (commonly an analgesic and an anti-emetic) are used, further criteria must be met:

(1) The drugs must be compatible with each other.

(2) The diluents must be compatible with each other.

(3) Each drug must be compatible with the diluent(s) of the other drug(s) in the combination.

Studies by Allwood (1984) and later work by Regnard & Davies (1986) have examined the stability and compatibility of analgesic/anti-emetic combinations. Regnard & Davies (1986) make the following recommendations:

(1) Protect the syringe from direct light whenever possible.

(2) Visual inspection of drug solutions should be made daily, and the syringe discarded if signs of crystallization, precipitation or discoloration occur.

(3) Avoid high concentrations of drugs if used in combination.

(4) Avoid mixing more than two drugs in one syringe.

(5) Do not infuse anti-emetics for more than 24 hours, particularly if part of a combination of drugs.

However, it remains the responsibility of each individual practitioner to ensure that the drug(s) prescribed are suitable for continuous subcutaneous infusion, and are stable under these conditions. If in any doubt, seek advice from an appropriate professional.

References and further reading

Allwood, M. C. (1984) Diamorphine mixed with antiemetic drugs in plastic syringes. *British Journal of Pharmaceutical Practice*, 6, 88–90.

Auty, B. & Protheroe, D. T. (1986) Syringe pumps: a review. *British Journal of Parenteral Therapy*, 7, 72–7.

Badger, C. & Regnard, C. (1986) Pumping in pain relief. *Nursing Times*, 82, 52–4.

Baines, M. (1981) Drug control of common symptoms. *World Medicine*, 7(4), 47–59.

Beswick, D. T. (1987) Use of syringe driver in terminal care. *Pharmaceutical Journal*, 239, 656–8.

Blackwell, N. et al. (1993) Subcutaneous ketorolac – a new development in pain control. *Palliative Medicine*, 7, 63–5.

Brenneis, C. et al. (1987) Local toxicity during the subcutaneous infusion of narcotics (SCIN). *Cancer Nursing*, 10(4), 172–6.

Bruera, E. et al. (1987) Continuous SC infusion of narcotics using a portable disposable device in patients with advanced cancer. *Cancer Treatment Reports*, 71(6), 635–7.

Cox, P. & Potter, M. (1984) Controlling pain. *Journal of District Nursing*, 3(4), 4–3, 9.

Coyle, N. et al. (1986) Continuous subcutaneous infusions of opiates in cancer patients with pain. *Oncology Nursing Forum*, 13(4), 53–7.

Dover, S. B. (1987) Syringe driver in terminal care. *British Medical Journal*, 294, 553–5.

Doyle, D. et al. (1993) *Oxford Textbook of Palliative Medicine*. Oxford University Press, Oxford.

Hanks, G. W. et al. (1987) Diamorphine stability and pharmacodynamics. *Anaesthesia*, 42, 664–73.

Hawkett, S. & Nicholson, R. (1987) Syringe drivers (drug administration for the terminally ill in the community). *Journal of District Nursing*, 5(8), 4–6.

Hoskin, P. et al. (1988) Syringe drivers *Anaesthesia*, 43, 708

Hoskin, P. et al. (1988) Sterile abscess formation by continuous subcutaneous infusion of diamorphine. *British Medical Journal*, 296, 1605.

Jones, V. A. & Hanks, G. W. (1986) New portable infusion pump for prolonged administration of opioid analgesics in patients with advanced cancer. *British Medical Journal*, 292, 1496.

Jones, V. A. et al. (1985) Solubility of diamorphine. *Pharmaceutical Journal*, 235, 426.

Jones, V. A. et al. (1987) Diamorphine stability in aqueous solution for subcutaneous injection. Proceedings of the BPS, 17–19 December. *British Journal of Clinical Pharmacology*, 23, 651.

Latham, J. (1987) Syringe drivers in pain control. *Professional Nurse*, 2(7), 207–9.

Ledger, T. (1986) Administering heparin with syringe pumps. *Professional Nurse*, 1(7), 176–7.

Leggett, A. (1990) Looking at infusion devices (advantages and disadvantages of syringe pumps and drivers). *Nursing Standard*, 4(18), 29–31.

Mercadante, S. (1992) Treatment of diarrhoea due to enterocolic fistula with octreotide in a terminal cancer patient. *Palliative Medicine*, 65, 257–9.

Nicholson, H. (1986) The success of the syringe driver. *Nursing Times* 82, 49–51.

Oliver, D. J. (1988) Syringe drivers in palliative care: a review. *Palliative Medicine*, 2, 21–26.

Oliver, D. J. & Sykes, C. (1988) Histopathological study of subcutaneous drug infusion sites in patients dying with cancer. *Lancet*, 1, 478.

Regnard, C. F. & Davies, A. (1986) *A Guide to Symptom Relief in Advanced Cancer*. Haigh & Hochland, Manchester.

Regnard, C. & Newbury, A. (1983) Pain and the portable syringe pump. *Nursing Times*, 79, 25–8.

Regnard, C. *et al.* (1968) Anti-emetic/diamorphine mixture compatibility in infusion pumps. *British Journal of Pharmaceutical Practice*, 8, 218–20.

Russell, P. S. B. (1979) Analgesia in terminal malignant disease. *British Medical Journal*, 1(6177), 1561.

Storey, P. *et al.* (1990) Subcutaneous infusions for control of cancer symptoms. *Journal of Pain and Symptoms Management*, 5(1), 33–41.

Tiffany, R. (ed.) (1988) *Oncology for Nurses and Health Care Professionals, Vol. I. Pathology, Diagnosis and Treatment*, 2nd edn. Harper & Row, London.

Twycross, R. G. & Lack, S. A. (1984) *Therapeutics in Terminal Cancer*. Pitman, London.

Vere, D. W. (1978) Pharmacology of morphine drugs used in terminal care. In: *Topics in Therapeutics*, (ed. D. W. Vere). Pitman Medical, London.

Weston, A. (1989) Graseby syringe driver (brief research project). *Nursing Times and Nursing Mirror*, 85, 60–61.

Wright, B. M. & Callam, K. (1979) Slow drug infusions using a portable syringe driver. *British Medical Journal*, 2, 582.

GUIDELINES: SUBCUTANEOUS ADMINISTRATION OF DRUGS USING A SYRINGE DRIVER (E.G. GRASEBY MEDICAL MS16A)

EQUIPMENT

1 Syringe driver MS16A.
2 Battery (PP3 size, 9 volt alkaline).
3 Winged infusion set (for example, Vygon microflex PVC infusion set tube 100 cm, 0.5 mm G25).
4 Luer lock syringe of suitable size (5 ml or larger).
5 Swab saturated with isopropyl alcohol 70%.
6 Transparent adhesive dressing.
7 Drugs and diluent.
8 Needle (to draw up drug).
9 Drug additive label.
10 Patient's prescription.

CALCULATING THE RATE SETTING FOR ADMINISTRATION OF DRUGS USING A SYRINGE DRIVER (E.G. GRASEBY MEDICAL MS16A) OVER A 12-HOUR PERIOD

1 Measure stroke length in mm. The stroke length is the *length* of fluid to be infused, i.e. the distance the plunger has to travel (irrespective of the number of ml) (Fig. 40.2).
2 Check the delivery time (previously prescribed) in hours.

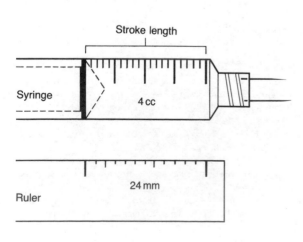

Figure 40.2   Measuring the stroke length.

3 Calculate:

$$\frac{\text{Stroke length (mm)}}{\text{Delivery time (h)}} = \text{Rate setting}$$

Example:

Stroke length = 24 mm
Delivery time = 12 h
Rate setting = 2 mm/h

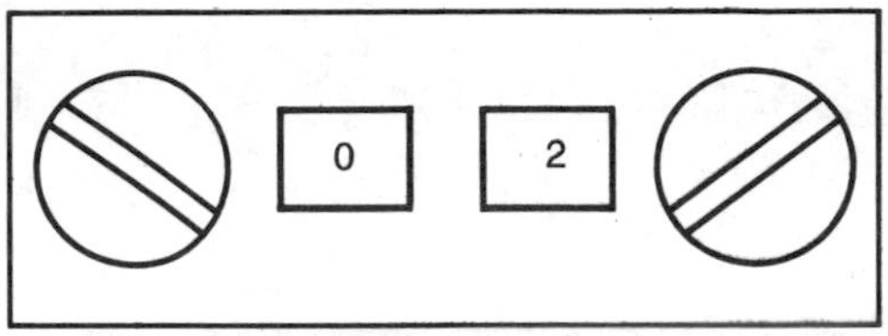

Figure 40.3   Setting the rate.

Set rate using screwdriver provided.
If the set rate is a single figure, e.g. 2, this must be preceded by 0 (Fig. 40.3).
See instruction booklets provided with individual syringe pumps.

GUIDELINES: PREPARATION OF THE SYRINGE FOR 12-HOUR DRUG ADMINISTRATION USING GRASEBY MEDICAL MS16A SYRINGE DRIVER

Action

1   Calculate dosage of drugs and minimum volume of diluent required over 12 hours (use at least 1 ml diluent per 250 mg diamorphine hydrochloride injection).

2   Draw up drugs with diluent, withdrawing the plunger until the stroke length corresponds with a number divisible by 12, e.g. 24, 36 or 48 mm.

3   Establish the rate setting of the pump and check (or where appropriate educate the patient to check) the rate 4- to 6-hourly.

Rationale

This is more comfortable for the patient.
Smaller volumes reduce the risk of inflammation at infusion site.

Ensures accuracy as the infusion rate can only be set in whole numbers.

Ensures drug is given over the prescribed time period.

GUIDELINES: PRIMING THE INFUSION SET

Action

1   Using previously prepared syringe, connect a 100 cm winged infusion set.

2   Gently depress the plunger until the infusion tubing is filled up to the needle end.

3   Having previously calculated the rate setting, allow time for speedier first infusion rate.

Rationale

This length of tubing allows patient greater freedom of movement.

This removes extraneous air from the system. Adding further diluent to syringe reduces the potency and therefore the effect of drug to be infused.

Ensures patient receives drugs immediately and accurately. (Usually priming the line reduces delivery time by approximately half an hour.) Do not alter previously calculated rate setting despite volume reduction in barrel of syringe.

GUIDELINES: INSERTING THE WINGED INFUSION SET

Action	Rationale
 **1** Explain and discuss the procedure with the patient.	To ensure that the patient understands the procedure and gives his/her valid consent.
2 Assist the patient into a comfortable position.	
3 Expose the chosen site for infusion (see skin site selection under 'Reference material', above).	
4 Clean the chosen site with a swab saturated with 70% isopropyl alcohol. Wait until the alcohol evaporates.	To reduce the risk of infection.
5 Grasp the skin firmly.	To elevate the subcutaneous tissue.
6 Insert the infusion needle into the skin at an angle of 45° and release the grasped skin.	Shallower positioning than 45° may shorten the life of the infusion site.
7 Tape the infusion wings firmly to the skin using transparent adhesive dressing (see 'Care of the skin site' under 'Reference material', above).	Transparent dressing allows observation of the infusion site and maintains the correct position of the needle.
8 Connect the syringe to the syringe driver (see instructions below).	To ensure the syringe is connected correctly to the syringe driver.
9 Record, in the appropriate documents, that the infusion has been commenced.	To comply with local drug administration policies.

CONNECTING THE SYRINGE TO THE SYRINGE DRIVER

(1) Place the syringe on the syringe driver along the grooved lines, with barrel clamp firmly in position.

(2) Secure in place with rubber strap.

(3) Slide the actuator assembly along the lead screw by pressing white release button as shown in Fig. 40.4, until it rests against the end of the plunger.

(4) Secure plunger with additional safety clamp (Fig. 40.5).

(5) Press start/test button to commence infusion. The indicator light should flash to indicate functioning syringe pump.

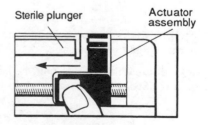

Figure 40.4 Connecting the syringe to the syringe driver.

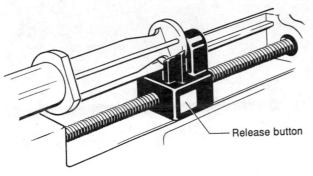

Release button

Figure 40.5 Securing the plunger.

ADDITIONAL NOTES

(1) Different manufacturers of syringes have different barrel sizes, i.e. 4 ml in a 10 ml syringe made by one company may yield a different stroke length to 4 ml in a 10 ml syringe made by another.

(2) If more than one drug is to be administered, for example, analgesic and antiemetic, it is important not to increase the rate of the syringe driver to yield more pain relief, as this will increase the antiemetic dose.

(3) If 'breakthrough' analgesia is required, it is prefer-able to administer the equivalent of a 4-hourly dose as a separate extra statim subcutaneous injection. Bolus pushes using the boost button are not recommended, for the following reasons.

(a) Those outlined in point 2 above.

(b) A 'boost' push yields only 0.2 mm of extra analgesia.

(c) Pain assessment is more difficult and evaluation of pain control is hindered.

(d) Inaccuracies of infusion time may occur as a result.

CHAPTER 41
Tracheostomy Care and Laryngectomy Voice Rehabilitation

TRACHEOSTOMY CARE

The care of patients with a tracheostomy varies from one hospital to another. The changing of a tracheostomy tube will usually be undertaken by a doctor or a trained nurse who has been instructed in this procedure. It is important, however, that nurses are aware of the procedures and basic principles and know how to respond in an emergency situation.

Definition
A tracheostomy is an artificial opening made into the trachea through the neck (Fig. 41.1a) (Stell & Moran, 1978).

Indications
Tracheostomy may be carried out:

(1) To provide and maintain a patent airway.
(2) To enable the removal of tracheobronchial secretions.

A tracheostomy may be performed as a temporary, permanent or emergency procedure (Stell & Moran, 1978).

General care of tracheostomy patients

(1) When caring for a tracheostomy patient the following should always be at the bedside or accessible if the patient is self-caring or ambulant.
  (a) Humidified oxygen with tracheostomy mask.
  (b) Suction machine with a selection of suction catheters.
  (c) Covered bowl of sodium bicarbonate (1 teaspoon to 500 ml sterile water) to clear suction tubing of secretions when suctioning has been performed.
  (d) Clean disposable gloves (Watson, 1979).
  (e) Two cuffed tracheostomy tubes, one the same size as the patient is wearing, the other a size smaller, in the event of an emergency tracheostomy tube change.
  (f) One 10 ml syringe to inflate cuff on tracheostomy tube.
  (g) One clamp to ensure that air stays in cuff.
  (h) Tracheal dilators, in the event of tracheostomy tube falling out or being removed and inability to insert another tube. Tracheal dilators can be used to keep stomal opening patent until medical assistance arrives.
(2) Tracheostomy tube changes are mostly dependent on the type of secretions the patient has, for example, a patient with copious, tenacious secretions will need a daily tube change, sometimes twice a day, as this will be the only way of ensuring that the stoma and tube are free from any accumulation of secretions. If the patient has minimal secretions then the necessity to change the tube decreases until some patients need to have their tube changed only weekly.

Sometimes if the patient has a wound area up to the stoma edge, the tracheostomy tube has to be removed to gain access for cleaning the wound and observing its general status.

The tracheostomy dressing can be renewed without removing the tube and this should be done daily or twice a day to ensure that any secretions are cleared, and do not lay wet against the skin and cause any excoriation (Jeter & Tintle, 1988).

REFERENCE MATERIAL

Types of tracheostomy

Temporary
A temporary tracheostomy (Fig. 41.1b) is performed for patients as an elective procedure, e.g. at the time of major surgery.

(a)

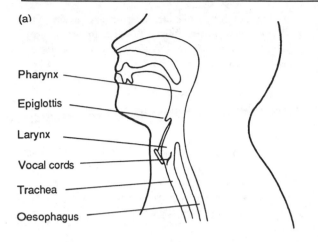

(b)

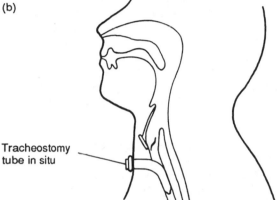

(c)

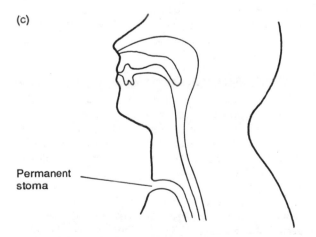

Figure 41.1 (a) Anatomy of the head and neck. (b) Temporary tracheostomy. (c) Permanent tracheostomy (total laryngectomy).

Permanent

A permanent tracheostomy is the creation of a tracheostomy following a total laryngectomy (Fig. 41.1c). The top three tracheal cartilages are brought to the surface of the skin and sutured to the neck wall to form a stoma. The 'end' tracheostomy is permanent and the rigidity of the tracheal cartilage keeps the stoma open. The patient will breathe through this stoma for the remainder of his/her life. As a result, there is no connection between the nasal passages and the trachea.

Emergency

A tracheostomy may be performed as an emergency procedure when a patient has an obstructed airway. Among the more common conditions causing obstruction are trauma to the airway or neck, poisoning, infections or neoplasms.

Types of tubes

Experience has shown that the choice of tracheostomy tube depends on the type of operation performed; the patient's ability to tolerate the tube depends on various external factors. A selection of tubes is listed below.

Portex cuffed tracheostomy tube

This is a disposable plastic tracheostomy tube with an introducer and inflatable cuff to give an airtight seal (Fig. 41.2a). The cuff prevents blood from reaching the lungs and the seal facilitates ventilation at the time of surgery.

It is an anaesthetic tube which is usually in site for 24–48 hours. Depending on the patient's condition, the Portex tube will be removed and the stoma left exposed, or a more suitable sturdier tube will be inserted, such as a Shiley tracheostomy tube.

Portex uncuffed tracheostomy tube

This is a disposable plastic tracheostomy tube (Fig. 41.2b) used, for example, during radiotherapy to the neck area when a metal tube would cause tissue reaction (Holmes, 1988).

Shiley plain tracheostomy tube (Fig. 41.3a)

This is a plastic tube with an introducer and two inner tubes. One inner tube has an extension at its upper aspect. This facilitates connection to other equipment, e.g. nebulizers and speaking valves.

This tube is usually used for the following reasons:

(1) To keep the tracheostomy tract patent if the patient is going to have further surgery.
(2) In place of a metal tracheostomy tube if the patient is going to have radiotherapy to the neck area when a metal tube would cause tissue reaction.
(3) For a laryngectomy patient who has a benign or malignant stenosis of the trachea and requires a

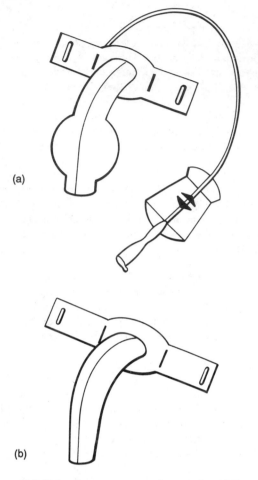

(a)

(b)

Figure 41.2 Tubes for temporary tracheostomies. (a) Portex cuffed tube. (b) Portex uncuffed tube.

longer tube than the regular length laryngectomy tube to keep the stenosis patent.

(4) As a weaning method. For example, the patient could occlude the tube with a cap for certain periods of time to get used to breathing normally again, until the cap can be worn for a full uninterrupted 24 hours, breathing comfortably via the oral airway.

Alternatively, the cuffless tube can be used to assist with maintaining a patent airway while the patient is learning to swallow without aspirating food.

These weaning methods can also be used with the Shiley plain fenestrated tube, and the cuffed fenestrated tube.

Shiley cuffed tracheostomy tube (Fig. 41.3b)

This is a plastic tube with an introducer and two inner tubes. One inner tube has an extension at its upper as-

pect to facilitate connection to other equipment. The outer tube has an inflatable cuff to give an airtight seal. The cuff prevents secretions from reaching the lungs. The seal facilitates ventilation.

Shiley plain fenestrated tube (Fig. 41.3c)

This is a plastic tube with an introducer and two inner tubes. One inner tube has an extension at its upper end to facilitate connection to other apparatus. The outer tube has a fenestration in the middle of the cannula. This is to encourage the passage of air and secretions into the oral and nasal passages. It is useful when attempting to encourage a return to normal function following long-term use of a temporary tracheostomy.

Shiley cuffed fenestrated tube (Fig. 41.3d)

This is a plastic tube with an introducer and two inner tubes. One inner tube has an extension at its upper aspect to facilitate connection to other apparatus. The outer tube has a fenestration in the middle of the cannula, again to encourage a return to normal function. The outer tube also has an inflatable cuff to give an airtight seal. The cuff prevents secretions from reaching the lungs. This tube is useful for patients with swallowing problems but who are starting to return to normal function.

Jackson's silver tracheostomy tube

This is a silver tube with an introducer and inner tube (Fig. 41.4a). The inner tube is locked in position by a small catch on the outer tube and may be removed and cleaned as necessary without disturbing the outer tube.

Negus's silver tracheostomy tube

This is a silver tracheostomy tube with an introducer and a choice of inner tubes, with and without speaking valves (Fig. 41.4b). The outer tube does not have a safety catch, consequently the inner tube may be coughed out inadvertently.

Rusch speaking valve

This is a plastic device with a two-way valve which fits onto the extended aspects of the Shiley inner tube (Fig. 41.5a). When breathing, the valve stays open but when the patient attempts to speak the valve closes, thus redirecting air up through the normal air passages and allowing the production of voice.

Shiley decannulation plug

This is a plastic inner tube with a red blind and or a small red plastic plug (Fig. 41.5b) which fits in the tracheostomy tube. It should be used when encouraging patients to breath via normal air passages before removal of the tracheostomy tube.

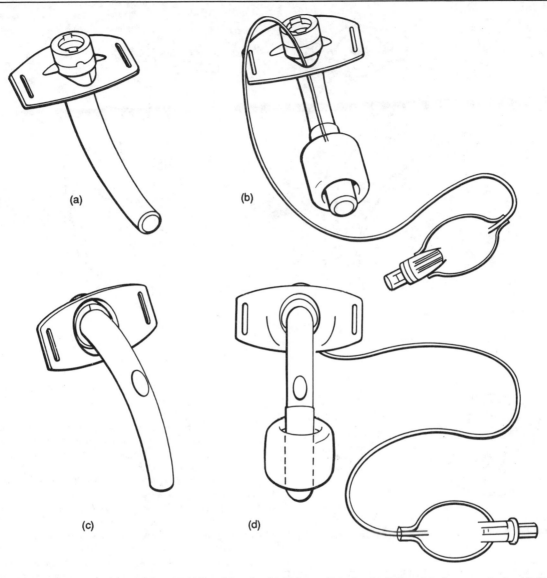

Figure 41.3 Shiley's tracheostomy tubes. (a) Shiley plain tube. (b) Shiley cuffed tube. (c) Shiley plain fenestrated tube. (d) Shiley cuffed fenestrated tube.

It is not advisable to leave the red decannulation plug in a fenestrated tube for periods longer than 2 or 3 hours at a time due to the risk of granulation tissue forming in the fenestration. For longer periods the red, blind-ended decannulation inner tube should be used.

Colledge silver laryngectomy tube
This is a silver laryngectomy tube with an introducer (Fig. 41.6a). It is an old-fashioned tube and clinical experience has shown it is often preferred by laryngectomy patients who dislike their stoma being exposed.

Shiley laryngectomy tube
This is a plastic tube with an introducer and inner tube (Fig. 41.6b). The inner tube may be removed and cleaned frequently without disturbing the outer tube. It is sometimes worn postoperatively while the stoma is healing to help facilitate a good shaped stoma.

Shaw's silver laryngectomy tube
This is a silver laryngectomy tube with an introducer and an inner tube beyond both lower and upper aspects of the outer tube (Fig. 41.6c). Thus pressure dressings

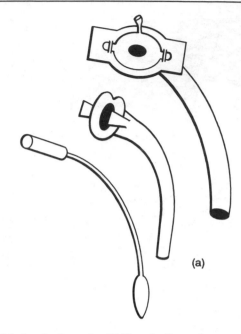
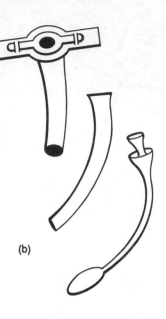

Figure 41.4 (a) Jackson's silver tube. (b) Negus's silver tube.

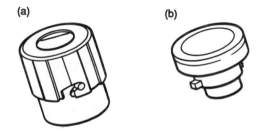

Figure 41.5 (a) Rusch speaking valve. (b) Shiley decannulation plug.

may be secured without occluding the stoma. The lower extension of the tube has demonstrated in clinical experience that crusting does not occur when the tube is changed regularly. The silver catch on the outer tube keeps the inner tube in position.

Stoma button

This is a soft Silastic 'button' (Fig. 41.6d). It may be used in place of a laryngectomy tube. It is very light and comfortable to wear and is the appliance of choice when the patient has a Blom–Singer speaking valve *in situ*.

References and further reading

Allan, D. (1987) Making sense of tracheostomy. *Nursing Times*, 83(45), 36–8.

Ballantyne, J. C. *et al.* (1987) *Otolaryngology*, 3rd edn. John Wright, Bristol.

Cox, S. & Jones, G. (1980) Head and neck nursing care. In: *Cancer Nursing: Surgical*, (ed. R. Tiffany). Faber & Faber, London.

Davis, J. (1980) Surgical treatment – preparation of the patient. I. By the nurse. In: *Laryngectomy Rehabilitation Seminars*, (eds Poole (1978) & Abindon (1980)), pp. 67–72. National Society for Cancer Relief.

Edels, Y. (1983) *Laryngectomy – Diagnosis to Rehabilitation*. Croom Helm, London.

Freud, R. H. (1979) *Principles of Head and Neck Surgery*. Appleton Century Crofts, New York.

Golding-Wood, D. (1989) Disorders of the nose, throat and larynx. *MIMS Magazine*, 1 November, 37–47.

Harris, R. B. & Hyman, R. B. (1983) Clean vs sterile tracheostomy care and level of pulmonary infection. *Nursing Research*, 33(2), 80–5.

Holmes, S. (1988) *Radiotherapy*, Chapter 6. Austin Cornish, London.

Iveson-Iveson, J. (1981) Students' forum. Tracheostomy. *Nursing Mirror*, 153(4), 30–1.

Jeter, K. F. & Tintle, T. (1988) Principles of wound cleaning and wound care. *Journal of Home Health Care Practice*, 1, 43–7.

Kuzenski, B. M. (1978) Effect of negative pressure on tracheobronchial trauma. *Nursing Reseach*, 27, 260–63.

Law, J. H. *et al.* (1993) Increased frequency of obstructive airway abnormalities with long-term tracheostomy. *Chest: The Cardiopulmonary Journal*, 104(1), 67–76.

McKelvie, P. L. (1980) Surgical aspects of laryngectomy. In: *Laryngectomy Rehabilitation Seminars*, (eds Poole (1978) & Abindon (1980)), pp. 80–1. National Society for Cancer Relief.

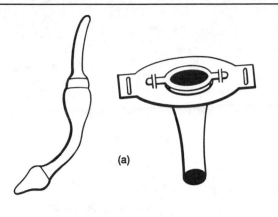

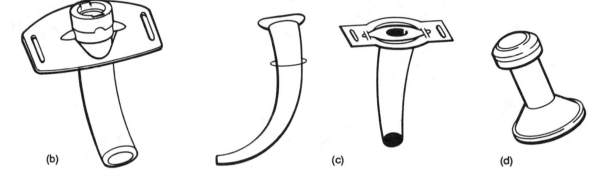

Figure 41.6 Tubes for permanent tracheostomics. (a) Colledge silver tube. (b) Shiley laryngectomy tube. (c) Shaw's laryngectomy tube. (d) Stoma button.

McMinn, R. M. H. *et al.* (1981) *A Colour Atlas of Head and Neck Anatomy*. Wolfe Medical, London.

Moore, G. V. & Stafford, N. (1987) *Aids to Ear, Nose and Throat*. Churchill Livingston, Edinburgh.

Nursing (US) (1976) Up to date survey of tracheal tubes. *Nursing* (US), 5(11), 66–72.

Schoeffel, R. B. *et al.* (1981) Bronchial hyperreactivity in response to inhalation of ultrasonically nebulised solutions of distilled water and saline. *British Medical Journal*, 283, 1285.

Serra, A. *et al.* (1986) *Ear, Nose and Throat Nursing*. Blackwell Scientific Publications, Oxford.

Stell, P. M. & Moran, A. G. D. (1978) *Head and Neck Surgery*. Heinemann Medical Books, London.

Thurston-Hookway, F. & Seddon, S. (1989) Care after laryngectomy. *Ear, Nose and Throat*, 3(35).

Tiffany, R. (1979) *Cancer Nursing: Surgical*. Faber & Faber, London.

Turner, A. L. (1988) *Nose, Throat and Ear*, (ed. A. G. D. Moran), 10th edn. J. Wright, Bristol.

Watson, J. E. (1979) *Medical–Surgical Nursing and Related Physiology*, pp. 381–472. W. B. Saunders, Philadelphia.

Young, C. (1984) Recommended guidelines for suction. *Physiotherapy*, 70(3), 106–8.

LARYNGECTOMY VOICE REHABILITATION

Definition

A voice prosthesis is a one-way silicone valve that slots into a surgically created fistula reconnecting the trachea to the pharynx following surgical removal of the larynx. The valve, once fitted, allows air to be directed from the lungs and trachea into the pharynx when the patient wishes to speak. This airflow causes the pharyngeal muscles to vibrate, producing the sound or voice for speech (Fig. 41.7). Since the valve is one-way it also prevents food and drink passing from the pharynx into the trachea and down the airway. A valve which begins to leak food and/or drink may be defective, worn-out, or ill-fitting.

The fistula for the voice valve may be created at the time of the total laryngectomy operation. Hence the terms *primary surgical voice restoration* (at the time of laryngectomy) and *secondary surgical voice restoration* (i.e. procedure carried out later) are used.

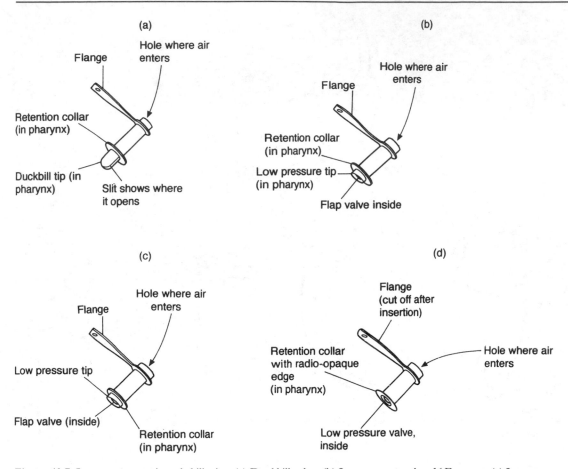

Figure 41.7 Laryngectomy voice rehabilitation. (a) Duckbill valve. (b) Low pressure valve, 16 Fr gauge. (c) Low pressure valve, 20 Fr gauge. (d) Indwelling valve, 20 Fr gauge.

REFERENCE MATERIAL

Voice prostheses for patients undergoing laryngectomy have been available in Britain since the early 1980s (Blom & Singer, 1980). There are a number of different types of prosthesis on the market, including Blom–Singer, Bivona, Provox and Gröningen. All work according to the same principle. The Blom–Singer prosthesis, developed in the USA by Eric Blom, a speech pathologist, and Mark Singer, an otolaryngologist, will be described in detail here.

Types of valves (Fig. 41.7)

Although there are many different makes of voice valve, most have a diameter of either 16 Fr or 20 Fr. All makes of valve are available in a series of different lengths (1.4–

3.6 cm) to fit the depth of the tracheo-pharyngeal wall, which varies from patient to patient. Initially, the patient should be measured and fitted with a prosthesis by an experienced and specialized practitioner who will select the most suitable type of valve, taking into account the patient's fitness and individual needs.

Duckbill valve/Blom–Singer type
voice prosthesis

This prosthesis is named after its design: the valved end of the prosthesis opens like a duck's bill to allow air to pass into the pharynx. Talking with the prosthesis requires a little more effort than talking prior to laryngectomy. The device has a rounded end making it easy to insert, and is less susceptible to infection by

Candida albicans than the low pressure model. The low pressure valve requires less effort to use than the duckbill type as it creates less resistance to the airflow.

Low pressure valve/Blom–Singer type voice prosthesis

The Blom–Singer low pressure device has a flatter posterior aspect than the duckbill with a small hinged flap acting as the one-way valve. It can sometimes be more difficult to insert though new insertion techniques help to minimise problems. Its design makes it more susceptible to infection with *Candida albicans*. Talking with the prosthesis requires approximately the same amount of effort as talking prior to laryngectomy.

Low pressure valve/Blom–Singer type voice prosthesis (20 Fr gauge)

This is a special wide diameter prosthesis recommended for patients with specialized needs. The decision to fit this lies with the specialist ENT doctor and/or specialist speech and language therapist.

Indwelling valve/Blom-Singer type voice prosthesis (20 Fr gauge)

This type of prosthesis has been available in Britain since late 1994. The main advantage is that it can last for about 6 months, providing the patient uses prophylactic antifungal treatment to counteract fungal infection of the valve. It has to be inserted and removed by a specialist speech and language therapist, ENT doctor experienced in fitting and managing voice prostheses or a nurse trained in the procedure.

Economy duckbill valve/Bivona type voice prosthesis (economy)

This is another duckbill valve, similar to the Blom–Singer device. It is made of flesh-tone silicone and is available in a full range of sizes, including the extra long 4 cm size.

Bivona type voice prosthesis (ultra-low resistance)

The Bivona ultra-low voice prosthesis functions with little resistance like the Blom–Singer type, low pressure model. The valved part of the prosthesis is a small, blue, hinged flap within the main body of the device. The posterior aspect is hooded to divert food and drink away. This device is susceptible to infection by *Candida albicans*.

Provox type in-dwelling voice prosthesis

This device is more difficult to insert as it has to be passed through the mouth and pharynx. This can be done under local anaesthetic, although for some patients a general anaesthetic is preferable. Once inserted it remains in place for an average of 4–6 months. This device is susceptible to infection by *Candida albicans*.

Gröningen type voice prosthesis

In most cases this prosthesis is inserted under general anaesthetic. It is currently used at only one centre in the UK. Once inserted it remains in place for approximately 6 months. This device is susceptible to infection by *Candida albicans*.

Stoma buttons and vents

To prevent stenosis of the stoma created for the voice prosthesis, patients may need to wear a stoma button, especially in the first few weeks after surgery. Although the stoma would not close completely, it may become so narrow that breathing is restricted and care of the voice prosthesis difficult.

Stoma buttons, made of soft Silastic, are available in a range of diameters: 10 mm, 12 mm and 14 mm. For patients with voice prostheses, 12 mm or 14 mm is most suitable, so that the stoma is wide enough for the patient to clean the prosthesis. If a voice prosthesis is used with a stoma button, a hole is cut in the button to allow air to pass through the valve during speech. An experienced, specialized practitioner is required to adapt the button in this way. (For further information see 'Stoma button' above.)

Bivona type vent and Forth Medical type laryngectomy tube for use with a voice prosthesis

These devices are made of a softer plastic than the traditional Shiley type laryngectomy tube, making them more comfortable and more appropriate for long-term use (beyond the post-operative period and on a continuing basis providing they are kept clean). Some patients find the stoma consistent enough in diameter to dispense completely with a vent or button some 6 months to 1 year after the laryngectomy. Other patients need to continue wearing either a vent or a button all the time. They are available in a range of three diameters, and two different lengths: 36 mm or 55 mm. If a voice prosthesis is used at the same time as either of these two devices, an aperture is made in the upper side to allow air to pass through the valve. The Forth tube is made with an indentation to mark the site of the aperture.

Indications for replacing a voice prosthesis

(1) *The voice prosthesis showing signs of wear and tear.* In most cases, experience indicates that a voice prosthe-

sis will last for 6–8 weeks. After that time patients may find it harder to use it to make voice, when previously they had no difficulty. This deterioration is gradual.

(2) *The voice prosthesis is leaking.* Valves are made of silicone and are therefore susceptible to fungal infection by *Candida albicans*. Micro–organisms burrow into the silicone and interfere with the functioning of the posterior (internal) end of the prosthesis. The effect of this is to cause saliva and drinks to leak in small drops through it, causing the patient to cough. Leakage such as this is a very common problem and can shorten the life of the prosthesis considerably.

(3) *Drink and/or food are leaking around the valve.* This problem is less common. It indicates that the diameter of the fistula has become greater than the diameter of the valve, probably as a result of infection. A specialist speech and language therapist or a nurse or doctor with the ENT training required to fit and manage voice prostheses should be contacted for advice.

(4) *The patient cannot make any sound with the voice prosthesis.* It is possible that patients may suddenly find that they can no longer make any sound with the prosthesis, or sound may be intermittent. The prosthesis must be removed and inspected, and almost certainly needs to be changed. A specialist speech and language therapist, or a nurse or doctor with the ENT training required to fit and manage voice prostheses should be contacted for advice.

Indications for replacing a 'lost' or dislodged voice prosthesis

The voice prosthesis is held in position by a silicone retention collar which is an integral part of the whole device. It is therefore possible for it to become accidentally dislodged. Patients are told that this might happen, and shown how to insert a Jacques 14 Fr red rubber catheter or a white Silastic 14 Fr Foley catheter through the fistula to keep it open. If patients are able to perform this procedure when a voice prosthesis is accidentally dislodged, the fistula remains open and a new prosthesis is inserted after removal of the catheter. If the voice prosthesis is ejected and the patient is unable to insert a catheter satisfactorily a speech and language therapist or doctor with experience in fitting and managing voice prostheses should be contacted for advice.

References and further reading

Blom, E. D. & Singer, M. (1980) An endoscopic technique for the restoration of voice after laryngectomy. *Annals of Otology, Rhinology and Laryngology*, 89(6), 529–33.

Blom, E. D. (1988) Tracheo-oesophageal valves: problems, solutions and directions for the future. *Head and Neck Surgery*, 10, 5142–5.

Edels, Y. (1983) *Laryngectomy: Diagnosis to Rehabilitation.* Croom Helm, London.

Evans, E. (1990) *Working with Laryngectomees.* Winslow, Oxford.

Garth, R. J. N. *et al.* (1991) Tracheo-oesophageal puncture: a review of problems and complications. *Journal of Laryngology and Otology*, 105, 750–4.

Lund, V. *et al.* (1987) Blom–Singer puncture: practicalities in everyday management. *Journal of Laryngology and Otology*, 101, 164–8.

GUIDELINES: CHANGING A TRACHEOSTOMY DRESSING

EQUIPMENT

1 Sterile dressing pack.
2 Tracheostomy dressing or a keyhole dressing.
3 Cleaning solution, such as 0.9% sodium chloride.
4 Tracheostomy tape.
5 Bactericidal alcohol hand rub.

PROCEDURE

Action	Rationale
1 Explain and discuss the procedure with the patient.	To ensure that the patient understands the procedure and gives his/her valid consent.
2 Screen the bed or cubicle.	To ensure the patient's privacy.

3	Wash hands using bactericidal soap and water or bactericidal alcohol hand rub, and prepare the dressing tray or trolley.	To reduce the risk of infection.
4	Perform the procedure using aseptic technique.	To prevent infection.
5	Remove the soiled dressing around the tube and clean around stoma with 0.9% sodium chloride.	To avoid discomfort to the patient. To remove secretion and crusts.
6	Replace with a tracheostomy dressing or a comfortable keyhole dressing.	To ensure the patient's comfort. To avoid pressure from the tube.
7	Renew tracheostomy tapes.	To secure the tube.

GUIDELINES: SUCTION AND TRACHEOSTOMY PATIENTS

The aim of suction is to maintain an airway and to prevent the formation of crusts. The frequency of suction varies with individual patients, according to their needs.

EQUIPMENT

1 Suction machine (wall source or portable).
2 Aero-flow sterile suction catheters (assorted sizes; see notes below).
3 Disposable gloves.
4 Jug of sodium bicarbonate solution (1 teaspoon in 500 ml water).
5 ENT spray containing sterile 0.9% sodium chloride.
6 Disposable plastic apron.
7 Bactericidal alcohol hand rub.

Note: it is advisable to use the right size of catheter for the lumen of the tracheostomy tube; a 10FG catheter is appropriate for a 27–30FG tube, a 12FG catheter for a 33–36FG tube, a 14FG catheter for a 39FG tube.

PROCEDURE

Action	Rationale
1 Instruct the patient to use the spray every 2 hours or more frequently if secretions are tenacious, i.e. two or three sprays directly into the tracheostomy.	Suction will not be achieved if the secretions become too tenacious or dry. Regular spraying minimizes this occurrence (Schoeffel *et al.*, 1981).
2 Suctioning should be taught if the patient is able to perform his/her own suction. Otherwise inform the patient what is to be done.	To obtain the patient's co-operation and to help them relax. The procedure is unpleasant and can be frightening for the patient. Reassurance is vital. Self-control of the patient's suction is preferable if the patient is able to manage it.
3 Wash hands with bactericidal soap and water or bactericidal alcohol hand rub, and put on a disposable plastic apron.	To reduce the risk of cross-infection. Some patients may accidently cough directly ahead at the nurse; standing to one side with tissues at the patient's tracheostomy minimizes this risk.

Guidelines: Suction and tracheostomy patients (cont'd)

Action	Rationale
4 Check that the suction machine is set to the appropriate level.	Sputum which is more tenacious requires more powerful suction. The maximum level being 200 mmHg. If pressures up to and above 200 mmHg are used, then vacuum-interrupted suctioning techniques are recommended to prevent pressure build-up should the catheter become occluded (Young, 1984). For thin or moderate secretions, a vacuum pressure of 70–100 mmHg is suggested (Kuzenski, 1978).
5 Open the end of the suction catheter pack and use the pack to attach the catheter to the suction tubing. Keep the rest of the catheter in the sterile packet.	To reduce the risk of transferring infection from hands to the catheter and to keep the catheter as clean as possible. The size of suction catheter is dependent on tenacity and volume of secretions, that is, the thicker the secretion and the larger the volume, the greater the bore of the tube.
6 Put on disposable gloves and withdraw the catheter from the sleeve.	Gloves minimize the risk of infection transfer to the catheter or from the sputum to the nurse's hands.
7 Introduce the catheter to about one-third of its length and apply suction by placing the thumb over the suction port control.	Gentleness is essential; damage to the tracheal mucosa can lead to trauma and respiratory infection. The catheter should go no further than the carina to prevent trauma. The catheter is inserted with the suction turned off so as not to irritate mucous membrane.
8 Withdraw the catheter gently with a rotating motion. Do not suction the patient for more than 15 seconds at a time.	To remove secretions from around the mucous membranes. Prolonged suction will result in infection if the mucous membranes are traumatized, and the patient may experience a choking sensation.
9 Wrap catheter around gloved hand then pull back glove over soiled catheter, thus containing catheter in glove, then discard.	Catheters are used only once to reduce the risk of introducing infection.
10 Rinse the connection by dipping its end in the jug of sodium bicarbonate solution with the suction turned on to clear secretions into the receptacle.	To loosen secretions which have adhered to the inside of the tube.
11 If the patient requires further suction, repeat the above actions using new gloves and a new catheter.	
12 Repeat the suction until the airway is clear.	

HUMIDIFICATION

Definition

Humidification may be defined as increasing the moisture content of air. In health, inspired air is filtered, warmed and moistened by the ciliated lining, and mucus is produced in the upper respiratory pathways. Because the upper respiratory pathways are bypassed in patients with a tracheostomy, they need artificial humidification to ensure that these pathways remain moist (Watson, 1979).

GUIDELINES: HUMIDIFICATION

PROCEDURE

Immediate post-operative care, i.e. the first 24–48 hours

Action

1 Fill a suitable nebulizer with sterile water and attach it to the air or oxygen supply. Set the air or oxygen rate as recommended by manufacturer. Give a constant supply of humidified air or oxygen for 24–48 hours.

2 Spray 0.9% sodium chloride into the trachea as necessary, using a spray or a syringe.

3 For patients in cubicles, a room humidifier may be placed at the bedside.

Rationale

Constant humidification is required while new stoma adapts to the outside environment (especially for laryngectomy patients).
Humidification also prevents the formation of crusts which are liable to obstruct the airway. The use of sterile water reduces the risk of infection.

To loosen secretions prior to suction and to stimulate the cough reflex. To keep secretions moist.

Subsequent care

Action

1 Give humidified oxygen as required. Usually, patients need about 10–15 minutes of humidification every four hours. This may be adapted according to the patient's needs, e.g. throughout the night, according to time.

2 If the patient does not require oxygen, blow humidifiers may be used.

3 Teach the patient to keep the tracheostomy moist by using a spray containing 0.9% sodium chloride, before suctioning.

4 Provide laryngeal stoma protectors, e.g. Lyofoam, Buchanan bib or Romet covers.

Rationale

Patients begin to adapt to breathing through their tracheostomy after the first 24–48 hours. Some humidification is required according to individual needs and to prevent crust formation in the airway.

These provide humidified air without the need for an oxygen supply.

To loosen secretions and to prevent crust formation. To prevent contamination. 0.9% sodium chloride is supplied in small bottles which, if not used within 24 hours, should be changed to prevent infection. If a spray is used, this should be washed and dried each day and resterilized once the patient is discharged.

To protect the airway.

GUIDELINES: CHANGING A TRACHEOSTOMY TUBE

EQUIPMENT

1 Sterile dressing pack.
2 Tracheostomy dressing or a keyhole dressing.
3 Tracheostomy tape.
4 Cleaning solution, such as 0.9% sodium chloride.
5 Barrier cream.

Guidelines: Changing a tracheostomy tube (cont'd)

6 Lubricating jelly.
7 Disposable plastic apron.
8 Bactericidal alcohol hand rub.

PROCEDURE

Action	Rationale
1 Explain and discuss the procedure with the patient.	To ensure that the patient understands the procedure and gives his/her valid consent.
2 Wash hands using bactericidal soap and water or bactericidal alcohol hand rub, and prepare a dressing trolley.	To prevent cantamination.
3 Screen the patient's bed.	To ensure the patient's privacy.
4 Perform the procedure using clean technique.	To prevent contamination.
5 Assist the patient to sit in an upright position, supported by pillows with the neck extended.	To ensure the patient's comfort and to maintain a patent airway. If the neck is not extended, skin folds may occlude the tracheostomy when the tube is removed.
6 Remove the dressing pack from its outer wrappings and open the tracheostomy dressing.	Technique should be clean to reduce the risk of cross-infection.
7 Put on a disposable plastic apron.	
8 Clean hands with bactericidial alcohol hand rub.	
9 Put on clean disposable plastic gloves.	To prevent infection.
10 Prepare the tracheostomy tube as outlined in steps 11–14.	So that the tube is ready for immediate insertion when required.
11 Thread on piece of tape through the slits in the flanges so that the tape passes behind the flange next to the stoma.	The tape is kept behind the flange to prevent it occluding the passage of air into the tracheostomy tube.
12 Put the tracheostomy dressing around the tube.	To prevent abrasion of the patient's skin by the tube.
13 Lubricate the tube sparingly with a lubricating jelly.	To facilitate insertion.
14 Remove the soiled tube from the patient's neck while asking the patient to breathe out.	Conscious expiration relaxes the patient and reduces the risk of coughing. Coughing can result in unwanted closure of the tracheostomy.
15 Clean around the stoma with 0.9% sodium chloride and dry gently. Apply barrier cream with topical swabs. (An aqueous cream may be used if the patient is having the site irradiated.)	To remove superficial organisms and crusts. Skin should not be left moist as this provides an ideal medium for the growth of micro-organisms (Watson, 1979).

16	Insert a clean tube with introducer in place, using an 'up and over' action.	Introduction of the tube is less traumatic if directed along the contour of the trachea.
17	Remove the introducer immediately.	The patient cannot breathe while the introducer is in place.
18	Place the inner tube in position.	The inner tube may be changed several times when the outer tube is in position, thus minimizing the risk of trauma to trachea and stoma. The quantity of secretions present will determine the frequency with which the inner tube is changed.
19	Tie the tape securely at the side of the neck.	To secure the tube. Place the tie in an accessible place, at the same time ensuring that it will not cause discomfort to the patient.
20	Remove gloves and ask the patient to breathe out onto the palm of your hand.	Flow of air will be felt if the tube is in the correct position.
21	Ensure that the patient is comfortable.	
22	Clear away the trolley and equipment.	
23	Scrub the soiled tube with a brush under cold running water. If the tube is very soiled then use sodium bicarbonate to remove debris. The tube must be rinsed thoroughly and stored dry at the patient's bedside.	To remove debris that may occlude the tube and/ or become a source of infection.

Note: plastic tubes should not be soaked in solutions as there is a danger that the material may absorb the solution which could then cause irritation of the trachea.

NURSING CARE PLAN

Problem	Cause	Suggested action
Profuse tracheal secretions.	Local reaction to tracheostomy tube.	Suction frequently, e.g. every 1–2 hours.
Lumen of tracheostomy tube occluded	Tenacious mucus in tube.	Spray frequently with normal saline e.g. every 1–3 hours, and suction. Change the inner tube regularly, e.g. 1- to 3-hourly.
	Dried blood and mucus in the tube, especially in the postoperative period.	Provide humidified air. (For further information, see 'Guidelines: Humidification', above.)
Tracheostomy tube dislodged accidentally.	Tapes not secured adequately.	Put in spare tube. This should be clean and ready at the bedside. *Note*: tracheal dilators must be kept at the bedside of patients with tracheostomies.

Nursing care plan (cont'd)

Problem	Cause	Suggested action
Unable to insert clean tracheostomy tube.	Unpredicted shape or angle of stoma.	Remain calm since an outward appearance of distress may cause the patient to panic and lose confidence. Lubricate the tube well and attempt to reinsert at various angles.
	Tracheal stenosis due to patient coughing, very anxious or because the tube has been left out too long.	Insert a smaller-size tracheostomy tube. If insertion still proves difficult, do not leave the patient but ask for a tube to be brought to the bed. Keep the tracheostomy patent with tracheal dilators if stenosis is pronounced until the tube is reinserted.
Tracheal bleeding following or during change of the tube.	Trauma due to suction or to the tube being changed. Presence of tumour. Granulation tissue forming in fenestration of tube.	Change the tube as planned if bleeding is minimal. For profuse bleeding, insert a cuffed tube and inflate. Inform the doctor. Suction the patient to remove the blood from the trachea.
Infected sputum.	Nature of surgery and condition of patient often predispose to infection.	Encourage the patient to cough up secretions and/or suction regularly. Change the tube and clean the stoma area frequently, e.g. 4-hourly. Protect permanent stomas with a bib or gauze.
		Following result of sputum specimen, commence appropriate antibiotics as needed.

GUIDELINES: CHANGING A BLOM–SINGER TYPE NON-INDWELLING VOICE PROSTHESIS

Nurses must wear gloves and eye protection (to prevent phlegm/blood entering the eyes) when carrying out this procedure. The area must be well lit to illuminate the stoma.

EQUIPMENT

1 Clinically clean tray or receiver.
2 Correct replacement voice prosthesis and introducer.
3 Red rubber Foley catheter (16 Fr gauge).
4 White plastic stent or dilator with correct diameter.
5 KY jelly or similar.

6 Tissues.
7 Blenderm transparent hypoallergenic tape or Micropore tape.

PROCEDURE

Action	Rationale
1 Explain and discuss the procedure with the patient.	To ensure that the patient understands the procedure and gives his/her valid consent.
2 Settle the patient in a chair and arrange lighting to illuminate stoma.	To ensure the patient is comfortable and well supported.
3 Place a little KY jelly on the tip of the red rubber catheter and/or stent, and on the voice valve and introducer.	To ease insertion.
4 Ask the patient to keep his/her lips apart as the old valve is removed; hold flange where it joins the body of the valve.	To minimize amount of saliva entering fistula and reduce the risk of coughing.
5 Swiftly insert red rubber catheter (or dilator) 20 cm into the fistula.	To keep fistula open. To ascertain the shape and direction of the fistula.
6 Place valve on introducer, securing with flange.	To prevent valve dislodging from introducer during insertion.
7 Remove catheter or stent and replace with valve. A slight click will be felt as the retention collar on the valve passes into the pharynx.	To insert valve.
8 Check valve is correctly inserted by pulling it gently: it will move slightly, then resist.	To ensure valve is correctly positioned.
9 Place 5 cm length of Blenderm tape over flange to secure it to the patient's neck.	To keep flange neatly out of way.

CHAPTER 42

Traction

Definition

Traction may be defined as a treatment modality in which a pulling force is applied to separate parts of an injured or diseased portion of the body or extremity (Davis, 1994). The opposite pulling force is counter-traction, the resistance to the traction pull. Most often it is the patient's own body weight that provides this countertraction. In other cases it can be achieved or increased by adjusting the angle of the patient's bed (Styrcula, 1994a). Traction and countertraction work together to achieve a type of balance. This is essential to overcome muscle spasm and to prevent the patient being pulled in the direction of the traction force (Fig. 42.1) (Heywood-Jones, 1990).

Indications

Traction will control the movement of the injured part, thereby enabling bone and soft tissue to heal. It can be used in a variety of conditions to achieve one or more of the following:

(1) Restore and maintain alignment of bone ends following fracture.
(2) Relieve pain and/or muscle spasm.
(3) Provide immobilisation to prevent soft tissue damage.
(4) Correct, lessen, or prevent deformities.
(5) Reduce and treat subluxations.
(6) Rest an inflamed, diseased, or injured body part.
(7) Prevent or correct the development of soft tissue contracture.
(8) Expand joint spaces prior to surgery.
(9) Maintain the desired position post-operatively.

(From Ceccio, 1991; Davis, 1994.)

REFERENCE MATERIAL

Types of traction

Traction is divided into two main categories:

(1) Manual.
(2) Mechanical.

Manual traction

Manual traction is accomplished by an individual exerting a temporary, steady pull on another's extremity or joint, using the former's hands. This type of traction may be used to reduce stable fractures or dislocations prior to casting, splinting, or application of skin and skeletal traction, as well as before surgical reductions and arthroscopies (Styrcula, 1994a). In manual traction a smooth, steady pull is preferred to a quick jerking motion, and therefore should not be attempted by a novice. Its main use is as a primary form of traction within an accident and emergency department.

Mechanical traction

Mechanical traction uses mechanical devices and is further classified depending on the nature of attachment and the nature of the pulling force. Attachment may be to either:

(1) skin, or
(2) skeleton.

The pulling force may be exerted by a variety of systems of weights and pulleys, examples of which are given here.

(1) *Sliding or balanced traction*. Weights and pulleys are used to apply and direct the pull of the traction. The counter traction is exerted by the weight of the patient's body, aided by gravity when the bed is tilted away from the pull of the traction (Fig. 42.2).
(2) *Fixed traction*. This is traction between two fixed points. If used, weights and pulleys elevate the limb, rather than create the pull. The patient is attached to traction apparatus at one point and the affected part is pulled away from the point of fixation by extensions and cords which are tied to the traction apparatus. The fixation point is the counter traction and the pulling extensions are the traction. This type of

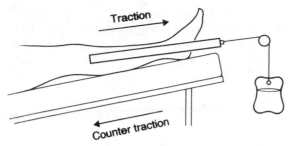

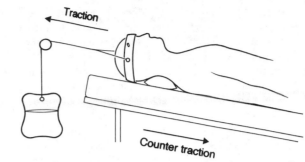

Figure 42.1   Traction and counter traction forces.

Figure 42.2   Balanced skeletal traction.

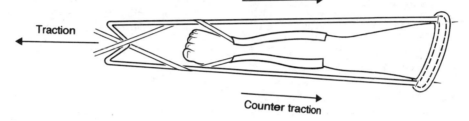

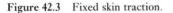

Figure 42.3   Fixed skin traction.

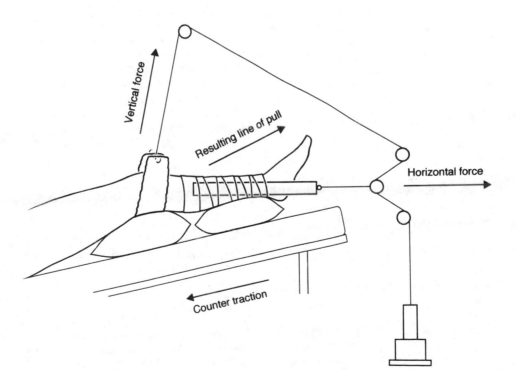

Figure 42.4   Hamilton–Russell traction.

traction has the advantage of requiring a small degree of force. It is frequently used to reduce or eliminate muscle spasm or as a temporary measure when transporting an individual on sliding traction. An example of this type of traction would be the application of a Thomas' splint to a leg using skin extensions tied to the end of the splint (Taylor, 1987) (Fig. 42.3).

(3) *Weight and pulley systems.* A pulley is a wheel with a grooved edge suspended on an axle around which it rotates in a framework or block. It is used to support traction rope and direct the line of pull of the weight that it suspends. A pulley block is a grouping of two or three pulleys on a single common axle in a frame. This type of traction may be a simple system using a single pulley to alter the direction of the force so that weights can be suspended conveniently, or a compound system using a number of pulleys in combination to increase the efficiency of the force applied as well as altering the direction (Fig. 42.4). Pulleys need regular maintenance to ensure optimal function. They need to be clean and receive regular lubrication to allow the pulley to spin easily. Always check this before use. Never lubricate a pulley after setting up traction. This could affect the force of the pull (Styrcula, 1994b).

SKIN TRACTION

In skin traction, the traction force is applied over a large area of skin from where it is transmitted to the musculoskeletal structures. This pull can be achieved through the use of various materials. Extensions, slings or splints can be applied to the limbs; belts, halters and slings can be used for the spine or pelvis. A light constant pull is achieved by weights that can be removed and reapplied.

Because the skin is susceptible to damage from large traction forces, skin traction is limited to conditions where a relatively light or intermittent pull is required. It is not suitable for long-term use when a strong pull must be exerted, for example in the case of an unstable fracture or when control of limb rotation is necessary. The maximum pull should not exceed that recommended by the manufacturers of the traction appliance: usually 4.5–6.7 kg (10–15 lb) depending on the area of the body involved (Davis, 1994).

Application of skin traction
The application of skin traction is generally contraindicated in the presence of an existing skin condition, e.g. wounds, sores, abrasions, where the skin is thin and friable, where there is circulatory impairment or loss of normal skin sensation (Morris *et al.*, 1988a).

The application of skin traction may be painful. To minimize the patient's pain, the following principles should be adhered to:

(1) Skill and gentleness are required when handling the affected part.
(2) Manual traction must be maintained.
(3) The traction should be applied with speed and dexterity.
(4) The skin extension to which the traction will be attached should be applied on both sides of the limb, leaving a strip of skin free in order to prevent a constrictive tourniquet effect; when applied to a fractured limb the extension should not extend above the fracture or traction will be exerted at the wrong site (Taylor, 1987).

There are two different types of skin extension:

(1) Adhesive.
(2) Non-adhesive.

Non-adhesive extensions are used on fragile skin. They are preferred if the traction is in place only for a short period of time, for example to reduce muscle spasm due to a fracture of the neck of femur in the few hours prior to surgery. They consist of soft-vented foam rubber attached to a traction cord and weight, held in place by bandages. The weight applied is usually limited to 3.2 kg because the grip is less secure than that obtained by adhesive skin extensions (Taylor, 1987).

Adhesive skin extensions are used on intact skin in good condition. They consist of 'non-stretch' Elastoplast with padding to protect bony prominences. They are attached in a similar way but are more secure.

Most self-adhesive skin traction kits contain zinc oxide. A disadvantage of these is that some patients develop a reaction in the form of contact dermatitis. Hypo-allergenic kits are available and it is worth checking with the patient for previous allergies before application (Taylor, 1987).

References and further reading
Apley, G. (1993) *Apley's System of Orthopaedics and Fractures*, 7th edn. Butterworth-Heinemann, Oxford.
Brunner, L. & Suddarth, D. (1989) *The Lippincott Manual of Medical–Surgical Nursing*, 2nd edn. Harper & Row, London.
Cameron, S. & Leaper, D. (1988) Antiseptic toxicity in open wounds. *Nursing Times*, 84(25), 77–9.
Cassels, C. J. (1983) Fundamentals of long bone traction. *Critical Care Update*, 10(5), 38–9.
Ceccio, M. (1991) Key concepts in the care of patients in traction. In: *An Introduction to Orthopaedic Nursing*, (eds D.

Syle & L. Theis). National Associaion of Orthopaedic Nurses, Pitman, New Jersey.

Davis, P. (1989) The principles of traction. *Nursing*, 3(34), 5–8.

Davis, P. (1994) *Nursing the Orthopaedic Patient*. Churchill Livingstone, Edinburgh.

Heywood Jones, I. (1990) Making sense of traction. *Nursing Times*, 86(23), 40–1.

Hines, N. & Bates, M. (1987) Discharging the patient in skeletal traction. *Orthopaedic Nursing*, 6(4), 21–4.

Jones-Walton, P. (1988) Effects of pin care on pin reactions in adults with extremity fracture treated with skeletal traction and external fixation. *Orthopaedic Nursing*, 7(4), 28–9.

Jones-Walton, P. (1991) Clinical standards in skeletal traction pin site care. *Orthopaedic Nursing*, 10(2), 12–16.

Magnum, S. & Sutherland, P. (1993) A comprehensive guide to the halo brace. *AORN Journal*, 58(3), 534–46.

Mooney, N. (1991) Orthopaedic complications. *Nursing Clinics of North America*, 26(1), 113–32.

Morris, L. *et al.* (1988a) Special care for skeletal traction. *Registered Nurse*, February, 24–9.

Morris, L. *et al.* (1988b) Nursing the patient in traction. *Registered Nurse*, January, 26–31.

Nance, D. & Mardjetko, S. (1994) Technical aspects and nursing considerations on limb lengthening. *Orthopaedic Nursing*, 13(1), 21–33.

Nichol, D. (1993) Preventing infection. *Nursing Times*, 89(13), 78–80.

Osborne, L. & Digiacomo, I. (1987) Traction: a review with nursing diagnoses and interventions. *Orthopaedic Nursing*, 6(4), 13–19.

Powell, M. (1986) *Orthopaedic Nursing and Rehabilitation*, 9th edn. Churchill Livingstone, Edinburgh.

Quain, M. & Tecklin, S. (1985) Lumbar traction: its effect on respiration. *Physical Therapy*, 65(9), 1342–3.

Resnick, B. (1994) Die from a broken hip? *Registered Nurse*, July, 22–6.

Sproles, K. (1985) Nursing care of skeletal pins: a closer look. *Orthopaedic Nursing*, 4(1), 11–19.

Styrcula, L. (1994a) Traction basics: part I. *Orthopaedic Nursing*, 13(2), 17–74.

Styrcula, L. (1994b) Traction basics: part II. Traction equipment. *Orthopaedic Nursing*, 13(3), 55–9.

Styrcula, L. (1994c) Traction basics: part III. Types of traction. *Orthopaedic Nursing*, 13(4), 34–44.

Taylor, I. (1987) *Ward Manual of Orthopaedic Traction*. Churchill Livingstone, Edinburgh.

Wallis, S. (1991) An agenda to promote self-care: nursing care of skeletal pin sites. *Professional Nurse*, September, 715–20.

GUIDELINES: SKIN TRACTION

There are different types of skin traction, and different mechanical devices may be used to apply traction. This section is intended to give an overview. If in doubt about any procedure, a more exhaustive orthopaedic text should be consulted (Powell, 1986; Taylor, 1987; Davis, 1994).

PROCEDURE

Adhesive

Action	Rationale
1 Explain and discuss the procedure with the patient.	To ensure that the patient understands the procedure and gives his/her valid consent.
2 Ensure privacy for the patient while carrying out the procedure.	To maintain patient's dignity.
3 Ensure that the affected part is clean and the skin intact.	To reduce risk of infection developing. Adhesive strips may cause further damage to friable or damaged skin.
4 Shave any limb covered by thick, tough hairs.	To ensure that adhesive sticks to the skin and not to the hairs. The part affected will be sore if the traction is applied to the hair follicles only.
5 If possible, leave the ankle joint free.	To allow full plantar flexion and dorsiflexion in the foot in order to prevent stiffness and deformity.
6 If the lower limb is for traction, apply pieces of felt or latex foam to the malleoli and other bony prominences.	To protect them from friction. To prevent the development of pressure ulcers.

Guidelines: Skin traction (cont'd)

Action	Rationale
7 Leave the patellae and the knee 10–15° off full flexion.	To prevent limb deformity and joint stiffness.
8 The limb may be painted or sprayed with tincture of benzoin compound (Taylor, 1987).	To reduce moisture through perspiration. To increase the adhesive quality of the material used. To act as a barrier to the adhesive in the event of the patient developing contact dermatitis.
9 Apply the extension strapping and bandage without folds or creases.	To prevent discomfort. To prevent skin deterioration under the strapping.
10 Ensure that the part affected is in the correct anatomical position, e.g. feet and patellae pointing upwards when patient is in the supine position.	To prevent limb deformity.
11 Check the temperature and colour of the extremity affected as required, together with the degree of sensation and movement.	To ensure that the tension of strapping is correct, and that circulation and nerve pathways to the extremity are not being compromised. To ensure early detection of allergic reactions to the adhesives.

Non-adhesive

As above, but omit steps 4 and 8.

Removing skin traction

Care must be taken to avoid skin damage during removal of adhesive extensions. Peeling the edges back slowly while pulling the skin taut is less damaging than trying to remove the adhesive quickly. Analgesia may be required. Adhesive solvents should be used where necessary. Manual traction should be maintained unless treatment is to be discontinued.

SKELETAL TRACTION

Skeletal traction applies force directly to bone using aseptically inserted pins, wires or traction screws. It affords a greater degree of comfort than skin traction and is the preferred method when traction is required over long periods. More weight can be applied as this is a direct pull on bone (Taylor, 1987). It is important to note that skeletal traction is not applied directly to broken bone but to a bone on the other side of the joint, e.g. with a fractured femur the pin is applied through the tibia, not the femur. This allows a continuous pull to be exerted along the long axis of the bone (Apley, 1993).

Some of the most common uses of skeletal traction include management of fractures of the lower limbs, pelvis and cervical spine. It is used for:

- Unstable and fragmented fractures.
- Fractures which can only be reduced with weights of 4.5 kg (10 lb) and over.
- Muscle spasms.
- Control of rotation.
- Fractures that require long-term traction.

More recently skeletal traction has been used during ankle arthroscopies (Styrcula, 1994a). Weights of up to 18 kg can be used, depending on the fracture and the density of the bone at the site of insertion (Taylor, 1987). Skeletal traction can be applied to the skull, the proximal end of the ulna, the distal end of the femur, the proximal and distal ends of the tibia and the calcaneus (Morris *et al.*, 1988b). Lighter weights can be used instead of skin traction when the latter is contraindicated.

The insertion of skeletal traction is a surgical procedure performed under strict aseptic conditions. It is important that subsequent dealings with entry sites are also performed using aseptic techniques.

Complications

The prevention of pin tract infections is of paramount importance. Infection at the insertion site can easily spread to bone and lead to osteomyelitis (Morris *et al.*, 1988a). This can be debilitating and difficult to eradicate. A predisposing factor to pin site infection, in addition to poor insertion technique, is the loosening of the pin or wire causing movement between the pin and surrounding tissues. Use of partially threaded pins, for example the Denham pin, may prevent this (Nichol, 1993).

It is difficult to state conclusively which way of preventing infection is the most effective: nursing and medical staff within a unit should identify an appropriate strategy consensually (Wallis, 1991; Nichol, 1993). Some antiseptics, however, may delay healing (Cameron & Leaper, 1988).

Following insertion a sterile keyhole dressing may be applied to absorb any leakage. This can be taped in place, but contact with the pin and the wound must be avoided (Nichol, 1993). After initial oozing from the site has ceased, the site may either be covered or left exposed (Davis, 1994). Cleaning the site to remove crusts and clots is not recommended for single skeletal pins as the crust provides a barrier to the external environment (Wallis, 1991; Davis, 1994). If serous discharge persists, or if pus is present, a swab should be taken for culture and sensitivity and the appropriate antibiotic prescribed.

Research to date has not conclusively established what is the most effective cleaning solution for pin sites. The three most commonly used products, hydrogen peroxide, chlorhexidine in spirit and povidone-iodine, are not necessarily the most appropriate (Jones-Walton, 1988; Wallis, 1991; Davis, 1994). Variables such as fracture and traction type, underlying illness, amount of surrounding muscle tissue and duration of pin insertion may have an impact on pin reaction development (Sproles, 1985; Jones-Walton, 1988; Wallis, 1991).

Irrespective of the regime adopted, technique should be aseptic and the incidence of pin tract infection closely monitored. Signs of pin infection include redness, swelling, local warmth and purulent exudate. Gentle percussion of the bone over the pin may be painful in cases of infection. (See also Chapter 48, Wound Management.)

Other complications which can occur with skeletal traction include:

(1) *Movement of pins.* Traction on a pin may be sufficient to bend it. This in itself is not important, but makes the removal of pins more difficult (Nichol, 1993).

Bending of pins can, however, result in local tissue damage such as necrosis or tearing. It may be possible for a surgeon to make an incision in the skin to allow for a small amount of pin migration. The skin will then usually heal behind the pin (Cassels, 1983).

Although it is unusual, pins or wires can break, particularly if the patient is very restless or if heavy weights are used (Taylor, 1987). Pins can be protected by incorporating them into a cast (Davis, 1989). Pins improperly placed, or placed in osteoporotic bone, can actually pull out of the bone and create a new small fracture (Cassels, 1983). Pin attachments must be checked daily for signs of skin pressure and to ensure that they are firmly secured. Observations must include a check on the pin guards which are attached to either side of the pin, protecting the patient and the nurse from accidental injury (Davis, 1989).

(2) *Overpull and distraction.* Excess traction force can lead to over-distraction of bone fragments. This is more likely to occur with skeletal traction than with skin traction because skeletal traction involves heavier weights. Over-distraction can lead to delayed healing or non-union (Heywood Jones, 1990).

(3) *Neurovascular damage.* The original injury, traction equipment and surgery can cause temporary or permanent neurovascular damage as a result of increased pressure on nerves and blood vessels (Davis, 1994). External rotation of a leg in traction can put pressure on the head of the fibula, with the risk of peroneal nerve injury and subsequent foot drop (Apley, 1993). Increasing pain, numbness, tingling or the inability to flex and extend the toes could indicate nerve compression (Morris *et al.*, 1988a). The limb should be checked regularly to see that it does not roll into external rotation during traction.

The same symptoms can also herald the onset of compartment syndrome. This is a serious neurovascular complication that can occur after trauma or following excessive traction through a calcaneal pin (Apley, 1993). Oedema in the affected limb increases the pressure in tissue compartments, muscle groups that are surrounded by inelastic connective tissue or fascia. Since the compartments cannot expand to accommodate the swollen tissues, nerves and blood vessels are compressed and muscle cells die. The end result is a binding down of tendons and nerve tissues with permanent paralysis and loss of sensation (Mooney, 1991).

Early detection of compartment syndrome is the key to preventing permanent disability. It is essential that the neurovascular status of the injured and treated limb is evaluated at regular intervals so that later observations can highlight any progressive dysfunction. Taylor (1987) suggests that, as a general guideline, checks should be carried out hourly for 24 hours after: initial injury, surgery, application of cast, splinting or traction. If there is no evidence of neurovascular compromise after 24 hours, checks should be carried out at least 2–4-hourly, and more frequently if required, and should include evaluation of:

(a) *Circulation.* Assessment of circulatory status involves monitoring colour, temperature, capillary refill in nail beds, and pulses. This should be compared with the unaffected limb.

(b) *Movement.* This assessment involves the ability to contract muscle groups below the level of injury. Inability to do so may indicate compromised nerve function.

(c) *Sensation.* Changes in sensation can also indicate compromised nerve function or compromised circulation (Brunner & Suddarth, 1989).

Most important, never ignore a patient who complains of pain.

Removing skeletal traction
Skeletal traction should not be discontinued except under medical orders or in an emergency situation (e.g. cardiac arrest). Premature discontinuation can lead to muscle spasm and displacement of bone at fracture site causing delayed healing (Morris *et al.*, 1988a).

Removing skeletal traction pins
Removal technique will depend on the type of pin used, for example, a Denham pin will need to be unscrewed until the threaded section is free of the bone, whereas a Steinmann's pin is simply pulled out. Analgesia will be necessary. Skeletal traction is generally removed on the ward, using aseptic technique.

Taylor (1987) suggests that scarring at pin removal sites can be minimized by firmly pinching the pin tract at time of removal so that the adhesion of skin to deeper tissue is broken, giving a better cosmetic result.

GENERAL PRINCIPLES FOR THE CARE OF PATIENTS ON TRACTION

All traction systems should be regularly checked, particularly after interventions, when the system may be inadvertently altered. To maintain the therapeutic effects of traction, the principles set out below should be considered.

(1) *Provide traction and countertraction.* Countertraction must be present for any type of traction to be effective. This can be maintained by using the patient's body, the position of the bed, or the pull of weights, as dictated by the specific type of traction (Osborne & Digiacomo, 1987).

(2) *Maintain the prescribed direction of pull.* The part of the patient's body which is in the traction system must be correctly aligned and the patient's body correctly positioned. Interrupting or altering the line of pull, especially in fractures, can change the bone alignment resulting in muscle spasm, pain and disrupted or delayed healing (Ceccio, 1991). The patient with balanced traction may be elevated, turned slightly and moved as desired, whereas the patient with fixed traction must not be turned without disrupting the line of pull.

(3) *Maintain traction continuously.* Traction must be continuous to be effective. The only exception is intermittent traction which may be used for the

pelvis. Both continuous and intermittent traction is maintained by applying the prescribed weights.

(4) *Prevent or reduce friction.* Friction interferes with the pull of the traction and reduces its therapeutic effect. Friction can be avoided by ensuring that:

(a) Weights are hanging freely and not resting on the floor, bed, or chair.

(b) Traction ropes are unobstructed and move freely through pulleys. Cords should not be frayed.

(c) Bedclothes or other materials do not interfere with traction pull (bed cradles should be used).

(d) Both weights and traction knots are hanging free of the pulleys.

(e) The extremity and/or the soft goods in traction are not resting on the head or foot board.

(f) Countertraction is sufficient to prevent shearing forces from damaging the patient's skin.

(From Davis, 1994; Styrcula, 1994b).

Care of the patient
As well as traction-related needs, patients in traction have needs associated with long- or short-term immobility and bed rest. Elderly and/or frail patients are particularly at risk of deep vein thrombosis with or without pulmonary embolus, chest infection, pressure ulcers, urinary stasis and constipation, joint stiffness, muscle wasting and deformity. Nursing care should include actions aimed at preventing these complications (Styrcula, 1994b).

A routine exercise programme should be devised by the nurse in conjunction with the physiotherapy department. This should include active and passive exercises of all extremities, including isometric exercise for the involved extremity, if permitted (Osborne & Digiacomo, 1987). Special attention should be given to the arms, thighs and feet.

As well as physical needs, patients in traction have social and psychological needs. Equipment can seem both confining and threatening. Patients may experience loss of independence, feelings of frustration, boredom and depression, and social, family and occupational disruption. Magnum & Sutherland (1993) offer an overview of some of the psychological needs associated with wearing a halo brace.

NURSING CARE PLAN

Problem	Cause	Suggested action
Irritation or burning of skin under skin extensions.	Allergic reaction to skin extensions.	Inform appropriate personnel. Remove supporting material if appropriate. Use non-adhesive skin extensions.
Inadequate traction and potential skin excoriation.	Slipping skin extensions.	Reapply.
Pressure ulcers over bony prominences.	Inadequate padding of vulnerable areas.	Provide adequate padding; ensure bandages are not too tight.
Nerve palsy.	Leg rolled into lateral rotation compressing common peroneal nerve against supporting slings.	Check alignment of leg regularly. Assess patient's ability to dorsiflex the ankle. Check sensation.
Paraesthesia or coldness of affected part.	Supporting material bound too tightly.	Re-bandage.
Joint irritation or displacement of bone at fracture site.	Insufficient traction.	Ensure sufficient traction.
Delayed union or non-union of fracture.	Over-distraction at fracture site.	Inform appropriate personnel. Realign.
Pin slipping from side to side, carrying an area of non-sterile pin into the bone or tissue.	Pin is loose. Perhaps an area of necrotic or osteoporotic bone around the pin.	Report to medical staff.
Joint stiffness or muscle wasting.	Poor positioning and prolonged inactivity.	Report to medical staff and physiotherapist. Liaise about exercises.
Low-grade osteomyelitis.	Infection at site of entry.	Inform appropriate personnel. Ensure strict aseptic technique when attending to lesion.

(From Osborne & Digiacomo, 1987; Taylor, 1987; Mooney, 1991; Davis, 1994.)

CHAPTER 43

Transfusion of Blood and Blood Products

Definition

A transfusion consists of the administration of whole blood or any of its components to correct or treat a clinical abnormality.

REFERENCE MATERIAL

Blood donation and testing

Safety of both the donor and the potential recipient are important criteria in the selection of blood donors. As well as microbiological testing of the donated blood, reliance is placed on the donor to answer questions on his or her general health, medical history and any drugs taken (Hewitt *et al.*, 1990). Prevention of transmission of infection is determined by donor selection criteria and laboratory testing. In the UK mandatory screening is done for antibodies to HIV 1 and 2, *Treponema pallidum* (syphilis) and hepatitis C and hepatitis B surface antigen (Mims, 1994).

Following donation blood products have varying shelf lives. Red blood cell products have a shelf life of 35 days if kept at 4°C (Mims, 1994), whereas platelets can only be stored for up to 96 hours at room temperature after donation and concentration (Mims, 1994). Table 43.1 describes the different blood products.

Cross matching – ABO and Rh

Landsteiner in 1901 discovered that human blood groups (the ABO system) existed and this marked the beginning of safe blood transfusion (Waters, 1991). There are four main blood groups: A, B, AB and O. These are based on antigens on the red cells and antibodies in the serum. There is racial variation in the frequency of these within a population (Waters, 1991). Apart from the ABO system most of the other red cell antigens are detected by antibodies stimulated by transfusion or pregnancy (Waters, 1991). Previous transfusions or pregnancies may immunize the patient against blood group antigens (Mims, 1994). The introduction of cells carrying A or B antigens results in immediate intravascular lysis in anyone with IgM antibodies to these antigens (Mims, 1994).

In 1940 the rhesus system was discovered. This is the second most important system in transfusion therapy (Weinstein, 1993) and is also an antigen found on the red cell. Approximately 15% of the UK population do not express the Rhesus antigen on their red blood cells (Mims, 1994). Transfusion of positive cells will result in immunization and the appearance of anti-D antibodies (Mims, 1994).

Full laboratory compatibility testing for cross matching of red blood cell transfusion can usually be done within one hour (Mims, 1994) (Table 43.1).

Blood groups in haemopoietic stem cell transplantation

The human lymphocyte antigen (HLA) is used to determine compatibility for organ transplantation including bone marrow and peripheral blood stem cells. Unfortunately, because ABO blood groups and HLA tissue types are determined genetically independently, it is not uncommon to find a well matched HLA donor who is ABO incompatible with the recipient. Major transfusion reactions can be avoided by red cell and/or plasma depletion of the donor cells in the laboratory before re-infusion. Very occasionally if the recipient has a very high titre of anti-A or anti–B lytic antibody and the donor marrow or peripheral blood stem cells are blood group A, V or AB, then plasmapheresis of the recipient is performed to lower the titre of this antibody to safe limits. This is necessary because it is not possible to remove all the red cells from the donor product and those remaining may cause a major transfusion reaction in this situation.

Indications

The range of products currently available, those most widely used, indications for use and recommendations for administration are listed in Table 43.1.

It may be unnecessary to correct a cytopenia or clotting deficiency to normal levels. Instead physiological

Table 43.1 Blood and products used for transfusion.

Type	Description	Indications	Cross-matching	Shelf life	Average infusion time	Technique	Special considerations
Whole blood	Complete unadulterated blood, approx. 510 ml including anticoagulant	To restore blood volume lost due to massive, acute haemorrhage whatever the cause	ABO and Rh	28–35 days at 4–6°C (dependent on anticoagulant)	2–4 hours/unit	Give via a blood administration set	If loss and replacement exceed twice the blood volume abnormalities of haemostasis may occur
*Plasma reduced blood (packed red blood cells)	Whole blood minus approx. 200 ml plasma, and anticoagulant; haematocrit 60–65%	To correct red blood cell deficiency and improve oxygen-carrying capacity of the blood	ABO and Rh	21 days at 4–6°C	2–4 hours/unit	As above	–
Red cells in optimal additive solutions	Red cells minus all plasma: 100 ml fluid used as replacement to give optimal red cell preservation; haematocrit 60–65%	As above	ABO and Rh	35 days at 4–6°C	1–2 hours/unit	As above	An example of a replacement solution is saline/adenine/glucose/mannitol
*Concentrated red cells	Plasma removed to produce a haematocrit of 70% plus	To correct anaemias when expansion of blood volume will not be tolerated	ABO and Rh	21 days at 4–6°C	1–2 hours/unit	As above	Availability varies
*Washed red blood cells	Red cells centrifuged free of plasma and resuspended in saline	To increase red cell mass and prevent tissue antigen formation in: (1) Immunosuppressed patients (2) Patients with previous transfusion reactions	ABO and Rh	Use within 12 hours or preferably immediately	1–2 hours/unit	As above	–
Frozen red blood cells	(1) Cells from normal healthy donor with very rare blood group (2) Patient's own cells taken in anticipation of later illness (autologous blood transfusion)	To treat transplant patients or patients with atypical antibodies which react with almost the entire population To increase safety of tranfusion therapy	ABO and Rh	Stored frozen cells: 3 years. Use within 12 hours of thawing	2–3 hours/unit	As above	Available from a few centres. Freezing process and recovery are time consuming and expensive
Leucocyte-poor blood	Red cells from which accompanying leucocytes have been removed	To prevent further reactions in patients who have had febrile attacks when receiving whole or plasma reduced blood	ABO and Rh	4–6°C. Time stated on pack. Usually within 12 hours of preparation, preferably immediately	2–3 hours/unit	As above	Frozen red cells may be used as an alternative
*White blood cells (leucocyte concentrate)	Mainly granulocytes obtained by	To treat patients with life-threatening	ABO and HLA (human leucocyte	24 hours after collection. Stored at 5°C	60–90 minutes/unit	Administer via a blood administration	White blood cell infusion *induces* fever, may cause

Table 43.1 *Continued.*

Type	Description	Indications	Cross-matching	Shelf life	Average infusion time	Technique	Special considerations
	leucophoresis or by 'creaming off' the buffy layers from packs of fresh blood	granulocytopaenia, e.g. due to chemotherapy	group A antigen)			set. Usually 1 unit only	hypertension, rigors and confusion. Treat symptoms and reassure patient. Preparation may be irradiated to prevent initiation of graft versus heart (GVH) disease in bone marrow transplant patients. Do not give to patients receiving amphotericin B
*Platelets	Platelet sediment from platelet-rich plasma, resuspended in 40–60 ml plasma	To treat thrombocytopaenia due to (1) Decreased production (2) Increased destruction (3) Functionally abnormal platelets (4) Dilutional problems following massive transfusions	ABO and rhesus compatibility preferred	Up to 5 days after collection at 22°C, with continuous gentle agitation; best within 6 hours	20–30 minutes/unit	Administration using a component set is preferred. Flush the line with 100 ml 0.9% sodium chloride after the infusion to ensure full dose is delivered. Do not use micro–aggregate filters	General guide to use: (1) Count less than 10×10^9/litre (2) Count 10–20 × 10^9/litre with haemorrhage (3) Count 20–50 × 10^9/litre or on chemotherapy may need platelets Prophylactic use in the absence of haemorrhage is controversial
Plasma: fresh or fresh, frozen (FFP)	Citrated plasma separated from whole blood. All coagulation factors preserved for several months	To treat a clotting factor deficiency, when specific concentrates are unavailable or precise deficiency is unknown, e.g. DIC	ABO compatibility; Rh preferred	Fresh: within 6 hours after collection. FFP: 12 months at −25°C. Use immediately after thawing	15–45 minutes/unit (approximately 200 ml)	Administer rapidly via a blood administration set	500 ml of FFP should be transfused after 8 units of blood (when massive transfusions given) to prevent dilutional hypocoagulability
Albumin 4.5% (plasma protein fraction)	Solution of selected proteins from pooled plasma in a buffered, stabilized saline diluent. Usually 400-ml bottle	To treat hypovolaemic shock or hypoproteinaemia due to burns, trauma, surgery or infection	Unnecessary	5 years at 2°C, 3 years at 25°C; store in the dark	30–60 minutes/unit	Administer via a blood administration set	Heated at 60°C for 10 hours to inactivate hepatitis virus. The solution should be crystal clear with no deposits
Salt poor human albumin 20%	Heat treated, aqueous chemically processed fraction of pooled plasma	To treat hypovolaemic shock or hypoproteinaemia due to burns, trauma, surgery or infection. To maintain appropriate electrolyte balance	Unnecessary	5 years at 2°C, 3 years at 25°C; store in the dark	30–60 minutes/unit	Administer via a blood administration set undiluted or diluted with saline or 5% glucose solution. Slower administration is advised if a cardiac disorder is present to avoid gross fluid shift	Heated at 60°C for 10 hours to inactivate hepatitis virus. The solution should be crystal clear with no deposits
Factor VIII (cryoprecipitates, dried anti-	Cold-insoluble portion of plasma recovered from	To control bleeding disorders due to lack of	ABO compatibility between	Cryoprecipitates at −30°C for 1 year. Use	15–30 minutes via infusion, 10–15 minutes	Administer rapidly via syringe or	Heat treated 80°C for 72 hours to eliminate risk of hepatitis or

Table 43.1 *Continued.*

Type	Description	Indications	Cross-matching	Shelf life	Average infusion time	Technique	Special considerations
haemophilic globulin concentrates)	FFP – amount of factor VIII varies. Potency in freeze-dried concentrates can be assayed more reliably	factor VIII or fibrinogen, e.g. haemophilia, Von Willebrand's disease	donor plasma and recipient's red blood cells	immediately after thawing. Freeze-dried concentrates at +4°C. Reconstitute at room temperature and use immediately	via intravenous push	component set. Flush each unit with saline to obtain maximum dose	HIV contamination, as multiple donors and imported preparation; limited availability
Dried factor IX concentrate	Preparation contains factor IX, prothrombin and factor X. Some may contain factor VII	To correct bleeding disorders due to lack of these factors, e.g. Christmas disease	Unnecessary	Refer to indivdual expiry dates	15–30 minutes	Administer via a blood administration set. Dose varies	As above. Limited availability

* Most commonly used blood products.

levels should be restored (Kickler & Ness, 1993). A rise of approximately 10 g/l of haemoglobin may be expected from each transfused unit of red blood cells (Davies & Brozovic, 1990).

Delivery of blood and blood products
The transfusion of stored blood exposes the patient to the possible infusion of particulate matter (Lowe, 1981a). After only a few hours of storage the presence of fibrin particles, clumps of white blood cells, disintegrating platelets and small clots can be detected (Fantus & Schirmir, 1938). After transfusion this may result in clinical problems including non-haemolytic febrile reactions and respiratory impairment caused by pulmonary micro-emboli. These problems are more commonly associated with large transfusions of 6 units and above and the use of blood stored for a long time.

The variable size (between 10 and 200 microns) and number of micro-aggregates are dependent on two main factors:

(1) The storage time: in general the older the blood the more micro-aggregates it contains.
(2) The anticoagulant used to prevent the blood clotting.

Inline blood filters
Filters are used to remove micro–aggregates and leucocytes present in the blood to be transfused.

Micro-aggregate filters
Micro-aggregate or micro-particle filters are used mainly to filter out red cell debris, platelets, white blood cells and fibrin strands that have clumped together. The filter compartment of commonly used blood administration sets will only remove particles of 170–200 microns and above.

Three types of filter are available:

(1) Screen or surface filters, which effectively sieve the blood. The size of the particle removed will depend on the pore size on the surface. These filters tend to become more efficient the more blood flows through them. They remove particles of 40 microns or above.
(2) Depth filters: these work by absorbing the particles into the layers of fibre. They tend to be effective for the removal of smaller particles but their efficiency diminishes as the number of units used increases. They also tend to slow the rate at which blood can be administered. These filters remove particles of 10–20 microns or above.
(3) Combination filters, which consist of a surface filter above and a depth filter below.

The use of additional inline blood filters is not indicated for the majority of transfusions, and is contraindicated with certain products such as platelets, to avoid the removal of desired components.

Leucocyte depletion filters
The main problem for the patient associated with the transfusion of leucocytes is sensitization due to white cells or HLA antigens. Leucocyte depletion filters may be used prospectively for patients who are to undergo many transfusions, e.g. the bone marrow transplant patient. There are specific filters designed for use in red cells and platelet transfusions, and it is important that the correct type is used.

Blood warmers

The warming of blood and blood products is not recommended as it is of limited benefit and is potentially dangerous. The use of blood warmers is indicated when:

(1) Massive, rapid transfusion could result in cooling of cardiac tissue, causing dysfunction.
(2) Frozen plasma or other components are prescribed and must be thawed before administration.
(3) Transfusion is required by patients with potent cold agglutinins.
(4) Exchange transfusion is indicated in the newborn (Weinstein, 1993).

Both waterbaths and dry heat blood warmers are available. Whatever device is chosen, the temperature should be maintained below 38°C, as warming in excess of this can cause haemolysis of red cells and can denature proteins.

The optimum effectiveness of dry heat blood warmers is reached when the rate of delivery to the patient is 150–160 ml per minute. This means that their use is restricted, and because of the greater flexibility of water baths these are more frequently used.

Wherever there is water, there is the risk of bacterial contamination of blood products, particularly with *Pseudomonas*. For the patient this could result in a fatal systemic infection. Therefore, certain safety measures must be adhered to:

(1) Waterbaths must be cleaned before and after use with disinfectant.
(2) They must be stored dry and empty.
(3) When needed, they should be refilled with sterile water.
(4) A protective overbag should be considered for the blood produce to be thawed, to prevent entry of contaminants through microscopic punctures or breaks in the seal.
(5) The blood warmer should be drained after each use.
(6) The blood product should be used immediately after it has been thawed.

All devices should be serviced at regular intervals.

Problems associated with administration of red blood cells, granulocytes and platelets

Red blood cells

Circulatory overload

This may occur when the blood is transfused too rapidly for compensatory fluid redistribution (Mims, 1994). Clinical features include pulmonary oedema, fullness in the head and a dry cough (Hoffbrand & Pettit, 1993).

Iron overload (transfusion haemosiderosis)

Each unit of blood contains 250 mg of iron that the body is unable to excrete. In recipients who require regular frequent transfusion iron chelation should be considered as a build up of iron may lead to pigmentation, poor growth, hepatic cirrhosis and cardiac failure (Davies & Brozovic, 1990).

Haemolytic reactions

Haemolytic transfusion reactions may be immediate or delayed (Hoffbrand & Pettit, 1993). These may result from ABO incompatibility. Clinical features include tachycardia, loin pain and hypotension and the onset is usually severe and immediate (Mims, 1994), with the haemolytic shock phase potentially occurring after only a few millilitres of blood have been transfused (Hoffbrand & Pettit, 1993). The patient may also experience nausea, shaking, chills, chest pain and pain at the infusion site (Pittiglio & Green, 1987). Intravascular haemolysis may lead to renal insufficiency, disseminated intravascular coagulation (DIC) and possibly death (Kickler & Ness, 1993). The severity of the reaction depends on the recipient's titre of antibody (Hoffbrand & Pettit, 1993). Occasionally the only clinical sign is no increase in the patient's haemoglobin post-transfusion (Pritchard & David, 1988). Red cell lysis resulting from ABO mismatch almost always arises from clerical errors at the time of sampling or errors when infusing (Mims, 1994). Secondary immune reactions can occur in patients immunized by pregnancy or previous transfusion (Mims, 1994).

Febrile non-haemolytic reactions

These occur usually as the result of antileucocyte antibodies in the recipient directed against the donor leucocytes (Weinstein, 1993). A febrile reaction is classified as a rise in temperature of 1°C usually occurring within 1–6 hours after the initiation of the transfusion (Weinstein, 1993). This may be accompanied by features such as flushing, chest tightness, tachycardia and palpitations.

Citrate and potassium intoxication

Acid citrate dextrose (ACD) or citrate phosphate dextrose (CPD) is used to prevent blood from clotting during storage. Potassium leaks out of red blood cells during storage and this process is exacerbated if the blood is kept for too long at room temperature (Davies & Brozovic, 1990). If blood is transfused in large quantities or if the patient has hepatic or renal disease the citrate and potassium levels in the patient's blood may become toxic and could lead to cardiac damage.

Allergic reactions

These are often caused by the development of anti-immunoglobulin A antibodies in the patient's plasma reacting against immunoglobulin A (IgA) protein in the transfused blood. The reaction may be mild with a rash soon appearing, or severe with the development of oedema around the eyes and/or around the larynx with accompanying dyspnoea.

Granulocytes

Leucocyte mediated transfusion reactions

Leucocyte antigens are complex and are mainly linked with the human leucocyte antigen (HLA) system. The recipient may become immunized to leucocyte antigens through multiple transfusions or through pregnancy. The patient may experience fever, chills and dyspnoea.

Transmission of cytomegalovirus (CMV)

The risk of transmitting the CMV is high with granulocyte transfusions. If the recipient is at risk of becoming infected with the CMV virus granulocytes should only be given from CMV seronegative donors (Hows & Brozovic, 1990).

Pulmonary infiltration

Antibody mediated granulocyte sequestration in the lungs together with pulmonary oedema and exacerbation of pre-existing pulmonary infection is a serious complication of granulocyte transfusions (Hows & Brozovic, 1990).

Platelets

Platelet refractoriness

This is where there is a consistent lack of response to platelet transfusions (Kickler & Ness, 1993). It can be defined as the failure of two consecutive transfusions to give a corrected increment of greater than $7.5 \times 10^9/l$ one hour after the transfusion in the absence of fever, infection, severe haemorrhage, splenomegaly or DIC (Hows & Brozovic, 1990). The cause may be non-immune or immune. Non-immune causes include hypersplenism, fever, infection and DIC. These may affect platelet survival (Kickler & Ness, 1993). HLA antigen alloimmunization occurs in patients who receive multiple transfusions (Kickler & Ness, 1993). Other immune causes include autoimmune thrombocytopenia and post transfusion purpura (Kickler & Ness, 1993).

Infectious complications of blood transfusion

Bacterial

Bacterial infections are now rare due to good collection methods. When they do occur they can be rapidly fatal. Reactions to contaminated blood usually develop quickly and include chills, rigors, fever, nausea, vomiting, pain and hypotension (Barbara et al., 1990a). The two bacterial diseases that have in the past been spread via blood transfusion are brucellosis and syphilis (Treponema pallidum).

Parasitic

Plasmodium falciparum is the most dangerous of the human malarial parasites (Barbara et al., 1990a). Prevention of transmission via blood transfusion is dependent on careful questioning of donors about foreign travel and the postponement of donation by those who have recently visited areas in which the disease is endemic (Hewitt et al., 1990).

Viral

Viruses which are transmissible via blood transfusion may be either plasma-borne or cell-associated (Barbara et al., 1990b). Plasma-borne viruses include hepatitis B and delta agent, hepatitis A (rarely), hepatitis C, serum parvovirus B19 and HIV1 and HIV2. Cell-associated viruses include cytomegalovirus (CMV), Epstein–Barr virus, HTLV1 and HTLV2, HIV1 and HIV2.

Hepatitis B

Screening for hepatitis B surface antigen (HBsAg) is mandatory. In the UK, hepatitis B virus is detected in 1 in 1000 donors or less because donors at risk of having HIV or hepatitis B are now excluding themselves (Barbara et al., 1990a).

Hepatitis C

Hepatitis C virus is a single-stranded RNA virus, which was discovered in 1989, and is reported to be the cause of 90–95% of cases of transfusion-associated non-A non-B hepatitis (Mims, 1994). It is transmitted primarily via contact with blood and blood products (Crowe, 1994). Screening for antibodies to the hepatitis C virus began in 1991 (Department of Health, 1995). This will have a significant impact on the prevention of post-transfusion hepatitis C virus infection (Teo, 1992). Recipients of blood or blood components from donors now known to be carriers of the hepatitis C virus are being traced with the view to providing counselling, testing and specialist referral as appropriate (Department of Health, 1995).

Human immunodeficiency virus (HIV1)

Before mandatory screening in 1985, HIV had been transmitted by most blood products including red cells, platelets, fresh frozen plasma and factor VIII and factor IX concentrates. Consequently a large number of haemophiliacs were infected with HIV, as were a smaller number of people receiving the other blood products. The prevalence is now 1 in 70 000 of UK donors, and the risk of infection being transmitted by blood components is 1 in 3 000 000 units transfused in the UK. The virus can be inactivated in plasma products such as factor VIII and factor IX with heat at 80°C for 72 hours and chemicals, but red cells and platelets cannot be treated by these methods (Barbara & Contreras, 1986a,b).

CMV

CMV is a member of the herpes family and as such has the ability to establish a latent infection and reactivate during periods of immunosuppression (Barnes, 1992). Approximately 50% of the UK population have antibodies to CMV; these persons are therefore capable of transmitting the infection through blood donation, although those most recently infected appear to be more likely to do so (Barbara *et al.*, 1990b). Primary infection occurs when a previously seronegative patient acquires the virus from blood products. Re-infection can occur with a different strain of CMV. CMV infection in vulnerable patient groups can cause significant morbidity and mortality. CMV pneumonitis carries a mortality rate of 85% in bone marrow transplant patients (Barnes, 1992). Screening of donors for cytomegalovirus is only necessary for neonates and immunocomprimised recipients who remain CMV negative.

Irradiation of blood products

Irradiation of blood products is used to prevent the transfusion of cells capable of replication (Patterson, 1992). If the recipient is immunocompromised (such as the bone marrow transplant patient) lymphocytes may proliferate and cause graft versus host disease.

Infusion of cryopreserved bone marrow and peripheral blood stem cells

Bone marrow and peripheral blood stem cells may be cryopreserved between harvesting and infusion. Thawing takes place in a large volume waterbath at 40°C and the cells are infused within 15 minutes. The cryoprotectant dimethylsulphoxide (DMSO) together with the haemoglobin released from lysed red blood cells may cause toxic effects such as nausea, abdominal pain, renal failure and anaphylaxis (Smith *et al.*, 1987; Davis *et al.*, 1990).

Autologous blood

Autologous transfusion (using the patient's own blood) is primarily intended to avoid the transmission of infection. Blood may be taken by a predeposit programme collecting during the weeks prior to the operation. Up to four units of blood can be taken at weekly intervals or by pre-operative haemodilution where the patient may have about a quarter of their blood withdrawn and replaced by a volume expander in the 48 hours prior to surgery (Lee & Napier, 1990). Blood salvage procedures may also be used to recover shed blood for reinfusion.

References and further reading

AIDS Newsletter (1991) *Survey Findings Transmission*, April, p. 2. Abbott Diagnostics Division.

Barbara, J. A. J. *et al.* (1990a) Infectious complications of blood transfusion: bacteria and parasites. In: *ABC of Transfusions*, (ed. M. Contreras), pp. 45–8. British Medical Journal Publications, London.

Barbara, J. A. J. *et al.* (1990b) Infectious complications of blood transfusion: viruses. In: *ABC of Transfusions*, (ed. M. Contreras), pp. 42–9, 45–52. British Medical Journal Publications, London.

Barbara, J. & Contreras, M. (1986a) Bacterial and parasitic diseases transmitted by blood transfusion. *Hospital Update*, 12, 629–31.

Barbara, J. & Contreras, M. (1986b) Viral diseases transmitted by blood transfusion. *Hospital Update*, 12, 697–708.

Barnes, R. (1992) Infections following bone marrow transplantation. In: *Bone Marrow Transplantation in Practice*, (eds J. Treleavan & J. Barrett), pp. 281–8. Churchill Livingstone, Edinburgh.

Brozovic, B. (1986) Blood and blood products: availability and indications. *Hospital Update*, 12, 445–58.

Canadian Red Cross Society Blood Transfusion Service (1982) *Clinical Guide to Transfusion*. Canadian Red Cross Society, Toronto.

Crowe, H. M. (1994) Forum: A perspective on hepatitis. *Asepsis*, 16(2), 13–17.

Davies, S. & Brozovic, M. (1990) Transfusion of red cells. In: *ABC of Transfusions*, (ed. M. Contreras), pp. 9–24. British Medical Journal Publications, London.

Davis, J. *et al.* (1990) Clinical toxicity of cryopreserved bone marrow graft infusion. *Blood*, 75, 781–6.

Department of Health and Social Security, National Blood Transfusion Service, Scottish National Blood Transfusion Service (1984) *Notes on Transfusion*. DHSS, London.

Department of Health (1995) *Hepatitis C and Blood Transfusion Look Back 1995*. PL CMO (95)1. Department of Health, London.

Editorial (1985) Warming of blood and blood products. *Canadian Intravenous Nurses Association Journal*, 1(2), 5.

Fantus, B. & Schirmir, E. H. (1938) The therapy of the Cook County Hospital – blood preservation technique. *Journal of the American Medical Association*, 111, 317.

Hewitt, P. E. *et al.* (1990) The blood donor and tests on donor blood. In: *ABC of Transfusions*, (ed. M. Contreras), pp. 1–4.

British Medical Journal Publications, London.

Hoffbrand, A. V. & Pettit, J. E. (1993) *Essential haematology*, 3rd edn. Blackwell Science, Oxford.

Hows, J. M. & Brozovic, B. (1990) Platelet and granulocyte transfusion. In: *ABC of Transfusions*, (ed. M. Contreras). British Medical Journal Publications, London.

Huws, J. & Brozovic, B. (1990) Platelet and granulocyte transfusions. In: *ABC of Transfusions*, (ed. M. Contreras), pp. 14–17. British Medical Journal Publications, London.

Kaberry, S. (1991) Blood simple. *Nursing Times*, 87(2), 56.

Kickler, T. S. & Ness, P. M. (1993) Blood component therapy. In: *Hematological and Oncological Emergencies*, (ed. W. R. Bell), pp. 125–40. Churchill Livingstone, Edinburgh.

Lee, D. & Napier, J. A. F. (1990) Autologous transfusion. In: *ABC of Transfusions*, (ed. M. Contreras), pp. 18–21. British Medical Journal Publications, London.

Lloyd, G. M. & Marshall, L. (1986) Blood micro-aggregates: their role in transfusion reactions. *Intensive Care World*, 3(4), 119–22.

Lowe, G. D. (1981a) Filtration in IV therapy. Part III: Clinical aspects of blood filtration. *British Journal of Intravenous Therapy*, September, 28–38.

Lowe, G. D. (1981b) Filtration in IV therapy: blood filters. *British Journal of Intravenous Therapy*, 2(6), 24–38.

Mims Handbook of Haematology (1994) Haymarket Medical Imprint Ltd.

Patterson, K. (1992) Bone marrow harvesting and preparation of harvested marrow. In: *Bone Marrow Transplantation in Practice*, (eds J. Treleavan & J. Barrett), pp. 219–26. Church-ill Livingstone, Edinburgh.

Pittiglio, D. H. & Green, R. L. B. (1987) Hemolytic anemias: extracorpuscular defects. In: *Clinical Haematology and Fundamentals of Hemostasis*, (eds D. H. Pittiglio & R. A. Sacher). F. A. Davis, Philadelphia.

Pritchard, A. P. & David, J. A. (1988) *The Royal Marsden Hospital Manual of Clinical Nursing Procedures*, 2nd edn. Harper & Row, London.

Smith, D. S. (1987) The appropriate use of diagnostic services: a guide to blood transfusion practice. *Health Trends*, 19, 12–16.

Smith, D. *et al.* (1987) Acute renal failure with autologous bone marrow transplantation. *Bone Marrow Transplantation*, 2, 195–201.

Swaffield, L. (1987) Circulating the blood. *Nursing Times*, 83(11), 16–17.

Teo, C. G. (1992) The virology and serology of hepatitis: an overview. *Communicable Disease Report*, 10(2), 109–13.

Waters, A. H. (1991) Platelet and granulocyte antigens and antibodies. In: *Practical Haematology*, (eds J. Dacie & S. M. Lewis), 7th edn, pp. 441–54. Churchill Livingstone, Edinburgh.

Watson, J. E. & Royale, J. A. (1987) Blood transfusion. In: *Watson's Medical–Surgical Nursing and Related Physiology*, 3rd edn., p. 293. Ballière Tindall, London.

Webster, A. (1987) Banking your own blood. *Nursing Times*, 83(31), 36–7.

Weinstein, S. M. (1993) *Plumer's Principles and Practice of Intravenous Therapy*, 5th edn. J. B. Lippincott, Philadelphia.

NURSING CARE PLAN

The problems identified in this section are those associated specifically with blood or blood products transfusion. Common problems associated with delivery of these substances are similar to those encountered in intravenous administration of any therapy and reference should be made to Chapter 23, Intravenous Management.

Examples of problems frequently encountered are:

1 The infusion slows or stops shortly after commencing the unit of blood. The most likely cause for this is venous spasm due to a cold solution being infused. The preventive or corrective measure would be to apply a warm compress to soothe and dilate the vein and increase blood flow.

2 The infusion slows or stops due to occlusion of the cannula. Maintenance of continuous flow is important here. If this problem is recognized early, then flushing the cannula gently with 0.9% sodium chloride may resolve this. However, if some minutes have elapsed it may be necessary to prime a new administration set with 0.9% sodium chloride to re-establish flow as clotting may have occurred in the tubing. Keeping the patient warm and relaxed will also increase the peripheral circulation and prevent problems.

Potential problem	Cause	Preventive measure	Suggested action
Elevated temperature after the commencement of a unit of blood with temperature falling if the blood is slowed.	Pyrogenic reaction.	Observation of the patient's temperature, pulse and blood pressure during the transfusion dependent on patient's condition and especially at the start of each unit.	Slow blood transfusion rate. Inform medical staff.

Nursing care plan (cont'd)

Potential problem	Cause	Preventive measure	Suggested action
		If patient has had multiple transfusions or experienced this type of reaction previously, ensure 'cover' of hydrocortisone and chlorpheniramine is written up and administered before commencement of therapy.	
A high temperature associated with fever and rigor during a transfusion.	White cell antibody reaction.	Observation as above.	Stop transfusion. Change giving set and commence 0.9% sodium chloride slowly to keep vein open. Inform medical staff.
Slightly elevated temperature with associated rash, may be severe with oedema round the eyes and larynx and shortness of breath.	Allergic reaction to protein in the plasma.	Observation as above. Ensure patient is aware of symptoms to report, e.g. appearance of a rash or breathlessness. Close observation of patient for swollen eyes and signs of breathlessness.	If mild, slow the rate of transfusion. Inform medical staff. If severe, stop transfusion. Change giving set and commence 0.9% sodium chloride to keep vein open, or hepflush cannula. Lie patient flat, treat as for shock. Inform medical staff.
Patient complains of feeling hot with chest and abdominal pain. Fall in blood pressure, patient's temperature subnormal at first and later rising to a pyrexia.	Infection introduced either from bacteria in the blood or during the cannulation or connection set changes.	Adhere to strict aseptic technique when handling the blood bags and intravenous line. Use blood within 30 minutes of removal from refrigerator. Regular observations, as above. Adhere to recommended delivery time for each unit of blood; discard if hanging for 8 hours.	Stop transfusion. Change giving set and commence 0.9% sodium chloride slowly to keep vein open. Inform medical staff and institute prescribed treatment, e.g. steroids, antibiotics. Return remaining blood for examination by the bacteriology department.
Patient complaining of feeling a hot flush along the vein, facial flushing and lumbar pain. The patient may become shocked with a fall in the	Blood not cross-matched. Urgent cross-match completed and blood not fully compatible. Blood administered to wrong patient.	Ensure blood cross-matching forms are completed correctly. If taking blood sample, check carefully that the name and number on the	Stop transfusion. Change giving set and commence 0.9% sodium chloride to keep vein open. Lay patient flat and treat

blood pressure and the urine output may fall.

Cross-matched blood sample wrongly labelled or taken from wrong patient.

form matches the patient. Ensure that a unit is checked against the cross-match form for blood group, patient's name, patient's number, ward, Rh factor, unit number of blood, when blood taken, and expiry date.
Begin transfusion slowly and observe the patient carefully at the start of each unit.

as for shock.
Inform medical staff.

Note: transfusion risks associated with administration of massive amounts of blood include:

1 Abnormal bleeding tendencies.
2 Hypocalcaemia.
3 Risk of development of adult respiratory distress syndrome.
4 Potassium intoxication.
5 Elevated blood ammonia level.
6 Haemosiderosis.
7 Hypothermia.

Massive transfusion refers to quantities in excess of six units and specific texts should be consulted in these circumstances.

CHAPTER 44

The Unconscious Patient

Definition

In coma an individual's awareness, as well as those responses essential to comfort and self-preservation, no longer operate (Wong *et al.*, 1984).

Introduction

Complete care of the unconscious patient presents a special challenge to the nurse because the patient is totally dependent on the nurse's skills – for his/her comfort needs and indeed for his/her life. This inability to respond must spur efforts to include the patient and the family or close friends in re-orientation programmes, by using stimuli associated with the patient's previous physiological and social experiences.

The normal reflexes protecting the conscious person are lost and their protective function is assumed by the nurse until the patient can function to maximum potential. In order to do so it would be necessary to:

(1) Establish and maintain a clear airway.
(2) Assess the level of consciousness (see Chapter 28, Neurological Observations).
(3) Record and evaluate vital signs.
(4) Maintain fluid and electrolyte balance.
(5) Carry out nursing care as appropriate to the patient's condition.
(6) Involve relatives and/or friends in care from the beginning.

REFERENCE MATERIAL

Causes of unconsciousness

Causes of unconsciousness are many and may dictate the length of the coma period. Some patients may recover spontaneously, e.g. after a seizure, while others remain unconscious until their death. This chapter deals mainly with the patient who is unconscious for some time and not with the anaesthetized and post-anaesthetic patient whose coma is controlled. The following list of causes of unconsciousness is not exhaustive, nor can it indicate the outcome of the comatosed state.

Poisons and drugs

(1) Alcohol.
(2) General anaesthetics.
(3) Overdose of drugs, including solvents.
(4) Gases, e.g. carbon monoxide.
(5) Heavy metals, e.g. lead poisoning.

Vascular causes

(1) Post–cardiac arrest.
(2) Ischaemia.
(3) Hypertensive encephalopathy.
(4) Haemorrhage – intracerebral or subarachnoid.
(5) Sudden reduction in circulating blood volume.

Infections

(1) Septicaemia.
(2) Viruses, e.g. herpes, encephalitis, HIV.
(3) Meningitis.
(4) Protozoan infections, e.g. malaria.
(5) Fungal, e.g. aspergillosis.

Seizures

(1) Idiopathic or post-traumatic epilepsy.
(2) Eclampsia.
(3) Metabolic disorders.

Other causes

(1) Neoplasm, primary, e.g. glioma, or secondary tumour from other body primary, e.g. lung.
(2) Trauma, e.g. head injury or trauma resulting in hyper/hypothermia, dehydration.
(3) Liver, renal, cardiac or lung failure.
(4) Tetany.

(5) Metabolic causes, e.g. diabetic coma, myxoedema.
(6) Degenerative diseases, e.g. multiple sclerosis.

Recording the level of consciousness

There are many methods of assessing and recording a patient's level of consciousness. One of the most commonly used in the UK is the Glasgow Coma Scale (Jennett & Teasdale, 1974; Allan, 1986). An extensive description of this scale can be found in Allan (1986). Terms such as 'semiconscious' should be avoided since they mean different things to different people and can be misleading. It is more appropriate to describe the patient in terms of the responsiveness to environmental stimuli (Mangiardi, 1990).

Attitudes of nurses

Leon & Snyder (1980) explored the psychosocial problems in caring for head-injured patients and concluded that, in general, nurses accepted unconscious patients and were challenged by them. The phase of management appears to affect the attitude of the nursing staff, e.g. critical care, post-emergent care and continuing care. Bell (1986) discusses the hopelessness, guilt, ambivalence, frustration and depression felt by nurses in some situations. The involvement of families and friends of the patient may lead the nurse to experience professional, moral and ethical problems, depending on the likely outcome of the coma and the length of the comatosed state.

All nurses must recognize that 'it is difficult to provide constant and continuous excellent care to the comatosed (head-injured) patient when the professional rewards are minimal' (Flaherty, 1982). Peer support in units or wards caring for the unconscious patient is vital, particularly perhaps where the patient is a child, or the patient is brain dead (Rudy, 1982; Pallis, 1983). The needs of the patient's family and friends must also be addressed by the nursing staff. Grieving is a natural and necessary process for family and friends of the terminally ill or long-term unconscious patient, and they must be supported through and prepared for the eventual outcome (Allan, 1988; Penson, 1988).

References and further reading

Ackerman, L. L. (1993) Alterations in level of responsiveness. *Nursing Clinics of North America*, 28(4), 729–45.

Allan, D. (1986) Nursing the unconscious patient. *Professional Nurse*, 2(1), 15–17.

Allan, D. (1988) The ethics of brain death. *Professional Nurse*, 3(8), 295–8.

Bell, T. N. (1986) Nurses' attitudes in caring for comatose head-injured patients. *Journal of Neurological Nursing*, 18(5), 279–89.

Flaherty, M. (1982) Care of the comatose: complex problems faced alone. *Nursing Management*, 13(10), 44–6.

Fuller, G. (1993) *Neurological Examination Made Easy*. Churchill Livingstone, Edinburgh.

Gooch, J. (1985) Mouth care. *Professional Nurse*, 1(3), 77–9.

Hickey, J. V. (1986) *The Clinical Practice of Neurological and Neurosurgical Nursing*, 2nd edn. Lippincott, Philadelphia.

Jennett, B. & Teasdale, G. (1974) Assessment of coma and impaired consciousness. A practical scale. *Lancet*, 2, 81–3.

Leon, M. & Snyder (1980) The psychosocial aspects of the care of long-term comatose patients. *Journal of Neurosurgical Nursing*, 11(4), 235–7.

Lindsay, K. W. et al. (1991) *Neurology and Neurosurgery Illustrated*, 2nd edn. Churchill Livingstone, Edinburgh.

Mangiardi, J. R. (1990) Initial management of head injury. *Topics in Emergency Medicine*, 11(4), 11–23.

Nikas, D. (1982) Altered states of consciousness. Part I. *Focus and Critical Care*, 10(5), 10–14; Part II – 10(6), 10–13; Part III – (1984), 11(1), 54–8.

Pallis, C. (1983) *ABC of Brain Stem Death*. British Medical Association, London.

Payne-James, J. et al. (eds) (1995) *Artificial Nutritional Support in Clinical Practice*. Arnold, London.

Penson, J. (1988) The needs of the terminally ill patient's family. *Professional Nurse*, 3(5), 153–5.

Podurgiel, M. (1990) The unconscious experience: a pilot study. *Journal of Neuroscience Nursing*, 22(1), 52–3.

Rudy, E. (1982) Brain death. *Dimensions of Critical Care Nursing*, 1(3), 178.

Scherer, P. (1986) Assessment: the logic of coma. *American Journal of Nursing*, 86(5), 542–9.

Taylor, S. J. (1988) A guide to nasogastric feeding. *Professional Nurse*, 3(11), 439–43.

Taylor, S. J. (1989) Preventing complications in internal feeding. *Professional Nurse*, 4(5), 247–9.

Taylor, S. J. (1989) A guide to internal feeding. *Professional Nurse*, 4(4), 195–8.

Wong, J. et al. (1984) Care of the unconscious patient: a problem-orientated approach. *Journal of Neurosurgical Nursing*, 16(3), 148–50.

de Young, S. (1987) Coma recovery program. *Rehabilitation Nursing*, 12(3), 121–4.

GUIDELINES: CARE OF THE UNCONSCIOUS PATIENT

EQUIPMENT

At the bedside:

Guidelines: Care of the unconscious patient (cont'd)

1 Airway (of correct size).
2 Suction.
3 Oxygen.
4 Intravenous infusion equipment.
5 Personal hygiene equipment:
   (a) Eye toilet pack.
   (b) Oral toilet pack.
   (c) Catheter care pack.
6 Cot sides (to be assessed on an individual basis).
7 Observation charts:
   (a) Neurological.
   (b) Intake and output.
8 Feeding equipment (as necessary).

Easy access to:

1 Ambu-bag with valve and mask; or intubation (and tracheostomy) equipment.
2 Neurological observation tray, thermometer and sphygmomanometer.

PROCEDURE

Action	Rationale
1 Call the patient by preferred name. Introduce yourself, explain each procedure before starting; talk to patient; tell patient date, time, etc.	Hearing often remains intact in the unconscious patient. To prevent sensory deprivation.
2 The room or ward area should be warm and well lit, and adequately ventilated with easy access to the patient.	To facilitate rapid assessment of the patient at a glance, e.g.: (a) Colour of skin – cherry red after carbon monoxide poisoning, frost in uraemia, yellow in hepatic failure, blue in cyanosis. (b) Smell – alcohol; 'toasted almonds' after cyanide poisoning, the sickly sweet smell of diabetic ketoacidosis (Mangiardi, 1990).
3 Nurse the patient in a bed with a firm base, a detachable bed head (and cot sides if deemed necessary).	To facilitate cardiac massage and intubation if required. (To prevent self-injury to the restless patient.)
4 Insert a bed cradle, if required.	To allow unhampered limb movements. To enhance view of limbs if leg is in plaster or on traction (as in multiple injuries).
5 Place patient in lateral or semi-prone position (if condition allows).	To prevent occlusion of airway by tongue falling back against the pharyngeal wall. To encourage drainage of respiratory secretions, and prevent pooling of same in throat.

Note: if a patient's injuries or other conditions prevent him/her from being nursed from side to side or prone, then a nurse should be in attendance at all times while there is an airway hazard.

6 Pass nasogastric tube.	To empty gastric contents regularly. Paralytic ileus occurs frequently in the unconscious patient and this may lead to aspiration of stomach contents.

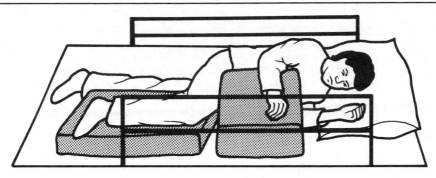

Figure 44.1 Positioning the unconscious patient.

7 Place the limbs as follows (Fig. 44.1):

(a) Head: put the patient's head on a pillow.

(b) Trunk: keep the spine straight and place pillows at the patient's back for support.

To promote comfort and maintain proper alignment of the body.

(c) Upper limb: bring the uppermost arm forward in front of the patient. Bend the elbow slightly, but keep the wrist extended. Support the arm on a pillow and bring the bottom arm alongside the face with the palm facing upwards.

To prevent oedema by inappropriate pressure on venous flow.

(d) Lower limbs: flex the uppermost leg and bring it forward. Support it on pillows.

To prevent internal rotation of the hip.

Keep the lower leg extended straight and in line with the spine.

To avoid pressure ulcers.

Make sure the patient's uppermost leg does not rest on the lower leg.

(e) Consult with physiotherapist and anaesthetist about positioning exercises to enhance pulmonary function.

To effect optimal respiratory function and gaseous exchange.

(f) Institute passive physiotherapy exercises and observe colour, temperature and pulses of limbs.

To prevent deep vein thrombosis formation; to recognize early signs of limb deformity.

(g) Apply anti-embolism stockings as ordered.

To aid venous return to the heart.

8 (a) Remove all dental prostheses and note caps, loose teeth, bleeding gums etc.

To obtain and maintain clear airway.

(b) Clean patient's nostrils.

(c) Insert an airway (either oral or nasal) as appropriate.

9 Perform neurological assessment as frequently as physician or patient's condition dictates.

To note changes in condition and act on changes as appropriate.

10 (a) Administer intravenous fluids as prescribed and record.

To maintain electrolyte and fluid balance.

(b) Strict asepsis must be maintained when carrying out proceedings involving puncture sites of cannulae or sterile ends of intravenous infusion sets.

To prevent infections – local or systemic.

Guidelines: Care of the unconscious patient (cont'd)

Action

11	Maintain feeding regime either by nasogastric tube – by fine bore continuous tube feeding – by central venous catheter (see Chapter 11)

12	Touch the patient gently and describe boundaries and environment, e.g. place patient's hand on the bedside, blankets, locker and explain what each item is, describe the room.

13	Give the patient daily baths (or as required).

14	Carry out eye care (see procedure on eye care, Chapter 20).

15	Carry out mouth care (see procedure on mouth care, Chapter 26).

16	Observe the patient for signs of bladder distension (or urinary bypass of catheter; see Chapter 45, Urinary Catheterization).

(a) Read catheter information carefully.

(b) Perform regular catheter care.

17	Carry out bowel care.

18	Change the patient's position every two hours or as dictated by condition.

19	Keep relatives and friends informed of changes in the patient's condition and involve them in caring for the patient as appropriate.

Rationale

To maintain metabolic stasis.
To prevent weight loss (Taylor, 1988; Taylor, 1989; Payne-James *et al.*, 1995).

Through touch, individuals establish (and maintain) their body boundaries and relationships with others, and their environment. Being denied opportunities to touch can impair physiological, psychological and social development (de Young, 1987; Podurgiel, 1990).

To ensure patient's skin is kept clean, dry and supple (Gooch, 1985).

The blink reflex is absent during unconsciousness (or the patient's eyes may be open all the time). This may lead to corneal drying, irritation and ulceration (see Chapter 20).

To maintain a clean, moist mouth, to prevent the accumulation of oral and postnatal secretions and to prevent the development of mouth infections (Gooch, 1985).

To prevent urinary complication. In males an external sheath may be used and catheterization may become necessary. In females, catheterization may be immediately necessary.
To prevent over-distending the balloon and damaging urethra.
To prevent infection.

To prevent constipation and/or diarrhoea.

To relieve pressure areas. To prevent respiratory complications by allowing for postural drainage, and for each side of the chest to receive a period free of compression by body weight when it can expand fully.

To help family and friends adjust to the situation and (depending on prognosis) facilitate 'anticipatory grief' (Penson, 1988).

NURSING CARE PLAN

Problem	Cause	Suggested action
Restlessness and/or confusion.	A degree of restlessness may indicate that the patient is	Ascertain, where possible, the cause of the discomfort and

	regaining consciousness. During this time there may be a clouding of consciousness with confusion, aggression, uncooperative behaviour and disorientation. Restlessness may also indicate brain damage, cerebral anoxia (when there is a partially obstructed airway), a full bladder, bowel pain, discomfort or generalized pain.	rectify as appropriate. Summon help if the patient becomes aggressive or violent. Ensure the patient does not inflict self-injury, e.g. place cot sides in position on the bed.
Seizures	An unconscious patient is a potential candidate for seizures.	Maintain a clear airway. Protect the patient from self-injury. Observe the patient during the seizure and record observations on a seizure chart. Administer prescribed drugs.
Cerebrospinal fluid leakage through nose or ears.	May be indicative of base of skull fracture, or some dural damage (Nikas, 1982).	Place sterile swab against nose and ears and collect fluid. Test drainage for sugar (it will be positive if CSF is present). Inform medical staff.
Vomiting.	The unconscious patient is prone to paralytic ileus, or medulla oblongata may be involved.	Maintain a clear airway. Keep stomach empty until ileus resolves.
Distended bladder.	See Chapter 45, Urinary Catheterization, for problems associated with catheterization.	
Inability to maintain own nutritional intake.	See Chapter 29, Nutritional Support, for problems associated with this type of nutrition.	

CHAPTER 45
Urinary Catheterization

Definition
Urinary catheterization is the insertion of a special tube into the bladder, using aseptic technique, for the purpose of evacuating or instilling fluids.

Indications

Male
In the male, urinary catheterization may be carried out for the following reasons:

(1) To empty the contents of the bladder, e.g. before or after abdominal, pelvic or rectal surgery and before certain investigations.
(2) To determine residual urine.
(3) To allow irrigation of the bladder.
(4) To bypass an obstruction.
(5) To relieve retention of urine.
(6) To introduce cytotoxic drugs in the treatment of papillary bladder carcinomas.
(7) To enable bladder function tests to be performed.
(8) To measure urinary output accurately, e.g. when a patient is in shock, undergoing bone marrow transplantation or receiving high-dose chemotherapy.
(9) To relieve incontinence when no other means is practicable.

Female
In the female, urinary catheterization may be carried out for the nine reasons listed above and for two further reasons:

(10) To empty the bladder before childbirth, if thought necessary.
(11) To avoid complications during intracavitary insertion of radioactive caesium.

REFERENCE MATERIAL

Catheter selection
New materials and improvements in design have allowed manufacturers to offer a wide range of urinary catheters.

Careful assessment of the most appropriate material, size and balloon capacity will ensure that the catheter selected is as effective as possible, and that complications are minimized. Types of catheters are listed in Table 45.1, together with their applications.

Balloon size
A catheter with a 30 ml balloon was designed by Dr Frederick Foley in the 1920s. The sole purpose of this catheter was to prevent haemorrhage following prostatectomy. The 30 ml balloon has become associated with leakage of urine (Kennedy *et al.*, 1983), and a study by Kristiansen *et al.* (1983) found that the large balloon caused damage to the neck of the bladder.

Consequently, a 5–10 ml balloon is recommended for adults, and a 3–5 ml balloon for children. Care should be taken to use the correct amount of water to fill the balloon because too much or too little may cause distortion of the catheter tip, leading to irritation and trauma to the bladder wall. One or more of the drainage eyes may also become occluded (Bard Ltd, 1987).

Catheter size
Urethral catheters are measured in charrières (ch). The charrière is the outer circumference of the catheter in millimetres and is equivalent to three times the diameter. Thus a 12 ch catheter has a diameter of 4 mm.

Potential side-effects of large gauge catheters include:

• Pain and discomfort;
• Pressure sores, which may lead to stricture formation;
• Blockage of paraurethral ducts; and
• Abscess formation (Edwards *et al.*, 1983; Crow *et al.*, 1986; Roe & Brocklehurst, 1987; Blandy & Moors, 1989).

The most important guiding principle is to choose the smallest size of catheter necessary to maintain adequate drainage (McGill, 1982). If the urine to be drained is likely to be clear, a 12 ch catheter should be considered.

Table 45.1 Types of catheter.

Catheter type	Material	Uses
Balloon (Foley) two-way catheter: two channels, one for urine drainage; second, smaller channel for balloon inflation	Various (see below)	Most commonly used for patients who require bladder drainage (short-, medium- or long-term)
Balloon (Foley) three-way irrigation catheter: three channels, one for urine; one for irrigation fluid; one for balloon inflation	Latex, Teflon, silicone, plastic	To provide continuous irrigation (e.g. after prostatectomy). The potential for infection is reduced by minimizing need to break the closed drainage system
Non-balloon (Nelaton) or Scotts, or intermittent catheter (one channel only)	PVC and other plastics	To empty bladder or continent urinary reservoir intermittently; to instil solutions into the bladder

Larger gauge catheters may be necessary if debris or clots are present in the urine.

Length of catheter

Until 1979 only one length of urethral catheter (41–45 cm) was available for both men and women (Crummey, 1989). A shorter catheter (20–25 cm) is now available for women. It is more discrete than the longer catheter, and less likely to cause trauma or infections because movement in and out of the urethra is reduced. Infection may also be caused by the longer catheter looping or kinking. In obese women, however, the inflation valve of the shorter catheter may cause soreness by rubbing against the inside of the thigh, and the catheter is more likely to pull on the bladder neck (Britton & Wright, 1990).

Tip design

Several different types of catheter tip are available in addition to the standard round tip. Each tip is designed to overcome a particular problem:

(1) *Tieman-tipped catheter* – has a curved tip with one to three drainage eyes to allow greater drainage. This catheter has been designed to negotiate the membranous and prostatic urethra in patients with prostatic hypertrophy.
(2) *Whistle-tipped catheter* – has a lateral eye in the tip and eyes above the balloon to provide a large drain-

age area. This design is intended to facilitate drainage of debris.
(3) *Roberts catheter* – has an eye above and below the balloon to facilitate drainage when leakage is a problem.

Catheter material

A wide variety of materials is used to make catheters. The key criterion in selecting the appropriate material is the length of time the catheter is expected to remain in place. Three broad time scales have been identified:

(1) Short-term (1–14 days);
(2) Short- to medium-term (2–6 weeks);
(3) Medium- to long-term (6 weeks–3 months).

The principle catheter materials are as follows:

(1) *Latex*. Latex is a purified form of rubber and is the softest of the catheter materials. It has a smooth surface, with a tendency to allow crust formation. Latex has been shown to cause urethral irritation (Wilksch et al., 1983) and therefore should only be considered when catheterization is likely to be short-term.
(2) *Teflon or silicone elastomer coatings*. A Teflon or silicone elastomer coating is applied to a latex catheter to render the latex inert and reduce urethral irritation (Slade & Gillespie, 1985). Teflon or silicone elastomer coated catheters are recommended for short- or medium-term catheterization.
(3) *All silicone*. Silicone is an inert material which is less likely to cause urethral irritation. Silicone catheters are not coated, and therefore have a wider lumen and block less easily. Because silicone permits gas diffusion, balloons may deflate and allow the catheter to fall out prematurely (Studer, 1983). Silicone catheters are recommended for long-term use.
(4) *Hydrogel coatings*. Catheters made of an inner core of latex encapsulated in a hydrophilic polymer coating have recently been developed. The polymer coating is well tolerated by the urethral mucosa causing little irritation. Hydrogel coated catheters become smoother when rehydrated, reducing friction with the urethra. They are inert (Nacey & Delahunt, 1991), and are reported to be resistant to bacterial colonization and encrustation (Roberts et al., 1990). Hydrogel coated catheters are recommended for long-term use.

The *conformable catheter* is designed to conform to the shape of the female urethra, and allows partial filling of the bladder. The natural movement of the urethra on the catheter, which is collapsible, is intended to prevent obstructions (Brocklehurst et al., 1988). Conformable catheters are approximately 3 cm longer than conventional catheters for women.

Anaesthetic lubricating gel

The use of anaesthetic lubricating gels is well recognized for male catheterization, but there is some controversy in its use for female catheterization. In males the gel is instilled directly into the urethra and then external massage is used to move the gel down its length. In female patients the anaesthetic lubricating gel or plain lubricating gel is applied to the tip of the catheter only if it is used at all. It has been suggested that most of the lubricant is wiped off the catheter at the urethral introitus so therefore it fails to reach the urethral tissue (Muctar, 1991).

These differences in practice imply that catheterization is a painful procedure for men but is not so for women. This assumption is not based on any empirical evidence or on any biological evidence. Other than the differences in length and route the male and female urethra are very similar except for the presence of lubricating glands in the male urethra (Tortora & Grabowski, 1993). The absence of these lubricating glands in the female urethra suggests that there is perhaps a greater need for the introduction of a lubricant. Women have complained of pain and discomfort during catheterization procedures (Mackenzie & Webb, 1995), suggesting that the use of anaesthetic lubricating gels must be reconsidered. Since there is a lack of research to clarify the efficacy of lubricating gels, practice must be based on the research evidence that is available and the physiology and anatomy of the urethra.

Common sites of cross-infection

The common sites of cross-infection in a catheterized patient are illustrated in Fig. 45.1. To reduce the risk of cross-infection, particular care should be taken when obtaining urine specimens. All specimens should be taken from the rubber cuff which is specially designed to occlude the puncture hole when the needle is withdrawn. Reference should be made to the manufacturer's instructions as to the number of times the cuff can be punctured safely. Some manufacturers indicate that cuffs can be punctured up to 50 times (e.g. Simpla). With other drainage systems this may not be possible.

Meatal cleansing

Cleaning the urethral meatus, where the catheter enters the body, is a nursing procedure intended to minimize infection of the urinary tract. There is no consensus about the value of this procedure, or about which cleansing solutions, if any, should be used. Antiseptics do not appear to check the development of urinary tract infections, indeed they have been implicated in the development of multi-resistant organisms (Dance *et al.*, 1987). Roe (1992) recommends soap, water and clean wash cloths, particularly for patients with long-term catheters.

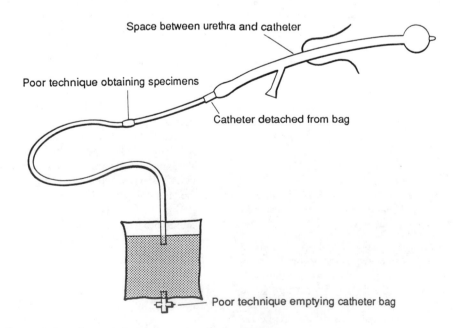

Space between urethra and catheter

Poor technique obtaining specimens

Catheter detached from bag

Poor technique emptying catheter bag

Figure 45.1   Common sites of cross-infection in a catheterized patient.

Drainage bags

A wide variety of drainage systems are available. Selecting a system involves consideration of the reasons for catheterization, the intended duration, the wishes of the patient and infection control issues.

The highest risk of cross-infection occurs when the bag is emptied or changed (Crow *et al.*, 1986). Reid *et al.* (1982) recommend weekly bag changes, on the grounds that more frequent changes do not positively influence infection rates. The Department of Health drug tariff (Department of Health, 1992) recommends changing bags every 5–7 days.

At home, patients re-use their drainage bags (Roe, 1993). This practice is currently the subject of research. Until further research evidence is available, it is recommended that patients be given a choice between disposing of used drainage bags and re-using them after thorough cleaning and drying (Roe, 1993).

Leg drainage bags

A variety of supports are available for use with these bags, including sporran waist belts, leg holsters, knickers/pants, and leg straps (Roe, 1992).

Catheter valves

Catheter valves, which eliminate the need for drainage bags, are becoming increasingly popular. The valve allows the bladder to fill and empty intermittently, and is particularly appropriate for patients who require long-term catheterization, as they do not require a drainage bag. Little research into the advantages and disadvantages of catheter valves has been completed.

Intermittent self-catheterization (ISC)

This is not a new technique, although it has become noticeably more popular in recent years.

This procedure involves the episodic introduction of a catheter into the bladder to remove urine. After this the catheter is removed, leaving the patient catheter-free between catheterizations. The patient should perform the catheterization as often as necessary to prevent incontinence or to prevent prolonged retention of urine (usually four or five times a day) (Seth, 1987).

Patients suitable for intermittent self-catheterization include:

(1) Those who can comprehend the technique.
(2) Those with a reasonable degree of manual dexterity.
(3) Those who are highly motivated.
(4) Those who have a willing partner to perform the technique (i.e. if agreeable to both).
(5) Those who can position themselves to attain reasonable access to the urethra (especially females) (Seth, 1987).

In 1970, Lasides, in the USA, found that patients using a clean rather than a sterile technique did not encounter problematic urinary tract infection. The catheters used for intermittent self-catheterization are technically described as semi-disposable, i.e. they are designed to be washed and re-used for a limited period only, usually one week.

They should always be rinsed in running water and properly dried after use; between uses they should be kept in a container such as a plastic envelope (Simcare booklet).

References and further reading

Bard Ltd (1984) *Guidelines for the Management of the Catheterized Patient.* Bard Ltd.

Bard Ltd (1987) *You, Your Patients, and Urinary Catheters.* Bard Ltd.

Bielski, M. (1980) Preventing infection in the catheterized patient. *Nursing Clinics of North America*, 15, 703–13.

Blandy, J. P. & Moors, J. (1989) *Urology for Nurses.* Blackwell Science, Oxford.

Blannin, J. P. & Hobden, J. (1980) The catheter of choice. *Nursing Times*, 76, 2092–3.

Britton, P. M. & Wright, E. S. (1990) Catheters: making an informed choice. *Professional Nurse*, 5(4), 194, 196–8.

Brocklehurst, J. C. *et al.* (1988) A new urethral catheter. *British Journal of Medicine*, 296, 1691–3.

Brunner, L. S. & Suddarth, D. S. (1986) *The Lippincott Manual of Nursing Practice*, 4th edn. J. B. Lippincott, Philadelphia.

Chilman, A. M. & Thomas, M. (1987) *Understanding Nursing Care*, 3rd edn. Churchill Livingstone, Edinburgh.

Crow, R. A. *et al.* (1986) *A Study of Patients with an Indwelling Catheter and Related Nursing Practice.* Nursing Practice Unit, University of Surrey.

Crow, R. *et al.* (1988) Indwelling catheterization and related nursing practice. *Journal of Advanced Nursing*, 13(4), 489–95.

Crummey, V. (1989) Ignorance can hurt. *Nursing Times and Nursing Mirror*, 85, 67–8, 70.

Dance, D. A. B. *et al.* (1987) A hospital outbreak caused by chlorhexidine and antibiotic resistant *Proteus mirabilis. Journal of Hospital Infection*, 10, 10–16.

Department of Health (1992) *Drug Tariff.* HMSO, London.

Edwards, L. E. *et al.* (1983) Post-catheterisation urethral strictures: a clinical and experimental study. *British Journal of Urology*, 55, 53–6.

Gupta, J. (1988) Effectiveness of different methods: effectiveness of three methods of periurethral hygiene in urinary catheterized surgical female patients. *Nursing Journal of India*, 79(10), 257–8, 280.

Heenan, A. (1990) Indications for long-term catheterization. *Nursing Times*, 86, 70–1.

Kennedy, A. P. *et al.* (1983) Factors related to the problems of long-term catheterisation. *Journal of Advanced Nursing*, 8, 207–12.

Kristiansen, P. *et al.* (1983) Long-term urethral catheter drainage and bladder capacity. *Neurology and Urodynamics*, 2, 135–43.

Lowthian, P. (1989) Preventing trauma (in patients with

indwelling catheters). *Nursing Times and Nursing Mirror*, 85, 73–5.

McGill, S. (1982) Catheter management: it's size that's important. *Nursing Mirror*, 154, 48–9.

Mackenzie, J. (1993) Questioning the assumption that urinary catheterisation is a pain free event for women. *Journal of Clinical Nursing*, 2, 64–5.

Mackenzie, J. & Webb, C. (1995) Gynopia in nursing practice: the case of urethral catheterization. *Journal of Clinical Nursing*, 4, 221–6.

MacSweeney, P. (1989) Self-catheterization – a solution for some incontinent people. *Professional Nurse*, 4(8), 399–401.

Muctar, S. (1991) The importance of a lubricant in transurethral interventions. *Urologue [B]*, 31, 153–5 [translation].

Mulhall, A. (1990) Bacteria, biofilm and bladder catheters. *Nursing Times*, 86, 57.

Nacey, J. N. & Delahunt, B. (1991) Toxicity study of first and second generation hydrogel-coated latex catheters. *British Journal of Urology*, 67, 314–16.

Oliver, H. (1988) Continence supplement. The treatment of choice. *Nursing Times and Nursing Mirror*, 84, 70.

Phipps, W. J. *et al.* (1986) *Medical-Surgical Nursing: Concepts and Clinical Practice*, 3rd edn. C. V. Mosby, St Louis.

Reid, R. I. *et al.* (1982) Comparison of urine bag changing regimes in elderly catheterised patients. *Lancet*, 2, 754–6.

Roberts, J. A. *et al.* (1990) Bacterial adherence to urethral catheters. *Journal of Urology*, 144, 264–9.

Roe, B. H. (1992) Use of indwelling catheters. In: *Clinical Nursing Practice: The Promotion and Management of Continence*, (ed. B. H. Roe). Prentice Hall, Hemel Hempstead.

Roe, B. H. (1993) Catheter associated urinary tract infection: a review. *Journal of Clinical Nursing*, 2(4), 197–203.

Roe, B. H. & Brocklehurst, J. C. (1987) Study of patients with indwelling catheters. *Journal of Advanced Nursing*, 12, 713–18.

Seth, C. (1987) Catheters ring the changes. *Nursing Times and Nursing Mirror*, 84, *Community Outlook*, 12, 14.

Sibley, L. (1988) Confidence with incontinence. *Nursing Times and Nursing Mirror*, 84, 42–3.

Simcare (undated) *Intermittent Self-Catheterization – A Guide For Patients' Families*. Simcare, Lancing.

Slade, N. & Gillespie, W. A. (1985) *The Urinary Tract and the Catheter: Infection and Other Problems*. John Wiley, Chichester.

Stickler, D. J. & Chawla, J. C. (1987) The role of antiseptics in the management of patients with long-term indwelling bladder catheters. *Journal of Hospital Infection*, 10(3), 219–28.

Studer, U. E. (1983) How to fill silicone catheter balloons. *Urology*, 22, 300–302.

Tortora, G. V. & Grabowski, S. R. (1993) *Principles of Anatomy and Physiology*, 7th edn. Harper Collins College Publishers, New York and San Francisco.

Wilksch, J. *et al.* (1983) The role of catheter surface morphology and extractable cytotoxic material in tissue reactions to urethral catheters. *British Journal of Urology*, 55, 48–52.

Wright, E. (1988) Catheter care: the risk of infection. *Professional Nurse*, 3(12), 487–8, 490.

Wright, E. (1988) Minimising the risks of UTI. *Professional Nurse*, 4(2), 63–4, 66–7.

GUIDELINES: URINARY CATHETERIZATION

EQUIPMENT

1 Sterile catheterization pack containing gallipots, receiver, low-linting swabs, disposable towels.
2 Disposable pad.
3 Sterile gloves.
4 Selection of appropriate catheters.
5 Sterile anaesthetic lubricating jelly.
6 Universal specimen container.
7 0.9% sodium chloride or antiseptic solution.
8 Bactericidal alcohol hand rub.
9 Gate clip.
10 Hypo-allergenic tape.
11 Scissors.
12 Sterile water.
13 Syringe and needle.
14 Disposable plastic apron.
15 Drainage bag and stand or holder.

PROCEDURE

Male

Action	Rationale
1 Explain and discuss the procedure with the patient.	To ensure that the patient understands the procedure and gives his valid consent.
2 (a) Screen the bed.	To ensure patient's privacy. To allow dust and airborne organisms to settle before the field is exposed.
(b) Assist the patient to get into the supine position with the legs extended.	
(c) Do not expose the patient at this stage of the procedure.	To maintain patient's dignity and comfort.
3 Wash hands using bactericidal soap and water or bactericidal alcohol hand rub.	To reduce risk of infection.
4 Put on a disposable plastic apron.	To reduce risk of cross-infection from micro-organisms on uniform.
5 Prepare the trolley, placing all equipment required on the bottom shelf.	The top shelf acts as a clean working surface.
6 Take the trolley to the patient's bedside, disturbing screens as little as possible.	To minimize airborne contamination.
7 Open the outer cover of the catheterization pack and slide the pack onto the top shelf of the trolley.	To prepare equipment.
8 Using an aseptic technique, open the supplementary packs.	To reduce the risk of introducing infection into the bladder.
9 Remove cover that is maintaining the patient's privacy and position a disposable pad under his buttocks and thighs.	To ensure urine does not leak onto bedclothes.
10 Clean hands with a bactericidal alcohol hand rub.	Hands may have become contaminated by handling the outer packs.
11 Put on sterile gloves.	To reduce risk of cross-infection.
12 Place sterile towels across the patient's thighs and under buttocks.	To create a sterile field.
13 Apply the nozzle to the tube of anaesthetic lubricating jelly.	In preparation for applying the lubricating jelly.
14 Wrap a sterile topical swab around the penis. Retract the foreskin, if necessary, and clean the glans penis with 0.9% sodium chloride or an antiseptic solution.	To reduce the risk of introducing infection to the urinary tract during catheterization.
15 Insert the nozzle of the lubricating jelly into the urethra. Squeeze the gel into the urethra, remove the nozzle and discard the tube. Massage the gel along the urethra.	Adequate lubrication helps to prevent urethral trauma. Use of a local anaesthetic minimizes the discomfort experienced by the patient.

Guidelines: Urinary catheterization (cont'd)

Action	Rationale
16 Grasp the shaft of the penis, raising it until it is almost totally extended. Maintain grasp of penis until the procedure is finished.	This manoeuvre straightens the penile urethra and facilitates catheterization. Maintaining a grasp of the penis prevents contamination and retraction of the penis.
17 Place the receiver containing the catheter between the patient's legs. Insert the catheter for 15–25 cm until urine flows.	The male urethra is approximately 18 cm long.
18 If resistance is felt at the external sphincter, increase the traction on the penis slightly and apply steady, gentle pressure on the catheter. Ask the patient to strain gently as if passing urine.	Some resistance may be due to spasm of the external sphincter. Straining gently helps to relax the external sphincter.
19 Either remove the catheter gently when urinary flow ceases, or:	
(a) When urine begins to flow, advance the catheter almost to its bifurcation.	Advancing the catheter ensures that it is correctly positioned in the bladder.
(b) Inflate the balloon according to the manufacturer's direction, having ensured that the catheter is draining properly beforehand.	Inadvertent inflation of the balloon in the urethra causes pain and urethral trauma.
(c) Withdraw the catheter slightly and attach it to the drainage system.	
(d) Tape the catheter laterally to the thigh or on the abdomen.	This smoothes out the urethral curve and eliminates pressure on the penoscrotal junction which can lead to the formation of a fistula.
(e) Ensure that the catheter is not taut on the skin.	This allows room for movement should spontaneous erection occur.
20 Ensure that the glans penis is clean and then reduce or reposition the foreskin.	Retraction and constriction of the foreskin behind the glans penis (paraphimosis) may occur if this is not done.
21 Make the patient comfortable. Ensure that the area is dry.	If the area is left wet or moist, secondary infection and skin irritation may occur.
22 Measure the amount of urine.	
23 Take a urine specimen for laboratory examination, if required (see Chapter 38, Specimen Collection).	For further information, see the procedure on collection of a catheter specimen of urine, below.
24 Dispose of equipment in a yellow plastic clinical waste bag and seal the bag before moving the trolley.	To prevent environmental contamination. Yellow is the recognized colour for clinical waste.
25 Draw back the curtains.	
26 Record information (e.g. catheter type and size, balloon size, date) in relevant documents.	To provide a point of reference or comparison in the event of later queries.

Female

Action	Rationale
1 Explain and discuss the procedure with the patient.	To ensure that the patient understands the procedure and gives her valid consent.
2 (a) Screen the bed.	To ensure patient's privacy. To allow dust and airborne organisms to settle before the sterile field is exposed. To enable genital area to be seen.
(b) Assist the patient to get into the supine position with knees bent, hips flexed and feet resting about 60 cm apart.	
(c) Do not expose the patient at this stage of the procedure.	To maintain the patient's dignity and comfort.
3 Ensure that a good light source is available.	To enable genital area to be seen clearly.
4 Wash hands using bactericidal soap and water or bactericidal alcohol hand rub.	To reduce risk of cross-infection.
5 Put on a disposable apron.	To reduce risk of cross-infection from micro-organisms on uniform.
6 Prepare the trolley, placing all equipment required on the bottom shelf.	To reserve top shelf for clean working surface. (Also, see section on catheter selection.)
7 Take the trolley to the patient's bedside, disturbing screens as little as possible.	To minimize airborne contamination.
8 Open the outer cover of the catheterization pack and slide the pack on the top shelf of the trolley.	To prepare equipment.
9 Using an aseptic technique, open supplementary packs.	To reduce risk of introducing infection into the urinary tract.
10 Remove cover that is maintaining the patient's privacy and position a disposable pad under the patient's buttocks.	To ensure urine does not leak onto bedclothes.
11 Clean hands with a bactericidal alcohol hand rub.	Hands may have become contaminated by handling of outer packs, etc.
12 Put on sterile gloves.	To reduce risk of cross-infection.
13 Place sterile towels across the patient's thighs.	To create a sterile field.
14 Separate the labia minora so that the urethral meatus is seen. Using low-linting swabs, one hand should be used to maintain labial separation until catheterization is completed.	This manoeuvre helps to prevent labial contamination of the catheter and provides better access to the urethral orifice.
15 Clean around the urethral orifice with 0.9% sodium chloride or an antiseptic solution, using single downward strokes. Change gloves.	Inadequate preparation of the urethral orifice is a major cause of infection following catheterization. To reduce the risk of cross-infection.
16 Insert the nozzle of the lubricating jelly into the urethra. Squeeze the gel into the urethra, remove the nozzle and discard the tube.	Adequate lubrication helps to prevent urethral trauma. Use of a local anaesthetic minimizes the patient's discomfort.

Guidelines: Urinary catheterization (cont'd)

Action	Rationale
17 Place the catheter, in the receiver, between the patient's legs.	To provide a temporary container for urine as it drains.
18 Introduce the tip of the catheter into the urethral orifice in an upward and backward direction. Advance the catheter until 5–6 cm have been inserted.	The direction of insertion and the length of catheter inserted should bear relation to the anatomical structure of the area.
19 Either remove the catheter gently when urinary flow ceases, or: (a) Advance the catheter 6–8 cm. (b) Inflate the balloon according to the manufacturer's directions, having ensured that the catheter is draining adequately. (c) Withdraw the catheter slightly and connect it to the drainage system. (d) Tape the catheter and drainage system to the thigh.	This prevents the balloon from becoming trapped in the urethra. Inadvertent inflation of the balloon within the urethra is painful and causes urethral trauma. This prevents traction and tension on the bladder and friction in the urethra.
20 Make the patient comfortable and ensure that the area is dry.	If the area is left wet or moist, secondary infection and skin irritation may occur.
21 Measure the amount of urine.	
22 Take a urine specimen for laboratory examination if required.	For further information, see the procedure on collection of a catheter specimen of urine (below).
23 Dispose of equipment in a yellow plastic clinical waste bag and seal the bag before moving the trolley.	To prevent environmental contamination. Yellow is the recognized colour for clinical waste.
24 Draw back the curtains.	
25 Record information (e.g. catheter type and size, balloon size, date) in relevant documents.	To provide a point of reference or comparison in the event of later queries.

Note: when the bladder is very distended a gate clip should be applied to the drainage bag tubing to regulate the flow rate after 500 ml of urine have been drained. This prevents shock due to sudden reduction in intra-abdominal pressure. However, the catheter should not be left clamped because this allows bacteria, if present, to multiply above the clamp, increasing the risk of ascending infection.

An alternative way of preventing sudden emptying of the bladder on catheterization in the patient with a long history of urinary outflow obstruction would be to place the urinary collection bag at the height of the patient's bladder. This allows urine drainage to be gradual and controlled. However, once emptying has occurred, the bag should be placed below the level of the bladder to pevent pooling and potential ascending bacterial contamination.

GUIDELINES FOR PATIENTS: INTERMITTENT SELF-CATHETERIZATION

EQUIPMENT

1 Mirror (for female patients).

2 Appropriately sized catheters for male/female patients.
3 Lubricating gel.
4 Clean container (e.g. plastic envelope) for catheter.

PROCEDURE

Female

Action	Rationale
1 Wash hands using bactericidal soap and water or bactericidal alcohol hand rub, and dry them.	To reduce risk of cross-infection.
2 Take up a comfortable position, depending on mobility (e.g. sitting on toilet; standing with one foot placed on toilet seat).	To facilitate insertion of intermittent catheter.
3 Spread the labia and wash the genitalia from front to back with soap and water, then dry and insert the catheter, using lubricant if necessary. A mirror may be used to make genitalia more visible.	To reduce risk of introducing infection. For ease of insertion.
4 Drain the urine into a toilet or suitable container.	
5 Remove the catheter when flow has ceased.	
6 If catheter is to be re-used, wash through with tap water. Allow to drain and dry. Store in dry container.	To remove urine.
7 Wash hands, using bactericidal soap and water.	To reduce the risk of infection.

Male

Action	Rationale
1 Wash hands using bactericidal soap and water or bactericidal alcohol hand rub.	To prevent infection.
2 Stand in front of a toilet or a low bench with a suitable container if it is easier.	To catch urine.
3 Clean glans penis with plain water. If the foreskin covers the penis it will need to be held back during the procedure.	To reduce risk of infection.
4 Hold penis with left hand (if right handed), three forefingers underneath and the thumb on top. The penis should be held straight out. Coat the end of the catheter with lubricating gel.	To prevent trauma to the penoscrotal junction, also allows easier observation of procedure.
5 Pass the catheter gently with the right hand (or left, if left-handed); it can be felt as it passes the fingers holding the penis. There will be a change of feeling as the catheter passes through the prostrate gland and into the	The prostate gland surrounds the urethra just below the neck of the bladder and consists of much firmer

Guidelines for patients: Intermittent self-catheterization (cont'd)

Action

bladder. It may be a little sore on the first few occasions only. If there is resistance do not continue; withdraw the catheter and contact a nurse or doctor.

6 Urine will drain as soon as the catheter enters the bladder, so have the end positioned over the toilet or a suitable container.

7 Withdraw catheter slowly so that all the urine is drained. The catheter will slide out easily.

8 Wash catheter through if it is reusable and store in a clean container.

9 Wash hands and dry them.

10 A mirror to stand in front of is helpful for patients with a large abdomen.

11 Beware of patient having a vasovagal attack.

Rationale

tissue. Can enlarge and cause obstruction, especially in older men.

To keep the area clean.

To prevent stasis of residual urine.

To reduce risk of infection.

To reduce risk of infection.

For ease of observation.

This is caused by the vagal nerve being stimulated so that the heart slows down, leading to a syncope faint. If it happens, lie the patient down in the recovery position. Inform doctors.

GUIDELINES: COLLECTION OF A CATHETER SPECIMEN OF URINE

EQUIPMENT

1 Swab saturated with isopropyl alcohol 70%.
2 Gate clip.
3 Sterile syringe and needle.
4 Universal specimen container.

PROCEDURE

Action

1 Explain and discuss the procedure with the patient.

2 Screen the bed.

3 Only if there is no urine in the tubing, clamp the tubing below the rubber cuff until sufficient urine collects. (An access point is now available on catheter bags.)

  Wash hands using bactericidal soap and water or bactericidal alcohol hand rub.

Rationale

To ensure that the patient understands the procedure and gives his/her valid consent.

To ensure the patient's privacy.

To obtain an adequate urine sample.

To reduce risk of infection.

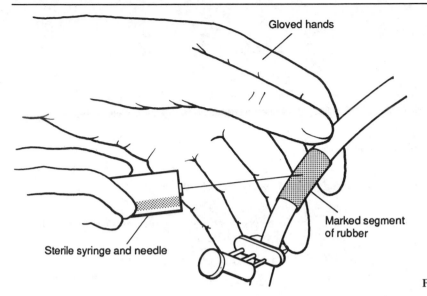

Gloved hands

Marked segment
of rubber

Sterile syringe and needle

Figure 45.2 Taking a specimen.

5	Clean the rubber cuff or access point with a swab saturated with isopropyl alchohol 70%.	To reduce risk of cross-infection.
6	Using a sterile syringe and needle, aspirate the required amount of urine from the rubber cuff or access point (Fig. 45.2).	If the catheter bag or tubing is punctured it causes leakage of urine and aspiration of air inwards, carrying organisms with it. Specimens collected from the catheter bag may give false results due to organisms proliferating there.
7	Place the specimen in a sterile container.	
8	Wash and dry hands with bactericidal soap and water.	To reduce risk of cross-infection.
9	Unclamp if necessary.	To allow drainage to continue.
10	Make the patient comfortable.	
11	Label the container and dispatch it (with the completed request form) to the laboratory as soon as possible after sample is taken to allow more accurate results from culture.	To ensure the best possible conditions for laboratory tests.

GUIDELINES: EMPTYING A CATHETER BAG

EQUIPMENT

1 Swabs saturated with 70% isopropyl alcohol.
2 Clean jug.
3 Disposable gloves.
4 Sterile jug.

Guidelines: Emptying a catheter bag (cont'd)

PROCEDURE

Action	Rationale
1 Explain and discuss the procedure with the patient.	To ensure that the patient understands the procedure and gives his/her valid consent.
2 Wash hands using bactericidal soap and water or bactericidal alcohol hand rub, and put on disposable gloves.	To reduce risk of cross-infection.
3 Clean the outlet valve with a swab saturated with isopropyl alcohol 70%.	To reduce risk of infection.
4 Allow the urine to drain into the appropriate jug.	To empty drainage bag and accurately measure volume of contents.
5 Close the outlet valve and clean it again with a new alcohol-saturated swab.	To reduce risk of cross-infection.
6 Cover the jug and dispose of contents in the sluice, having noted the amount of urine if this is requested for fluid balance records.	To reduce risk of environmental contamination.
7 Wash hands with bactericidal soap and water.	

GUIDELINES: REMOVING A CATHETER

EQUIPMENT

1 Dressing pack containing sterile towel, gallipot, foam swab or non-linting gauze.
2 Disposable gloves.
3 Needle and syringe for urine specimen, specimen container.
4 Syringe for deflating balloon.
5 Chlorhexidine solution to clean gloves.

PROCEDURE

Action	Rationale
1 Catheter usually removed early in the morning.	So that any retention problems can be dealt with during the day.
2 Explain procedure to patients and inform them of post-catheter symptoms, i.e. urgency, frequency and discomfort which are often caused by irritation of the urethra by the catheter. Symptoms should resolve over the following 24–48 hours. If not, further investigation may be needed. Encourage patient to exercise and to drink 2–3 litres of fluid per day.	So that patient knows what to expect, and can plan daily activity.
	For adequate flushing of bladder, especially to dilute and expel debris and infected urine, if present.

3	Wearing gloves, use saline to clean the meatus and catheter, always swabbing away from the urethral opening.	To reduce risk of infection.

In women, never scrub from the perineum/vagina towards the urethra.

To help reduce the risk of bateria from the vagina and perineum contaminating the urethra.

4	Clean/change gloves. Take a catheter specimen of urine using specimen port hole.	To assess if post-catheter antibiotic therapy is needed.

Curve catheter tubing so that the urine sample is taken from the top of the curve.

The catheter should not be clamped for this.

In case the catheter is left clamped for an excessive period of time, allowing bacteria to accumulate, and thus increasing the risk of infection.

5	Release leg support.	For easier removal of catheter.

6	Having checked volume of water in balloon (see patient documentation), use syringe to deflate balloon.	To confirm how much water is in the balloon. To ensure balloon is completely deflated before removing catheter.

7	Ask patient to breathe in and then out; as patient exhales, gently – but quickly – remove catheter. Male patients should be warned of discomfort as the deflated balloon passes through the prostate gland.	To relax pelvic floor muscles.

8	Clean meatus, tidy away equipment, and make the patient comfortable.

NURSING CARE PLAN

With the catheter in place

Problem	Cause	Suggested action
Urinary tract infection introduced during catheterization.	Faulty aseptic technique. Inadequate urethral cleansing. Contamination of catheter tip.	Inform a doctor. Obtain a catheter specimen of urine.
Urinary tract infection introduced via the drainage system.	Faulty handling of equipment. Breaking the closed system. Raising the drainage bag above bladder level.	Inform a doctor. Obtain a catheter specimen of urine.
No drainage of urine.	Incorrect identification of external urinary meatus (female patients). Blockage of catheter.	Check that catheter has been sited correctly. In the female if catheter has been wrongly inserted in the vagina, leave the catheter in position to act as a guide, re-identify the urethra and recatheterize the patient.

Nursing care plan (cont'd)

Problem	Cause	Suggested action
		Remove the inappropriately sited catheter.
	Empty bladder.	When changing the catheter, clamp the catheter 30 minutes before the procedure. On insertion of the new catheter, urine will drain.
Urethral mucosal trauma.	Incorrect size of catheter. Procedure not carried out correctly or skilfully. Movement of the catheter in the urethra.	Recatheterize the patient using the correct size of catheter. Check the strapping and reapply as necessary.
	Creation of false passage as a result of too rapid insertion of catheter.	Nurse may need to remove the catheter and wait for the urethral mucosa to heal.
Inability to tolerate indwelling catheter.	Urethral mucosal irritation.	Nurse may need to remove the catheter and seek an alternative means of urine drainage.
	Psychological trauma.	Explain the need for and functioning of the catheter.
	Unstable bladder. Radiation cystitis.	
Inadequate drainage of urine.	Incorrect placement of a catheter.	Resite the catheter.
	Kinked drainage tubing.	Inspect the system and straighten any kinks.
	Blocked tubing, e.g. pus, urates, phosphates, blood clots.	If a three-way catheter, such as Foley, is in place, irrigate it. If an ordinary catheter is in use, milk the tubing in an attempt to dislodge the debris; then replace it with a three-way catheter.
Fistula formation.	Pressure on the penoscrotal angle.	Ensure that correct strapping is used.
Penile pain on erection.	Not allowing enough length of catheter to accommodate penile erection.	Ensure that an adequate length is available to accommodate penile erection.
Paraphimosis.	Failure to retract foreskin after catheterization or catheter toilet.	Always retract the foreskin.
Formation of crusts around the urtheral meatus.	Infection involving urea-splitting organisms that cause deposits of salts to form around the catheter.	Correct catheter toilet.
Leakage of urine around catheter.	Incorrect size of catheter.	Replace with the correct size, usually 2 ch smaller.
	Incorrect balloon size.	Select catheter with 10 ml balloon.

	Bladder hyper-irritability.	Use Roberts tipped catheter. As a last resort bladder hyper-irritability can be reduced by giving diazepam or anticholinergic drugs.
Unable to deflate balloon.	Valve expansion. Valve displacement.	(1) Check the non-return valve on the inflation/deflation channel. If jammed, use a syringe and needle to aspirate by means of the inflation arm above the valve.
	Channel obstruction.	(2) Obstruction by a foreign body can sometimes be relieved by the introduction of a guidewire through the inflation channel. (3) Inject 3.5 ml of dilute ether solution (diluted 50/50 with sterile water or normal saline) into the inflation arm. (4) Alternatively, the balloon can be punctured suprapubically using a needle under ultrasound visualization. (5) Following catheter removal the balloon should be inspected to ensure it has not disintegrated leaving fragments in the bladder. *Note*: steps 2 to 4 should be attempted by or under the directions of a urologist. The patient may require cystoscopy following balloon deflation to remove any balloon fragments and to wash the bladder out.

After removal of the catheter

Problem	Cause	Suggested action
Dysuria.	Inflammation of the urethral mucosa.	Ensure a fluid intake of 2–3 litres per day. Advise the patient that dysuria is common but will usually be resolved once micturition has occurred at least three times. Inform medical staff if the problem persists.
Retention of urine.	May be psychological.	Encourage the patient to increase fluid intake.

Nursing care plan (cont'd)

Problem	Cause	Suggested action
		Offer the patient a warm bath. Inform medical staff if the problem persists.
Urinary tract infection.		Encourage a fluid intake of 2–3 litres a day. Collect a specimen of urine. Inform medical staff if the problem persists. Administer prescribed antibiotics.

Definition
Venepuncture is the term used for the procedure of entering a vein with a needle.

Indications
Venepuncture is carried out for two reasons:

(1) To obtain a blood sample for diagnostic purposes.
(2) To monitor levels of blood components.

REFERENCE MATERIAL
Venepuncture is the most commonly performed invasive procedure for hospital patients in the UK (Peters *et al.*, 1984). It is now becoming more routinely performed by nursing staff (Rowland, 1991). In order to do this safely the nurse must have a basic knowledge of the following:

(1) The relevant anatomy and physiology.
(2) The criteria for choosing both the vein and device to use.
(3) The potential problems which may be encountered.
(4) The correct disposal of equipment.

Certain principles, such as adherence to an aseptic technique, must be applied throughout. The circulation is a closed sterile system and a venepuncture, however quickly completed, is a breach of this system providing a method of entry for bacteria.

The nurse must be aware of the physical and psychological comfort of the patient (Sager & Bomar, 1980; Middleton, 1985; Weinstein, 1993). He/she must appreciate the value of adequate explanation and simple measures to prevent haematoma formation – a complication of venepuncture, not a natural consequence of it.

Anatomy and physiology
The superficial veins of the upper limb are most commonly chosen for venepuncture. These veins are numerous and accessible, ensuring that the procedure can be performed safely and with minimum discomfort (Carola *et al.*, 1992; Marieb, 1994). Occasionally, the veins of a lower limb may be utilized. This should be avoided if possible as blood flow in this region is diminished and the risk of ensuing complications is higher (Weinstein, 1993).

Criteria for choosing a site for venepuncture

Condition and accessibility of the peripheral veins
Veins may be tortuous, sclerosed, fibrosed or thrombosed, inflamed or fragile and unable to accommodate the device to be used. If the patient complains of pain or soreness over a particular site, this should be avoided, as should areas that are bruised in order to prevent further trauma to the vein. Veins adjacent to foci of infection must not be considered.

Preference is given to a vessel which is unused, easily detected by inspection and/or palpation, patent and healthy. These veins feel soft, bouncy and will refill when depressed (Weinstein, 1993).

Anatomical considerations
The venous anatomy of each individual differs, but care must always be taken to avoid adjacent structures, e.g. arteries and nerves. Accidental puncture of an artery may cause painful spasm and could result in prolonged bleeding. If a nerve is touched, this can result in severe pain and the attempted venepuncture at this site should be stopped (Yuan & Cohen, 1987).

Palpation is of value in distinguishing structures clinically, e.g. arteries and tendons, due to the presence of a pulse or resistance, and detecting deeper veins (Weinstein, 1993).

Use of veins which cross joints or bony prominences and those with little skin or subcutaneous cover, e.g. the inner aspect of the wrist, will subject the patient to more discomfort.

The sites of choice (Fig. 46.1) are branches of:

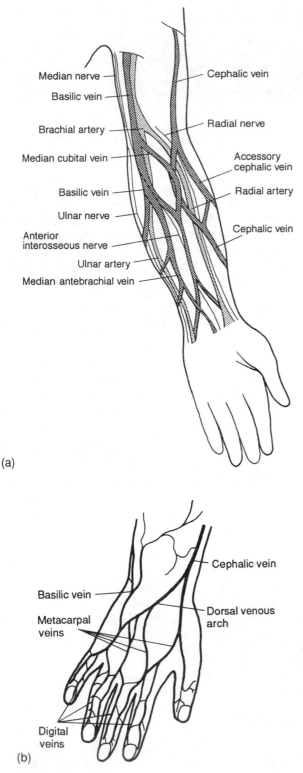

(a)

(b)

Figure 46.1   (a) Superficial veins of the forearm. (b) Superficial veins of the dorsal aspect of the hand. (Reproduced by permission from Becton Dickinson and Company.)

(1) The basilic vein.
(2) The cephalic vein.
(3) The median cubital vein in the antecubital fossa.

These are chosen because they are sizeable veins capable of providing copious and repeated blood specimens (Weinstein, 1993). The brachial artery and median nerve are in close proximity and must not be damaged.

The choice of vein, however, must be that which is best for the individual patient. When using other sites it is advisable to avoid junctions within the venous network. Another feature in veins is the presence of valves. These are folds of the endothelium present in larger vessels to prevent a backflow of blood to the extremity. If detected, a puncture should be performed above the valve in order to facilitate collection of the sample (Weinstein, 1993).

Clinical status of the patient

Injury or disease may prevent the use of a limb for venepuncture by reducing the venous access, e.g. amputation, fracture and cerebrovascular accident. Use of a limb may be contraindicated because of an operation on one side of the body, e.g. mastectomy. This can lead to impairment of lymphatic drainage which can influence venous flow regardless of whether there is obvious lymphoedema (Rowland, 1991). An oedematous limb should be avoided as there is danger of stasis of lymph, predisposing to such complications as phlebitis and cellulitis. Positioning of the patient may also dictate the site of the venepuncture (Rowland, 1991; Millam, 1992).

Physiological factors

The tunica media, the middle layer of the vein wall, is composed of muscle fibres capable of constricting or dilating in response to stimuli from the vasomotor centre in the medulla via the sympathetic nerves. The nurse must be aware of the factors which can influence venous dilation. These are:

(1) Anxiety.
(2) Temperature.
(3) Mechanical or chemical irritation.
(4) The clinical state of the patient, e.g. hypovolaemia due to dehydration.

Anxiety may be reduced by presenting a confident manner together with an adequate explanation of the procedure. Careful preparation and an unhurried approach will help to relax the patient and this in turn will increase vasodilation (Middleton, 1985; Millam, 1992; Weinstein, 1993).

The temperature of the environment will influence venous dilation. If the patient is cold, no veins may be evident on first inspection. Application of heat, e.g. in the form of a hot compress or soaking the arm in hot water will increase the size and visibility of the veins, thus increasing the likelihood of a successful first attempt. Ointment or patches containing small amounts of glyceryl trinitrate have been used to cause local vasodilatation to aid venepuncture (Hecker *et al.*, 1983; Gunawardene & Davenport, 1989).

Venepuncture may cause the vein to collapse or go into a spasm. This will produce discomfort and a reduction in blood flow. Careful preparation and choice of vein will reduce the likelihood of this and stroking the vein or applying heat will help resolve it.

The practitioner can prevent trauma to the tunica intima (the lining of the vein) by ensuring a smooth, atraumatic venepuncture and avoiding multiple or through punctures (Weinstein, 1993). Roughening of the smooth endothelium encourages the process of thrombus formation (Weinstein, 1993).

Choice of device

The intravenous devices commonly used to perform a venepuncture for blood sampling are a straight steel needle and a steel winged infusion device. The optimum gauge to use is 21 swg (standard wire gauge, which measures internal diameter – the smaller the gauge size, the larger the diameter. Standard wire gauge measurement is determined by how many cannulae fit into a tube with an inner diameter of 1 inch, and uses consecutive numbers from 13 to 24). This enables blood to be withdrawn at a reasonable speed without undue discomfort to the patient or possible damage to the blood cells.

The nurse must choose the device dependent on the condition and accessibility of the individual patient's veins (Table 46.1).

Given the concern about possible contamination of the practitioner by blood, a number of new systems of collection are now available commercially. The equipment available will depend on local policy.

Skin preparation

Asepsis is vital when performing a venepuncture as the skin is breached and an alien device is introduced into a sterile circulatory system. The two major sources of microbial contamination are:

(1) Cross-infection from practitioner to patient.
(2) Skin flora of the patient.

Good hand washing and drying techniques are essential on the part of the nurse; gloves should be changed between patients.

To remove the risk presented by the patient's skin flora, firm and prolonged rubbing with an alcohol-based solution, such as chlorhexidine 70% in spirit, is advised. This cleaning should continue for at least 30 seconds, although some authors state a minimum of 1 minute or longer (Rowland, 1991; Millam, 1992; Weinstein, 1993). The area that has been cleaned should then be allowed to dry to facilitate coagulation of the organisms, thus ensuring disinfection. The skin must not be touched or the vein repalpated before puncture.

Skin cleansing is a controversial subject and it is acknowledged that a cursory wipe with an alcohol swab does more harm than no cleaning at all as it disturbs the skin flora. Good cleaning techniques in a hospital environment, where transient pathogens abound, are of value in controlling infection (Weinstein, 1993).

Safety of the practitioner

With the increase over the past few years of blood-borne viruses, it is no longer appropriate to protect staff only when a disease is suspected or identified. Adherence to universal safe technique and practice is necessary, thus protecting staff from any potential blood spills.

While performing venepuncture, which is an invasive and therefore potentially hazardous procedure, manual

Table 46.1 The choice of intravenous device.

Device	SWG	Advantages	Disadvantages	Use
Needle	21	Cheaper than winged infusion devices. Easy to use with large veins	Rigid. Difficult to manipulate with smaller veins in less conventional sites. May cause more discomfort	Large, accessible veins in the antecubital fossa. When small quantities of blood are to be drawn
Winged infusion device	21	Flexible due to small needle shaft. Easy to manipulate and insert at any site. Causes less discomfort	More expensive than steel needles	Veins in sites other than the antecubital fossa. When quantities of blood greater than 20 ml are required from any site
	23	As above. Smaller swg and therefore useful with fragile veins	As above, plus there can be damage to cells which can cause inaccurate measurements in certain blood samples, e.g. sodium, potassium	Small veins in more painful sites, e.g. inner aspect of the wrist, especially if measurements are related to plasma and not cellular components

dexterity and sensitivity are required which may be reduced when wearing gloves (British Medical Association, 1991). The Department of Health (1990) have recommended that gloves should be worn when taking blood in the following circumstances:

* When the venepuncturist is inexperienced.
* When the health care worker has cuts or abrasions on the hands which cannot be covered by dressings alone.
* When the patient is restless.
* When the patient is known to be infected with HIV or hepatitis.

There is no substitute for good technique. It must always be remembered that although the use of gloves will protect practitioners from unexpected spillage, they will not prevent a needlestick injury if practice is not safe. Thus practitioners must always work carefully when performing this procedure.

Vacutainer systems should be used whenever possible, thus further reducing the risk of blood spillage. Used needles should always be discarded directly into an approved sharps container, without being resheathed.

Specimens from patients with known or suspected infections such as hepatitis or HIV should be double-bagged in clear polythene bags with a biohazard label attached. Only the required amount of blood should be drawn. The accompanying request forms should be kept separately from the specimen to avoid contamination. All other non-sharp disposables should be placed in a universal yellow clinical waste bag.

Summary

In order to perform a safe and successful venepuncture, it is important that the practitioner (a) considers carefully the choice of vein and device, and (b) applies the principles of asepsis, and adheres to and understands safe technique and practices.

Appropriate training, supervision and assessment by an experienced member of staff are essential when a nurse begins to practise venepuncture (Millam, 1992). It is important to remember that patients often dread venepuncture (Johnston-Early *et al.*, 1981) and the nurse's manner and approach may have a direct bearing on the patient's experience (Weinstein, 1993; Dougherty, 1994).

References and further reading

British Medical Association (1991) *A Code of Practice for the Safe Use and Disposal of Sharps*, pp. 20, 21. BMA, London.

Carola, R. *et al.* (1992) *Human Anatomy*, p. 533. McGraw Hill, USA.

Department of Health (1990) *Guidance for Clinical Health Care Workers: Protection against Infection with HIV and Hepatitis Viruses: Recommendations of the Expert Advisory Group on AIDS*. HMSO, London.

Dougherty, L. (1994) *A study to discover cancer patients' perceptions of the cannulation experience*. MSc thesis, University of Surrey, Guildford.

Dyson, A. & Bogod, D. (1987) Minimizing bruising in the antecubital fossa after venepuncture. *British Medical Journal*, 294, 1659.

Gunawardene, R. D. & Davenport, H. T. (1989) Local application of EMLA and glyceryl trinitrate ointment before venepuncture. *Anaesthesia*, 45, 52–4.

Hecker, J. F. *et al.* (1983) Nitroglycerine ointment as an aid to venepuncture. *Lancet*, 12 February, 332–3.

Johnston-Early, A. *et al.* (1981) Venepuncture and problem veins. *American Journal of Nursing*, September, 1636–40.

Marieb, E. N. (1994) *Essentials of Human Anatomy and Physiology*, 4th edn., p. 322. Benjamin/Cummings Publishing Company, California.

Middleton, J. (1985) Don't needle the patient. *Nursing Mirror*, 161(4), 22–3.

Millam, D. A. (1992) Starting IVs – how to develop your venepuncture skills. *Nursing*, 92, 33–46.

Peters, J. L. *et al.* (1984) Peripheral venous cannulation: reducing the risks. *British Journal of Parenteral Therapy*, March, 56–68.

Weinstein, S. M. (1993) *Plumer's Principles and Practice of Intravenous Therapy*, 5th edn. J. B. Lippincott, Philadelphia.

Rowland, R. (1991) Making sense of venepuncture. *Nursing Times*, 87(32), 41–3.

Sager, D. & Bomar, S. (1980) *Intravenous Medications – A Guide to Preparation, Administration and Nursing Management*. J. B. Lippencott, Philadelphia.

Sim, A. J. (1988) Intravenous therapy and HIV infection. *Intensive Therapy & Clinical Monitoring*, July/August, 140–5.

White, J. *et al.* (1970) Skin disinfection. *Johns Hopkins Medical Journal*, 126, 169–70.

Yuan, R. T. W. & Cohen, M. D. (1987) Lateral antebrachial cutaneous nerve injury as a complication of phlebotomy. *Journal of Canadian Intravenous Nurses Association*, 3(3), 16–17.

GUIDELINES: VENEPUNCTURE

EQUIPMENT

1 Clinically clean tray or receiver.
2 Tourniquet or sphygmomanometer and cuff.
3 21 swg multiple sample needle or 21 swg winged infusion device and multiple sample luer adaptor.

4 Plastic shell to hold specimen tubes.
5 Appropriate vacuumed specimen tubes.
6 Swab saturated with chlorohexidine in 70% alcohol.
7 Low-linting swabs.
8 Sterile adhesive plaster or hypoallergenic tape.
9 Specimen requisition forms.
10 Gloves, if necessary.
11 Plastic apron (optional).

There are a number of vacuum systems available that can be used for taking blood samples. These are simple to use and cost-effective. The manufacturer's instructions should be followed carefully if one of these systems is used. Vacuum systems reduce the risk of health care workers being contaminated, and are the method of choice for collecting blood samples using venepuncture. If not available, the following items replace the vacuum system:

(a) 21 swg needle or 21 swg winged infusion device.
(b) Syringe(s) of appropriate size.
(c) Appropriate blood specimen bottle(s).

PROCEDURE

Action	Rationale
1 Approach the patient in a confident manner and explain and discuss the procedure with the patient.	To ensure that the patient understands the procedure and gives his/her valid consent.
2 Allow the patient to ask questions and discuss any problems which have arisen previously.	A relaxed patient will have relaxed veins.
3 Check the identity of the patient matches the details on the requisition form.	To ensure the sample is taken from the correct patient.
4 Assemble the equipment necessary for venepuncture.	To ensure that time is not wasted and that the procedure goes smoothly without unnecessary interruptions.
5 Carefully wash hands using bactericidal soap and water or bactericidal alcohol hand rub, and dry before commencement.	To minimize risk of infection.
6 Check hands for any visibly broken skin, and cover with a waterproof dressing.	To minimize the risk of contamination, by blood, of the practitioner.
7 Check all packaging before opening and preparing the equipment on the chosen clinically clean receptacle.	To maintain asepsis throughout and check that no equipment is damaged.
8 Take all the requirements to the patient, exhibiting a competent manner.	To help the patient feel more at ease with the procedure.
9 In both an inpatient and an outpatient situation, lighting, ventilation, privacy and positioning must be checked.	To ensure that both patient and operator are comfortable and that adequate light is available to illuminate this procedure.
10 Consult the patient as to any preferences and problems that may have been experienced at previous venepunctures.	To involve the patient in the treatment. To acquaint the nurse fully with the patient's previous venous history and identify any changes in clinical status, e.g. mastectomy, as both may influence vein choice.

Guidelines: Venepuncture (cont'd)

Action

Rationale

11 Support the chosen limb.

To ensure the patient's comfort.

12 (a) Apply a tourniquet to the upper arm on the chosen side, making sure it does not obstruct arterial flow. The position of the tourniquet may be varied, e.g. if a vein in the hand is to be used it may be placed on the forearm. A sphygmomanometer cuff may be used as an alternative.

To dilate the veins by obstructing the venous return.

(b) The arm may be placed in a dependent position. The patient may assist by clenching and unclenching the fist.

To increase the prominence of the veins.

(c) The veins may be tapped gently or stroked.

(d) If all these measures are unsuccessful, remove the tourniquet and apply moist heat, e.g. a hot compress, soak limb in hot water or, with medical prescription, apply glyceryl trinitrate ointment/patch.

To promote blood flow and therefore distend the veins.

13 Select the vein using the afore-mentioned criteria.

14 Select the device, based on vein size, site, etc.

To reduce damage or trauma to the vein.

15 Wash hands with bactericidal soap and water or bactericidal alcohol hand rub.

To maintain asepsis.

16 Put on gloves, if appropriate.

To prevent possible contamination of practitioner.

17 Clean the patient's skin carefully for at least 30 seconds using an appropriate preparation and allow to dry. Do not repalpate the vein or touch the skin.

To maintain asepsis.

18 Inspect the device carefully.

To detect faulty equipment, e.g. bent or barbed needles. If these are present, discard them.

19 Anchor the vein by applying manual traction on the skin a few centimetres below the proposed insertion site.

To immobilize the vein.
To provide countertension, which will facilitate a smoother needle entry.

20 Insert the needle smoothly at an angle of approximately 30°. The shaft of a straight needle may be bent slightly at the hub, against the inside of the lid, to enable the entry to be as flush with the skin as possible.

To facilitate a successful, pain-free venepuncture.

21 Level off the needle as soon as a flashback of blood is seen in the tubing of a winged infusion device or when puncture of the vein wall is felt. If you are using a needle and syringe, pull the plunger back slightly prior to venepuncture and a

To prevent advancing too far through vein wall and causing damage to the vessel.

flashback of blood will be seen in the barrel on vein entry.

22	Slightly advance the needle into the vein, if possible.	To stabilize the device within the vein and prevent it becoming dislodged during venepuncture.
23	Do not exert any pressure on the needle.	To prevent a through puncture occurring.
24	Withdraw the required amount of blood using a vacutainer system or syringes.	
25	Release the tourniquet. In some instances this may be requested at the beginning of sampling as inaccurate measurements may be caused by haemostasis, e.g. blood calcium levels.	To decrease the pressure within the vein.
26	Withdraw a small amount of blood into the syringe.	To reduce the amount of static blood in the vein and therefore the likelihood of leakage.
27	Pick up a low-linting swab and place it over the puncture point.	
28	Remove the needle, but do not apply pressure until the needle has been fully removed.	To prevent pain on removal.
29	Discard the needle immediately in sharps bin.	To reduced the risk of accidental needle stick injury.
30	Apply digital pressure directly over the puncture site. Pressure should be applied until bleeding has ceased, approximately one minute longer may be required if current disease or treatment interferes with clotting mechanisms.	To stop leakage and haematoma formation. To preserve vein by preventing leakage or haematoma formation.
31	The patient may apply pressure with the finger but should be discouraged from bending the arm if a vein in the antecubital fossa is used (Dyson & Bogod, 1987).	To prevent leakage and haematoma formation.
32	Where a syringe has been used, transfer the blood to appropriate specimen bottles as soon as possible, making sure that the correct quantity is placed in each container.	To prevent clotting in the syringe. To ensure that an adequate amount is available for each test.
33	Mix well if the bottle contains a chemical to prevent clotting or aid accurate measurements.	To ensure that the blood is correctly presented to the laboratory and that the patient does not have to have a repeat specimen taken.
34	Label the bottles with the relevant details.	To ensure that the specimens from the right patient are delivered to the laboratory, the requested tests are performed and the results returned to the correct patient's records.
35	Inspect the puncture point before applying a dressing.	To check that the puncture point has sealed.
36	Ascertain whether the patient is allergic to adhesive plaster.	To prevent an allergic skin reaction.
37	Apply an adhesive plaster or alternative dressing.	To cover the puncture and prevent leakage or introduction of bacteria until healing is complete.

Guidelines: Venepuncture (cont'd)

Action	Rationale
38 Ensure that the patient is comfortable.	To ascertain whether patient wishes to rest before leaving (if an outpatient) or whether any other measures need to be taken.
39 Discard waste, making sure it is placed in the correct containers, e.g. 'sharps' into a designated receptacle.	To ensure safe disposal and avoid laceration or other injury of staff. To prevent re-use of equipment.
40 Follow hospital procedure for collection and transportation of specimens to the laboratory.	To make sure that specimens reach their intended destination.
41 Remove gloves and discard in appropriate clinical waste bag.	

NURSING CARE PLAN

Problem	Cause	Suggested action
Excessive pain.	Anxiety, fear, low pain tolerance.	Confident, unhurried approach. Use all methods, including heat, to dilate veins. Use of local anaesthetic cream. Avoid hesitancy and skin 'tickling'. Consider use of winged infusion device, as is may cause less discomfort on insertion.
	Frequently used vein.	Avoid this site, if possible, otherwise proceed as above.
	Nerve touched.	Remove the needle immediately and proceed to a different site.
Very anxious patient.	Previous trauma. Needle phobia.	Confident unhurried approach. Make sure the patient is comfortable, perhaps reclining/lying down. Use all methods such as heat, relaxation techniques, etc. to dilate veins. Consider use of winged infusion device.
Limited venous access.	Repeated use, e.g. prolonged cytotoxic therapy. Phlebitis.	Confident, unhurried approach. Use all methods including heat to dilate veins. Use a winged infusion device of 21 swg or 23 swg. Only proceed if sure of a successful first attempt. Consider referral to a more experienced colleague.

	Bruising due to: (1) Fragile veins in the elderly; (2) Anticoagulant therapy or low platelet levels.	As above plus apply tourniquet gently or do not use. Ensure adequate pressure to puncture site to prevent further damage.
	Peripheral shutdown.	Use all methods to dilate veins as listed. A sphygmomanometer and cuff may enable more effective restriction of the venous return. Work quickly if the patient is in a collapsed state. Pull blood back into the veins by massaging above the venepuncture site.
Infection.	Poor aseptic technique.	Practise good hand washing and skin cleansing and take particular care with immune-compromised patients.

Practical problems

Problem	Cause	Suggested action
Missed vein.	Inadequate anchoring. Wrong positioning. Poor lighting. Less than 100% concentration. Difficult venous access.	Withdraw the needle almost to the bevel and manoeuvre gently to realign needle and vein. Readvance, but if it becomes painful, remove. After two attempts seek assistance from more experienced colleague. Better preparation will minimize this problem.
Spurt of blood on entry.	Bevel tip of needle entering vein before entire bevel is under the skin, due to vein being very superficial.	Ignore. Reassure the patient if a small blood blister develops.
Blood flow stops.	Overshooting vein or advancing needle while withdrawing blood. Vein collapse due to contact with valve or vein wall.	Gently ease needle back and continue. Manoeuvre gently. Release and retighten tourniquet and continue.
	Poor blood flow.	As above and massage above the needle tip to pull blood into vein.
Haematoma.	Perforation of opposite wall of vein.	Insert needle at correct angle and stop when a flashback is seen in syringe or tubing of winged fashion infusion device. Do not advance needle during taking of sample.
	Forgetting to remove tourniquet before removing needle.	Remember next time.

Nursing care plan (cont'd)

Problem	Cause	Suggested action
	Inadequate pressure on puncture site.	Press. Supervise the patient doing the same.
Hardening of the veins due to scarring and thrombosis.	Prolonged use of one site.	Alternate venepuncture sites to prevent this. Do not use hard veins as this is often not successful and will cause the patient pain.
Mechanical problems.	Faulty equipment, e.g. bent needle tips, cracked syringes.	Check carefully before use and discard.
Transmittable diseases.	Viruses pose the major risk, causing hepatitis B, cytomegalovirus, acquired immune deficiency syndrome.	All blood should be handled with care and caution used when handling specimens from infected patients, e.g. Hepatitis B. Gloves should be worn when taking blood and handling samples. Hospital policy should be strictly observed.
Needle inoculation.	Lack of caution. Overfilling of 'sharps' containers.	Dispose of equipment safely to prevent inoculation. If it does occur, follow accident procedure and report the incident immediately. An injection of hepatitis B immunoglobulin may be required.

CHAPTER 47

Violence: Prevention and Management

Definition

Stuart & Sundeen (1991) define violence as 'an act of destructive aggression which may involve injury to the self, assaulting people or objects in the environment'.

Robinson (1983) defines aggression as 'an assertive force which may be expressed through attitude or behaviour and is usually directed to external objects, though it may be turned inward, as reflected in self-destructive behaviour'. She states that 'aggression is a healthy force which sometimes needs to be channelled'.

Indications

Management of violence is necessary:

(1) When the patient shows a predisposition to violence.
(2) When a patient makes a physical attack on another person.
(3) When a patient becomes disturbed to the extent that his/her behaviour is considered a threat to his/her own safety or the safety of others.

REFERENCE MATERIAL

Violent crime is increasing steadily on both sides of the Atlantic (Golding, 1995; Shepherd & Farrington, 1995). Similarly, violence and threats of violence against health care workers are increasing at alarming rates (Casseta, 1993). Incidents range from threats and abuse to permanently disabling injuries and, rarely, loss of life. This chapter is confined to the prevention and management of violence in the hospital setting.

Principles

The following principles underlie the management of violent patients:

(1) Prevention of violent incidents is the foremost principle.
(2) Restraint is always therapeutic, never punitive. As far as possible the therapeutic regime should be maintained.
(3) The risk of physical injury should be minimized.

Any restraint applied must be of a degree appropriate to the actual danger or resistance shown by the patient. This is particularly important with children and the elderly.

(4) The agreed procedure for the nursing care of violent patients should be adhered to.

Theories of violence

Mechanisms which may combine to explain or produce a violent act are reviewed by Harrington (1972) and Gunn (1973). Generally, theories of violence may be classified as biological (Lorenz, 1966; Gray, 1971; Montague, 1979), psychological (Freud, 1955; Dollard & Miller, 1961) or sociocultural (Bandura & Walters, 1963; Wertham, 1968; Gelles, 1972). Recent studies have shown associations between combat experience, posttraumatic stress disorder, anger and hostility, and involvement in violence (Reilly et al., 1994). Incidents of verbal or physical abuse are more likely to happen in extended care and emergency areas and may be directed towards nurses and nursing assistants rather than doctors. Staff gender is not strongly associated with the risk of abuse (Binder & McNeil, 1994; Graydon et al., 1994). Violence may be viewed as a behaviour influenced by various factors including personality, environment and social culture. Each perspective may add to the development of a body of knowledge about the problem of violence in the hospital setting.

Agitation and aggression preceding violent behaviour have been identified particularly among elderly confused patients, and nursing interventions such as feeding, dressing and bathing represented the most common antecedents (Campbell et al., 1989).

Physiological considerations

Under certain circumstances patients may have little or no ability to exercise control over their aggression. In these instances aggression may be related to pathological physiology. Internal stressors may include endocrine imbalance as in hyperthyroidism, hypoglycaemia, convulsive disorders, dementia and brain tumours. Krakowski & Czobor (1994) confirmed an association between persistent violence and neurological impairment. The effects of alcohol and substance abuse should also be considered. Preventive measures may not be appropriate and the policy for the management of violence should be adhered to.

In patients with HIV, there may be nervous system involvement (Royal College of Nursing, 1986). Between 50 and 60% of AIDS patients are estimated to develop neurological complications, and 60–70% of patients contract HIV encephalopathy. Symptoms include memory and concentration impairment and, less frequently, organic psychosis with agitation, inappropriate behaviour and/or hallucinations (McArthur et al., 1988). Although there have been no reported cases of violent incidents in hospitals involving patients with HIV or AIDS, the general principles for the management of such patients who become violent are no different to those for the management of other violent patients.

Policy formation for the care of violent patients or visitors

At present there are no national guidelines for nurses caring for violent patients. However, 'care and responsibility' is a method of training which has been adapted from techniques taught by Home Office personnel, which is appropriate to the requirements of a therapeutic regime. It is based upon a therapeutic value system and is concerned with returning autonomy and control to the individual rather than the simple and efficient control of 'difficult' individuals (Swan, 1994). The focus should therefore be on assessment of the individual and prevention of violent incidents.

In forming a policy for managing aggression, Miller (1990) suggests considering the following factors:

(1) The general philosophy of the unit and specific considerations like staff support, training, health and safety, service provision and systems of review.
(2) Psychological methods.
(3) Self-defence.
(4) Restraint.
(5) Seclusion.

Vousden (1987) describes methods of control and restraint as used in the prison service. However, it is important to stress that seclusion, control and restraint must only be used as a last resort (Vousden, 1987; McHugh et al., 1995). Nurses should therefore choose the most appropriate option according to the circumstances (McHugh et al., 1995). At all times the Code of Professional Conduct must be adhered to (UKCC, 1992). T. Swan (personal communication) advocates that it may be dangerous for health professionals to practise

control and restraint techniques without adequate training and that hospital managers need to be supportive in encouraging staff training and staffing levels.

Leiba (1980) isolates four aspects that need to be considered in the management of violence in the hospital setting:

(1) Organization of the ward, department, etc.
(2) Prevention.
(3) Management.
(4) Follow-up.

These are considered below.

Organization

The way in which staff are deployed influences the likelihood and outcome of any violent incident. There must be adequate staff to deal with the violence and there must be a hospital policy for the management of violence. All hospital personnel should know what to do and how to do it. Teaching sessions on the management of violence should be held on a regular basis so that staff benefit from controlled practice of the required techniques for avoiding and containing violence. Topics may include alternatives to violent behaviour, appropriate expression of emotions or stress reduction techniques (Green, 1989). Paterson et al. (1992) found that after a training course in the short-term management of violence, staff reported increased levels of success and confidence in their ability to manage violent incidents and reduced stress levels. It is helpful if there is a team in the hospital that can be called if an emergency occurs (Brayley et al., 1994). Teamwork is essential and the leader must be seen to be confident in making the necessary decisions. It is advisable to work in teams of three wherever possible, but where a one-to-one violent confrontation arises, using a breakaway technique is usually the safest option for staff and patient (T. Swan, personal communication). It is the responsibility of individual members of staff to state whether they have a physical condition, such as a back injury or pregnancy, which would render them incapable of performing procedures.

Prevention

Identify high-risk patients, examples of whom may be those with physiological conditions as previously discussed or patients with a previous history of violent behaviour. A multidisciplinary approach may be helpful in establishing this. Violent incidents may be spontaneous, without apparent provocation, for example with a patient suffering from a psychotic illness or cerebral lesions which affect behaviour. However, there may be warning signs which would alert staff to a potentially violent situation and give opportunity for prevention of violence.

Physical signs may include increased motor agitation, verbal content such as aggressive language, change in voice tone or volume, thigh tapping, fist clenching or sudden cessation of activity (Smith, 1987; Benson & Den, 1992). Responding to these cues to violence with verbal interaction can prevent escalation of an incident (Brennan & Swan, 1995). Stuart & Sundeen (1991) see violence as the culmination of an escalating process, where anger and aggression are considered as precursors to violence. They suggest that preventive therapeutic interventions can be used to intercept this process, thus deferring a potentially violent situation. Ritter (1989) suggests prevention of violence requires:

(1) Detailed individual assessment of patients.
(2) Close cooperation between multidisciplinary team members.
(3) Attention to the methods of communication used by the patient.
(4) Clearly defined systems for decision-making which allow the patient a degree of control.

Familiarity with risk indicators enables health care providers to intervene early when needed (Roberts & Quillian, 1992). Environmental measures can be taken to reduce aggression. Lighting, noise levels, furnishings and routine can be taken into consideration, while simple solutions such as providing information can alleviate frustration in waiting areas (Shuttleworth, 1989). Three steps have been identified in calming an agitated or aroused person:

(1) Diminish the anger as the person cannot deal appropriately with the problems while remaining aroused.
(2) Work at problem solving which involves clarifying the problem, providing solutions and aiming to evaluate them with the person.
(3) Carry out the actions decided upon with the person. Communication is vital and questions should be open, using 'how' and 'when' rather than 'why', which may be perceived as provocative. It should not be seen as a weakness of staff if they try to avoid violence (Brennan & Swan, 1995).

Knowledge of the propensities of individual patients will enable a nurse to recognize many of the signs of impending violence, thus allowing steps to be taken to help patients find alternative outlets for their aggressive feelings.

Management

The Overt Aggression Scale (Yudofsky *et al.*, 1986) can be used to identify patterns of aggression, support the use of medication and compare rates of seclusion, restraints, and 'as needed' medication at different facilities.

However, Hoff & Rosenbaum (1994) found that after developing a victimization assessment tool, staff viewed patients with a history of assault as less deserving of sympathy than those with no such history. McHugh *et al.* (1995) describe a model of 'de-escalation' in which physical restraint is a last resort. The aim is to foster autonomy in the patient and encourage one-to-one discussion with the nurse. Gould & Charlton (1994) found that substituting a controlling approach to patients with a supporting and valuing one had a positive effect on reducing levels of violence.

Once violence has occurred, the following may be regarded as among the important management decisions that need to be implemented:

(1) All medical and nursing personnel must be involved immediately, the former because medication may be required as part of the management of the situation.
(2) Some nurses must be delegated to attend to the needs of the remaining patients, to telephone for help and to prepare any required medication.
(3) If immobilization is needed, the agreed policy for restraining a patient must be implemented.

Follow-up

Following the incident, staff should be given an opportunity to discuss their feelings about the patient, other members of staff involved and the way the incident was managed. This should happen as soon as possible after the incident has resolved and with as many of the staff concerned as possible. Some staff view incident reporting as admission of failure, especially if violence is rare in the area in which they work (Drummond *et al.*, 1989), therefore debriefing becomes particularly relevant.

Staff injured as a result of their involvement in the incident may be entitled to industrial injuries benefit or a payment under the criminal injuries compensation scheme and will need to be informed of their rights by the appropriate body. All documentation required by law or hospital policy should be completed and forwarded to the appropriate departments. If restraints have been used, how and by whom they were applied should be documented. Specific written records will aid recall if it is required, perhaps years later (Navis, 1987).

Summary

Violent incidents often arise from a patient feeling vulnerable. Attack may become the preferred means of defence. The manner in which a patient is approached may be crucial in determining whether the patient will feel secure enough to cease the behaviour or continue to feel threatened, perhaps leading on to violent behaviour. The need for physical restraint should be seen as the application of the appropriate technique in a particular situation and not as a failure of other methods. Protection against any administrative or legal problems lies in following the appropriate guidelines and applying them in good faith and with due restraint.

References and further reading

Bandura, A. & Walters, R. (1963) *Social Learning and Personality Development*. Holt, Rinehart & Winston, New York.

Benson, S. & Den, A. (1992) Monitoring violence. *Nursing Times*, 88(41), 46–8.

Bethlem Royal and Maudsley Hospital (1976) *Guidelines for the Nursing Management of Violence*. Bethlem Royal and Maudsley Hospital, London.

Binder, R. & McNeil, D. (1994) Staff gender and risk of assault on doctors and nurses. *Bulletin of the American Academy of Psychiatry and Law*, 22(4), 545–50.

Blackburn, R. (1970) *Personality Types Among Abnormal Homicides. Special Hospitals Research Report No. 1*. Broadmoor Hospital, Special Hospitals Research Unit.

Brayley, J. *et al.* (1994) The violence management team: An approach to aggressive behaviour in a general hospital. *Medical Journal of Australia*, 161(4), 254–8.

Brennan, W. & Swan, T. (1995) Managing violence and aggression. In: *Royal College of General Practitioners, Members Reference Book*, pp. 443–5. Sabrecrown Publishing, London.

Campbell, B. *et al.* (1989) A high-risk occupation? *Nursing Times*, 85(13), 37–9.

Casseta, R. (1993) Group calls attention to violence against health care workers. *The American Nurse*, 3, 13.

Dollard, J. & Miller, N. E. (1961) *Frustration and Aggression*. Yale University Press, New Haven.

Drummond, D. J. *et al.* (1989) Hospital violence reduction among high-risk patients. *Journal of the American Medical Association*, 261(17), 2531–4.

Freud, S. (1955) *The Complete Psychological Works of Sigmund Freud*, Vol. 18. Hogarth Press, London.

Gelles, R. J. (1972) *The Violent Home*. Sage, Beverly Hills and London.

Golding, A. (1995) Leading article: Understanding and preventing violence: a review. *Public Health*, 109(2), 91–7.

Gould, J. & Charlton, S. (1994) The impact of change on violent patients. *Nursing Standard*, 8(19), 38–40.

Gray, J. A. (1971) Sex differences in emotional behaviour in mammals including man: endocrine basis. *Acta Psychologica*, 35, 29–44.

Graydon, J. *et al.* (1994) Verbal and physical abuse of nurses. *Canadian Journal of Nursing Administration*, 7(4), 70–89.

Green, E. (1989) Patient care guidelines: management of violent behavior. *Journal of Emergency Nursing*, 15(6), 523–8.

Gunn, J. (1973) *Violence*. David & Charles, Newton Abbot.

Harrington, J. A. (1972) Violence: a clinical viewpoint. *British Medical Journal*, 1, 228–31.

Hoff, L. & Rosenbaum, L. (1994) A victimization assessment tool: instrument development and clinical implications. *Journal of Advanced Nursing*, 20(4), 627–34.

Krakowski, M. & Czobor, P. (1994) Clinical symptoms, neurological impairment, and prediction of violence in psychiatric inpatients. *Hospital Community Psychiatry*, 45(7), 711–13.

Leiba, P. A. (1980) Management of violent patients. *Nursing Times*, Occasional Papers, 76(23), 101–4.

Lorenz, K. (1966) *On Aggression*. Harcourt, Brace & World, New York.

McArthur, J. H. *et al.* (1988) Human immunodeficiency virus and the nervous system. *Nursing Clinics of North America*, 23(4), 823–41.

McHugh, A. *et al.* (1995) Handle with care. *Nursing Times*, 91(6), 62–3.

Miller, R. (1990) *Managing Difficult Patients*. Faber & Faber, London.

Montague, M. C. (1979) Physiology of aggressive behaviour. *Journal of Neurosurgical Nursing*, 11, 10–15.

Navis, E. S. (1987) Controlling violent patients before they control you. *Nursing*, 17(9), 52–4.

Paterson, B. *et al.* (1992) An evaluation of a training course in the short-term management of violence. *Nurse Education Today*, 12, 368–75.

Reilly, P. *et al.* (1994) Anger management and temper control: critical components of post traumatic stress disorder and substance abuse treatment. *Journal of Psychoactive Drugs*, 26(4), 401–7.

Ritter, S. (1989) *The Bethlem Royal and Maudsley Hospitals Manual of Clinical Psychiatric Nursing Principles and Procedures*. Harper & Row, London.

Roberts, C. & Quillian, J. (1992) Preventing violence through primary care intervention. *Nurse Practitioner: American Journal of Primary Health Care*, 17(8), 62–70.

Robinson, L. (1983) *Psychiatric Nursing as a Human Experience*. W. B. Saunders, Philadelphia.

Royal College of Nursing (1986) *Nursing Guidelines on the Management of Patients in Hospitals and the Community Suffering from AIDS*. Royal College of Nursing, London.

Royal College of Psychiatrists and Royal College of Nursing (1979) *Principles of Good Medical and Nursing Practice in the Management of Acts of Violence in Hospitals*. Royal College of Psychiatrists/Royal College of Nursing, London.

Shepherd, J. & Farrington, D. (1995) Preventing crime and violence (editorial). *British Medical Journal*, 310(6975), 271–2.

Shuttleworth, A. (1989) Violence: is enough being done to protect you? *Professional Nurse*, 4(5), 227–8.

Smith, D. (1987) Preventing violence in nursing. *New Zealand Nursing Journal*, 80(12), 18–19.

Stuart, G. W. & Sundeen, S. J. (1991) *Principles and Practice of Psychiatric Nursing*, 4th edn. C. V. Mosby, St Louis.

Surrey Area Health Authority (1979) *Guidelines to Staff on the Management of Violent or Potentially Violent Patients*. Surrey Area Health Authority.

Swan, T. (1994) Definition of care and responsibility. In: *Guidance Document, Centre for Aggression Management*. Ashworth Hospital, Liverpool.

United Kingdom Central Council for Nursing, Midwifery and Health Visiting (1992) *Code of Professional Conduct*. UKCC, London.

Vousden, M. (1987) Are you safe? *Nursing Times*, 83(26), 28–33.

Wertham, D. J. (1968) *A Sign For Cain*. Hale, New York.

Yudofsky, S. *et al.* (1986) The Overt Aggression Scale for the objective rating of verbal and physical aggression. *American Journal of Psychiatry*, 143(1), 35–9.

GUIDELINES: PREVENTION AND MANAGEMENT OF VIOLENCE

PROCEDURE

Assessment of violence

Action

1 Involve all multidisciplinary staff concerned to assess if the patient is at risk of becoming violent. Some considerations are:
- (a) Endocrine imbalance, e.g. hyperthyroidism, hyperglycaemia.
- (b) Convulsive disorders.
- (c) Dementia.
- (d) Neurological impairment.
- (e) Alcohol and substance abuse.
- (f) HIV encephalopathy.
- (g) Pharmacological factors, e.g. drug toxicity.
- (h) Previous history of violence or aggressive behaviour, combat experience or post-traumatic stress disorder.
- (i) Social or psychological factors such as extreme stress.

2 Physical signs:
Increased motor agitation.
Verbal content such as aggressive language.
Change in voice tone or volume.
Thigh tapping.
Fist clenching.
Sudden cessation of activity.

3 Assess any nursing interventions which may be antecedents to aggression in individual patients, e.g. feeding, dressing and bathing.

Rationale

To prevent a violent situation. If the patient is at risk of becoming violent, steps should be taken to avoid violence arising.

Prevention of violence

Action

1
- (a) It is important that the nurse makes other staff aware of a potentially violent situation and does not enter it unobserved.
- (b) Try not to encroach upon the patient's personal space. Keep at arm's length.
- (c) If possible ask other patients to leave the area.
- (d) Ensure that there is a clear exit from the situation.
- (e) Avoid cornering the patient.
- (f) Observe the area around the patient for potential weapons.

Rationale

To maintain a safe environment for all patients, staff and visitors present and to avoid aggravating the situation further.

Guidelines: Prevention and management of violence (cont'd)

Action

Rationale

(g) Try to appear confident, calm and relaxed. Do not fold your arms, maintain an open posture. Move slowly, showing that you have nothing in your hands.

2 Talk quietly and clearly to the patient. Do not argue or become defensive.

The nurse may be able to gauge the patient's level of frustration and give an opportunity to express anger verbally by initiating conversation. Arguing or defensiveness may fuel the person's anger.

3 Ask open questions using 'how' and 'when' to help clarify the problem.

'Why' may be perceived as provocative.

4 Work at problem solving and carry out the actions decided upon with the patient.

This helps to diminish the anger as the problem is easier to deal with when the patient is less aroused.

5 Adopt an attentive expression but do not stare.

Staring could be interpreted as an attempt at domination (Brennan & Swan, 1995).

6 Address the patient by name and name yourself.

To help orientate the patient and demonstrate respect.

Management of violence

Action

Rationale

1 Consider carefully the accessories you wear. Be aware of the length of your fingernails and the way long hair is dressed. Pens, badges and other items should be removed beforehand.

To minimize the risk of physical injury to patients.

2 Call for assistance by shouting or using any signalling system. Ask another patient to summon help when appropriate.

It is easier to manage the situation with two or more people.

3 Other patients should be led away from the area where the patient is to be restrained.

Violent incidents are distressing and may trigger off more violence.

4 The person in charge of the ward or unit should assess whether or not there are enough staff, and inform the senior nurse if more are needed.

To contain the violence.

5 When help arrives, the staff should be organized. A leader should be nominated (e.g. the person in charge or patient's key worker) who should identify himself/herself to the patient as leader. He/she should give the other staff a brief history of the patient and an account of the circumstances and events leading up to the incident.

The staff will need to be informed to enable them to manage the situation.

6 A doctor, preferably the patient's own, should be called immediately. A nurse should be allocated to draw up medication and give injections if required.

Medication may be required in the management of the patient.

7	To restrain the patient, clear instructions should be given. The manager should indicate when the patient is to be restrained and coordinate staff during the procedure. Any disagreements between staff should not be voiced in front of the patient.	All staff must know the overall plan for restraint. Disagreements voiced in front of the patient are unprofessional and the patient may feel the staff are not in full control.
8	Each person should know which part of the patient's body is to be held and from where to approach the patient. (The policy for immobilization may vary from area to area.)	To achieve full immobilization of the patient.
9	Allocate one member of staff, preferably someone the patient knows, to talk to the patient throughout the procedure.	To inform the patient about what is happening and why.
10	Try to minimize discomfort. Restraint must be of a degree appropriate to the actual resistance given by the patient.	The procedure is not a punitive one.
11	As the patient calms down, the leader should indicate when restraint can be reduced. This should be done gradually, e.g. release one wrist at a time.	The patient may still be likely to strike.
12	The leader should withdraw staff from the patient gradually. Some staff should stay with the patient.	To observe mood and behaviour.

Follow-up

Action

Rationale

1	Attend to any patients and staff injured during the incident. Such people should be informed of their legal rights.	To provide care and to comply with legal obligations and hospital policy.
2	Record details of any violent incidents in the appropriate documents.	To comply with legal obligations and hospital policy.
3	The entire team should discuss the incident.	To ventilate feelings and evaluate care provided. Violent incidents are to be regarded as learning experiences and an opportunity for reflective practice.

CHAPTER 48
Wound Management

Definition of a wound

A wound can be defined as a cut or break in continuity of an organ or tissue caused by an external agent, such as injury or surgery (Cape & Dobson, 1978; *Dictionary of Nursing*, 1990), or a loss of continuity of the skin. Soft tissue, muscle and bone may or may not be involved (Milward, 1988). The first definition allows for tissue damage that occurs without a break in the skin, for example, 'bruising', the second includes the premise that a wound involves a break in skin.

Wounds are traditionally divided into four categories. These are:

(1) Contusion (bruise).
(2) Abrasion (graze).
(3) Laceration (tear).
(4) Incision (cut).

Puncture wounds may now also be incorporated into these groupings (Wingate & Wingate, 1988). Different causes of wounds include:

(1) External, e.g. burns (chemical, electrical, fire); hypoxia; mechanical; micro-organisms; radiation; temperature extremes.
(2) Internal, e.g. circulatory (venous, arterial, lymphatic); systemic (autoimmune, endocrine, haematological, neuropathies); local (infective, neoplastic) (David, 1986; Allen, 1988; Lawrence & Groves, 1988).

REFERENCE MATERIAL

Classification of wounds

Wounds can be classified in different ways depending on the information required and action to be taken on the data.

Classifications can be utilized to assess which treatment is most appropriate. These classifications most usefully contain an appraisal of the amount of tissue loss (Westaby, 1985). An example of such a system is that developed by the National Pressure Ulcer Advisory Panel (1989) which combines several of the most commonly used systems. There are four categories which begin with no tissue loss – 'non-blanchable erythema of intact skin' (stage one), and progress to 'full thickness skin loss with extensive destruction, tissue necrosis or damage to muscle, bone, or supporting structures' (stage four). The Panel also suggests that additional descriptions of these wounds, such as surface size, would assist in evaluation (National Pressure Ulcer Advisory Panel, 1989). Other gradings of pressure ulcers have been determined using a five-point scale (Dealey, 1988).

Further classifications that might prove valuable for assessment of treatment entail whether the wound is clean or infected or dry or wet. The following categories are described as worthwhile when considering the application of disinfectants to wounds:

(1) Dry, clean surgical wounds.
(2) Wet, oozing, clean surgical wounds.
(3) Open, contaminated wounds or lesions (Gustafsson, 1988).

A similar but more sophisticated system concerns both differing wounds and the various stages they pass through as they heal. This classification is designed for selection of a dressing:

(1) Black and necrotic – covered with a hard, dry layer of skin.
(2) Sloughy/necrotic – covered or filled with a soft yellow slough.
(3) Clean and granulating with a significant amount of tissue loss.
(4) Epithelializing (*The Dressing Times*, 1989).

In addition, surgical wounds can be identified as one of four types. These are: clean, clean contaminated, contaminated or dirty. This is dependent on the infection encountered (Cruse & Foord, 1980).

Some classifications consider the origin of the wound. For example: surgical trauma, accidental trauma or ulceration caused by pressure or vascular insufficiency (Turner, 1983); or intentional wounds and accidental wounds (Milward, 1988).

Although these classifications give an indication of the aetiology of the wound, from which some evaluation may be made of its likely nature, they are unsuitable for assessing relevant treatment. When treatment is deliberated, the most appropriate classifications will include those that consider both the degree of tissue loss and whether or not the wound is infected (Turner, 1983; Westaby, 1985).

Wound healing

Wound healing is the process by which tissues damaged or destroyed by injury or disease are restored to normal function (Cape & Dobson, 1978; Wingate & Wingate, 1988; Silver, 1994).

> 'Wound healing is only one aspect of the body's response to injury and the whole person, not just the visible injury, must be treated.'   (Torrance, 1985)

The latter statement reflects a holistic perspective and is, therefore, more appropriate as a framework for planning nursing care.

Healing may occur by first, second or third intention. Healing by first intention involves the union of the edges of a clean, incised wound under aseptic conditions without visible granulations (Cape & Dobson, 1978; *Dictionary of Nursing*, 1990; Dealey, 1994).

Healing by second intention signifies the process of contraction and epithelialization. The wound edges are separated and the cavity is gradually filled with granulation tissue from the bottom and the sides (Winter, 1972). Epithelial tissue grows over the granulations and forms fibrous tissue which contracts to form a scar (Cape & Dobson, 1978; Westaby, 1985; *Dictionary of Nursing*, 1990).

Healing by third intention occurs when the wound ulcerates and granulations are slow to form (*Dictionary of Nursing*, 1990).

Phases of wound healing

Wound healing is a complex series of physiological events which occur in a predictable sequence (Messer, 1989). Generally, the mechanism is described in three or four stages. These are:

(1) The inflammatory phase.
(2) The destructive phase.
(3) The proliferative or reconstructive phase or fibroplasia.
(4) The remodelling phase or maturation phase (Cooper, 1990; Jackson & Rovee, 1988; Johnson,

1988a; Messer, 1989; Torrance, 1985; Westaby, 1985; Silver, 1994).

These stages overlap to an extent but will be discussed individually to enhance clarity (see also Table 48.1). Contraction and epithelialization are also necessary to the wound healing process but are not usually included in the above stages. These will be considered separately.

Inflammatory stage (0–3 days)

Vasoconstriction occurs within a few seconds of tissue damage. This lasts approximately 5–10 minutes. During this time injured blood vessels bleed into the cavity and leucocytes arrive and marginate along the vessel walls. Platelets adhere to vessel walls and edges and are stabilized by a network of fibrin to form a clot. Bleeding ceases when the blood vessels thrombose. In the absence of noradrenaline (broken down by extracellular enzymes from damaged cells), and with the release of histamine, vasodilation begins. The liberation of histamine also increases the permeability of the capillary walls, and plasma proteins, leucocytes, antibodies and electrolytes exude into the surrounding tissues. The wound becomes red, swollen and hot.

Polymorphonuclear leucocytes and macrophages are chemotactically attracted to the wound to defend against infection and begin the process of repair. The macrophage is also known as the 'director cell' of wound healing. If the number and function of macrophages is reduced, as may occur in disease, e.g. diabetes (Tooke *et al.*, 1988), healing is seriously affected.

Destructive stage (2–5 days)

Polymorphonuclear leucocytes and macrophages combine to destroy and ingest bacteria, debris and devitalized tissue. This involves a great deal of cellular activity which requires up to 20 times the normal resting rate of oxygen of phagocytic cells. Patients with hypoxic wounds are, therefore, more susceptible to wound infection.

The degradation of unwanted material causes an increased osmolarity within the area resulting in further swelling by osmosis. This may increase pressure in restricted parts of the body thus precipitating ischaemia.

Proliferative stage (3–24 days)

Macrophages produce factors which are chemotactic to fibroblasts and angioblasts. The macrophage secretes a fibroblast-stimulating factor which in the presence of a growth factor released by the dead platelets causes the fibroplast to migrate into the wound soon after damage has occurred.

The fibroblasts are activated to divide and produce collagen by processes initiated by the macrophages. This develops a network of poorly organized collagen which increases the strength of the wound. Newly synthesized collagen creates a 'healing ridge' below an intact suture line, thus giving an indication of how wound healing is progressing. This mechanism is dependent on the presence of iron, vitamin C and oxygen. Therefore, appropriate levels of nutrition and oxygenation during this phase of wound healing are particularly necessary.

Angioblasts are required to form new blood vessels which grow into the wound under conditions of a hypoxic tissue gradient (Knighton *et al.*, 1981). The vessels branch and join other vessels forming loops. The fragile capillary loops are held within a framework of collagen. This complex is known as granulation tissue. Granulation tissue can grow into wound dressings such as gauze. On removal of the dressing any adhered delicate granulation tissue is also destroyed.

There is an acceleration of the inflammatory and proliferative phases in moist conditions compared to dry conditions (Dyson *et al.*, 1988).

Remodelling phase (24 days onwards)

In this stage the collagen is reorganized so the fibres are enlarged and oriented along the lines of tension in the wound (right angles to the wound margin). This occurs via a process of lysis and resynthesis. Intermolecular cross-linking aids to increase the tensile strength of the wound. Maximum strength (about 80%) is reached in approximately 3 months, although the scar never achieves the same strength as the original tissue.

(Winter, 1972; Torrance, 1985; Westaby, 1985; David, 1986; Jackson & Rovee, 1988; Johnson, 1988a; Pritchard & David, 1988; Messer, 1989; Cooper, 1990; Silver, 1994.)

Contraction

If the wound is clean and granulating, myofibroblasts round the edge of the wound contract in unison. This can reduce significantly the size of the wound and the area that the new tissue must cover. When the edges first contract (about 4 days from injury) the wound becomes larger but after 3 or 4 days the wound area begins to decrease, leaving a scar in approximately 3 weeks. The position of the wound is relevant to the success of healing by contracture. If the skin is attached to nearby structures this may result in its distortion and limitation of movement. However, wounds on the abdomen and breasts may close with a small amount of scarring (Torrance, 1985; Westaby, 1985; David, 1986; Johnson, 1988a; Messer, 1989; Thomas, 1990b).

Oxygen-treated burns have been found to increase contraction significantly and healing of the wound in animals. However, this was accompanied by thicker scar formation which could prove detrimental for aesthetic and rehabilitative reasons (Kaufman & Alexander, 1988).

Epithelialization

Epithelial cells will migrate across healthy granulation tissue only by 'leap-frogging' over each other and will burrow under contaminated debris and unwanted material. Splinters, dirt and sutures may be 'worked out' of the wound (Winter, 1972; Torrance, 1985; Westaby, 1985; David, 1986). Epidermal cells also secrete an enzyme which separates the scab from the underlying tissue. Dissolving the eschar requires nearly 50% of the cell's metabolic energy (Johnson, 1988a; Messer, 1989). Sources of epithelial cells include hair follicles, sweat glands and the perimeter of the wound (Johnson, 1988a; Torrance, 1985). As the epithelial cells migrate they begin to differentiate and cannot divide (Torrance, 1985). The ability of the epithelium to cover the wound surface is limited to approximately 2 cm. This means the process of contraction is of vital importance to healing in normal wounds (Messer, 1989).

Epithelialization (migration, mitosis and differentiation) is best achieved in moist conditions (Rovee *et al.*, 1972; Silver, 1994). Covering the wound in a polythene film accelerates epithelialization probably because hydration is maintained, while blowing air over wounds causes a deeper scab than normal to form and epidermal repair is delayed (Winter, 1972).

Raising oxygen tension in fluid in the wound has also been found to increase epidermal migration. This suggests that in normal wound healing the availability of oxygen may be the limiting factor (Winter, 1972). The epidermal migration under different types of films is perhaps directly related to their oxygen permeabilities (Winter, 1972). Oxygen breathing by man was not found to increase the partial pressure of oxygen in intact skin, while vasodilation produced by warming the body or limb did raise the oxygen tension (Silver, 1972). (Different results have been demonstrated in experiments involving animals (Knighton *et al.*, 1981).) This suggests that warming rather than giving oxygen may be of more clinical use, although this was probably not the limiting factor in the healthy subjects studied. Another trial is necessary in hypoxic patients.

Topical acidification has also been found to increase epidermal regeneration, and may prove to be of use therapeutically (Kaufman *et al.*, 1985; Glover, 1992).

Growth factors

Recent research has indicated that essential cellular activity that occurs during wound healing can be attributed to specific proteins known as growth factors (Cox, 1993). They are naturally occurring proteins secreted by cells in response to an injury and 'mediate, co-ordinate and con-

trol cellular interactions that occur during skin maintenance and wound healing' (Cox, 1993). This discovery
has led to advances in wound therapeutics (Devel, 1987;
Brown *et al.*, 1991; Robson *et al.*, 1992; Robson *et al.*,
1993). For example, a small study showed that a group of
patients with non-healing venous ulcers showed a significantly faster healing rate following treatment with
TGF-β2 growth factors (Robson *et al.*, 1993). This area
requires further research.

Only by understanding the different stages of wound
healing will the health carer be able to provide the appropriate treatment to produce the optimum wound
environment.

Factors affecting wound healing

The rate of healing of a wound varies depending on the
general health of the individual, the location of the
wound, the degree of the damage (David, 1986) and
the treatment applied.

Factors which may delay healing include systemic
variables such as disease, poor nutritional state and
infection. Other influences involve the local micro-
environment of the wound including temperature, pH,
humidity, air gas composition (Dyson *et al.*, 1988;
Kaufman and Berger, 1988; Kaufman & Hirshowitz,
1982; Rovee *et al.*, 1972), oxygen tension (Kaufman
& Alexander, 1988; Silver, 1972), blood supply,
inflammation, etc. Whether this influence is positive
or negative may depend on the stage of wound healing
that has been reached. Other important considerations
are external variables such as continuing trauma – possibly caused by treatment, the presence of foreign
bodies, etc.

It is necessary when treating a wound to appraise all
potential detrimental factors and minimize them, where
possible, in order to provide the optimum systemic, local
and external conditions for healing. Wound care begins
with the care of the patient.

Factors known to affect wound healing are listed in
Table 48.1.

Promotion of wound healing

General care of the patient

Promotion of wound healing concerns optimizing the
local, internal and external environments. This includes
the control of disease or underlying pathology, reduction
of external risk factors such as infection and maintaining
an ideal microclimate for healing in the wound (Table
48.1). Many factors need to be considered when assessing a patient with a wound.

Where possible, health care should be aimed at preventing wounding, for example, prevention of pressure
ulcers by regular turning and adequate nutrition. In addition, hydrocolloid dressings have been found to be
effective in preventing pressure ulcers in 'at risk' patients (Johnson, 1989).

The psychological care of the patient is important to
ensure acceptance of the wound and reduction in stress.
It is also imperative to assess and treat pain. Apart from
the obvious unpleasantness for the patient, this will also
lead to stress which will then delay wound healing.

Table 48.1 Factors that may delay wound healing.

Disease, disorders and syndromes	Addison's disease; anaemia; arteriosclerosis; auto-immune disorders; Buerger's disease; diabetes; cardiopulmonary disease; Crohn's disease; Cushing's syndrome; hepatic failure; hypovolaemia; hypoxia; immune disorders; infection; inflammatory bowel disease; jaundice; leucopenia; malignancy; protein losing enteropathy; Raynaud's disease; renal failure; respiratory conditions; rheumatoid arthritis; thyroid deficiency; uraemia; vascular diseases; venous stasis
Drugs	Alcohol; antimicrobials; cytotoxics; immunosuppressives; nicotine; non-steroidal anti-inflammatories; penicillamine and penicillin; steroids
Poor nutritional state	Anaemia; malnutrition; mineral deficiency (particularly zinc); protein deficiency; vitamin deficiency (particularly A and C)
Microenvironment of wound	Blood supply; gas composition; humidity; infection; inflammation; high pH; low temperature; oxygen tension
Other	Aetiology of wound; age; fibrous ring round open wound; foreign body in wound; obesity; radiation; stress; suture materials; suture technique; trauma/mechanical stress; treatment (including use of antiseptics and/or linting materials)

Note: some conditions may affect the healing process via several mechanisms.
(From: Silver, 1972; Kaufman & Hirshowitz, 1982; Rovee *et al.*, 1972; Kaufman *et al.*, 1985; Westaby, 1985; David, 1986; Deas *et al.*, 1986; Dyson *et al.*, 1988; Kaufman & Alexander, 1988; Kaufman & Berger, 1988; Tubman Papantonio, 1988a; Lycarotti & Leaper, 1989; Messer, 1989; Cooper, 1990; Cutting, 1994.)

Attention must be given to adequate nutrition of the patient since this is necessary for wound healing (Roberts, 1988). A dietitian's assessment is advisable. Patients are considered 'at risk' for wound healing if they have lost 20% or more of their body weight within the previous 6 months or 10% in the previous 2 months (Messer, 1989).

Protein and calorie malnutrition are possible in patients with chronic or acute malabsorption. This includes diabetes, Crohn's disease, alcohol abuse, gastrointestinal surgery, liver disease and long-term steroid therapy. Malignancy, major trauma, fever, inflammatory disease, smoking, drug use, stress and iatrogenic starvation are associated with deficient intake or high energy demands (Messer, 1989).

Patients at risk of inadequate vitamin A levels include those with severe diabetes and rheumatoid arthritis (Messer, 1989). Vitamin A supplementation in these patients has been found to improve wound healing and should be considered as a supplement in steroid-dependent patients for at least 5 days post-wounding (Messer, 1989). This may be related to the fact that vitamin A is a potent immune stimulant which, when administered topically or orally, will reverse much of the steroid suppression of wound healing. However, it is not as effective in reversing the effects of non-steroidal anti-inflammatory drugs (Hunt et al., 1969; Cohen & Cohen, 1973; Ehrlich et al., 1973; Hunt and Dunphy, 1979).

Patients with sepsis and those having undergone major trauma are also at risk of depletion of vitamin A. Supplementation of vitamin A should be contemplated for these groups (Messer, 1989). Vitamin C is necessary for collagen synthesis during the proliferative stage of the wound healing process. Deficiency of vitamin C is also associated with lowered resistance to infection (Morison, 1992). Patients with poor nutritional status may benefit from zinc supplements because of the role of zinc in DNA synthesis and the immune response (Wells, 1994).

In the absence of any malabsorption aetiology, the provision of adequate nutrition by diet or supplement is the easiest and often the cheapest method of ensuring the patient is nourished (Roberts, 1988). A thorough nutritional assessment is essential to identify actual or potential problems and to guide treatment.

The majority of chronic non-malignant wounds are hypoxic wounds (Messer, 1989). The major conditions that predispose to this are diabetes, venous stasis, vascular insufficiency, cardiopulmonary disease, irradiation, oedema, hypovolaemia and smoking (Messer, 1989). It is possible that hyperbaric oxygen therapy may be helpful for healing wounds in these patients. This involves the patient breathing 100% oxygen while in a chamber where the pressure is elevated above atmospheric pressure, and enables the amount of oxygen in solution to be increased. This has been used to successfully treat chronic unhealed wounds (Barr et al., 1990).

However, it is not always possible to overcome the deleterious effects of smoking with hyperbaric oxygen therapy while the patient continues to smoke (Messer, 1989). It is, therefore, important to educate patients and assist them in this aspect of their care by helping them to reduce or stop smoking.

Drugs that may delay wound healing should be reduced or withdrawn where therapeutically possible. This includes penicillamine which prevents collagen cross-linking (Messer, 1989).

Other factors that require consideration are: the necessity to maintain adequate fluid replacement post-operatively or post-trauma to prevent hypovolaemia (Messer, 1989); containing and removing infection (both local and systemic); use of measures to assist healing (for example, using mattresses which can reduce the healing time of sores) (Andrews & Balai, 1989), etc.

Physical and psychological rehabilitation may be necessary if the result of wounding and wound healing are debilitating and disfiguring and adjustment to changes in body image are necessary. This includes physiotherapy, counselling and occupational therapy.

Care of the microscopic wound environment

A considerable percentage of nurses' time is spent carrying out dressing procedures. Although research has examined wound physiology (Winter, 1971; Johnson, 1984; Ayton, 1985; Torrance, 1985; Westaby, 1985; Leaper, 1986; Turner et al., 1986) and wound dressings (Johnson 1984; Draper, 1985; Harkiss, 1985a, b; Ayton, 1985; Silver, 1994) there is little that appraises different dressing packs and procedures.

Packs and procedures should be designed for safety, comfort and ease and speed of use. Opinion and research indicate that forceps (especially those made of plastic) are clumsy, can cause pain and damage and are difficult to use (Wells 1984; Mallett, 1988). Gloves are a more suitable alternative and, in addition, should assist in reducing the risk of cross-infection.

Cotton wool or gauze used in cleaning can leave fibres in the wound. This may stimulate foreign body reaction and lengthen the inflammatory phase. Not only will this act as a focus for infection and damage new epidermis, but it will also retard wound healing (Winter, 1971, 1972; Turner, 1979; Johnson, 1984). Medical foam or low-linting material may be used instead. Appropriate use of hydrotherapy via a whirlpool, shower or a water or 0.9% sodium chloride stream can be utilized to remove debris or for debridement (Zederfeldt et al., 1980; Gogia et al., 1988; Jeter & Tintle, 1988; Trelstad & Osmundson, 1989).

Introduction of a less complicated wound dressing procedure and new pack containing medical foam and gloves instead of cotton wool and forceps was evaluated in one London hospital. This demonstrated that it was not only quicker to use but also that nurses preferred the new pack to the original pack (Mallett, 1988).

The implications of research suggest that traditional packs are likely to be detrimental to the patient and are also more difficult to use by the health care professional. Studies of new packs and procedures indicate that foam and gloves may be suitable subsitutes. Further research in this area is necessary.

Evaluation of the wound

The wound should be evaluated each time a dressing is applied or if it gives rise for concern. The aim of evaluating the wound is to assess healing and to establish which treatment will best provide the ideal environment for healing. The different classifications of wounds that relate to tissue loss and regeneration and absence or presence of infection may be of assistance in this process.

Factors that should be appraised include the underlying pathology of the wound. For example, if an ulcer is present on the leg, is it venous, arterial, lymphatic, malignant, etc? In addition, the surface area or volume of the wound should be measured. This can be carried out using a number of methods (Fincham Gee, 1990; McTaggart, 1994), and is necessary to ascertain the rate of healing. The amount and type of drainage is also

Table 48.2 Assessment of wounds.

Factor	Variables
General	Aetiology; location; presence of haematoma, seroma, oedema; amount of necrosis; open/closed; number of times requires dressing per unit time
Pain	Amount; at change of dressing; only when traumatized; intermittent; continuous; time of day; type of pain (e.g. sharp, stabbing, dull, etc.)
Stage of healing	Original tissue loss; amount of granulation and epithelial tissue; area/volume/depth of wound; temperature; sensation; inflammation
Drainage	Colour; consistency; nature/type; volume over time; odour
Area surrounding wound	Colour; oedema; erythema; sensation; turgor; other skin conditions
Infection	Amount of pus; pain; temperature; positive swab culture; inflammation

important, both in traumatic and surgical wounds.

A list of variables that require regular assessment is shown in Table 48.2.

Principles of cleaning the wound

The aim of wound cleansing is to help create the optimum local condition for wound healing by removal of excess debris, exudate, foreign and necrotic material, toxic components, the food source of potential infecting micro-organisms, bacteria and other micro-organisms (Wells, 1984; Turner et al., 1986; Gustafsson, 1988; Jeter & Tintle, 1988; Morison, 1989). Debridement is necessary to remove necrotic tissue which provides the ideal environment for bacterial growth and can hinder the healing process (Jackson & Rovee, 1988).

If the wound is clean and little exudate is present, repeated cleansing is contraindicated since it may damage new tissue, decrease the temperature of the wound unnecessarily and remove exudate (Morison, 1989). A fall in the temperature of the wound of 12°C is possible if the procedure is prolonged or the lotions are cold. This can take 3 hours or longer to return to normal warmth, during which time the cellular activity is reduced and therefore the healing process slowed (Stronge, 1984).

Sodium chloride (0.9%) used at body temperature is the safest and best cleansing solution for non-contaminated wounds (Ferguson, 1988; Jeter & Tintle, 1988; Tubman Papantonio, 1988b; Morgan, 1990). Although sodium chloride has no antiseptic properties it dilutes bacteria and is non-toxic to tissue (Morgan, 1990).

A number of other solutions have been used traditionally to clean wounds, some of which need to be used with caution (Table 48.3). An example of this is povidone-iodine. This is sometimes used in a weak aqueous solution (1%) as an antiseptic. However, solutions of 5% povidone-iodine, have been found to reduce blood flow in granulation tissue (Brennan & Leaper, 1985).

Some compounds used to clean wounds have documented deleterious effects on tissue or have been found to have detrimental effects in mammals. These include the much discussed sodium hypochlorite which is found in several wound cleansing solutions (Table 48.3). Eusol is a particularly well known solution containing sodium hypochlorite. Debate about its use has continued for a number of years. Many clinicians and researchers have recommended that it should not be used (Ferguson, 1988; Johnson, 1988b; Morgan, 1990; Spanswick et al., 1990) or not be used routinely (Morison, 1989). In view of the mounting evidence against sodium hypochlorite (Bloomfield & Sizer, 1985; Brennan and Leaper, 1985; Deas et al., 1986; Thorp et al., 1987) and the availability of a range of alternatives, the use of sodium hypochlorite

Table 48.3 Suitability of products used on wounds.

Suitable	Sodium chloride (0.9%) (safe, non-irritant and non-toxic)
	Tap water (used more frequently, especially on areas already colonized. Patients prefer to shower prior to dressing changes)
Not ideal, use with caution	Chlorhexidine – antiseptic (can cause sensitization and irritation; do not use alcoholic solutions)
	Hydrogen peroxide – antiseptic (use on dirty, infected, necrotic wounds only; do not use on large or deep wounds as may cause air embolism; may be caustic to skin and wound)
	Metronidazole – antibacterial (anaerobes only) (can cause nausea, neuropathy if used systemically)
	Potassium permanganate (0.01%) – mild antiseptic properties (causes staining of skin)
	Povidone-iodine (1%) antiseptic (do not use alcoholic solution; rarely causes skin reactions; some sources suggest that it should not be used on severe or extensive burns; if non-toxic goitre is present; or in pregnancy; or on lactating women)
Not suitable	Cetrimide – antibacterial and antifungal (toxic to wound tissue and causes skin hypersensitivity)
	Gentian violet – astringent, antiseptic (carcinogenic; is sometimes used on excoriating radiotherapy burns)
	Mercurochrome – weak bacteriostatic agent (toxic to tissue)
	Sodium hypochlorite – antiseptic (powerful oxidizing agent which is toxic to tissue)

(From: Valdes-Dapena & Arey, 1962; Bloomfield & Sizer, 1985; Brennan & Leaper, 1985; Deas *et al.*, 1986; Thorp *et al.*, 1987; *Nurses' Drug Alert*, 1987; Johnson, 1988a; Morison, 1989; Morgan, 1990; Farrow & Toth, 1991.)

is not recommended in this manual except for short-term use in exceptional circumstances, such as in recent war wounds and some patients' wounds in accident and emergency departments. Its use should be defined only by the clinical specialist.

Principles of dressing the wound

It is not possible or appropriate to describe here which dressing is most suitable for which types of wound, as each wound needs to be assessed individually. An ideal wound dressing may be described in general terms as follows:

> 'A material which, when applied to the surface of a wound, provides and maintains an environment in which healing can take place at the maximum rate.'
> (Turner *et al.*, 1986)

More specifically, to provide such an environment the dressing must be capable of fulfilling the following functions:

(1) To remove excess exudate and toxic components.
(2) To maintain a high humidity at the wound–dressing interface.
(3) To allow gaseous exchange.
(4) To provide thermal insulation.
(5) To be impermeable to bacteria.
(6) To be free from particulate or toxic components.
(7) To allow change without trauma (Turner, 1985).

In addition, the dressing should minimize pain, odour and bleeding and be comfortable and acceptable to the patient.

Occlusive dressings achieve many of these criteria. They affect the wound and healing in several ways.

Occlusive dressings have the ability to maintain hydration and prevent the formation of an eschar. This leads to a more rapid epithelial migration. The lag phase before epithelial cell proliferation and the time for epidermal differentiation is reduced. Wound contraction occurs more quickly and there is a decrease in some signs of inflammation (redness, oedema) as well as pain. Dermal repair is also accelerated (Rovee *et al.*, 1972; Dyson *et al.*, 1988; Jackson & Rovee, 1988; Winter & Hewitt, 1990).

Protocols have been developed which suggest different types of treatment depending on whether the wound is clean, infected or necrotic or shallow or deep (Johnson, 1988d). Dry dressings do not afford most of the criteria for an ideal dressing and should not be used as a primary contact layer (Dealey, 1991). Care should be taken with wounds that are difficult shapes to treat. These include long, narrow cavities which require a dressing that can be comfortably inserted into the space but removed easily without leaving any fibres behind (Bale, 1991) and without trauma. (See Table 48.4 for details of groups of dressings.)

Other treatments

Other treatments for wounds include the possibility of topical acidification (Kaufman *et al.*, 1985) and active treatment using growth factors or autologous platelet-derived factors (Jackson & Rovee, 1988).

Small, full-thickness skin loss can be repaired easily using skin grafts (Westaby, 1985). Where possible, it is preferable to use autografts. However, if donor sites are limited, homografts can be utilized. Muscle, tendon and bone may also be used to replace lost tissue (Pritchard & David, 1988).

Table 48.4 Dressing groups.

Dressing	Advantages	Disadvantages
Polymeric films	Only suitable for shallow wounds; prophylactic use against pressure sores; retention dressings; cool the surface of the wound; allow passage of water vapour; allow monitoring of wound	Possibility of adhesive trauma on removal; cool the surface of the wound
Dextranomers	Form stiff hydrophillic paste; useful in the treatment of infected wound cavities	Require retaining dressing
Hydrogels	Suitable for light to medium exuding wounds; reduce pain; cool the wound surface; desloughing abilities allow monitoring of wound; carrier for medications; good permeability gas profile; low trauma at change; non-allergenic; non-sensitizing; easy to use	Cool the surface of the wound; some hydrogels cannot be used on infected wounds. Please refer to manufacturers' recommendations with regard to particular products.
Hydrocolloids	Provide a moist wound environment suitable for assisting debridement of wound; swelling of hydrocolloid increases pressure on the base of the wound, *may* aid healthy granulation; pain relief; waterproof; provide thermal insulation; most provide a barrier to micro-organisms; low trauma at change; non-allergenic; non-sensitizing; easy to use	May release degradation products into the wound; strong odour produced as dressing interacts with exudate; some hydrocolloids cannot be used on infected wounds. Please refer to manufacturers' recommendations with regard to particular products.
Alginates	Suitable for heavily exuding wounds; highly absorbent; can be used on infected wounds; useful for sinus and fissure drainage; hydrophillic gel formed in the presence of sodium ions provides a moist wound environment; sodium chloride (0.9%) can be used to flush away some alginates; fibres trapped in the wound are biodegradable; some alginates are haemostatic in action; odour remission	Cannot be used on wounds that are not exuding or exuding lightly; cannot be used on wounds with hard necrotic tissue; sometimes a mild burning sensation occurs on application
Polyurethane foams	Suitable for use with open, exuding wounds; provide high thermal insulation; left *in situ* for long time	May be difficult to use in wounds with deep tracks

(From: Fraser & Gilchrist, 1983; Gilchrist & Martin, 1983; Lawrence, 1985; Mertz *et al.*, 1985; Pottle, 1987; Johnson, 1988c; Dealey, 1989; Goren, 1989; Piper, 1989; Margolin *et al.*, 1990; Thomas & Loveless, 1992; Benbow, 1994.)

PARTICULAR WOUNDS: LEG ULCERATION

REFERENCE MATERIAL

'Ulceration of the skin of the lower limb has been an affliction of the human race since the time of Hippocrates. It is almost certainly the price we pay for having emerged from the ocean and learnt to stand erect.'   (Burnand, 1990)

Prevalence and cost
Approximately 1% of the general population are affected by leg ulceration during their lifetime (Callam *et al.*, 1985). Ulceration is often recurrent (Callam *et al.*, 1987b), persistent (Dale & Gibson, 1986a), and affects more women than men (Anning, 1954; Dale & Gibson, 1986a; Callam *et al.*, 1987b; Ryan, 1987).

The annual cost of treatment to the National Health Service of leg ulceration is between £300 million and £600 million (Thomas, 1990a; West & Priestly, 1994). Leg ulceration treated by community nurses was estimated to use over £400 000 of resources in Paddington and North Kensington Health District in 1988 (Mallett & Charles, 1989); much of this is borne by the cost of the district nursing service (Callam *et al.*, 1987b).

Aetiology
The most common predisposing factors to leg ulceration are venous and arterial disease.

Venous disease
Venous disease has been found to be prevalent in 70–95% of cases (Fangrell, 1979; Callam *et al.*, 1987b; Williamson, 1988; Perkins, 1989). Venous hypertension

precipitating micro-oedema is probably the main cause of venous leg ulcers (Fangrell, 1979; Ryan, 1985b). This, in turn, can lead to lymphatic damage with resulting lymphoedema, fibrosis or liposclerosis (Robinson, 1988; Ryan, 1988a).

The reason that more women than men are prone to leg ulceration is due to the presence of varicose veins and episodes of deep vein thrombosis associated with pregnancy, which can lead to venous damage and ulceration in the affected leg (Dale & Gibson, 1986a; Ryan, 1987; Knight, 1990). In one study only 12% of women with varicose veins had never been pregnant, compared with 57% who had four or more pregnancies (Henry & Corless, 1989). In addition, further research indicates that multiple pregnancies enlarge the gonadal veins leading to vulvar, inner and posterior thigh and leg varicosities which do not follow the saphenous system. Symptoms are pain and heaviness in the thigh and legs and lateral aspects of the leg and foot (Lechter et al., 1987). Venous pathology is also related to the menstrual cycle, when the level of circulating oestrogens are at their lowest (Marcelon et al., 1988).

Warming can induce venous dilation resulting in decreased venous return and 'heavy legs' (Marcelon & Vanhoutte, 1988), and disorders relating to chronic venous insufficiency appear especially when the ambient temperature is high (Boccalon & Ginestet, 1988).

Venous ulcers are often described as occurring in the area around or on the medial malleolus, shallow and extensive and on the left leg (Falanga & Eaglstein, 1986; Matthews, 1986; Callam et al., 1987b; Ryan, 1987; Swanwick & MacLellan, 1988; Thomas, 1988a; Williamson, 1988). This may be associated to iliocaval syndrome which occurs when the left common iliac vein is compressed by the common iliac artery (Ryan, 1987; Taheri et al., 1987). These findings were not supported by the Paddington and North Kensington Health District survey, which suggested that significantly more ulcers were found on the anterolateral aspect of the lower leg. Ulceration was also statistically more likely to be on the right leg (Mallett & Charles, 1990). A larger, more recent survey has not strengthened either claim (Mallett and Charles, unpublished data).

Venous ulcers develop gradually and produce intermittent pain (Dale & Gibson, 1986a; Thomas, 1988a). Data from a survey in Parkside Health District do not support this.

Arterial disease

Between 4% and 30% of patients with leg ulceration have been reported to have arterial insufficiency. This proportion increases with age to 50% in the very elderly (Matthews, 1986; Callam et al., 1987a,b; Williamson, 1988; Perkins, 1989). Women are also more prone to arterial ulceration than men (Knight, 1990), although some research contradicts this (Callam et al., 1987a).

Arterial ulcers are deep and 'punched out' (Dale & Gibson, 1986b; Mani et al., 1988; Williamson, 1988; Perkins, 1989), and found on the feet or the anterior or lateral aspect of the ankle (Thomas, 1988a). These ulcers develop rapidly and give continuous or persistent pain, especially at night (Dale & Gibson, 1986c; Thomas, 1988a; Perkins, 1989). This is not supported by recent research.

Other predisposing and aggravating factors

Rheumatoid arthritis causes vasculitis which can lead to small, painful, 'punched out' ulcers (Williamson, 1988). In addition, treatment with steroids leads to thinning of the skin and susceptibility to trauma.

Diabetes is also associated with vasculitis and neuropathy, and has been found to be five times more common in patients with leg ulceration (Callam et al., 1987b).

Diastolic hypertension can lead to (usually) painful bilateral ischaemic ulceration, known as 'Martorell's ulcer' (Alberdi, 1988).

Blood disease, such as sickle cell anaemia or thalassaemia, can cause haematological ulcers (Hallows, 1987; Williamson, 1988).

Obesity, immobilization and dependency of the lower limb, limitation of ankle joint and poor gait due to ulceration (the last two both leading to an inadequately functioning calf muscle pump) can aggravate ulceration and contribute to its persistence (Callam et al., 1987b).

Treatment

It is imperative to distinguish between ulcers of varying pathologies as the management and treatment are very different. Assessment must be carried out to elicit which of the three vascular systems (arterial, venous and/or lymphatic) are diseased to provide the most appropriate care (Ryan, 1988a). Understanding and systematic management of the underlying disease, as well as topical wound care are necessary for a therapeutic approach (Falanga & Eaglstein, 1986). However, nurses and doctors may use the above factors associated with leg ulceration to appraise pathology. The problem arises when health care professionals are confronted with such concepts as 'shallow and extensive', 'develop rapidly', etc. Evaluation of the underlying pathology of ulceration must be underpinned where possible by definable and sound criteria.

Venous and lymphatic disease can be treated by improving the function of the calf muscle pump by graduated compression (Callam et al., 1987b; Dale & Gibson, 1987; Dale and Gibson, 1990; Blair et al., 1988b; Evans,

1988; Smith, 1988; Thompson, 1990). This has been found to be more important than certain types of dressing (Blair *et al.*, 1988a). The practical problems of applying compression stockings have been shown to adversely affect compliance with this treatment (Moffat & Dorman, 1995). Compression bandaging is detrimental to those with arterial insufficiency. Surgery may be necessary in these cases to increase the perfusion of the tissues, although it should be noted that arterial surgery can also lead to a decrease in the venous return time (Struckmann, 1988).

As with all wound care, it is important that nutritional requirements (especially vitamin A, vitamin C and zinc) are met and pain control is adequate (Cherry & Ryan, 1987; Hallows, 1987; Ryan, 1988a; Thomas, 1988b).

PRESSURE ULCERS OR DECUBITUS ULCERS

Definition
The terms 'decubitus ulcer' or 'pressure ulcer or sore' are used to describe any area of damage to the skin or underlying tissues caused by direct pressure or shearing forces. The extent of this damage can range from persistent erythema to necrotic ulceration involving muscle, tendon and bone.

REFERENCE MATERIAL

Cost
The cost of prevention and management of pressure sores has been a key issue in recent reports (e.g. Department of Health, 1994). It is estimated that the cost to the NHS may be as high as £400 million per year (McSweeney, 1994). There are no established criteria for assessing the cost of pressure ulcers, and whilst the cost of bed hire and wound care products can be calculated, it is difficult to estimate the cost of nursing care (West & Priestley, 1994).

A pressure sore prevention programme may be beneficial, but if comprehensive could also be costly. West & Priestly (1994) argue that although a prevention programme would involve costs in the short term, benefits would occur in the medium and long term (see also Taylor & Clark, 1994).

Aetiology of pressure ulcers
There are three major factors which have been identified as being significant contributory factors in the development of pressure ulcers. These are:

(1) Pressure. The blood pressure at the arterial end of the capillaries is approximately 30 mm Hg, while at the venous end this drops to 10 mm Hg (the average mean capillary pressure equals about 17 mm Hg (Guyton, 1984)). Any external pressures exceeding this will cause capillary obstruction. Tissues that are dependant on these capillaries are deprived of their blood supply. Eventually, the ischaemic tissues will die (David, 1986; Waterlow, 1988; Wyngaarden & Smith, 1988; Department of Infection Control, Memorial Hospital, 1989; Johnson, 1989). However, research has demonstrated that with constant pressure, even in denigrated tissues, a critical period of one to two hours exists before pathological changes occur (Kosiak, 1958, 1976).

(2) Shearing. This may occur when the patient slips down the bed or is dragged up the bed. As the skeleton moves over the underlying tissue the microcirculation is destroyed and the tissue dies of anoxia. In more serious cases lymphatic vessels and muscle fibres may also become torn, resulting in a deep pressure ulcer (Pritchard & David, 1988; Waterlow, 1988; Wyngaarden & Smith, 1988; Department of Infection Control, Memorial Hospital, 1989; Johnson, 1989).

(3) Friction. This is a component of shearing which causes stripping of the stratum corneum, leading to superficial ulceration (Waterlow, 1988; Wyngaarden & Smith, 1988; Johnson, 1989).

The most likely sites for pressure ulcer development are:

(1) Sacral area.
(2) Coccygeal area.
(3) Ischial tuberosities.
(4) Greater trochanters (Wyngaarden & Smith, 1988).

Identification of at-risk patients
Many predisposing factors are involved in the development of pressure ulcers:

(1) Immunosuppression (Waterlow, 1987).
(2) Immobility (Waterlow, 1988; National Pressure Ulcer Advisory Panel, 1989).
(3) Moisture (Wyngaarden & Smith, 1988).
(4) Inactivity (National Pressure Ulcer Advisory Panel, 1989).
(5) Faecal and urinary incontinence (Waterlow, 1988; Department of Infection Control, Memorial Hospital, 1989; National Pressure Ulcer Advisory Panel, 1989).
(6) Decreased level of consciousness (Department of Infection Control, Memorial Hospital, 1989; National Pressure Ulcer Advisory Panel, 1989).
(7) Infection (Waterlow, 1988).

(8) Circulatory diseases (for example, peripheral vascular disease, cardiac disease) (Barton, 1988; Department of Infection Control, Memorial Hospital, 1989).

(9) Personal hygiene (Waterlow, 1988).

(10) Neurological diseases (for example, multiple sclerosis) (Waterlow, 1988; Department of Infection Control, Memorial Hospital, 1989).

(11) Weight distribution (Waterlow, 1988).

(12) Treatment regimes (Waterlow, 1988).

(13) Malnutrition/nutritional status (Waterlow, 1988; Department of Infection Control, Memorial Hospital, 1989).

(14) Drugs which affect mobility (for example, sedatives) (Waterlow, 1988; Department of Infection Control, Memorial Hospital, 1989).

(15) Anaemia (Waterlow, 1988).

(16) Malignancy (Waterlow, 1988).

(17) Patient-handling methods (Waterlow, 1988; Department of Infection Control, Memorial Hospital, 1989).

(18) Shortage of nursing staff where patients require regular positioning (Department of Infection Control, Memorial Hospital, 1989).

(19) Design of beds, mattresses, chairs and wheelchairs (Department of Infection Control, Memorial Hospital, 1989).

(20) Advanced age (National Pressure Ulcer Advisory Panel, 1989).

(21) Fracture (National Pressure Ulcer Advisory Panel, 1989).

(22) Chronic systemic illness (National Pressure Ulcer Advisory Panel, 1989).

A patient's risk of developing a pressure ulcer should be assessed either on admission to hospital or in the community when they first come into contact with health services. The *UKCC Code of Professional Conduct* states that nurses have a responsibility to identify patients at risk (UKCC, 1993). Norton *et al.* (1985) and Waterlow (1991) developed 'at risk' scales, which are shown in Table 48.5 and Fig. 48.1. In Norton's scale, patients with scores of 14 or below are considered to run the greatest

risk of developing pressure ulcers. Patients with scores of 14–18 are not considered to be at risk, but they will require reassessment immediately any change in their condition is observed. Scores of 18–20 indicate patients at minimal risk. Waterlow's scale defines patients with a score of 11–15 as being 'at risk', 16–20 as 'high risk' and over 20 as 'very high risk' (Fig. 48.1, Waterlow, 1991). In one study (Smith, 1989), 22 (75.7%) of patients identified as being 'at risk' (scores of 10 and over) on admission using Waterlow's scale developed pressure ulcers. In the same study, 18 (62%) of patients with scores of 16 or less on the Norton scale developed ulcers. The author concludes that the Waterlow scale is more accurate at predicting formation of pressure ulcers. Further research in this area with a larger sample of patients is required.

Another study (Edwards, 1994) analysed the use of the Waterlow scale with elderly people in the community. The criteria for allocating scores do not have clear operational definitions and can be ambiguous. The risk factor was found to be overestimated in some cases, and therefore not an accurate guide to allocating resources. The author concludes that the Waterlow scale on its own is not a sufficient means of deciding how preventive resources are to be allocated to patients in the community.

Some departments have successfully devised their own risk assessment tools in response to local conditions (Birtwistle, 1994). Whilst assessment of risk is essential, the validity and reliability of tools should not be taken for granted (Nuffield Institute of Health, 1995).

Grades of pressure ulcers

If a pressure ulcer develops then classification of the wound will assist in determining the most appropriate treatment (see 'Reference material', above). There are, however, grading systems that have been produced specifically for use with pressure ulcers, such as that by David *et al.* (1983) (Table 48.6), or the National Pressure Ulcer Advisory Panel (1989). These are valuable in describing the state of the ulcer and the most pertinent care required by the patient.

A recent report suggested a new four stage classifica-

Table 48.5   The Norton Scale (Norton *et al.*, 1985).

Physical condition	Score	Mental condition	Score	Activity	Score	Mobility	Score	Incontinent	Score
Good	4	Alert	4	Ambulant	4	Full	4	Not	4
Fair	3	Apathetic	3	Walk/help	3	Slightly limited	3	Occasionally	3
Poor	2	Confused	2	Chairbound	2	Very limited	2	Usually/urine	2
Very bad	1	Stuporous	1	Bedfast	1	Immobile	1	Doubly	1

WATERLOW PRESSURE SORE PREVENTION/TREATMENT POLICY

RING SCORES IN TABLE, ADD TOTAL. SEVERAL SCORES PER CATEGORY CAN BE USED

BUILD/WEIGHT FOR HEIGHT	★	SKIN TYPE VISUAL RISK AREAS	★	SEX AGE	★	SPECIAL RISKS	★
AVERAGE	0	HEALTHY	0	MALE	1	TISSUE MALNUTRITION	★
ABOVE AVERAGE	1	TISSUE PAPER	1	FEMALE	2		
OBESE	2	DRY	1	14 - 49	1	e.g.: TERMINAL CACHEXIA	8
BELOW AVERAGE	3	OEDEMATOUS	1	50 - 64	2	CARDIAC FAILURE	5
		CLAMMY (TEMP↑)	1	65 - 74	3	PERIPHERAL VASCULAR	
CONTINENCE	★	DISCOLOURED	2	75 - 80	4	DISEASE	5
		BROKEN/SPOT	3	81+	5	ANAEMIA	2
COMPLETE/						SMOKING	1
CATHETERISED	0	**MOBILITY**	★	**APPETITE**	★		
OCCASION INCONT	1					**NEUROLOGICAL DEFICIT**	★
CATH/INCONTINENT							
OF FAECES	2	FULLY	0	AVERAGE	0	eg: DIABETES, M.S, CVA,	
DOUBLY INCONT	3	RESTLESS/FIDGETY	1	POOR	1	MOTOR/SENSORY	
		APATHETIC	2	N.G. TUBE/		PARAPLEGIA	4 - 6
		RESTRICTED	3	FLUIDS ONLY	2	**MAJOR SURGERY/TRAUMA**	★
		INERT/TRACTION	4	NBM/ANOREXIC	3		
		CHAIRBOUND	5			ORTHOPAEDIC -	5
						BELOW WAIST, SPINAL	
						ON TABLE > 2 HOURS	5

SCORE	10+ AT RISK	15+ HIGH RISK	20+ VERY HIGH RISK

MEDICATION	★
CYTOTOXICS, HIGH DOSE STEROIDS ANTI-INFLAMMATORY	4

© J Waterlow 1991 Revised May 1995

OBTAINABLE FROM: NEWTONS, CURLAND, TAUNTON, TA3 5SG

REMEMBER TISSUE DAMAGE OFTEN STARTS PRIOR TO ADMISSION, IN CASUALTY. A SEATED PATIENT IS ALSO AT RISK

ASSESSMENT: (See Over) IF THE PATIENT FALLS INTO ANY OF THE RISK CATEGORIES THEN PREVENTATIVE NURSING IS REQUIRED.
A COMBINATION OF GOOD NURSING TECHNIQUES AND PREVENTATIVE AIDS WILL DEFINITELY BE NECESSARY.

PREVENTION:
PREVENTATIVE AIDS:

Special Mattress/ Bed:
10+Overlays or specialist foam mattresses
15+Alternating pressure overlays, mattresses and bed systems.
20+Bed Systems: Fluidised, bead, low air loss and alternating pressure mattresses.
Note: Preventative aids cover a wide spectrum of specialist features. Efficacy should be judged, if possible, on the basis of independent evidence.

Cushions:
No patient should sit in a wheelchair without some form of cushioning. If nothing else is available - use the patient's own pillow.
10+ 4" Foam cushion.
15+ Specialist Gell and/or foam cushion
20+ Cushion capable of adjustment to suit individual patient.

Bed Clothing:
Avoid plastic draw sheets, inco pads and tightly tucked in sheets/sheet covers, especially when using Specialist bed and mattress overlay systems.
Use Duvet - plus vapour permeable cover

NURSING CARE

General: Frequent changes of position, lying/sitting. Use of pillows.
Pain: Appropriate pain control.
Nutrition: High protein, vitamins, minerals
Patient Handling: Correct lifting technique - Hoists - Monkey Pole - Transfer Devices
Patient Comfort Aids: Real sheepskins - Bed Cradle.
Operating Table: 4' cover plus adequate protection.
Theatre/A&E Trolley
Skin Care: General Hygiene, NO rubbing, cover with an appropriate dressing.

IF TREATMENT IS REQUIRED, FIRST REMOVE PRESSURE

WOUND CLASSIFICATION

Stirling Pressure Sore Severity Scale (SPSSS)
Stage 0 - No clinical evidence of a pressure sore.
0.1 - Healed with scarring.
0.2 - Tissue damage not assessed as a pressure sore. (a) see below

Stage 1 - Discolouration of intact skin.
1.1 - Non blanchable erythema with increased local heat.
1.2 - Blue/purple/black discolouration - The sore is at least Stage 1 (a or b).

Stage 2 - Partial-thickness skin loss or damage.
2.1 Blister   2.2 Abrasion
2.3 Shallow ulcer, no undermining of adjacent tissue.
2.4 Any of these with underlying blue/purple/black discolouration or induration. The sore is at least Stage 2 (a,b or c+d for 2.3, + e for 2.4)

Stage 3 - Full thickness skin loss involving damage/necrosis of subcutaneous tissue, not extending to underlying bone, tendon or joint capsule.
3.1 - Crater, without undermining adjacent tissue.
3.2 - Crater, with undermining of adjacent tissue.
3.3 - Sinus, the full extent of which is uncertain.
3.4 - Necrotic tissue masking full extent of damage.
The sore is at least Stage 3 (b, +/- e, f, g, +h for 3.4)

Stage 4 - Full thickness loss with extensive destruction and tissue necrosis extending to underlying bone, tendon or capsule.
4.1 Visible exposure of bone tendon or capsule.
4.2 Sinus assessed as extending to same. (b+/-e, f,g,h,i)

Guide to types of Dressings/Treatment
a. Semi-permeable membrane   f. Alginate rope/ribbon
b. Hydrocolloid   g. Foam cavity filler
c. Foam dressing   h. Enzymatic debridement
d. Alginate   i. Surgical debridement
e. Hydrogel

Figure 48.1 The Waterlow Pressure Sore Prevention/Treatment Policy (with permission).

Table 48.6 Pressure sore grades (David *et al.*, 1983).

Grade	Description
1	(a) Where the skin is likely to break down (red, black and blistered areas) (b) Healed areas still covered by a scab
2	Superficial break in the skin
3	Destruction of the skin without cavity (full skin thickness)
4	Destruction of the skin with cavity (involving underlying tissues)

tion scale. The scoring is dependent on observation alone and consists of four stages which relate to discoloration of skin, degree of tissue involvement, nature of the wound bed and infective complications. The user can choose the level of detail required, but it is recommended that at least two of the categories are used. The scale can be adapted for local conditions (Reid & Morrison, 1994).

Treatment of pressure ulcers

Treatment of pressure ulcers is the same as for any other wound. The aetiology and underlying or related pathology, as well as the wound itself, must be assessed in order to provide the most appropriate treatment. Care should be aimed at relief of pressure, the minimization of symptoms from predisposing factors and the provision of the ideal micro-environment for wound healing.

The most effective treatment for and prevention of pressure ulcers includes frequent turning or moving the patient (for example, at least every 2 hours), keeping the skin clean and using an air or foam mattress (David, 1986; Wyngaarden & Smith, 1988; Andrews & Balai,

1989). Of prime consideration in nursing care is the positioning and regular repositioning of the patient (Barbenel, 1990).

The affected area should not be rubbed as this causes maceration and degeneration of the subcutaneous tissues, especially in elderly patients (Dyson, 1978).

Devices used for relief of pressure

The most effective way of preventing pressure ulcers or facilitating healing is to minimize the pressure in the affected area(s). Usually it is sufficient for the patient to be nursed on alternating aspects of the body surface, provided they are repositioned regularly. Sometimes this is inappropriate or impossible due to individual patients' circumstances, for example, surgical intervention, body deformities, etc. (Barton & Barton, 1981).

A wide variety of devices are available to help relieve pressure over susceptible areas. These devices differ in function and complexity, and choice must be based on meeting the patient's individual need, sound criteria for decision-making, and effective use of available resources (Table 48.7) (Pritchard & David, 1988; Lockyer-Stevens, 1994). The research on the effectiveness of pressure relieving devices is largely insufficient and inconclusive and does not provide clear guidelines on which equipment is cost effective (Nuffield Institute for Health, 1995).

Taking into consideration all of the factors regarding wound pressure, prevention and management, it may be useful for nurses to collect and collate statistics and build up an accurate profile of patients and the nature of their problems. In this way it would be possible to evaluate the care given and provide information on potential areas of concern that further research could be based upon. This could result in an increase in the efficiency and cost effectiveness of wound and pressure sore management within a hospital or in the community.

FUNGATING WOUNDS

REFERENCE MATERIAL

Definition

A fungating wound is the result of a cancerous mass that infiltrates the epithelium and surrounding lymph and blood vessels. It can present as an ulcerating crater with a distinct margin or a raised fungating nodule (Moody & Grocott, 1993).

Aetiology

Fungating wounds can occur almost anywhere on the body. They arise most commonly from cancer of the

breast or head and neck, melanoma, soft tissue sarcoma and some cancers of the genito-urinary system (Thomas, 1992). No two fungating wounds are completely alike. Each patient responds individually to having such a wound, the consequences of which impinge on physical, psychological, social, sexual as well as spiritual well-being. The highest level of nursing expertise is required.

The incidence of fungating lesions is difficult to establish precisely. Thomas (1992), who conducted a survey of radiotherapy centres across the UK and received 114 completed questionnaires, reported that 295 patients with fungating wounds were seen in 1 month, and 2417 in 1 year; 62% of the wounds were breast lesions. He concludes that 'fungating wounds occur in sufficient numbers to represent a significant problem'.

Table 48.7 A selection of mechanical methods for relieving pressure.

Aid	Use	Advantages	Disadvantages
Sheepskin	Low risk patients. Norton score 14 or above. Good for under heels	Warm and comfortable. Decreases friction	Does *not* relieve pressure. Hardens and matts with washing. Needs to be changed frequently. *Not recommended* for regularly incontinent patients
Heel and elbow pads: sheepskin, foam, silicone	Norton score 14 or less or patients on prolonged bedrest	Reduce friction and shearing over the elbow and heel	Often have inadequate methods of keeping them on. Become hardened by washing
Silicone-filled mattress pad (e.g. Transoft)	Norton score 14 or less or patients on prolonged bedrest, able to move spontaneously	Relieves pressure by distributing it over a greater area. Comfortable. Machine (industrial) washable. Acceptable in community settings as well as in hospital. Can be used for incontinent patients. Relatively cheap purchase price. Plastic protective covers available	If the patient is very incontinent of urine, even if the plastic side is uppermost, there is seepage into the core material. Stitching comes undone after several launderings
Roho air-filled mattress	Norton score 10–14, high to medium risk. To wear off pressure equalizing beds	Interlinked air cells transfer air with movement. Patient can be nursed sitting or recumbent. Non-mechanical. Washable	Can be punctured and is expensive to repair. Often incorrectly inflated due to lack of understanding and education
Alternating pressure beds (Pegasus, ripple, Nimbus)	Medium risk, Norton score 12–14	Mechanical alteration of pressure. Reduce the frequency of (but not need for) repositioning. Available on hire at short notice	Older types prone to breakdown. Must be checked and maintained. May increase pressures in very thin patients. Punctures possible
Mechanaid netbed	Moderate risk patients. Norton score 14 or less	Fits any bed. Easy to assemble and dismantle. Easy to store. No servicing, maintenance or laundry difficulties. Patients can be repositioned by one nurse. Appears to encourage relaxation and sleep. Can be lowered on to the bed surface when a firm base is required	Patients do not always like it. Wedge of pillows needed to sit patient up. Patients may lose heat. Not always easy for patients to communicate with people sitting by bed
Water bed	Moderate risk, Norton score 12–16	Spreads pressure. Is warm and comfortable. Available on hire at short notice	Patient is supported on the skin of the water sac thus reducing the pressure-relieving properties. Difficult to get the patient in and out
Water flotation bed	Moderate to high risk patients. Norton score 14 or less	Equalizes pressure and weight. Heated	Expensive to buy, run and maintain. Makes some patients feel 'sea-sick'. Reduces self-motivated movement. Heavy to move. If not filled correctly can create more pressure than conventional bed. Not to be confused with water trough above
Fluidized air bed	High risk patients, Norton score 10 or less or indicated because of medical condition	As near to levitation as possible. Warm, sterile air produces a beneficial environment for healing wounds. One	Expensive to hire, run and in old buildings maintain. Need to reinforce floors before it

Table 48.7 *Continued.*

Aid	Use	Advantages	Disadvantages
		nurse can manage even very heavy or debilitated patients on his/her own. Can be used for incontinent patients or those with heavy wound exudate. May help to alleviate severe pain	can be installed. Minimizes self-motivation. Can be difficult for the patient to get in and out of bed even with help. Available on hire basis only
Low air loss bed	High risk patient, Norton score 10 or less. Orientated and immobile patients	Pressure-equalizing properties equal to the fluidized air bed. Patient can be nursed in any position including prone. (Patient can control position.) Mobilization easy	Expensive to buy but can be hired. Nurses need education in the use of the equipment

(From: Pritchard & David, 1988.)

Assessment

Assessment and evaluation of a wound are discussed earlier in the chapter, but it is important to emphasize that an accurate history of a malignant lesion should be taken, and that the management of the wound is documented clearly from the beginning. A wound assessment tool to record the amount and type of odour/exudate/pain, and the dressings used, is a helpful means of evaluating care strategies.

Problems associated with fungating wounds

Physical

(1) Wound is conspicuous.
(2) Pain/discomfort.
(3) Irritation/itching.
(4) Exudate.
(5) Odour.
(6) Bleeding/haemorrhage.
(7) Infection.
(8) Side-effects of treatment, e.g. radiotherapy.

Psychological/social/sexual

(1) Altered body image/relationship with partner.
(2) Embarrassment.
(3) Social isolation.
(4) Chronic nature of condition: situation may deteriorate.
(5) Impact on life: frequent dressing changes; hospital admissions/visits; treatment.

Aims of treatment

Malignant fungating lesions are an immense challenge. The aim of treatment is rarely to heal: care is focused on reducing the impact of symptoms and maximizing comfort (Saunders & Regnard, 1989; Fairburn, 1994). Quality of life is the guiding principle of care planning, which is undertaken in partnership with the patient.

Nurses must ensure that patients are aware that comfort, not cure is the aim, and respond to patients' needs sensitively. The chronic nature of malignant wounds means that patients are involved in an ongoing process of adjustment. Wounds are also a constant reminder to patients of advanced disease.

Management of symptoms

(1) *Pain.* Localized pain is sometimes experienced with wounds in addition to generalized pain which is addressed separately (see Chapter 31, Pain Assessment). A short-acting analgesic such as dextromoramide (e.g. Palfium) or nitrous oxide (e.g. Entonox) may be required to supplement the regular analgesic, for instance when dressings are changed.

(2) *Itching.* Irritation may occur around the margin of the wound (Fairburn, 1993). A gentle moisturising cream (e.g. Diprobase) or a barrier cream (e.g. Siopel) may provide relief. Irritation caused by radiotherapy may respond to topical hydrocortisone.

(3) *Exudate.* Exudate from a fungating lesion can act as a reservoir for infection (especially bacterial infection) (Collinson, 1992). Surgical debridement of necrotic and sloughy areas can control the production of exudate, but may be too extensive a procedure for some patients with advanced disease (Collinson, 1992; Fairburn, 1993). Plastic surgical procedures are often not feasible because of local invasion by the tumour (Moss, 1989). Less invasive measures (e.g. radiotherapy) may be beneficial in the

short term (Fairburn, 1993; Thomas, 1992). Wound dressings should be absorbent and non-adhesive (Fairburn, 1994), but can be bulky. The social and psychological effects of large, conspicuous dressings must be taken into account when selecting a suitable dressing (Thomas, 1992).

(4) *Malodour/infection.* Malodour is often an indication that a wound is infected (Dealey, 1994). Swabs should be taken to identify the causative organism before systemic and/or topical measures are adopted. Metronidazole as a gel has proved an effective agent for de-odourization of fungating lesions (Newman *et al.*, 1989; Thomas & Hay, 1991). It can be combined with a hydrogel for debridement of sloughy areas (Thomas & Hay, 1991). Charcoal dressings are also effective at controlling odour in less heavily exuding and less extensively infected wounds (Thomas, 1992; Fairburn, 1994). Small studies have been conducted on same other topical applications, but there is little substantial research evidence available:

- *Natural live yoghurt.* The wound is cleaned with 0.9% sodium chloride and the yoghurt applied for 10 minutes. The yoghurt is then rinsed away thoroughly, again with 0.9% sodium chloride. The wound is then dressed according to the plan of care. The process may be repeated three to four times daily (Welch, 1981; Schulte, 1993).
- *Sugar paste.* Useful for debridement and to aid regranulation of tissue. Twice daily application has been recommended for 'optimum antibacterial effect' (Middleton, 1990).
- *Icing sugar.* May be effective for de-odourizing lesions. The powder is sprinkled over the affected area, washed off and then re-applied as a viscid liquid (Thomlinson, 1980).

(5) *Bleeding/haemorrhage.* As the lesion increases in depth and extends at the margins, capillary bleeding may occur (Fairburn, 1994). Dressings should be loosened off by showering or soaking to prevent trauma. Alginate dressings may be useful for controlling capillary bleeding (Thomas, 1992). If bleeding is profuse, measures with an immediate effect may be taken:

- *Adrenaline 1 : 1000.* Acts as a vasoconstrictor when applied topically, but must be applied with caution because it is absorbed systemically (Dealey, 1994).
- *Transexamic acid.* Transexamic acid applied topically stems bleeding by inhibiting fibrinolysis (removal of clots from a wound). The literature on its mode of action refers only to cases of epistaxis (Jash, 1973).
- Haemostatic swabs are available which stimulate rapid capillary coagulation. They are most commonly applied in surgical procedures, but are becoming established in primary care to control bleeding in urgent cases (Twycross & Lack, 1990).

(6) *Dressings.* Numerous dressings are available to help overcome the problems associated with malignant wounds. Table 48.8 lists types of wound and recommended dressings according to Thomas's (1992) research data. The FP10 index is the drug tariff that general practitioners use to prescribe wound dressings for patients in the community. There are several limitations to this guide and it is important that hospital nurses are aware of dressing availability before they do their selection process (Dale, 1995).

Table 48.8 Dressings for the management of fungating wounds (adapted from Thomas, 1992).

Wound type	Recommended dressings
Bleeding wounds	Alginate sheet dressings (Kallostat or Sorbsan).
Lightly exuding wounds	Hydrocolloid sheets, semipermeable films, Lyofoam, Sorbsan SA or Kalloclude. Alternatively, Silicone NA or Tegapore used with a secondary dressing.
Heavily exuding wounds	Alginate sheets (e.g. Sorbsan, Kallostat) covered with an absorbent pad or Sorbsan Plus or Allevyn sheet may be applied.
Cavity wounds	Alginate rope or packing, Allevyn cavity wound dressing or Silastic foam.
Malodorous wounds	Dressings containing activated chareoal. e.g. Actisorb Plus, Kallocarb, Lyofoam C, topical metronidazole (Metrotop), Intrasite (Scherisorb) gel containing metronidazole, or sugarpaste.
Infected wounds	Topical metronidazole (Metrotop), or Intrasite (Scherisorb) gel with metronidazole, sugar paste. Sorbsan, products containing iodine or povidone-iodine, e.g. Inadine, Iodosorb.
Necrotic/sloughy wounds	Intrasite (Scherisorb) gel, Sorbsan, sugar paste, Debrisan paste, Iodosorb

(7) *Radiotherapy*. This can reduce the amount of exudate and control bleeding in malignant wounds. It is given either as a single fraction to avoid frequent hospital visits, or in divided doses over 2–3 weeks, in which case patients are admitted for the full course of treatment (Ashby, 1991). Occasionally radiotherapy is used prophylactically to prevent fungation if the skin is intact. If fungation has already occurred, radiotherapy may still be of value in reducing tumour bulk and enabling a degree of healing. Palliative radiotherapy of this kind is designed to spare healthy skin cells surrounding the wound and to avoid damage to the bed and margins of the wound (Horwich, 1992).

(8) *Hormone therapy*. Hormone therapy can reduce the rate at which a fungating wound progresses and deteriorates (Fairburn, 1993). Chemotherapy is occasionally used for this purpose, but hormone therapy has fewer side-effects and can enhance the patient's sense of well-being.

Fungating wounds pose a challenge in primary care, where district and Macmillan nurses are an invaluable resource in the important work of assessing wounds and liaising with hospitals and hospices about individual care plans. Clear, rational decision-making is vital to establishing trust with the patient and achieving maximum levels of comfort and quality of life.

Skilful communication is needed to help patients to adjust to the dependence that serious wounds may cause. Frequent hospital admissions and dressing changes, and deteriorating health, may leave patients and family feeling that their lives are being taken over by the illness. Psychological wounds, caused by embarrassment, changes in body image and, sometimes, social isolation, may never heal completely, but patients can be greatly helped by tact, understanding and supportive care.

References and further reading

Alberdi, J. M. Z. (1988) Hypertensive ulcer: Martorell's ulcer. *Phlebology*, 3, 139–42.

Allen, S. (1988) Ulcers: treating the cause. *Nursing Times*, 84(51), 62–3.

Andrews, J. & Balai, R. (1989) The prevention and treatment of pressure sores by use of pressure distributing mattresses. *Care – Science and Practice*, 7(3), 72–6.

Anning, S. T. (1954) Leg ulcers, their cause and treatment. Churchill, London. In: *The Management of Leg Ulcers* (1987), 2nd edn., (ed. T. J. Ryan). Oxford University Press, Oxford.

Ashby, M. (1991) The role of radiotherapy in palliative care. *Journal of Pain and Symptom Management*, 6(6), 380–88.

Ayton, A. (1985) Wounds that won't heal: wound care. *Community Outlook*, November 16–19.

Bale, S. (1991) A holistic approach and the ideal dressing. *Professional Nurse*, 6(6), 316–23.

Barbenel, J. C. (1990) Movement studies during sleep. In: *Pressure Sores – Clinical Practice and Scientific Approach*, (ed. D. L. Bader), pp. 249–60. Macmillan, London.

Barr, P. O. *et al.* (1990) Hyperbaric oxygen and problem wounds. *Care – Science and Practice*, 8(1), 3–6.

Barton, A. & Barton, M. (1981) *The Management and Prevention of Pressure Sores*. Faber & Faber, London.

Barton, A. A. (1988) Prevention of pressure sores. *Nursing Times*, 73, 1593–5.

Benbow, M. (1994) The benefits of hydrogel dressings. *Community Outlook*, October, 29–34.

Birtwistle, J. (1994) Pressure sore formation and risk assessment in intensive care. *Care of the Critically Ill*, 10(4), 154–5; 157–9.

Blair, S. D. *et al.* (1988a) Do dressings influence the healing of chronic venous ulcers? *Phlebology*, 3, 129–34.

Blair, S. D. *et al.* (1988b) Sustained compression and healing of chronic leg ulcers. *British Medical Journal*, 297(6657), 1159–61.

Bloomfield, S. F. & Sizer, T. J. (1985) Eusol BPC and other hypochlorite formulations used in hospitals. *Pharmaceutical Journal*, 3 August, 153–7.

Boccalon, H. & Ginestet, M. C. (1988) Influence of temperature variations on venous return: clinical observations. *Phlebology*, 3, Supplement 1, 47–9.

Brennan, S. S. & Leaper, D. J. (1985) The effect of antiseptics on the healing wound: a study using the rabbit ear chamber. *British Journal of Surgery*, 72, 780–2.

Brown, G. L. *et al.* (1989) Enhancement of wound healing by topical treatment with epidermal growth factor. *New England Journal of Medicine*, 321(2), 76–9.

Brown, G. L. *et al.* (1991) Stimulation of healing of chronic wounds by epidermal growth factor. *Plastic Reconstructive Surgery*, 88, 189–94.

Burnand, K. G. (1990) Aetiology of venous ulceration. *British Journal of Surgery*, 77, 483–4.

Callam, M. J. *et al.* (1985) Chronic ulceration of the leg: extent of the problem and provision of care. *British Medical Journal*, 290, 1855–6.

Callam, M. J. *et al.* (1987a) Arterial disease in chronic leg ulceration: an underestimated hazard? Lothian and Forth Valley Leg Ulcer Study. *British Medical Journal*, 294, 929–31.

Callam, M. J. *et al.* (1987b) *Lothian and Forth Valley Leg Ulcer Study*. Buccleuch Printers, Hawick.

Cape, B. F. & Dobson, P. (eds) (1978) *Baillière's Nurses' Dictionary*, 18th edn. Baillière Tindall, London.

Cherry, G. W. & Ryan, T. J. (1987) *Blueprint for the Treatment of Leg Ulcers and the Prevention of Recurrence*. Squibb Surgicare, Hounslow.

Cohen, B. E. & Cohen, I. K. (1973) Vitamin A: adjuvant and steroid antagonist in the immune response. *Journal of Immunology*, 3(5), 1376–1380. In: Messer, M. S. (1989) Wound care. *Critical Care Nursing Quarterly*, 11(4), 17–27.

Collinson, G. (1992) Improving quality of life in patients with malignant fungating wounds. In: *Proceedings of the 2nd European Conference on Wound Management*. Macmillan, London.

Cooper, D. M. (1990) Optimizing wound healing. *Nursing*

Clinics of North America, 25(1), 165–80.

Cox, B. D. *et al.* (1987) *The Health and Lifestyle Survey*, Health Promotion Trust, London.

Cox, D. A. (1993) Growth factors in wound healing. *Journal of Wound Care*, 12(6), 339–42.

Cruse, P. J. E. & Foord, R. (1980) The epidemiology of wound infection. *Surgical Clinics of North America*, 60(1), 27–40. In: Pritchard, A. P. & David, J. A. (eds) (1988) *The Royal Marsden Hospital Manual of Clinical Nursing Procedures*, 2nd edn. Harper & Row, London.

Cunliffe, W. J. (1990) Eusol – to use or not to use? *Dermatology in Practice* 8(2), 5–7.

Cutting, K. (1994) Factors influencing wound healing. *Nursing Standard*, 8(50), 33–7.

Dale, J. (1995) Wound dressings on the Drug Tariff. *Professional Nurse*, 10(7), 461–5.

Dale, J. J. & Gibson, B. (1986a) Leg ulcers: a disease affecting all ages. *Professional Nurse*, 1(8), 213–16.

Dale, J. J. & Gibson, B. (1986b) Leg ulcers: the nursing assessment. *Professional Nurse*, 1(9), 236–8.

Dale, J. J. & Gibson, B. (1986c) The treatment of leg ulcers. *Professional Nurse*, 1(12), 321–4.

Dale, J. J. & Gibson, B. (1987) Compression bandaging for venous ulcers. *Professional Nurse*, 2(7), 211–14.

Dale, J. J. & Gibson, B. (1990) Back-up for the venous pump. *Professional Nurse*, 5(9), 481–6.

David, J. A. (1983) Normal physiology from injury to repair. *Nursing*, 2(11), 296–7.

David, J. A. (1986) *Wound Management: A Comprehensive Guide to Dressing and Healing*. Martin Dunitz, London.

David, J. A. (1987) Beds. *Nursing*, 3(13), 503–5.

David, J. A. (1990) Recent venous ulcer treatments. *Nursing Standard*, 4(23), 24–6.

David, J. A. *et al.* (1983) *An Investigation of the Current Methods used in Nursing for the Care of Patients with Established Pressure Sores*. Nursing Practice Research Unit, University of Surrey.

Dealey, C. (1988) The role of the tissue viability nurse. *Nursing Standard*, 2(51), Supplement, 4–5.

Dealey, C. (1989) Management of cavity wounds. *Nursing*, 3(39), 25–7.

Dealey, C. (1991) Criteria for wound healing. *Nursing*, 4(29), 20–1.

Dealey, C. (1994) *The Care of Wounds*. Blackwell Science, Oxford.

Deas, J. *et al.* (1986) The toxicity of commonly used antiseptics on fibroblasts in tissue culture. *Phlebology*, 1, 205–9.

Department of Health (1994) *Pressure Sores: A Key Quality Indicator*. Department of Health, Leeds.

Department of Infection Control, Memorial Hospital (1989) *Blueprint for the Prevention and Management of Pressure Sores*. Convatec Ltd.

Devel. T. F. (1987) Polypeptide growth factors: roles in normal and abnormal cell growth. *Annual Review of Cell Biology*, 3, 443–64.

Dictionary of Nursing. Oxford Reference (1990) Consultant ed. P. Wainwright; general eds R. Fergusson *et al.* Oxford University Press, Oxford.

Draper, J. (1985) Make the dressing fit the wound. *Nursing*

Times, 81(41), 32–5.

Dyson, R. (1978) Bed sores – the injuries hospital staff inflict on patients. *Nursing Mirror*, 146(24), 30–2.

Dyson, M. *et al.* (1988) Comparison of the effects of moist and dry conditions on dermal repair. *Journal of Investigative Dermatology*, 91(5), 434–9.

Edwards, M. (1994) *The reliability and validity of the Waterlow pressure sore risk scale when used within district nursing to assess elders nursed in a domiciliary setting*. MSc dissertation, University of London.

Ehrlich, H. P. *et al.* (1973) The effects of vitamin A and glucocorticoids upon inflammation and collagen synthesis. *Annals of Surgery*, 2, 222–7. In: Messer, M. S. (1989) Wound care. *Critical Care Nursing Quarterly*, 11(4), 17–27.

Evans, P. (1988) Venous disorders of the leg. *Nursing Times*, 84(49), 46–7.

Fader, R. C. *et al.* (1983) Sodium hypochlorite decontamination of split-thickness cadaveric skin infected with bacteria and yeast with subsequent isolation and growth of basal cells to confluency in tissue culture. *Antimicrobial Agents and Chemotherapy*, 24(2), 181–5.

Fairburn, K. (1993) Towards better care for women. *Professional Nurse*, 9(30), 204–12.

Fairburn, K. (1994) A challenge that requires further research. *Professional Nurse*, 9(4), 272–7.

Falanga, V. & Eaglstein, W. (1986) A therapeutic approach to venous ulcers. *Journal of American Academy of Dermatology*, 14(5), 777–84.

Fangrell, B. (1979) Local microcirculaton in chronic venous incompetence and leg ulcers. *Vascular Surgery*, 13(4), 217–25.

Farrow, S. & Toth, B. (1991) The place of Eusol in wound management. *Nursing Standard*, 5(22), 25–7.

Ferguson, A. (1988) Best performer. *Nursing Times*, 84(14), 52–5.

Fincham Gee, C. (1990) Measuring the wound size. *Nursing*, 4(2), 34–5.

Flanagan, M. (1995) Who is at risk of a pressure sore? *Professional Nurse*, 10(5), 305–8.

Florey, C. du V. (1982) Diabetes mellitus (Chapter 25). In: *Epidemiology of Diseases*, (eds D. L. Miller & R. D. T. Farmer). Blackwell Scientific Publications, Oxford.

Forrest, R. D. (1980) The treatment of pressure sores. *Journal of International Medical Research*, 8, 430–5.

Fraser, R. & Gilchrist, T. (1983) Sorbsan calcium alginate fibre dressings in footcare. *Biomaterials*, 4, 222–4.

General Household Survey, 1986 (1989). HMSO, London, pp. 290–3.

Gilchrist, B. (1989) The treatment of leg ulcers with occlusive hydrocolloid dressings: a microbiological study, Chapter 6. In: *Directions in Nursing Research*, (eds J. Wilson-Barnett & S. Robinson) pp. 51–8. Scutari Press, London.

Gilchrist, T. & Martin, A. M. (1983) Wound treatment with Sorbsan – an alginate fibre dressing. *Biomaterials*, 4, 317–20.

Glover, M. (1992) Growth factors and wound healing. *Wound Management*, 2(1), 9–11.

Gogia, P. P. *et al.* (1988) Wound management with whirlpool and infrared cold laser treatment. *Physical Therapy*, 68(8), 1239–42.

Goren, D. (1989) Use of Omniderm in treatment of low-degree pressure sores in terminally ill cancer patients. *Cancer Nursing*, 12(3), 165–9.

Gould, D. (1984) Clinical forum. *Nursing Mirror*, 159(16), pp. iii–vi.

Griffin, T. (ed.) (1989) *Social Trends 19. Central Statistical Office*. HMSO, London.

Gustafsson, G. (1988) Guidelines for the application of disinfectants in wound care. *Nursing RSA Verpleging*, 3(11/12), 8–9.

Guttman, L. (1976) The prevention and treatment of pressure sores. In: *Bed Sore Biomechnics*, (eds R. M. Kenedi *et al.*). Macmillan, London.

Guyton, A. C. (1984) *Physiology of the Human Body*, 6th edn. CBS College Publishing, USA.

Hallows, L. (1987) Leg ulcers. An underlying problem. *Community Outlook*, September, 6–14.

Harkiss, K. J. (ed.) (1971) *Surgical Dressings and Wound Healing*. Bradford University Press, Bradford.

Harkiss, K. J. (1985a) Leg ulcers: cheaper in the long run. *Community Outlook*, August, 19–28.

Harkiss, K. J. (1985b) Wound management: cost analysis of dressing materials used in venous leg ulcers. *Pharmaceutical Journal*, 31 August, 268–9.

Henry, M. & Corless, C. (1989) The incidence of varicose veins in Ireland. *Phlebology*, 41, 133–7.

Holmes, S. (1990) Good food for long life. *Professional Nurse*, 6(1), 43–6.

Horwich, A. (1992) Radiotherapy update. *British Medical Journal*, 304, 1554–7.

Hunt, T. K. & Dunphy, J. E. (1979) *Fundamentals of Wound Management*. Appleton-Century-Crofts, New York. In: Messer, M. S. (1989) Wound care. *Critical Care Nursing Quarterly*, 11(4), 17–27.

Hunt, T. K. *et al.* (1969) Effect of vitamin A on reversing the inhibitory effect of cortisone on healing of open wounds in animals and man. *Annals of Surgery*, 170, 633–41. In: Messer, M. S. (1989) Wound care. *Critical Care Nursing Quarterly*, 11(4), 17–27.

Husian, T. (1953) An experimental study of some pressure effects on tissues, with reference to the bed-sore problems. *Journal of Pathology and Bacteriology*, 66, 347–58.

Ivetic, O. & Lyne, P. A. (1990) Fungating and ulcerating malignant lesions: a review of the literature. *Journal of Advanced Nursing*, 15, 83–8.

Jackson, D. S. & Rovee, D. T. (1988) Current concepts in wound healing: research and theory. *Journal of Enterostomal Therapy*, 15(3), 133–7.

Jash, D. K. (1973) Epistaxis: topical use of aminocapoic acid in its management. *Journal of Laryngology and Otology*, 87, 895–8.

Jeter, K. F. & Tintle, T. (1988) Principles of wound cleaning and wound care. *Journal of Home Health Care Practice*, 1, 43–7.

Johnson, A. (1984) Towards rapid tissue healing. *Nursing Times*, 80(48), 39–43.

Johnson, A. (1988a) Natural healing processes: an essential update. *Professional Nurse*, 3, 149–52.

Johnson, A. (1988b) The case against the use of hypochlorites in the treatment of open wounds. *Care – Science and Practice*, 6(3), 86–8.

Johnson, A. (1988c) Modern wound care products. *Professional Nurse*, 3, 392–8.

Johnson, A. (1988d) Standard protocols for treating open wounds. *Professional Nurse*, 3(12), 498–501.

Johnson, A. (1989) Granuflex wafers as a prophylactic pressure sore dressing. *Care – Science and Practice*, 7(2), 55–8.

Kaufman, T. & Alexander, J. W. (1988) Topical oxygen treatment promoted healing and enhanced scar formation of experimental full-thickness burns. In: *Beyond Occlusion: Wound Care Proceedings. Royal Society of Medicine International Congress and Symposium Series*, (ed. T. J. Ryan), pp. 61–6. Royal Society of Medicine, London.

Kaufman, T. & Berger (1988) Topical pH and burn wound healng: a review. In: *Beyond Occlusion: Wound Care Proceedings. Royal Society of Medicine International Congress and Symposium Series* (ed. T. J. Ryan), pp. 55–60. Royal Society of Medicine, London.

Kaufman, T. *et al.* (1985) Topical acidification promotes healing of experimental deep partial thickness skin burns: a randomized double-blind preliminary study. *Burns*, 12, 84–90.

Kaufman, T. & Hirshowitz, B. (1982) The influence of various microclimate conditions on the burn wound: a review. *Burns*, 9, 84–90.

Knight, A. (1990) The skin clinic. *Modern Medicine*, 35(8), 608–8.

Knighton, D. R. *et al.* (1981) Regulation of wound healing angiogenesis. Effect of oxygen gradients and inspired oxygen concentration. *Surgery*, 90(2), 262–70.

Kosiak, M. (1958) Evaluation of pressure as a factor in the production of ischial ulcers. *Archives of Physical Medicine and Rehabilitation*, 40, 62–9.

Kosiak, M. (1976) A mechanical resting surface: its effect on pressure distribution. *Archives of Physical Medicine and Rehabilitation*, 57, 481–3.

Lawrence, J. D. (1985) The physical properties of a new hydrocolloid dressing. In: *An Environment for Healing: The Role of Occlusion. Royal Society of Medicine International Congress and Symposium Series*, (ed. T. J. Ryan), pp. 69–76. Royal Society of Medicine, London.

Lawrence, J. D. & Groves, A. R. (1988) *Blueprint for the Management of Minor Burns*. Squibb Surgicare, Hounslow.

Leaper, D. (1986) Antiseptics and their effects on healing tissue. *Nursing Times*, 82(22), 45–6.

Lechter, A. *et al.* (1987) Pelvic varices and gonadal veins. *Phlebology*, 2, 181–8.

Lockyer-Stevens, N. (1994) A developing information base for purchasing decisions. *Professional Nurse*, 9(8), 534–42.

Lycarotti, M. E. & Leaper, D. J. (1989) Measurement in wound healing. *Care – Science and Practice*, 7(3), 68–71.

McSweeney, P. (1994) Assessing the cost of pressure sores. *Nursing Standard*, 8(52), 25–6.

McTaggart, J. H. (1994) An area of clinical neglect. *Professional Nurse*, 9(9), 600–6.

Maibach, H. I. & Rovee, D. T. (1972) *Epidermal Wound Healing*. Year Book Medical Publishers, Chicago.

Mallett, J. (1988) Wound dressing made easier. *Senior Nurse*,

8(5), 31–3.

Mallett, J. & Charles, H. (1989) *Survey of Clients with Leg Ulceration Treated by District Nurses in Paddington and North Kensington.* Report produced for Paddington and North Kensington Health Authority.

Mallett, J. & Charles, H. (1990) Defining the leg ulcer problem. *Journal of District Nursing*, 9(1), 5–10.

Mani, R. *et al.* (1988) Non-invasive oxygen measurements: have they a role in ulcer investigations? In: *Beyond Occlusion: Wound Care Proceedings. Royal Society of Medicine International Congress and Symposium Series*, (ed. T. J. Ryan). Royal Society of Medicine, London.

Marcelon, G. & Vanhoutte, P. M. (1988) Venotonic effect of ruscus under variable temperature conditions *in vitro*. *Phlebology*, 3, Supplement 1, 51–4.

Marcelon, G. *et al.* (1988) Oestrogens impregnation and ruscus action on the human vein *in vitro*, depending on preliminary results. *Phlebology*, 3, Supplement 1, 83–5.

Margolin *et al.* (1990) Management of radiation-induced moist skin desquamation using hydrocolloid dressing. *Cancer Nursing*, 13(2), 71–80.

Martindale, W. (1982) *The Extra Pharmacopoeia*, 28th edn. The Pharmaceutical Press, London.

Masi, A. T. & Medsger, T. A. (1979) Epidemiology of the rheumatic diseases. In: *Arthritis and Allied Conditions*, (ed. D. J. McCarty), pp. 11–35. Lea & Febiger, Philadelphia. In: Walker, J. M. *et al.* (1989) The nursing management of pain in the community: a theoretical framework. *Journal of Advanced Nursing*, 14, 240–7.

Matthews, R. N. (1986) Leg ulcers. *Surgery*, 1(33), 790–5.

Mertz, P. M. *et al.* (1985) Occlusive wound dressings to prevent bacterial invasion and wound infection. *Journal of the American Academy of Dermatology*, 12(4), 662–8.

Messer, M. S. (1989) Wound care. *Critical Care Nursing Quarterly*, 11(4), 17–27.

Middleton, K. (1990) Sugar pastes in wound management. *The Dressing Times*, 3(2). Available from the Surgical Materials Testing Laboratory, Bridgend.

Miller, D. L. & Farmer, R. D. T. (eds) (1982) *Epidemiology of Diseases*. Blackwell Scientific Publications, Oxford.

Milward, P. (1988) The healing process. *Care – Science and Practice*, 6(3), Educational Leaflet Supplement.

Moffat, C. J. & Dorman, M. C. R. (1995) Recurrence of leg ulcers within a community ulcer service. *Journal of Wound Care*, 4(2), 57–61.

Moody, M. & Grocott, P. (1993) Let us extend our knowledge base. *Professional Nurse*, 8(9), 586–90.

Morgan, D. A. (1990) *Formulary of Wound Management Products. A Guide for Health Care Staff*, 4th edn. Britcare Ltd.

Morison, M. J. (1989) Wound cleansing – which solution? *Professional Nurse*, 4, 220–5.

Morison, M. J. (1992) *A Colour Guide to the Nursing Management of Wounds*. Wolfe Publishing, London.

Moss, A. (1989) Treatment of terminal breast cancer. *British Medical Journal*, 298, 10.

National Pressure Ulcer Advisory Panel (1989) Pressure ulcers: incidence, economics and risk assessment. *Care – Science and Practice*, 7(4), 96–9.

Newman, V. *et al.* (1989) The use of metronidazole gel to control the smell of malodorous lesions. *Palliative Medicine*, 3, 303–5.

Nicholls, R. (1989) Leg ulcers: collecting the facts. *Nursing Standard*, Special Supplement, 6, pp. 12–13.

Nicholls, R. (1990) Leg ulcers: a study in the community. *Nursing Standard*, Special Supplement, 7, pp. 4–6.

Norton, D. *et al.* (1985) *An Investigation of Geriatric Nursing Problems in Hospital*. Churchill Livingstone, Edinburgh.

Nuffield Institute for Health (1995) *Effective health care: the prevention and treatment of pressure sores*, October, 2(1). NHS Centre for Reviews and Dissemination, University of York.

Nurses' Drug Alert (1987) *Avoid Use of Hydrogen Peroxide and Povidone-Iodine in Open Wounds*. M. J. Powers, Publishers, New Jersey.

Official Population Census Statistics (1983) *Midyear Population Estimates for Parkside Health District*. HMSO, London.

Pattie, A. H. & Gilleard, C. J. (1979) *Manual of the Clifton Assessment Procedures of the Elderly (CAPE)*. Hodder & Stoughton, London.

Perkins, P. (1989) A clinic to cope with leg ulcers. *Mims Magazine*, April, pp. 73–4.

Piper, S. M. (1989) Effective use of occlusive dressings. *Professional Nurse*, 4(8), 402–4.

Pottle, B. (1987) Trial of a dressing for non-healing ulcers. *Nursing Times*, 83(12), 54–8.

Pritchard, A. P. & David, J. A. (eds) (1988) *The Royal Marsden Manual of Clinical Nursing Procedures*, 2nd edn. Harper & Row, London.

Raiman, J. (1986) Pain relief – a two-way process. *Nursing Times*, 82(15), 24–8.

Reid, J. & Morrison, M. (1994) Towards a consensus: classification of pressure sores. *Journal of Wound Care*, 3(3), 157–60.

Roberts, G. (1988) Nutrition and wound healing. *Nursing Standard*, 2(51), Supplement, 8–12.

Robinson, B. (1988) Aetiology and treatment of leg ulcers. Focus on wound healing. Supplement to *Mims Magazine*, July, p. 23.

Robson, M. C. *et al.* (1992) Platelet derived growth factor BB for the treatment of chronic pressure ulcers. *Lancet*, 339(8784), 23–5.

Robson, M. C. *et al.* (1993) Transforming growth factor beta-2 accelerates healing of venous stasis ulcers in an open-label, placebo-controlled clinical study. *Wound Repair and Regeneration*, 1, 91.

Rovee, D. T. *et al.* (1972) Effect of local wound environment on epidermal healing, Chapter 8. In: *Epidermal Wound Healing*, (eds H. I. Maibach & D. T. Rovee), pp. 159–81. Year Book Medical Publishers, Chicago.

Royal College of General Practitioners (1986) *Alcohol: A Balanced View*. Royal College of General Practitioners (Report from General Practice, 24), Exeter.

Ryan, T. J. (ed) (1985a) *An Environment for Healing: The Role of Occlusion. Royal Society of Medicine, International Congress and Symposium Series*, pp. 5–14. Royal Society of Medicine, London.

Ryan, T. J. (1985b) Current management of leg ulcers. *Drugs*, 30(5), 461–8.

Ryan, T. J. (1987) *The Management of Leg Ulcers*, 2nd edn. Oxford University Press, Oxford.

Ryan, T. J. (1988a) Management of leg ulcers. *The Practitioner*, 232, 1014–21.

Ryan, T. J. (ed) (1988b) *Beyond Occlusion: Wound Care Proceedings. Royal Society of Medicine, International Congress and Symposium Series*. Royal Society of Medicine, London.

Saunders, C. M. (1978) *The Management of Terminal Disease*. Edward Arnold, Sevenoaks.

Saunders, J. (1989) Toilet cleaner for wound care? *Community Outlook*, pp. 11–13. *Nursing Times*, 85(10).

Saunders, Y. & Regnard, C. (1989) Management of malignant ulcers: a flow diagram. *Palliative Medicine*, 3, 153–5.

Schulte, M. (1993) Yoghurt helps to control wound odour. *Oncology Nursing Forum*, 20(8), 1262.

Silver, I. A. (1972) Oxygen tension and epithelialization, Chapter 17. In: *Epidermal Wound Healing*, (eds H. I. Maibach & D. T. Rovee), pp. 291–305. Year Book Medical Publishers, Chicago.

Silver, I. A. (1994) The physiology of wound healing. *Journal of Wound Care*, 3(2), 100–109.

Smith, I. (1989) Waterlow/Norton scoring system – a ward view. *Care – Science and Practice*, 7(4), 93–5.

Smith, S. (1988) Doing the leg work. *Community Outlook*, pp. 17–18. *Nursing Times*, 84(33).

Spanswick, A. *et al.* (1990) Eusol – the final word. *Professional Nurse*, 5(4), 211–14.

Stronge, J. L. (1984) Principles of wound care. *Nursing*, 2(26), Supplement, 7–10.

Struckmann, J. R. (1988) Venous muscle pump function following reconstructive arterial surgery. *Phlebology*, 3, 169–73.

Swanwick, T. & MacLellan, D. (1988) The treatment of venous ulceration. *Nursing*, 3(32), 40–3.

Taheri, S. A. *et al.* (1987) Iliocaval compression syndrome. *Phlebology*, 2, 173–9.

Taylor, A. & Clark, M. (1994) Management of pressure sore prevention: recent initiatives. *Nursing Standard*, 8(48), 54–5.

The Dressing Times (1988) 1(2). Welsh Centre for the Quality Control of Surgical Dressings, East Glamorgan Hospital, Glamorgan.

The Dressing Times (1989) 2(1). Welsh Centre for the Quality Control of Surgical Dressings, East Glamorgan Hospital, Glamorgan.

Thomas, L. (1988a) Treating leg ulcers. *Nursing Standard*, 2(18), 22–3.

Thomas, L. (1988b) Treating leg ulcers. *Nursing Standard*, 2(19), 28.

Thomas, S. (1990a) Cost-effective management of leg ulcers. *Community Outlook*, pp. 21–2. *Nursing Times*, 86(11).

Thomas, S. (1990b) *Wound Management and Dressings*. The Pharmaceutical Press, London.

Thomas, S. (1992) *Current Practices in the Management of Fungating Lesions and Radiation Damaged Skin*. The Surgical Materials Testing Laboratory, Bridgend.

Thomas, S. & Hay, N. (1991) The antimicrobial properties of 2 metronidazole-mediated dressings used to treat malodorous wounds. *Pharmaceutical Journal*, 2 March, 264–6.

Thomas, S. & Loveless, P. (1992) Observations on the fluid handling properties of alginate dressings. *Pharmaceutical Journal*, 248, 850–51.

Thomlinson, R. (1980) Kitchen remedy for necrotic malignant breast ulcers (letter). *Lancet*, 27 September, 707.

Thompson, J. (1990) Foot and leg care, *Community Outlook*, pp. 14–17. *Nursing Times*, 86(8).

Thorp, J. M. *et al.* (1987) Gross hypernatraemia associated with the use of antiseptic surgical packs. *Anaesthesia*, 42, 750–3.

Tomlinson, D. (1987) To clean or not to clean? *Journal of Infection Control/Nursing Times*, 83(9), 71–5.

Tooke, J. E. *et al.* (1988) Diabetes and wound healing: the skin response to injury, and white cell behaviour *in vivo* in diabetic patients. In: *Beyond Occlusion: Wound Care Proceedings. Royal Society of Medicine International Congress and Symposium Series*, (ed. T. J. Ryan), pp. 71–4. Royal Society Medicine, London.

Torrance, C. (1985) Wound care in accident and emergency. *Nursing*, 2(42), Supplement, 1–3.

Trelstad, A. & Osmundson, D. (1989) Water piks: wound cleansing alternative. *Plastic Surgical Nursing*, 9(3), 117–19.

Tubman Papantonio, C. (1988a) Holistic approach to healing: part I. *Home Healthcare Nurse*, 6(5), 31–4.

Tubman Papantonio, C. (1988b) Holistic approach to healing: part II. *Home Healthcare Nurse*, 6, 31–5.

Turner, T. D. (1979) Hospital usage of absorbant dressings. *Pharmaceutical Journal*, May, 421–2.

Turner, T. D. (1983) A practical guide to absorbant dressings. *Nursing*, 12, Supplement.

Turner, T. D. (1985) Semiocclusive and occlusive dressings. In: *An Environment for Healing: The Role of Occlusion. Royal Society of Medicine International Congress and Symposium Series*, (ed. T. J. Ryan). Royal Society of Medicine, London.

Turner, T. D. *et al.* (1986) Advances in Wound Management Symposium Proceedings. John Wiley, Cardiff. In: *Blueprint for the Treatment of Leg Ulcers and the Prevention of Recurrence*, (eds G. W. Cherry & T. J. Ryan, 1987). Squibb Surgicare, Hounslow.

Twycross, R. G. & Lack, S. A. (1990) *Therapeutics in Terminal Cancer*, 2nd edn. Churchill Livingstone, Edinburgh.

United Kingdom Central Council for Nursing, Midwifery and Health Visiting (1993) *UKCC Code of Professional Conduct*. UKCC, London.

Valdes-Dapena, M. A. & Arey, J. B. (1962) Boric acid poisoning. *Journal of Pediatrics*, 61(4), 531–46.

Walker, J. M. *et al.* (1989) The nursing management of pain in the community: a theoretical framework. *Journal of Advanced Nursing*, 14, 240–7.

Waterlow, J. (1987) Calculating the risk. *Nursing Times*, 83(39), 58–60.

Waterlow, J. (1988) Prevention is cheaper than cure. *Nursing Times*, 84(25), 69–70.

Waterlow, J. (1991) A policy that protects. *Professional Nurse*, 6(5), 258–64.

Welch, L. (1981) Simple new remedy for the odour of open lesion. *Registered Nurse*, February, 42–3.

Wells, L. (1994) At the front line of care. *Professional Nurse*,

9(8), 525–30.

Wells, R. J. (1984) Controversial issues in wound care. *Journal of Clinical Nursing*, Supplement, June, 10–11.

West, P. & Priestly, J. (1994) Money under the mattress. *Health Service Journal*, 104(5398), 20–2.

Westaby, S. (1985) *Wound Care*. Heinemann, London.

Williams, I. (1989) A company wraps up the bandage market with new deal for wounded. *The Guardian*, 13 March.

Williamson, D. (1988) Leg ulcers. Taking your time with leg ulcers. *Mims Magazine*, 1 May, 105–8.

Willington, F. L. (1977) The use of non-ionic detergents in sanitary cleansing: a report of a preliminary trial. *Journal of Advanced Nursing*, 3, 373–82.

Wilson-Barnett, J. & Robinson, S. (eds) (1989) *Directions in Nursing Research*. Scutari Press, London.

Wingate, P. & Wingate, R. (1988) *The Penguin Medical Enclyopedia*, 3rd edn. Penguin Books, West Drayton.

Winter, A. & Hewitt, H. (1990) Testing a hydrocolloid. *Nursing Times*, 86(50), 59–62.

Winter, G. D. (1971) Healing of skin wounds and the influence of dressings on the repair process. In: *Surgical Dressings and Wound Healing*, (ed. K. J. Harkiss), pp. 46–50. Bradford University Press, Bradford.

Winter, G. D. (1972) Epidermal regeneration studied in the domestic pig, Chapter 4. In: *Epidermal Wound Healing*, (eds H. I. Maibach & D. T. Rovee), pp. 71–112. Year Book Medical Publishers, Chicago.

Wood, P. H. N. (1977) In: *Epidemiology of Diseases*, (eds D. L. Miller & R. D. T. Farmer, 1982). Blackwell Scientific Publications, Oxford.

Wyngaarden, J. B. & Smith, L. H. (1988) *Cecil Textbook of Medicine*, 18th edn. W. B. Saunders, Philadelphia.

Zederfeldt, B. *et al.* (1980) *Wounds and Wound Healing*. Wolfe Medical Publications, New York.

GUIDELINES: CHANGING WOUND DRESSINGS

EQUIPMENT

1 As for 'Guidelines: Aseptic technique' (Chapter 4).
2 Cleansing fluid for irrigation (Table 48.3).
3 Appropriate dressing (Table 48.4).

PROCEDURE

See procedure for 'Aseptic technique' (Chapter 4) up to and including step 10, then loosen the dressing.

Action	Rationale
11 Where appropriate, loosen the old dressing.	The dressing can then be lifted off without causing trauma.
12 Clean hands with a bactericidal alcohol hand rub.	Hands may become contaminated by handling outer packets, dressing, etc.
13 Using the forceps in the pack, arrange the sterile field with the handles of instruments in one corner or around the edge of the sterile field. Where appropriate, swab along the 'tear area' of lotion sachet with chlorhexidine gluconate 0.5% and isopropyl alcohol. Tear open sachet and pour lotion into gallipots or an indented plastic tray (Table 48.3).	The time the wound is exposed should be kept to a minimum to reduce the risk of contamination. To minimize risk of contamination of lotion.
14 Remove dressing by placing a hand in the plastic bag, lifting the dressing off and inverting the plastic bag so that the dressing is now inside the bag. Thereafter use this as the 'dirty' bag.	To reduce the risk of cross-infection.
15 Attach the bag with the dressing to the side of the trolley below the top shelf.	Contaminated material is below the level of the sterile field.

Guidelines: Changing wound dressings (cont'd)

Action	Rationale
16 Assess the wound healing with reference to volume, amount of granulation tissue and epithelialization, signs of infection, underlying pathology etc (Table 48.2). (Record assessment in relevant documentation at the end of the procedure.)	To evaluate wound care.
17 Put on gloves, touching only the inside wrist end.	To reduce the risk of infection to the wound and contamination of the nurse. Gloves provide greater sensitivity than forceps and are less likely to traumatize the wound or the patient's skin.
18 If necessary, gently clean the wound with a gloved hand using 0.9% sodium chloride (unless another solution is indicated (Table 48.3)). If appropriate, irrigate by flushing with water or 0.9% sodium chloride.	To reduce the possibility of physical and chemical trauma to granulation and epithelial tissue.
19 Apply the dressing that is most suitable for the wound using the criteria for an ideal dressing (Table 48.4).	To promote healing and reduce symptoms.
20 Remove gloves and fasten with hypoallergenic tape/Netelast/bandaging as required.	To prevent irritation of skin and to avoid trauma to wound.
21 Make sure the patient is comfortable and the dressing is secure.	A dressing may slip or feel uncomfortable as the patient changes position.

Continue with steps 15–18 from the procedure for Aseptic technique.

GUIDELINES: REMOVAL OF SUTURES, CLIPS OR STAPLES

EQUIPMENT

1 As for 'Guidelines: Aseptic technique' (Chapter 4).
2 Sterile scissors, stitch cutter, Michel clip-removing forceps or staple remover.
3 Sterile adhesive sutures.

PROCEDURE

Action	Rationale
1 Explain and discuss the procedure with the patient.	To ensure that the patient understands the procedure and gives his/her valid consent.
2 Perform procedure using aseptic technique.	To prevent infection (for further information see procedure on aseptic technique, Chapter 4).
3 Clean the wound with an appropriate sterile solution such as 0.9% sodium chloride (Table 48.3).	To prevent infection.

For removal of sutures

| 4 | Lift knot of suture with metal forceps. Snip stitch close to the skin. Pull suture out gently. | Plastic forceps tend to slip against nylon sutures. To prevent infection by drawing exposed suture through the tissue. |

| 5 | Use tips of scissors slightly open or the side of the stitch cutter to gently press the skin when the suture is being drawn out. | To minimize pain by counteracting the adhesion between the suture and surrounding tissue. |

For removal of clips

| 6 | Squeeze wings of Kifa clips together with forceps to release from skin. For Michel clips use special forceps under the clips to flatten the loop. | To release clips atraumatically from the wound. |

| 7 | If the wound gapes use adhesive sutures to oppose the wound edges. | To improve the cosmetic effect. |

| 8 | When necessary, cover the wound with an appropriate dressing (Tables 48.4 and 48.8). | To provide the best possible environmemt for wound healing to take place. To reduce the risk of infection. To prevent the suture line from rubbing against clothing. |

For removal of staples

| 9 | Slide the lower bar of the staple remover with the V-shaped groove under the staple at an angle of 90°. Squeeze the handles of the staple removers together to open the staple. | To release the staple atraumatically from the wound. If the angle of the staple remover is not correct, the staple will not come out freely. |
| | If the suture line is under tension, use free hand to gently squeeze the skin either side of the suture line. | To reduce tension of skin around suture line and lessen pain on removal of staple. |

| 10 | If the wound gapes use adhesive sutures to oppose the wound edges. | To improve the cosmetic effect. |

For all suture lines

| 11 | Record condition of suture line and surrounding skin (for example, amount of exudate, pus, inflammation, pain, etc., see Table 48.2). | To document care and enable evaluation of the wound. |

GUIDELINES: DRAIN DRESSING (REDIVAC – CLOSED DRAINAGE SYSTEMS)

EQUIPMENT

1 As for Guidelines: Aseptic technique (Chapter 4).
2 Keyhole dressing.
3 Sterile padded dressing.

Guidelines: Drain dressing (cont'd)

PROCEDURE

Action   **Rationale**

1 Explain and discuss the procedure with the patient.   To ensure that the patient understands the procedure and gives his/her valid consent.

2 Perform procedure using aseptic technique.   To prevent infection (for further information on asepsis, see procedure on aseptic technique, Chapter 4).

3 Clean the surrounding skin with an appropriate sterile solution such as 0.9% sodium chloride (Table 48.3).   To prevent infection and remove excess debris.

4 Ensure that the skin suture holding the drain site in position is intact.   To prevent the drain from leaving the wound.

5 Cover the drain site with a keyhole dressing.   To protect the drain site, prevent infection entering the wound and absorb exudate.

6 Tape securely.   To prevent drain coming loose.

7 Ensure that the drain is primed or that the suction pump is in working order.   To ensure continuity of drainage.

GUIDELINES: CHANGE OF VACUUM BOTTLE (REDIVAC – CLOSED DRAINAGE SYSTEMS)

(See Chapter 22, Intrapleural Drainage.)

EQUIPMENT

1 Sterile topical swab.
2 Artery forceps.
3 Sterile drainage bottle.

PROCEDURE

Action   **Rationale**

1 Explain and discuss the procedure with the patient.   To ensure that the patient understands the procedure and gives his/her valid consent.

2 Wash hands using bactericidal soap and water or bactericidal alcohol hand rub.   To minimize the risk of infection.

3 Clean the nozzle of wall suction apparatus with an appropriate antiseptic solution (e.g. chlorhexidine gluconate 0.5% w/v in 70% v/v IMS) and prime a sterile vacuum bottle.   To ensure sterility and to prepare the bottle for attachment to the drainage tube.

4 Measure the contents of the bottle to be changed and record this in the appropriate documents.   To maintain an accurate record of drainage from the wound and enable evaluation of state of wound.

Action	Rationale
5 Clamp the tube with artery forceps and remove the bottle.	To prevent air and contamination entering the wound via the drain.
6 Put on clean gloves.	To prevent contamination from blood and body fluids.
7 Clean the end of the tube and attach it to the sterile bottle.	To maintain sterility.
8 Remove the artery forceps.	To re-establish the drainage system.
9 Ensure that the bottle is primed.	To ensure that drainage continues.
10 If the vacuum is constantly lost, take down the dressing and examine the entry site of the drain.	To ensure that the drain has not become dislodged.
11 If necessary, re-dress as drain dressing (above).	

GUIDELINES: REMOVAL OF DRAIN (REDIVAC – CLOSED DRAINAGE SYSTEMS, AND PENROSE, ETC. – OPEN DRAINAGE SYSTEMS)

EQUIPMENT

1 As for Guidelines: Aseptic technique (Chapter 4).
2 Sterile scissors or suture cutter.

PROCEDURE

Action	Rationale
1 Check the patient's operation notes.	To establish the number and site(s) of internal and external sutures.
2 Explain and discuss the procedure with the patient.	To ensure that the patient understands the procedure and gives his/her valid consent.
3 If appropriate (Redivac and closed drainage systems) release vacuum.	To prevent pulling at wound tissue.
4 Perform the procedure using aseptic technique.	To minimize the risk of infection. (For further information on asepsis, see Chapter 4.)
5 Where the wound is covered with an occlusive dressing (e.g. following lumpectomy in the breast), lift and snip the dressing from around the drain. Do not remove it from the entire wound.	To prevent disturbing the incision or contaminating the wound.
6 Only clean the wound if necessary, using an appropriate sterile solution, such as 0.9% sodium chloride (Table 48.3).	To reduce risk of infection.
7 Hold the knot of the suture with metal forceps and gently lift upwards.	Plastic forceps tend to slip against nylon sutures. To allow space for the scissors or stitch cutter to be placed underneath.

Guidelines: Removal of drain (cont'd)

Action	Rationale
8 Cut the shortest end of the suture as close to the skin as possible.	To prevent infection by allowing the suture to be liberated from the drain without drawing the exposed part through tissue.
9 Remove drain gently. If there is resistance place free gloved hand against the tissue to oppose the tugging of the drain being removed. If the resistance is felt to be excessive, nitrous oxide (e.g. Entonox) may be required.	To minimize pain and reduce trauma.
10 Cover the drain site with a sterile dressing and tape securely.	To prevent infection entering the drain site.
11 Measure and record the contents of the drainage bottle in the appropriate documents.	To maintain an accurate record of drainage from wound and enable evaluation of state of wound.
12 If disposable drainage bottle is used, dispose of in plastic yellow clinical waste bag.	To prevent environmental contamination. Yellow is the recognized colour for clinical waste.
13 If glass drainage bottle is used, empty contents into bedpan washer and send bottle to the sterile supplies department for cleaning and sterilizing.	To prevent environmental contamination. To ensure reusable bottles are cleaned and sterilized before use.

GUIDELINES: SHORTENING OF DRAIN (PENROSE, ETC. OPEN DRAINAGE SYSTEMS)

Action	Rationale
1 Follow steps 1–8 above (removal of drain), i.e. to the stage where the suture has been cut.	
2 Using gloved hand, gently ease the drain out of wound to the length requested by surgeons. Usually 3–5 cm.	Allows healing to take place from base of wound.
3 Using gloved hand, place a sterile safety pin through the drain as close to the skin as possible, taking great care not to stab either the nurse or patient.	To prevent retraction into the wound and minimize the risk of cross-infection.
4 Cut same amount of tubing from distal end of drain as withdrawn from wound.	So there is a convenient length of tubing to drain into the bag. To ensure patient comfort.
5 Place a sterile, suitably sized drainage bag over the drain site.	To allow effluent to drain into the bag. To prevent excoriation of the skin. To contain any odour.
6 Check bag is secure and comfortable for the patient.	For patient comfort.
7 Record by how much the drainage tube was shortened.	To ensure the length remaining in the wound is known.

GUIDELINES: DRAINAGE DRESSING (PENROSE AND CORRUGATED DRAINAGE SYSTEMS)

EQUIPMENT

1 As for Guidelines: Aseptic technique (Chapter 4).
2 Sterile padded dressings.
3 Stomahesive wafers.
4 Keyhole dressing.
5 Drainage stoma bag.

PROCEDURE

Minimum drainage

Action	Rationale
1 Explain and discuss the procedure with the patient.	To ensure that the patient understands the procedure and gives his/her valid consent.
2 Perform the procedure using aseptic technique.	To prevent infection. (For further information on asepsis, see Chapter 4.)
3 Clean the surrounding skin with an appropriate sterile solution (e.g. 0.9% sodium chloride).	To prevent infection.
4 Cut a hole slightly larger than the site in a Stomahesive wafer and apply the wafer to the skin surrounding the drain.	To protect the skin from the drainage which may cause excoriation. The wafer should fit as close as possible without interrupting the flow of effluent.
5 Leave the Stomahesive wafer in position until the drain is removed.	To continue to protect vulnerable skin.
6 Cover the drain site and the Stomahesive wafer with a keyhole dressing and sterile dressing pad. Tape securely.	To absorb drainage. To prevent infection.
7 Change the dressing whenever it becomes soiled.	To reduce risk of infection.
8 Describe the wound and type of drainage in appropriate documents and amend the care plan accordingly.	For accurate evaluation of progress of drainage.

Copious drainage

1 Follow steps 1–5 above, i.e. to the stage where the Stomahesive wafer has been applied.	
2 Cover the drain with a clinically clean drainage stoma bag preferably with a woven back. (If indicated a reservoir bag may be attached to stoma bag.)	To allow effluent to drain into the bag. To reduce sweating and so aid patient comfort. To reduce risk of stoma bag leaking.
3 Ensure that the drain is enclosed by the aperture of the bag.	To prevent excoriation of surrounding skin. To contain any odour.

Guidelines: Drainage dressing (cont'd)

Action	Rationale
4 Where necessary, pad under the bag and secure with Netelast.	To prevent bag rubbing skin and to keep it secure.
5 Empty the contents of the bag regularly and record the amount in appropriate documents.	To prevent accumulated fluid from detaching the bag from the skin due to its weight. To maintain an accurate record of drainage.

GUIDELINES: PREVENTION OF PRESSURE ULCERS

Action	Rationale
1 Assess every patient on admission using a recognized scale, such as the Norton (Table 48.5) or Waterlow (Fig. 48.1) Scale.	To identify the patient at risk of developing decubitus ulcers.
2 Reassess every patient on a regular basis and/or if there has been any deterioration or change in condition.	To provide appropriate data on which to base treatment.
3 Do not rub any area at risk.	Rubbing causes maceration and degeneration of subcutaneous tissues, especially in the elderly.
4 Wash areas at risk only if the patient is incontinent or sweating profusely. Use mild soap or a liquid detergent. Ensure that all detergent or soap is rinsed off and that the area is patted dry. Use moisturizer if the skin is very dry. Ask the patient what suits his/her skin.	To maintain skin integrity and prevent the formation of sores. Excessive use of soap can be harmful to the skin. Thorough gentle drying of the skin promotes comfort and discourages the growth of micro-organisms. Dry skin cracks allow entry of micro-organisms (Morison, 1992).
5 Use barrier creams only when indicated.	Barrier creams prevent damage to the epidermis. They are, however, occlusive and prevent moisture exchange from the skin (Pritchard & David, 1988).
6 Educate the patient to shift position, to pull or push up regularly and to examine the vulnerable areas.	After discharge the patient may be self-caring and possibly still vulnerable to sores. To encourage the patient to participate in own care.
7 Initiate a mobility programme for the patient. Call on the physiotherapist or occupational therapist as appropriate.	To reduce further tissue damage and improve the circulation.
8 Where possible relieve the pressure over areas vulnerable to tissue breakdown. Use appropriate pressure relief devices (Table 48.7). If necessary, turn the patient at least two-hourly and record the position on the relevant charts.	To reduce pressure where possible. Use of inappropriate aids may increase pressure to vulnerable areas.
9 Have the patient recumbent whenever possible. Support with bead bags or pillows in bed. Reduce period spent sitting in chair if pelvic sores develop.	Avoid the use of bedrests as these increase shearing.

Index